D1452289

JULIA K. TERZIS, M.D., Ph.D., F.R.C.S., (C)

Director, Microsurgical Research Center
Associate Professor, Department of Plastic and Reconstructive Surgery,
Eastern Virginia Medical School,
Norfolk, Virginia

MICRORECONSTRUCTION OF NERVE INJURIES

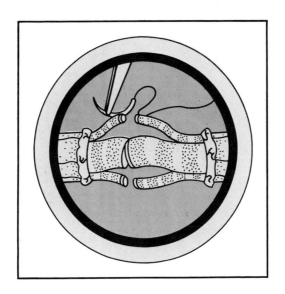

1987

W. B. SAUNDERS COMPANY

Philadelphia / London / Toronto / Mexico City
Rio de Janeiro / Sydney / Tokyo / Hong Kong

W. B. Saunders Company: West Washington Square
Philadelphia, PA 19105

Library of Congress Cataloging-in-Publication Data

Main entry under title:

Microreconstruction of nerve injuries.

1. Nerves, Peripheral—Wounds and injuries.   2. Nerves,
Peripheral—Surgery.   3. Microsurgery.   I. Terzis,
Julia K.   [DNLM: 1. Microsurgery.   2. Peripheral
Nerves—injuries.   3. Peripheral Nerves—surgery.
WL 500 M626]

RD595.M52   1987   617′.483   85–26203

ISBN 0–7216–1268–7

Editor: Dean Manke
Designer: Karen O'Keefe
Production Manager: Frank Polizzano
Manuscript Editor: Charlotte Fierman
Illustrator: Glenn Edelmayer
Illustration Coordinator: Peg Shaw
Indexer: Ellen Murray

Microreconstruction of Nerve Injuries   ISBN   0–7216–1268–7

Last digit is the print number: 9   8   7   6   5   4   3   2   1

CONTRIBUTORS

Y. ALLIEU, M.D.
Teaching Professor, Faculté de Médecine de Montpellier and Unité de Chirurgie
Orthopédique et de Chirurgie de la Main, C. H. U. Montpellier, Nimes, France.
Paralysis in Root Avulsions of the Brachial Plexus

J. Y. ALNOT, M.D.
Professor, Hospital Bichat, Paris, France.
Traumatic Paralysis of the Brachial Plexus; Infraclavicular Lesions

ROLFE BIRCH, F.R.C.S.
Recognized Teacher, St. Mary's Hospital Medical School, Consultant Ortho-
paedic Surgeon, St. Mary's Hospital and Royal National Orthopaedic Hospital,
London, England.
Experience with Vascularized Nerve Grafts

F. BONNEL, M.D.
Associate Professor, Laboratoire d'Anatomie Normale, Faculté de Médecine de
Montpellier, Nimes, France.
Paralysis in Root Avulsions of the Brachial Plexus

GEORGE BONNEY, M.S., F.R.C.S.
Hon. Consulting Orthopaedic Surgeon, St. Mary's Hospital, London, England.
Experience with Vascularized Nerve Grafts

WARREN C. BREIDENBACH, M.D., F.R.C.S.(C.)
Hand Scholar, Louisville Institute of Hand and Microsurgery; Clinical Instructor
in Orthopedic Surgery (Hand), University of Louisville Medical School, Louisville, Kentucky.
The Anatomy of Free Vascularized Nerve Grafts

KENNETH L. B. BROWN, M.Sc., M.D., F.R.C.S.(C.)
Assistant Professor, McGill University, Staff Orthopaedic Surgeon, The Mon-
treal Children's Hospital, The Shriner's Hospital for Crippled Children, The
Royal Victoria Hospital, Hôpital Sacré-Coeur, Montreal, Quebec, Canada.
Review of Obstetrical Palsies: Nonoperative Treatment

i

GIORGIO BRUNELLI, M.D., F.I.C.S., F.A.S.S.H.
Professor of Orthopaedics, Brescia University Medical School, Chairman of the
School of Specialisation in Clinical Orthopaedics, University of Brescia, Brescia,
Italy.
*Neurotization of Avulsed Roots of the Brachial Plexus by Means of Anterior Nerves of
the Cervical Plexus*

JAMES H. CARRAWAY, M.D.
Professor, Department of Plastic Surgery, Eastern Virginia Medical School,
Norfolk, Virginia.
Surgical Anatomy of the Facial Musculature and Muscle Transplantation

JOHN E. CASTALDO, M.D.
Clinical Instructor, Temple University, Philadelphia; Staff, Lehigh Valley Hos-
pital Center, Allentown, Pennsylvania.
Mechanical Injury of Peripheral Nerves

MARCUS CASTRO FERREIRA, M.D.
Associate Professor of Plastic Surgery, University of São Paulo Medical School,
Attending Surgeon, Plastic Surgery Division, University of São Paulo Medical
Center, Director, Microsurgical Laboratory, University of São Paulo Medical
School, São Paulo, Brazil.
Cross-Facial Nerve Grafting

L. CELLI, M.D.
Associate Professor, Orthopedic Clinic, and Aide in Orthopedic Surgery,
Orthopedic Clinic, University of Modena, Modena, Italy.
*Electrophysiologic Intraoperative Evaluations of the Damaged Root in Traction of the
Brachial Plexus*

LEO CLODIUS, M.D.
Docent, Plastic Surgery, and Head, Unit for Plastic and Reconstructive Surgery,
University Hospital, Zurich, Switzerland.
Irradiation Plexitis of the Brachial Plexus

A. LEE DELLON, M.D., F.A.C.S.
Assistant Professor of Plastic Surgery and Neurosurgery, Johns Hopkins University, Attending Hand Surgeon, Curtis Hand Center, Union Memorial Hospital, Attending Plastic Surgeon, Johns Hopkins Hospital, Children's Hospital,
and Union Memorial Hospital, Baltimore, Maryland.
Current Models for Nerve Research; Functional Sensation and Its Re-Education

VINKO V. DOLENC, M.D., Ph.D.
Professor of Neurosurgery and Chief, Department of Neurosurgery, University
Medical Centre, Ljubljana, Yugoslavia.
Intercostal Neurotization of the Peripheral Nerves in Avulsion Plexus Injuries

ROSEMARY A. EAMES, M.R.C.P., M.R.C.(Path.)
Consultant Histopathologist, Queen Elizabeth Hospital, King's Lynn, Norfolk,
England.
Experience with Vascularized Nerve Grafts

MILTON T. EDGERTON, M.D.
Chairman, Department of Plastic Surgery, University of Virginia, Charlottes-
ville, Virginia.
Quantitative Microanatomy of the Brachial Plexus

VICTORIA FRAMPTON, M.C.S.P., S.R.P.
Superintendent Physiotherapist, Rehabilitation Unit, Royal National Ortho-
paedic Hospital, London, England.
Rehabilitation of Patients Following Traction Lesions of the Brachial Plexus

ALAIN GILBERT, M.D.
Head, Microsurgical Laboratories, The Paris Hospitals, Staff, Institut Français
de la Main, Paris, France.
*Vascularized Sural Nerve Graft; Obstetrical Palsy: A Clinical, Pathologic, and
Surgical Review*

GEORGE E. GOODE, Ph.D.
Associate Professor of Anatomy, Eastern Virginia Medical School, Norfolk,
Virginia.
Modulation of Nociception and Analgesia

SEAN G. L. HAMILTON, M.B.B.S., F.R.A.C.S.
Clinical Lecturer, University of Western Australia, Plastic Surgeon, Royal Perth
and Sir Charles Gairdner Hospitals, Reconstructive Microsurgeon, Princess
Margaret Hospital for Children, Perth, Western Australia.
Surgical Anatomy of the Facial Musculature and Muscle Transplantation

KLAUS HESS, M.D.
Docent for Neurology, Department of Neurology, University Hospital, Zurich,
Switzerland.
Irradiation Plexitis of the Brachial Plexus

ALAN R. HUDSON, M.B., Ch.B., F.R.C.S.(Ed.), F.R.C.S.(C.)
Professor and Chairman, Division of Neurosurgery, University of Toronto,
Active Staff, St. Michael's Hospital, Toronto, Ontario, Canada.
Nerve Injection Injuries

IAN T. JACKSON, M.D., F.R.C.S., F.A.C.S.
Professor in Plastic Surgery, Mayo Medical School, Staff, St. Mary's Hospital,
and Mayo Clinic, Rochester, Minnesota.
Surgical Correction of Lagophthalmos

ANGUS M. JAMIESON, F.R.C.S.
Consultant Orthopaedic Surgeon, Robert Jones and Agnes Hunt Orthopaedic
Hospital, Oswestry, Shropshire, England.
Experience with Vascularized Nerve Grafts

S. J. JONES, M.A., Ph.D.
Medical Research Council, National Hospital, Queen Square, London, England.
Diagnostic Value of Peripheral and Spinal Somatosensory Evoked Potentials

KENNETH K. LEE, M.B.B.S., F.R.A.C.S.
Visiting Plastic Surgeon, The Royal Prince Alfred Hospital, Camperdown, Sydney, Australia.
Management of Acute Extratemporal Facial Palsy; Microsurgical Reanimation of the Eye Sphincter

RONALD LEVINE, M.D.
Microsurgical Fellow, Eastern Virginia Medical School, Microsurgical Research Center, Department of Plastic Surgery, Norfolk, Virginia.
Our Experience in Obstetrical Brachial Plexus Palsy

W. THEODORE LIBERSON, M.D. Ph.D.
Senior Lecturer in Rehabilitation Medicine, Downstate Medical Center College of Medicine; Attending in Rehabilitation, The Brooklyn Hospital, Brooklyn, New York; Consultant in Rehabilitation, Plastic Surgery Specialists, Norfolk, Virginia.
Motorcycle Brachial Plexopathy; Our Experience in Obstetrical Brachial Plexus Palsy; Contribution of Clinical Neurophysiology and Rehabilitation Medicine to the Management of Brachial Plexus Palsy

SUSAN E. MACKINNON, M.D., F.R.C.S.(C.)
Assistant Professor of Plastic Surgery, University of Toronto, Attending Plastic Surgeon and Hand Surgeon, Sunnybrook Hospital, Toronto, Ontario, Canada.
Current Models for Nerve Research

RALPH T. MANKTELOW, M.D., F.R.C.S.(C.)
Associate Professor, Department of Surgery, Division of Plastic Surgery, University of Toronto, Head, Division of Plastic Surgery, Toronto General Hospital, Toronto, Ontario, Canada.
Functioning Muscle Transplantation to the Arm; Free Muscle Transplantation for Facial Paralysis

HALLENE A. MARAGH, M.D.
Microfellow, Microsurgical Research Center, Eastern Virginia Medical School, Norfolk, Virginia.
Motorcycle Brachial Plexopathy

GRETCHEN L. MAURER, B.S., O.T.R.
Co-Director, Hand Therapy, Plastic Surgery Specialists, Inc., Norfolk, Virginia.
Rehabilitation of the Hand

HANNO MILLESI, M.D.
Professor of Plastic Surgery, Medical Faculty, University of Vienna, Chief of Plastic Surgery, 1st Surgical Clinic of the University of Vienna and Director of the Ludwig-Boltzmann Institute of Vienna, Austria.
Nomenclature in Peripheral Nerve Surgery; Nerve Grafting; Lower Extremity Nerve Lesions; Brachial Plexus Injuries: Management and Results

JEAN-CLAUDE MIRA, D.Sc.
Professor, René Descartes University of Biology, Paris, France.
Effects of Repeated Experimental Localized Freezings in the Distal Stump of Peripheral Nerves; Effects of Repeated Denervation on Muscle Reinnervation

ALISON MONTEITH, Dip., C.O.T., S.R.O.T.
Head Occupational Therapist, Royal National Orthopaedic Hospital, London, England.
Rehabilitation of Patients Following Traction Lesions of the Brachial Plexus

CHRISTINE A. MORAN, M.S., R.P.T.
Clinical Assistant Professor, Graduate Studies in Physical Therapy, Medical College of Virginia, Richmond; Adjunct Clinical Assistant Professor, Program in Physical Therapy, Old Dominion University, Norfolk; Director, The Richmond Upper Extremity Center, Richmond, Virginia.
Rehabilitation of the Hand

ALGIMANTAS O. NARAKAS, M.D.
Associate Professor, University of Lausanne Medical School, Surgeon in Chief, Longeraie Clinic for Reconstructive Surgery, Consultant Surgeon, University Hospital, Lausanne, Switzerland.
Thoughts on Neurotization of Nerve Transfers

JOSE L. OCHOA, M.D., Ph.D., D.Sc.
Professor of Neurology, University of Wisconsin, Madison, Wisconsin.
Mechanical Injury of Peripheral Nerves

GEORGE E. OMER, JR., M.D., M.Sc. (Orthop. Surg.)
Professor of Orthopaedics and Chairman, Department of Orthopaedics and Rehabilitation, Professor of Surgery and Chief, Division of Hand Surgery, University of New Mexico School of Medicine, Chief of Staff, University of New Mexico Hospital, Chief of Hand Clinics, Carrie Tingley Hospital for Crippled Children, Albuquerque, New Mexico.
Management Techniques for the Painful Upper Extremity

MICHAEL G. ORGEL, M.D., M.Sc.
Associate Professor of Surgery (Plastic), University of Massachusetts Medical School at the Berkshire Medical Center, Pittsfield Campus, Attending Plastic Surgeon, Berkshire Medical Center and Hillcrest Hospital, Pittsfield, Massachusetts.
Epineurial Versus Perineurial Repair of Peripheral Nerves

J. M. PRIVAT, M.D.
Assistant, Clinique de Neurochirurgie, C. H. U. Montpellier, Nimes, France.
Paralysis in Root Avulsions of the Brachial Plexus

NELSON G. PUBLICOVER, Ph.D.
Assistant Professor, University of Nevada School of Medicine, Reno, Nevada.
Physiologic Assessment of Nerve Injuries; Clinical Application of Electrophysiologic Recordings

JEAN RAIMBAULT, M.D.
Consultant in Clinical Neurophysiology, Clinical Neurophysiology Laboratory, Trousseau Hospital, Paris, France.
Electrical Assessment of Muscle Denervation

C. ROVESTA, M.D.
Assistant in Orthopedic Surgery, Orthopedic Clinic, University of Modena, Modena, Italy.
Electrophysiologic Intraoperative Evaluations of the Damaged Root in Traction Lesions of the Brachial Plexus

MADJID SAMII, M.D.
Professor of Neurosurgery, Institute of Neurosurgery, Chairman of Neurosurgical Clinic, City of Hanover, Nordstadt Hospital, Hanover, Germany.
Facial Nerve Grafting in Acoustic Neurinoma

LAURENT SEDEL, M.D.
Professor of Orthopaedic Surgery, University of Paris School of Medicine, Surgeon, Hospital St. Louis, Paris, France.
Surgical Management of Lower Extremity Nerve Lesions; Management of Supraclavicular Lesions

CRAIG L. SLINGLUFF, JR., M.D.
Resident, Department of Surgery, Duke University Medical Center, Durham, North Carolina.
Quantitative Microanatomy of the Brachial Plexus

J. L. TASSIN, M.D.
Department of Pediatric Orthopedics, Hôpital Trousseau, Paris, France.
Obstetrical Palsy: A Clinical, Pathologic, and Surgical Review

JULIA K. TERZIS, M.D. Ph.D., F.R.C.S.(C.)
Director, Microsurgical Research Center, Associate Professor, Department of Reconstructive and Plastic Surgery, and Assistant Professor, Departments of Anatomy and Physiology, Eastern Virginia Medical School, Norfolk, Virginia.
Nomenclature in Peripheral Nerve Surgery; Physiologic Assessment of Nerve Injuries; The Anatomy of Free Vascularized Nerve Grafts; Clinical Application of Electrophysiologic Recordings; Quantitative Anatomy of the Brachial Plexus; Motorcycle Brachial Plexopathy; Our Experience in Obstetrical Brachial Plexus Palsy; Contribution of Clinical Neurophysiology and Rehabilitation Medicine to the Management of Brachial Plexus Palsy; Surgical Anatomy of the Facial Musculature and Muscle Transplantation; Management of Acute Extratemporal Facial Palsy; Microsurgical Reanimation of the Eye Sphincter

GEORG UHLSCHMID, M.D.
Docent and Chief, Laboratory Division, Department of Surgery, University Hospital, Zurich, Switzerland.
Irradiation Plexitis of the Brachial Plexus

H. BRUCE WILLIAMS, M.D., F.R.C.S.(C.), F.A.C.S.
Professor of Surgery and Director of Plastic and Reconstructive Surgery, McGill University, Director, Plastic Surgery, Montreal General and Montreal Children's Hospitals, Montreal, Quebec, Canada.
The Painful Stump Neuroma and Its Treatment

C. B. WYNN PARRY, M.B.E., M.A., D.M., F.R.C.P., F.R.C.S.
Director of Rehabilitation, Royal National Orthopaedic Hospital, London, England.
Rehabilitation of Patients Following Traction Lesions of the Brachial Plexus

PREFACE

In my Foreword to Clinics in Plastic Surgery devoted to Peripheral Nerve Microsurgery (reprinted following this preface), I stated that in order to do justice to this important field, I was preparing a book in which all manuscripts (published briefly in the Clinics) would be included in an extended completed form. This volume is the fulfillment of this promise made 2 years ago.

Thus, finally, out of a cruise organized for the physicians and scientists, most of whom are pioneers of new micro-neuro-reconstructive procedures, an important contribution to the development of this surgical subspecialty is now presented in this book.

Not only are the brief papers that were previously published in the Clinics now completed, but they have been recently revised by their authors. In addition, 14 new contributions that were not included in the Clinics are now published in this book. These include:

A chapter on "Current Models for Nerve Research" by A. Lee Dellon and Susan Mackinnon, who have developed an animal model for peripheral neuropathy that appears to be reproducible in both rats and baboons. The reader will find in this chapter experimental data related to neuroma formation and nerve regeneration.

The chapter on "Modulation of Nociception and Analgesia—Localization of Spinal Mechanisms" by George Goode has reviewed recent research developments in the neurophysiological understanding of pain, covering 83 references. The reader will find in this chapter the present status of investigations of the role of substantia gelatinosa and other structures of the dorsal horn and brain stem and related biochemical research involving peptide neurochemistry, location of endogenous enkephalins, substance P, etc. The author describes the results of his own studies contributing to this new and exciting field of nociception.

The chapter "Rehabilitation of the Hand" written by Christine Moran and Gretchen Maurer, a physical therapist and an occupational therapist, respectively, offers the reader a discussion of current therapy techniques in this area. Both of these authors have extensive experience with patients who have traumatic neuropathies.

Two new chapters, one written by Hanno Millesi ("Lower Extremity Nerve Lesions") and the other by Laurent Sedel ("Surgical Management of Lower Extremity Nerve Lesions"), compare results obtained by microsurgery with those, much less favorable, obtained by classic techniques. Moreover, the reader will appreciate, I am sure, two different ways of describing essentially the same kind of surgery by two distinguished surgeons. Incidentally, in a later chapter (Chapter 40), Theodore Liberson and I describe a novel approach to localization of lesions in long nerves by the use of "electrical Tinel" techniques.

The detailed manuscript on "Quantitative Microanatomy of the Brachial Plexus" written by Craig Slingluff, Milton Edgerton, and myself, provides an exhaustive review of the anatomic background of the brachial plexus story, as well as a laboriously investigated new microanatomic study in a great number of cadavers. The initial goal was to quantify what is common to all of us, as well as to investigate individual variations of the anatomic patterns. Some novel aspects of these patterns are described and a number of laws are formulated governing these structures. These findings are projected onto the clinical problems of a surgeon. We were fascinated by the exchange between fascicles over only few millimeters of their trajectory, just as I was fascinated by analogous play in the median nerve intraneural organization during a recent study. Although the precise meaning of these exchanges remains elusive, one strongly feels that it must be of crucial importance for understanding of peripheral neuropathies. En passant, we could bring a new understanding of pre- and post-fixed plexuses by studying quantitative relationships between the constitutents of C5 and T1 roots, respectively.

In a monumental report on "Traumatic Paralysis of the Brachial Plexus: Preoperative Problems and Therapeutic Indications," based on some 400 individually studied cases, J. Y. Alnot supplies a great number of personal observations that are invaluable from both diagnostic and surgical viewpoints. The reader is invited to read and reread this chapter by an experienced microsurgeon (translated by Theodore Liberson), containing so many fruits of extensive experience and constant analysis of his anatomic and clinical observations.

In our own chapter on "Motorcycle Brachial Plexopathy," written in collaboration with Theodore Liberson, a clinical neurophysiologist and specialist in rehabilitation medicine, as well as with a fellow surgeon, Hallene Maragh, we have reported some puzzling clinical relationships between fascicular anatomy of spinal nerves and the frequency of their severe involvement during plexus injury. The reader will also find in this chapter an analysis of correlations between electromyography and intraoperative observations. Our clinical experience with microsurgery of the brachial plexus shows that we never downgraded a single patient. Return of function was graphically analyzed over time; this series showed that partial recovery was always initiated by a "silent period" of six months to one year. These observations, just as those of other surgeons, will generate some further research as to how one may promote a speedier recovery of these patients.

In the chapter on "Electrophysiologic Intraoperative Evaluations of the Damaged Root in Traction of the Brachial Plexus," L. Celli and C. Rovesta report a new technique of EMG segmental recordings from the cervical erector spinae muscle while the successive root is stimulated.

Chapter 38, "Our Experience in Obstetrical Brachial Plexus Palsy," was reviewed with Theodore Liberson and Ronald Levine, a fellow microsurgeon. Again, correlations between EMG and intraoperative findings are considered in detail, as well as some case histories involving both primary and secondary surgery.

It is also obstetrical brachial palsy that constitutes the subject of an authoritative report by Alain Gilbert and J. L. Tassin ("Obstetrical Palsy: A Clinical, Pathologic, and Surgical Review"). This longstanding experience in France thus becomes available to our readers.

In the chapter written by Theodore Liberson and myself on "Contribution of Clinical Neurophysiology and Rehabilitation Medicine to the Management of Brachial Plexus Palsy," a number of new techniques were applied to my patients: a novel diagnostic application of root stimulation with needle electrodes prior to surgery; a description of the methodology of "electrical Tinel" mentioned before; a possibility to take advantage of partial muscle reinnervation insufficient to give rise to a functional contraction but eventually sufficient to be used for electromechanical control of the muscles; new experiences with brief and slow pulse stimulation techniques for peripheral nerve injuries; new techniques of conditioned behavior therapies, etc.

Ian Jackson offers in his chapter on "Surgical Correction of Lagophthalmos" a historical review as well as different personal techniques addressing this difficult clinical problem.

Finally, a description of a novel technique of the "Microsurgical Reanimation of the Eye Sphincter" is the subject of a chapter written by Kenneth Lee, a fellow microsurgeon and myself. It contains a detailed original anatomic and physiologic study of the eye sphincter and clinical application of this investigation to restore eye sphincter reanimation by the use of either frontalis or platysma muscles in facial nerve palsies.

These new chapters, together with revised and extended previously published contributions, cover a sufficient territory of reconstructive microsurgery to constitute—we believe—an important contribution to our field.

The reader may be somewhat bewildered by a degree of diversity of opinions and techniques aiming at the solution to the same clinical problem—brachial plexus palsy, for example. However, I feel that such diversity is healthy at this stage of the progress of our young clinical science. Out of it, undoubtedly, a consensus will arise in the future, with additional knowledge, experience, and the number of operated cases with a longer follow-up.

It is only then that a real treatise of reconstructive microsurgery may be written with more certainty and, yet, perhaps, less gratification than felt now in doing pioneering work. At present, let us "stop, look, and listen," reading the contributions of the authors of this volume. I trust that it will be an exciting and useful reading.

It is therefore with a feeling of great fulfillment that I present this volume to the readers. My thanks go to all those who helped me in editing this book. Theodore Liberson shared with me some of the final labor in preparing this volume. I thank him for this.

JULIA K. TERZIS, M.D., Ph.D., F.R.C.S.(C.)

FOREWORD*

I am not born for one corner; the whole world is my native land.

SENECA

This issue of the Clinics in Plastic Surgery was conceived on the deck of a beautiful sailing ship, *The Sea Cloud*, where in January 1982 a small multinational group of reconstructive microsurgeons gathered and exchanged ideas on peripheral nerve microsurgery. This project was prompted by the realization that a great deal of excellent work on peripheral nerves is being accomplished in centers not readily accessible to the North American surgeon. Language barriers have maintained this gap during the past decade. Thus, it is a great pleasure for me to have initiated this exercise that brought together scientists and clinicians from several continents. For in peace, as in war, we are beneficiaries of knowledge contributed by people from every nation in the world.

Major advances in peripheral nerve surgery have occurred during the past two decades. In my opinion they include the following:

Introduction of magnification that allowed "atraumatic" intraneural invasion and popularization of techniques that optimally aligned corresponding fascicles of severed nerves; the ability through microsurgery to explore a nerve atraumatically without necessarily downgrading its function radically altered the timing of both exploration and repair of peripheral nerve injuries. Thus, the wait-and-see attitude of the past has been replaced by aggressive early exploration. In the case of proximal extremity lesions, such as brachial plexus lesions, early repair has spelled the difference between successful muscle reinnervation versus denervation atrophy.

Increased knowledge of peripheral nerve structure and function in health and disease; enhanced understanding of morphofunctional mechanisms of the regenerative process, axonal elongation, sprouting and central versus peripheral plasticity; introduction of powerful histochemical, immunochemical, and biochemical techniques that led to a complete redefinition of the central and the peripheral nervous system; factors that influence nerve growth, including electromagnetic fields and Nerve Growth Factor; the redefinition of factors that adversely affect regeneration, such as tension at the repair site.

---

*To Clinics in Plastic Surgery, January, 1984.

Morphologic and electrophysiologic proof of the functional supremacy of two interposed suture lines versus one under tension, a notion that led to the acceptance of nerve grafting as a legitimate procedure to substitute for shortening osteotomies and traction sutures.

Refinement of the nerve grafting technique based on a renewed awareness of fascicular group organization.

Introduction and refinement of intraoperative electrodiagnosis for lesions in continuity and assessment of functional transmission at the level of individual nerve fascicles.

Electrophysiologic depiction of cutaneous nerve territories, which led to the introduction of free neurovascular flaps for restoring sensation to blind cutaneous sheaths; a heightened understanding and a reevaluation of the nutritional requirements of nerve grafts versus recipient bed's blood supply, which led to nerve grafting procedures with immediate revascularization of the donor nerve from recipient vessels. Since then the vascular anatomy of several donor nerves has been described, and selected clinical trials have been accomplished.

Basic science research on the pathophysiology of normal, denervated, and reinnervated skeletal muscle, which led to the establishment of the notion that skeletal muscle survives microneurovascular transfer despite diminution of functional capability; the understanding of the importance of resting length muscle tension and its precise reproduction following transfer, a finding that greatly improved our results with free muscle transplantation in extremity and later facial palsy reconstructions.

I arbitrarily requested selective topics in peripheral nerve surgery where significant changes have been made and where I felt increased communication was needed. The introduction of magnification to the reconstruction of traumatic neuropathies led to the description of a plethora of new suture techniques. However, communication was hampered by the lack of a universally acceptable nomenclature. In the first article, the Committee Report of the International Society of Reconstructive Microsurgery is presented to address this need. This is followed by several articles on normal peripheral nerve ultrastructure and on ultrastructure subsequent to traumatic lesions. The topic of electrodiagnosis and the interpretation of the compound potential is discussed in experimental and clinical settings.

The mechanisms of muscle denervation and reinnervation precede the clinical application of free muscle for upper-extremity reconstruction. Three articles have been dedicated to the anatomy, rationale, and preliminary clinical applications of vascularized nerve grafts. Discussions on stump neuroma and upper extremity pain are included, followed by a paper on sensory reeducation.

End-to-end nerve repair techniques are described, as is the technique of interfascicular nerve grafting.

The management of brachial plexus injuries in infants and adults is covered by twenty experts from twelve centers and seven different countries. This I believe is the first time that such a multinational approach to brachial plexus injuries is offered to the reader. Finally, this Clinics issue concludes with five articles on the microsurgical reconstruction of acute and chronic facial palsies.

This effort was initially conceived to appear in two issues of the Clinics in Plastic Surgery because of the great number of participants whom I wanted to invite and whose work I have admired over the past decade. Unfortunately, long and unforeseeable delays in receiving the manuscripts almost made it necessary to cancel the project. I am truly grateful to Cynthia Fazzini, who agreed, after several discussions, to a new timetable for this topic, provided that the material could be presented in one issue. However, as my initial request to all the participating authors was for lengthy manuscripts, I had to edit manuscripts to the point of mutilation in some instances and even omit others.

In order to do justice to this very important field, I am preparing a book in which all manuscripts are included, along with the present papers in their complete form. Thus, the interested reader is greatly encouraged to refer to the book by W. B. Saunders that is forthcoming.

JULIA K. TERZIS, M.D., Ph.D., F.R.C.S.(C.)

CONTENTS

Part 3 MICRORECONSTRUCTION OF BRACHIAL PLEXUS INJURIES

Part 4   OBSTETRICAL BRACHIAL PLEXUS PALSY

Part **5** **COMBATING FACIAL PARALYSIS**

MORPHOFUNCTIONAL CHARACTERISTICS

PART

1

1

Nomenclature in Peripheral Nerve Surgery

■

Hanno Millesi, M.D.
Julia K. Terzis, M.D., Ph.D.

Microsurgery allows exposure and repair of tissue layers that were previously inaccessible. A clear terminology is mandatory to be able to describe the dissections, as existing terms are used in different ways by different surgeons. For example, *neurilemma* is defined by some authors as the external layer of the myelin sheath and the endoneurial sheath around the nerve fibers. Other surgeons use the term neurilemma synonymously with epineurium when describing epineurial nerve repair. Sometimes certain terms are clearly used incorrectly. Some surgeons have difficulties with the terms *epineurium* and *perineurium* and use them in a reversed way. Surgeons usually use the term epineurium to mean only that layer of connective tissue that surrounds the entire nerve trunk, not being aware that the epineurium also extends between the fascicles. Occasionally, two different terms are used to describe the same thing, which certainly does not facilitate understanding by a beginner in the field.

In the past only a few classic procedures were in common use. Neurorrhaphy was performed as an epineural or an epineurial nerve repair, uniting the entire nerve trunk with epineural or epineurial stitches, according to whether the stitches were placed in the epineurial tissue or in the more superficial (adventitial) layers (epineural). The alternative was the perineurial nerve repair, uniting individual fascicles by perineurial stitches. Nerve grafting was regarded as a last resort and did not become popular. Neu-

rolysis was performed only as an external procedure, and any attempt to extend the process of neurolysis to the nerve itself was rejected. A few terms were sufficient to describe and define these procedures, and everybody understood immediately what was meant. Therefore, variations in nomenclature were not important.

The development of microsurgery has brought about a significant change. There are now many more procedures available, and different steps of different procedures can be combined according to the particular situation. The layer where the stitches are placed has become less important in describing a procedure, as compared with the way the procedure is done, e.g., how lining of the fascicles was achieved. We must not forget that when epineural nerve repair was introduced in the 1870s, it became *the* decisive step and that use of the term epineural nerve repair to describe the entire procedure was therefore well justified. Before that time, surgeons did not dare to touch the nerve and tried to line up transected nerve trunks only by manipulating adjacent tissue, a process called "cum carne." Great progress was made when surgeons realized that they could manipulate a tissue layer on the surface of the nerve without touching the nerve tissue sensu strictori. Since then, more than 100 years have elapsed, but it is surprising to note that in many scientific papers the discussion concerning whether epineural or perineural repair is preferable is still kept alive,

3

without paying attention to the fact that over the past decades an enormous amount of knowledge about the intraneural composition of different nerve segments has been collected. This discussion is futile as long as no exact definition is given about the conditions under which the nerve repair had been performed, especially with respect to the fascicular pattern and the way the fascicles were managed.

General statements such as "an end-to-end nerve repair is better than a graft," or vice versa, are not justified today, if exact details are not given, since there are several different grafting procedures available and each step of grafting or of end-to-end nerve repair might have been performed in a different way and under different circumstances.

The International Society of Reconstructive Microsurgery has set up a committee to develop a more satisfactory terminology.* It was amazing to see how many terms were defined in different ways by this small group of experts, and that consensus could be achieved only after very long discussions. A committee report was presented to the Society of Reconstructive Microsurgery in May, 1979, at the meeting in Guaruja, Brazil, and the details were discussed thoroughly. A modified report was presented again in February, 1981, in Melbourne, Australia, and the recommendations were agreed upon after long discussions.

In the following pages, terms are used that were agreed upon by the committee. For other aspects of peripheral nerve repair, which were not covered by the committee, terms that have been used by the authors for many years are given.

GENERAL TERMS

The term *nerve repair* is used in many papers and books as a general term to cover all surgical efforts in connection with damaged peripheral nerves. Moberg[12] made the point that "nerve repair" does not define what really happens as far as functional return is concerned, since return of function always is far from normal. It is interesting to note that exact definitions are mandatory

---

*H. Millesi, Austria (Chairman); S. Sunderland, Australia; Y. Ykuta, Japan; G. Brunelli, Italy; J. Michon, France; R. D. Acland, United States; and J. K. Terzis, United States.

even for such general terms, in order to bring about mutual understanding. The term "repair" needs an object—to repair what. It is certainly true that the surgeon does not repair function. The surgeon repairs continuity (if it is lost) to create favorable circumstances for nerve regeneration, or he or she performs a repair by removing pathologic structures such as constricting bands, which prevent regeneration in a lesion in continuity. The amount of functional return will always depend on the quality of regeneration that follows the nerve repair.

The term *neurotization* describes the ingrowth of axons into a denervated peripheral nerve segment. Neurotization can occur at the level of a peripheral nerve stump after transection, when continuity was restored by a neurorrhaphy or nerve grafting, or it can occur at the level of the terminal branches of a peripheral nerve within a muscle. Consequently, we have to distinguish the following terms:

Nerve-to-nerve neurotization: This term is used if the continuity of a dissected nerve has been repaired by end-to-end approximation (i.e., *neurorrhaphy*), either by nerve grafts (i.e., *nerve grafting*) or by transposition of the proximal stump of another nerve, which is connected with the distal stump of the denervated nerve (i.e., *nerve transfer*).

Nerve-to-muscle neurotization: If the proximal stump of a peripheral nerve is inserted into a muscle at the level of the motor end-plates, the outgrowing axon sprouts are able to neurotize the motor end-plates.

Muscle-to-muscle neurotization: If the muscle belly of an innervated muscle is brought into direct contact with the muscle belly of a denervated muscle, the latter can be reinnervated by sprouting of axons from the innervated muscle.

MAIN COMPONENTS OF THE PERIPHERAL NERVE

The most important component of a peripheral nerve is the nerve fiber, which is responsible for the function of the nerve, i.e., transmitting stimuli. It can be myelinated or unmyelinated. All the other structures of the nerve are subordinated to provide optimal conditions for the nerve fibers. The fascicles provide the optimal milieu for the nerve fibers by their barrier function. Different numbers of fascicles are embedded in epineurial tissue to form the nerve trunk, which again provides optimal conditions against mechanical stress.

The Nerve Fiber

The main component of the nerve fiber is the *axon*, an extension of a neuron. It is surrounded by the *axolemma*. Since the axon is a part of a neuron, it degenerates after transection distal to the level of transection. The axon cannot survive without *Schwann cells*. In unmyelinated nerve fibers several axons are embedded in a Schwann cell (Fig. 1–1). In myelinated nerve fibers Schwann cells develop a *myelin sheath* around a single axon. A myelin sheath is axon-dependent because it degenerates with degeneration of the axon. The Schwann cell is not axon-dependent because it survives axon degeneration. By production of a myelin sheath, which does not occur without an axon, the Schwann cell becomes part of the nerve fiber. To summarize, the nerve fiber consists of an axon, an axolemma, and a myelin sheath (in myelinated nerve fibers) with Schwann cells. All these components are intact only as long as the connection with the neuron is preserved, and they are subject to Wallerian degeneration after transection (Committee report, Society of Reconstructive Microsurgery).

The nerve fiber is surrounded by the *endoneurial sheath*. The endoneurial sheath consists of a basal lamina and, on its external side, of collagen fibers and endoneurial fibroblasts (Committee report, Society of Recon-

structive Microsurgery). The components of the endoneurial sheath are not immediately affected after transection. The space within the endoneurial sheath after Wallerian degeneration is filled with mobile Schwann cells (Hanke Büngner bands). With prolonged denervation, the endoneurial sheath may become collagenized and may shrink.

In some older papers the myelin sheath and the endoneurial sheath together are referred to as the neurilemma. However, the above-mentioned committee held the view that the term neurilemma is confusing and should no longer be used.

The Fascicle

Many nerve fibers with their endoneurial sheath are surrounded by *perineurium*, forming the *fascicle*. The perineurium consists of several layers of mesothelial-like perineurial cells. A dense connective tissue layer surrounds the fascicle. Discussion is still going on as to whether the term perineurium should be used only for the mesothelial-like tissue layers or if it should also include the dense connective tissue sheath. Although this question is of great theoretical interest, it is not relevant for the surgeon. A surgeon is easily able to find a connective tissue layer in order to isolate the fascicle, leaving intact the perineurial sheath. Blood vessels, running longitudinally, are found between the different lamellae of the perineurium.[6, 7] Only capillaries are found inside the fascicle in the endoneural space; there are no blood vessels and also no lymphatics. The capillaries of the

Figure 1–1. *A,* Myelinated axon. Note the Schwann cell nucleus and its relation to the myelin sheath. Basal lamina surrounds the plasma membrane of this satellite cell. *B,* An unmyelinated fiber consisting of several unmyelinated axons enveloped from a single Schwann cell. (From Terzis, J. K., and Breidenbach, W. C.: Surgical treatment of peripheral nerve injuries in children. *In* Serafin, D., and Georgiade, N. G.: Pediatric Plastic Surgery. St. Louis, C. V. Mosby Co., 1984.)

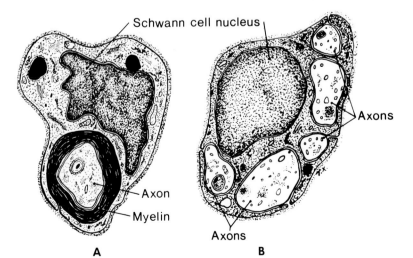

A

B

endoneural space are connected with the perineurial vessels just beneath the perineurial membrane. The perineurium maintains a higher pressure inside the fascicle. The perineurial membrane acts as a diffusion barrier, and the endothelium of the intrafascicular capillaries acts as a blood-nerve barrier.

It is important to note at this point that the term *perineurial* refers to everything that is part of the perineurium. The term *perineural* is a purely topographic designation, referring to something that is around the nerve. The same distinction is true for the term *endoneurial*, which means something belonging to the endoneurial space, and the term *endoneural,* which simply means "within the nerve." Likewise, *epineurial* refers to everything that is part of the epineurium, and *epineural* refers to something that is on the surface of the nerve.

The term *funicle* is synonymous with the term *fascicle*, but the committee members regarded the use of fascicle as more appropriate.

The Nerve Trunk

The nerve trunk consists of varying numbers of fascicles that are embedded in a loose connective tissue, the *epineurium*. Several layers of epineurium surround all the fascicles and are termed the outer or external layers of the epineurium by some members of our committee. The epineurium that extends between the fascicles is termed the inner or internal part of the epineurium. Since microsurgical dissection very often deals with these different tissue layers, clear distinction is mandatory. Since the outer or external or circumferential epineurium consists of several layers, the adjectives "outer" or "external" and "inner" or "internal" are misleading. For this reason the members agreed to use the adjectives "epifascicular" for the external layers and "interfascicular" for the internal layers. The term *epifascicular epineurium* is used to include the layers of the epineurium that surround the entire nerve trunk and are situated on top of the fascicles from whichever direction the surgeon looks at them. The term *interfascicular epineurium* includes all the extensions of the epineurium between the fascicles.

The outer nerve is enveloped by several layers of loose connective tissue that are superficial to the epineurium and contain fat

lobules. Some surgeons refer to this tissue as the *adventitia* of the nerve. Others do not distinguish these layers from the epifascicular epineurium.

The development of this system varies, according to the site and to the mechanical stress that the nerve is exposed to: For example, in the carpal tunnel three tissue layers surrounding the median nerve can be distinguished. These layers consist of loose connective tissue that corresponds to the lining of the tendon sheath.

1. After transection of the retinaculum flexorum a loose connective tissue layer can be defined, which corresponds to a *parietal* lining of the entire carpal tunnel.

2. The next layer envelopes both nerve and tendons as a *visceral* layer.

3. The median nerve itself is enveloped in a special layer that separates the nerve from the wall at the palmar and radial aspect and from the tendons at the dorsal and ulnar aspect. Only after transection of these three layers is the median nerve itself exposed, along with its epifascicular epineurium, which again consists of two or three superficial layers.

The interfascicular epineurium extends between the fascicles. It consists of loose and dense parts, the latter occurring around fascicles, sometimes including several fascicles to form a group. The committee members did not feel that it was necessary to have a special term for this structure.

The blood supply of peripheral nerves is provided by segmental vessels that enter the nerve within a double layer of loose connective tissue. The term *mesoneurium* was suggested for this double layer. Whether this double layer is formed as an extension of the epifascicular epineurium or of the more superficial adventitial tissue is open to discussion.

Fascicular Pattern

In very proximal levels the fibers of a particular type are diffusely distributed over a cross section,[10] but at peripheral levels the nerve fibers of different types are arranged in individual fascicles, according to the pending division of the nerve.[5] Sunderland studied this problem thoroughly[14, 16] and came to the conclusion that over a certain distance the changes in the fascicular pattern are so distinct that fascicular repair is not possible because the number and arrangement of fascicles no longer correspond. He recognized the fact that fascicles having a certain function might be arranged in a group before leaving the nerve (e.g., some sensory fibers of the ulnar nerve forming the dorsal branch), and he recommended the "fascicular exclusion" of such fascicles in order to avoid those fibers going into the main trunk of the ulnar nerve.

In spite of the great variations in a fascicular pattern, three types can be distinguished (Fig. 1–2):

1. Monofascicular pattern: The cross section of a nerve consists of one large fascicle, which is surrounded by perineurium and epifascicular epineurium. Consequently, there is no interfascicular epineurium and the cross section consists only of fascicular tissue, with the exception of the circumferential layers, as mentioned previously. The term unifascicular could also be used.

2. Oligofascicular pattern: The cross section of the nerve consists of a limited number of rather large fascicles (up to eight or ten). A synonymous term would be paucifascicular pattern. The use of a Latin prefix along with the Latin root word would satisfy linguistic considerations much better than mixing a Latin root with a Greek prefix (e.g., monofascicular or oligofascicular). However, the word paucifascicular would be pronounced in a different way in different languages and might therefore give rise to misunderstanding. Because of this the committee members decided to retain Greek prefixes, in spite of some linguistic impurity. Two subtypes can be distinguished.

   a. Oligofascicular pattern with a few large fascicles (two to five). Again there is only very little interfascicular tissue between these fascicles. The fascicles can be controlled easily by manipulating the epifascicular epineurial tissue, and these nerve segments are very similar to the monofascicular ones.

   b. If there are more than five but still a limited number of larger fascicles (six to ten), the amount of interfascicular tissue between the fascicles becomes a factor because there is danger of malalignment (fascicle to non-fascicular tissue) during repair. The larger size of the fascicles and their limited number allow independent manipulation.

3. Polyfascicular pattern: The cross section consists of many fascicles of different sizes with prevalence of small fascicles. (The alternative term for polyfascicular is pluri- or multifascicular). Two subtypes can be distinguished.

   a. Polyfascicular pattern with *diffuse arrangement* of fascicles. The large amount of non-fascicular tissue increases the danger of malalignment (fascicle to non-fascicular tissue). This can be avoided only by isolation of individual fascicles. However, the large number and small size of the fascicles make avoidance of malalignment very difficult. The identification of corresponding fascicles, especially if a defect is present, is almost impossible.

   b. Polyfascicular pattern with *group arrangement* of fascicles. Fascicles having

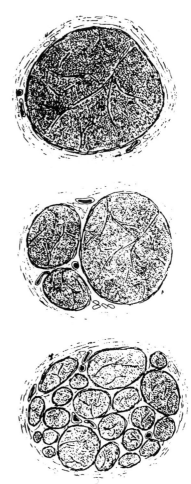

Figure 1–2. Diagrammatic representation of basic patterns of intraneural structure: monofascicular (*top*), oligofascicular (*center*), and polyfascicular (*bottom*).

a particular function are arranged in a group. Each group of fascicles maintains its integrity over a fairly long distance despite a changing fascicular pattern within the fascicle group and some exchange of fibers between the fascicle groups. One of this chapter's authors (H. M.) has utilized this concept of fascicle groups for nerve grafting since the mid-1960s.[11] The group pattern of different nerves was studied more recently by Williams[19] and by Jabaley et al.[3] It is evident that the presence of such a group pattern can be utilized for peripheral nerve surgery.

A monofascicular pattern (type 1) or an oligofascicular pattern with few fascicles (type 2a) was seen in the facial nerve at the stylomastoid foramen, in some roots of the brachial plexus, in proximal levels of the radial nerve, in the ulnar nerve in the upper arm, and in the axillary nerve. Mono- or oligofascicular arrangement (type 2a) can be combined with a group arrangement (type 3b) so that the main trunk of the nerve shows a mono- or oligofascicular pattern but one or two fascicle groups are present that correspond with branches that will shortly leave the nerve.

A polyfascicular pattern with a group arrangement is typical for the peripheral portions of peripheral nerves. A polyfascicular pattern without a group arrangement or an oligofascicular pattern with more fascicles (type 2b) is encountered in transient zones, e.g., the brachial plexus at the trunk and cord level, at the formation of the peripheral nerves, and in certain zones in the periphery where there is heavy fiber exchange. In these particular areas, identification of corresponding fascicles is very difficult. Between these zones, the arrangement remains rather constant.

At levels where the nerve is exposed to mechanical stress, a cross section usually consists of a greater number of fascicles compared with segments not exposed to mechanical stress. This adaptation to mechanical stress does not influence the group pattern if the pattern is present before and after the site of stress.

If a fascicle is starting to divide or if two fascicles are fusing, a perineurial septum dividing the fascicle can be seen. The fascicle should be considered as one structure if the separation is due to a single layer of perineurial tissue and as two fascicles if the dividing perineurium consists of two distinct layers with a layer of loose connective tissue in between.

LESION IN CONTINUITY AND LESION WITH LOSS OF CONTINUITY

Lesion in Continuity

In the two classification systems of nerve injuries by Seddon[13] and Sunderland,[15] the definition of the different degrees of injury is based on the amount of nerve tissue that has been lost and the nerve tissue that still preserves continuity. In a first-degree lesion (Sunderland), or neurapraxia (Seddon), the axon remains intact. A conduction block without morphologic consequences may develop and in addition a segmental demyelination may occur. In a second-degree lesion (Sunderland), or axonotmesis (Seddon), the axon is severed and Wallerian degeneration develops, but the endoneurial, perineurial, and epineurial tissues are still intact. In a third-degree lesion the damage in the endoneurial space is more extensive, but the perineurium, and consequently the fascicular pattern, is intact. In a fourth-degree lesion the fascicular pattern has been lost and continuity is preserved only by epineural tissue.

Sunderland's system classifies the acute situation very well, but it fails to include the reaction that develops with time. The reaction of the connective tissue of the peripheral nerve always involves fibrosis, but the degree of fibrosis differs in the various layers, according to the type of injury. Three different degrees of fibrosis can be distinguished.

1. Fibrosis of the epifascicular epineurium: This causes constriction of the fascicles (similar to constriction from a tight stocking). It can be present in first-, second-, or third-degree lesions and prevents or delays the spontaneous recovery that can be expected in first- or second-degree lesions and possibly in third-degree lesions.

2. Fibrosis of the epi- and interfascicular epineurium: This is due to extension of the fibrosis between the fascicles and can be found in first-, second-, and third-degree

lesions. A simple resection of the epifascicular epineurium does not correct the problem.

3. Fibrosis of the endoneural space: In this type of fibrosis, the fibrotic fascicles are solid and regeneration cannot be expected in spite of intact remnants of the fascicular pattern.

Neurolysis is a surgical procedure to release a nerve and to decompress the endoneural space. Based on the pathologic changes, the following steps in neurolysis can be distinguished:

1. Exposure of the involved nerve: Exposure should always start from normal tissue proximally and distally.
2. External neurolysis: A nerve that is adherent to other structures or is embedded in scar tissue must be released. Release is usually performed in a thickened layer that corresponds to the adventitial tissue and eventually to the external layers of the epifascicular epineurium. Internal layers of the epifascicular epineurium usually remain intact and the fascicles are not exposed after external neurolysis. Crossing fibrous bands, bony fragments, etc. that are causing external pressure are also removed.
3. Internal neurolysis: The term internal neurolysis is used if surgery is extended to the entire thickness of the epifascicular epineurium or to tissue layers that are surrounded by the epifascicular epineurium.
   a. If the pathologic tissue is restricted to the epifascicular epineurium, a longitudinal incision of this tissue layer is sufficient to provide decompression. This is called *epifascicular epineurotomy.* If removal of the epifascicular epineurium is necessary, an *epifascicular epineurectomy* (complete or partial) is performed.
   b. If the pathologic changes extend to the spaces between the fascicles or fascicle groups, a resection of the interfascicular epineurium is necessary, i.e., an *interfascicular epineurectomy.* This can be performed only as a partial procedure because it is impossible to remove all interfascicular epineurium. Epineurectomy is performed only when each fascicle is completely isolated and naked. Otherwise it is sufficient to excise as much of the tissue necessary to achieve decompression or to remove a

tumor, leaving all other parts of the epineurium intact. Some surgeons have claimed that this type of neurolysis may interfere with circulation and damage the connecting fibers between the fascicles. Theoretically, this may be true if all fascicles are isolated, but in clinical practice this is never done and interfascicular epineurectomy is always a partial procedure. The removal of fibrotic areas between the fascicles does not harm the circulation, because in these fibrotic areas the vessels are closed anyway and connecting fibers are already destroyed. Villas[18] demonstrated that epineurectomy did not impair blood flow.

   c. Neurolysis does not offer much chance of improvement in patients with fibrosis of the endoneural space. In these cases resection of the involved fascicles and restoration of continuity by nerve grafts are indicated. One could theoretically imagine a situation in which the perineurium has become fibrotic and shrunken but the endoneural space is still not completely fibrotic. In this case a perineurotomy could be considered. However, we have not yet encountered such a situation because if the perineurium is very much involved, the endoneural space is completely fibrotic as well.

Lesion with Loss of Continuity

In a lesion with loss of continuity, the continuity must be restored to offer a chance for regeneration. The repair can be performed by direct union of the cut ends of the nerve, i.e., *neurorrhaphy,* or by uniting the two cut ends indirectly using a nerve graft, i.e., *nerve grafting.*

Repairing the continuity of a peripheral nerve involves a number of different surgical maneuvers, which can be performed in different ways. These maneuvers include preparation of the stumps, approximation, coaptation, and maintenance of the coaptation. The various steps can also be combined in different ways. Thus, description of one basic step, e.g., describing the layer where the stitches are anchored (as in perineurial or epineurial nerve repair), does not define the entire procedure. Only a description of how these four basic steps have been performed, along with some additional information, provides a clear definition of what was really done.

Preparation of Stumps. At present the two stumps can be prepared in two different ways:

1. Resection of slices until normal tissue is reached: This technique is preferred in cases of monofascicular nerve segments (type 1), oligofascicular nerve segments with few fascicles (type 2a), and polyfascicular nerve segments without group arrangement (type 3a).

2. Interfascicular dissection of the two stumps: Individual fascicles or fascicle groups can be isolated by interfascicular dissection starting in normal tissue. This is done by resection of much of the epineurium and can be used in oligofascicular nerve segments with more fascicles (type 2b) and in polyfascicular nerve segments with a group arrangement. The technique should not be used for a mono- or oligofascicular nerve segment with only two to five fascicles (type 2a), because in both instances no or only very little interfascicular epineurial tissue is present. Its use in a polyfascicular nerve segment without group arrangement would require the isolation of the many small fascicles, resulting in possible extensive surgical trauma. This disadvantage may outweigh the eventual advantage of a more exact coaptation and a reduction of the epineural tissue.

Approximation. The two nerve stumps are brought into contact. This means that the *distance* between the two nerve stumps at time of surgery has to be overcome. We are used to talking about a gap between the two stumps and do not really think about the factors responsible for this gap. The distance between the two stumps at a given moment depends on: (a) defect of nerve tissue caused by trauma, (b) elastic retraction, (c) retraction by fibrosis (in secondary repairs), (d) defect of nerve tissue caused by resection (during preparation of stumps), (e) difference in distance according to joint position (i.e., increases with extension, decreases with flexion), and (f) difference in distance caused by mobilization, transposition, stretching, and eventual bone resection. The factors a, b, c, and d have to be added together, and they must be equal to f + e.

In an *ideal neurorrhaphy* without a defect (a

= 0), without damage to nerve tissue and therefore no resection (d = 0), and performed as a primary procedure (c = 0), only the elastic retraction has to be overcome. Mobilization has to be done to the extent necessary to achieve this goal: b = f. It is not important to flex the joints and therefore e can also equal zero. Immobilization in the flexed position is performed more as a protective measure than as a necessary step to achieve approximation.

In a secondary repair under *ideal conditions* there would be some retraction by fibrosis in addition to the elastic retraction, and we would have the formula b + c = f. In the case of a *small defect* (a) and *limited damage* to nerve tissue (d), the formula would be a + b + c + d = f + e. Since a and d are not extensive, mobilization (f) and flexion (e) can also be limited.

In a nerve lesion with a *marked defect* and *severe* trauma, a and d are extensive and consequently f and e (mobilization and flexion of the adjacent joints) must be extensive as well. Under these circumstances, some surgeons would perform only a limited resection to keep d small, which would mean that damaged nerve tissue is coapted with damaged nerve tissue.

A surgeon who decides to perform a nerve graft has two options. An *ideal nerve grafting* can be attempted, which would mean that the length of the relaxed nerve graft is selected according to the distance between the two stumps (a + b + c + d) without significant mobilization (f = 0) and with neutral position of the joint (e = 0). The surgeon can also try to *minimize the length of the graft*, i.e., the distance between the two stumps (a + b + c + d) is reduced by maximal flexion (±e) and by maximal mobilization (±f). This would mean that a shorter graft has to be used, but the site of coaptation will be exposed to problems similar to those encountered when an end-to-end repair has been attempted. It is evident that the outcome of a grafting procedure will be completely different according to the way selected of measuring the necessary length of the graft.

To be able to evaluate a procedure, the following information is necessary:

1. What was the distance between the two stumps at the time of exposure in neutral position of the joints (a + b + c)? In clinical practice, especially in secondary repairs, it

will not be possible to estimate the contributions of each of these three factors (a + b + c) to the distance achieved as the final result.

2. What was the extent of resection of the two stumps (d)?

3. In which position were the joints when approximation was achieved (e)?

4. What was done to achieve or facilitate approximation (f)?

As additional information, it would be helpful to know how approximation was achieved: by a stay stitch, by approximating the stumps using hooks, or by touching the nerve stumps using a forceps, etc.

Coaptation. The term coaptation is used here to mean "to bring together." We can coapt the two stumps of a transected nerve trunk. We can coapt the two stumps of a fascicle group and we can coapt individual fascicles. Independent of the level at which coaptation is performed, the term coaptation *implies the effort of the surgeon to bring the cross section of the transected fascicles into as good contact as possible.*

In the case of a monofascicular nerve segment, a *stump-to-stump coaptation* (truncal coaptation) is automatically a fascicular coaptation because the monofascicular nerve trunk consists of only one large fascicle. In an oligofascicular nerve segment with two to five fascicles (type 2a), it is usually easy to achieve optimal coaptation of the five fascicles by manipulation of the two nerve stumps, and again a *stump-to-stump coaptation* will provide good coaptation of the fascicles. In an oligofascicular nerve segment with six to ten fascicles (type 2b), it might be difficult to achieve the coaptation of the centrally situated fascicles simply by handling the two nerve stumps by their surface. In this case even an optimal stump-to-stump coaptation does not secure an optimal coaptation of the individual fascicles, especially in the center. It might be worthwhile, therefore, to isolate this limited number of large fascicles and perform a *fascicular coaptation* of each fascicle.

In the case of a polyfascicular nerve segment without group arrangement, a fascicular coaptation can be attempted as long as there is no defect. However, extensive manipulation is necessary, and the damage caused by surgical trauma might outweigh the advantage of a more exact coaptation. A fascicular coaptation is impossible if a defect

is present because the number of fascicles does not correspond. Since there are so many fascicles, the risk of coaptation of non-corresponding fascicles is high. Stump-to-stump coaptation with special attempts to secure a coaptation of the individual fascicles by interfascicular guide stitches might be an acceptable solution. In a polyfascicular nerve segment with group arrangement, a *group-to-group coaptation* (i.e., *interfascicular coaptation*) is performed after isolation of the fascicle group. If a defect is present, the number of fascicles within corresponding groups differs, and therefore an ideal coaptation cannot be achieved. However, the procedure is sufficient to provide a useful result.

If *direct coaptation* is not possible, *indirect coaptation* by the use of nerve grafts is performed.

A grafting procedure is defined based on the following three criteria:

1. According to the type of graft
   a. *Trunk graft:* Trunk grafts can be used as free trunk grafts, as pedicled trunk grafts, or as vascularized trunk grafts.
   b. *Cutaneous nerve graft:* Cutaneous nerve grafts can be used as free grafts and as vascularized nerve grafts.[2, 16]
2. According to the preparation of the stumps
   a. Preparation by resection: If a *trunk graft* is used, the two stumps are coapted similar to a stump-to-stump coaptation. If cutaneous nerve segments are used as grafts, each cutaneous nerve segment is connected with a certain sector of the nerve trunk (sectoral coaptation).
   b. Preparation by interfascicular dissection: If the nerve trunks are prepared by interfascicular dissection into individual fascicles or fascicle groups, the cutaneous nerve segment is connected with a fascicle of corresponding size (*fascicular grafting*) or with a fascicle group of corresponding size (*interfascicular grafting*).
3. According to the relative size between fascicles and grafts in cases of fascicular nerve grafting. Three possibilities can be distinguished:
   a. Large fascicle to several cutaneous nerves, if one nerve graft is not sufficient to cover the cross section.
   b. Medium fascicle to one cutaneous

nerve, if the fascicle and the nerve correspond in size.

c. Small fascicle to isolated fascicle or fascicles of the graft, if the fascicles are smaller than the nerve graft.

Maintaining the Coaptation. It is important to know what type of procedure was done in order to maintain the coaptation. This is very much influenced by the amount of tension that exists at the suture site or that has to be expected when the patient begins to move the limb. If there is no tension, the few stay stitches to approximate the two stumps and to achieve coaptation may be sufficient to maintain coaptation. Otherwise more stitches have to be used. The number of stitches, their size, and the material of which they are made have to be noted. Where the stitches are anchored must also be known. This can be in the:

1. Tissue surrounding the nerve (i.e., epineural stitch).

2. Epifascicular epineurium (i.e., epineurial stitch).

3. Interfascicular epineurium (i.e., interfascicular stitch).

4. Perineurium (i.e., perineurial stitch).

5. Epi- and perineurium (i.e., epi- and perineurial stitches).

6. In addition, removable stitches going across the fascicles have been used (intrafascicular stitches).

To maintain coaptation, tissue glues have been used with or without wrapping of the suture site. Concentrated solutions of fibrinogen have been used for gluing.[8, 9] Since this preparation contains fibrinolytic agents[4] and therefore antifibrinolytic treatment is necessary,[1] exact information about how the solution was prepared is necessary.

Additional Information. The site and extent of the lesion have to be noted. Information about the condition of the wound bed, the skin cover, and the skin closure is also necessary. Since the age of the patient and time interval since the accident are extremely important, an adequate history must be obtained. One would also like to know the tourniquet time, the time of immobilization, and the position of immobilization.

SUMMARY

These remarks are not intended to make simple things complicated. What we want to do is draw attention to the need for generally accepted terms and generally accepted definitions. Only if all the surgeons who want to investigate their results scientifically and researchers who want to study nerve regeneration under different conditions use the same terms and the same definitions will it be possible to compare the results of different groups. To promote this universal usage was the aim of the committee of the International Society of Reconstructive Microsurgery, and this was also our aim, if we have suggested some additional definitions that may be open to discussion and criticism.

References

1. Duspiva, W., Blümel, G., Haas–Denk, S., and Wriedt–Lübbe, I.: Eine neue Methode zur Anastomisierung durchtrennter peripherer Nerven. Chir. Forum, *100*, 1977.
2. Fachinelli, A., Masquelet, A., Restrepo, J., and Gilbert, A.: The vascularized sural nerve. Anatomy and surgical approach. Int. J. Microsurg., *3*:57, 1981.
3. Jabaley, M. E., Wallace, W. H., and Heckler, F. R.: Internal topography of major nerves of the forearm and hand: A current review. J. Hand Surg., *5*:1, 1980.
4. Kuderna, H.: Discussion. Symposium on Indications, Technique and Results of Nerve Grafting, May 22, 1977, in Vienna. Handchirurgie, Sonderheft No. 2.
5. Langley, J. N., and Hashimoto, M.: On the suture of separate nerve bundles in a nerve trunk and on internal nerve plexuses. J. Physiol. (Lond.), *51*:318, 1917.
6. Lundborg, G.: Problems of circulation. *In* Gorio, A., Millesi, H., and Mingrino, S. (eds.): Posttraumatic Peripheral Nerve Regeneration: Its Experimental Basis and Clinical Implications. New York, Raven Press, 1981, p. 79.
7. Lundborg, G.: Mechanical effects on circulation and nerve function. *In* Gorio, A., Millesi, H., and Mingrino, S. (eds.): Posttraumatic Peripheral Nerve Regeneration: Its Experimental Basis and Clinical Implications. New York, Raven Press, 1981, p. 157.
8. Matras, H., Dinges, H. P., Lassmann, H., and Mamoli, R.: Zur nahtlosen interfaszikulären Nerventransplantation im Tierexperiment. Wien. med. Wschr., *122*:527, 1972.
9. Matras, H., and Kuderna, H.: The principle of nervous anastomosis with clotting agents. Transactions of the 6th International Congress of Plastic and Reconstructive Surgery, Paris, August 24–29, 1975, Paris, New York: Masson, 1976, p. 143.
10. McKinnley, J. C.: Intraneural plexus of fasciculi and fibers in sciatic nerves. Arch. Neurol. Psychiatr., *6*:377, 1921.
11. Millesi, H.: Zum Problem der Überbrückung von Defekten peripherer Nerven. Wien. med. Wschr., *118*:182, 1968.

12. Moberg, E.: Paper presented at the 1st International Meeting of the International Confederation of the Societies for Surgery of the Hand, Rotterdam, May, 1980.
13. Seddon, H. J.: Three types of nerve injury. Brain, 66:237, 1943.
14. Sunderland, S.: The intraneural topography of the radial, median and ulnar nerves. Brain, 68:243, 1945.
15. Sunderland, S.: A classification of peripheral nerve injuries producing loss of function. Brain, 74:491, 1951.
16. Sunderland, S. L., and Ray, J.: The intraneural topography of the sciatic nerve and its popliteal divisions in man. Brain, 7:242, 1948.
17. Townsend, P.: Microvascular nerve grafts. Paper presented at the 4th Congress of the European Section of the International Confederation for Plastic and Reconstructive Surgery, Athens, May 10–15, 1981.
18. Villas, C.: Vascular alterations after epineurium removal. A qualitative and quantitative experimental study in rabbits. Int. J. Microsurg., 3:227, 1981.
19. Williams, H. B.: Peripheral nerve injuries in children. In Kerushen, D. A. et al. (eds.): Proceedings Symposium on Pediatric Surgery. St. Louis, C. V. Mosby, 1982, p. 266.

2

Mechanical Injury of Peripheral Nerves: Fine Structure and Dysfunction

■

John E. Castaldo, M.D.
Jose L. Ochoa, M.D., Ph.D., D.Sc.

When a peripheral nerve suffers mechanical injury, the character, degree, and duration of malfunction depend on the type of nerve fiber damage and the efficiency of repair processes. The mechanical injury may act acutely or chronically, and the type of structural pathology differs significantly for each. The morphologic features of these lesions, as studied in animal models of acute and chronic nerve compression, provide a fundamental look at the nature and mechanism of nerve injuries as well as a scientific approach to their management.

The early clinical manifestations of nerve injury (numbness, paralysis, paresthesiae and pain) may, in themselves, give little clue to the type or severity of nerve damage or the possibility of functional recovery. Specific electrophysiologic tests and a clear understanding of the pathophysiology of acute and chronic nerve compression are the physician's most powerful tool in assessing a nerve injury and successfully predicting its outcome. In selected cases, early surgical intervention may save months of unnecessary disability and suffering and may maximize the regenerative potential. What, then, are the anatomic substrates that account for disordered sensation, muscle weakness, and wasting? How might the clinician predict the outcome and increase the chances for recovery knowing the pathophysiology of such lesions? What follows is an attempt to (1)

compare and contrast the structural pathology of acute and chronic nerve compression as assessed by modern histopathologic techniques, (2) interpret the mechanisms of production, and (3) correlate abnormal structure with abnormalities of nerve function in producing positive or negative sensorimotor symptoms.

NERVE MORPHOLOGY

In order to understand the structural consequences of physical injury to nerves, it is useful to have a clear mental picture of their normal anatomy. Motor, sensory, and autonomic nerve fibers are composed of axons, satellite cells, and various connective tissue support elements. Mature fibers may be classified into myelinated or unmyelinated types on the basis of their diameter and type of axonal investment by Schwann cells. Groups of unmyelinated axons cohabitate Schwann cells to form well-defined units that are interspersed among myelinated fibers in a nerve trunk.[16, 57]

In myelinated fibers, multiple layers of the cell membrane of a Schwann cell are wrapped around a single axon to form a myelin sheath over a definable segment of axon known as the internode. The internode length varies in direct proportion to the diameter of the myelinated fiber and may range from 0.1 to 1.8

15

mm in length.[5, 28, 82] For a short distance (0.3 to 2.0 μm) between internode segments, the axon is not invested with myelin. This region is known as the node of Ranvier and is instrumental for saltatory conduction of the nerve impulse.[39, 40] Individual nerve fibers are separated from each other by a basal lamina and then by a surrounding endoneurium composed of collagen fibrils, fibroblasts, and blood vessels. Bundles of nerve fibers are in turn defined into fascicles by a multilayered cellular sheath known as the perineurium. The epineurium consists of connective tissue that binds several nerve fascicles into a single nerve trunk.[5, 78]

The paranodes of a nerve fiber are the regions at the extremities of the myelin internodal segments.[78] They are characterized by a slight increase in axonal caliber for a short distance on either side of the node of Ranvier.[48] The axon cylinder and its myelin investment become crenated in this region, and myelin lamellae end in terminal loops containing Schwann cell cytoplasm.[4, 40, 62]

At the nodes of Ranvier, the axon is without myelin investment and is smaller in caliber. The relative degree of axonal narrowing at the nodes is greater for large-diameter fibers.[30, 32] The length of the nodal gap and the diameter of the nodal axon are inversely proportional, such that the surface area of the axon in this region remains within very narrow limits.[30]

Peripheral nerves are abundantly supplied by a rich anastomotic network of longitudinal and segmental blood vessels that constitute the vasa nervorum. The caliber and course of the individual vessels may vary considerably; the largest are found in the epineurium. From these, fine branches pass internally and are lost in a complex intraneural vascular plexus.[1, 78]

CLASSIFICATION OF MECHANICAL NERVE INJURIES

There are at least three fundamental morphophysiologic types of lesions associated with local mechanical nerve injury. The classification was originally introduced by Seddon[75] in 1943 and was later amplified by Sunderland[78] in 1978.

1. *Local conduction block.* This lesion, the mildest recognized form of injury, abolishes propagation of the nerve impulse along a defined stretch of nerve. There is preservation of axonal continuity and of nerve impulse conduction above and below the lesion. The structural damage to the nerve is comparatively minor, affecting largely the myelin sheath. There is full recovery of impulse conduction after a period of weeks or a few months, and Wallerian degeneration of the distal segment does not necessarily take place.

This type of injury occurs as a result of any number of mechanical insults to a nerve. The most common, and best studied experimentally, is due to nerve compression. However, as we shall see in some detail, compressive injury to limbs may block nerve conduction either by transient ischemia of the nerve (*rapidly reversible physiologic block*) or by physical damage to nerve myelin (*neurapraxia*).

2. *Axonotmesis:* A more severe nerve injury may be sufficient to damage the anatomic integrity of axons without disrupting continuity of the nerve trunk. This is typical of crush injuries, and the term axonotmesis is used to indicate that the portion of axon distal to the lesion is separated from the neuronal cell body. This is usually associated with local hyperemia and endoneurial edema at the site of the lesion, retrograde axonal degeneration for a few millimeters proximal to the injury, and chromatolysis of the parent cell body.[46, 47, 67, 85] Schwann cells proliferate along the course of this segment to form bands of Büngner or cellular columns within the basal lamina tube that guide the regenerating axons. Nerve sprouts, emerging from the intact proximal axons, advance down the Schwann cell tubes with ameboid activity at a rate of approximately 1 mm per day.[45, 52, 69, 78]

Myelination proceeds centrifugally down the fiber soon after, and Schwann cells reorganize to re-establish one cell per internode segment.[32, 46, 73, 82] Prognosis for functional recovery is favorable because regeneration of nerve fibers to their original peripheral targets is accurate in this setting. If the basal lamina scaffold is destroyed, the alignment of the regenerating fiber of the proximal stump with its original distal channel is not warranted.

3. *Neurotmesis:* The third type of focal nerve injury is known as neurotmesis. This refers to disruption of the normal architecture of nerve fibers with division of the axon and destruction of the anatomic integrity of the

endoneurium, perineurium, and epineurium. The result is that following Wallerian degeneration, in this setting, regeneration of axons to their original targets is unlikely, and hence functional outcome is poor. When the nerve integrity is severed or obstructed by scarring, regenerating fibers may be unable to proceed beyond the site of injury and may instead become entwined in a painful neuroma.[33, 69, 75, 77]

After the first week, electrodiagnostic tests distinguish between local nerve block (indicating neurapraxia) and total inexcitability of the distal nerve segment (indicating axonal division). However, electrophysiologic tests cannot distinguish axonotmesis from neurotmesis and therefore cannot predict outcome of the repair process following axonal damage. It is often assumed that the survival of some excitable fibers in the nerve distal to the site of injury (after sufficient time for Wallerian degeneration has elapsed) is evidence against neurotmesis and the need for exploration. This obviously can be deceiving, however, in that a nerve can be partially cut, severing some fascicles, while leaving others untouched. In such a case of presumed axonotmesis, recovery falls short of expectations. For this reason, if the nature and force of the physical injury are compatible with neurotmesis and if the electrophysiologic tests 5 days later are consistent with significant Wallerian degeneration, early surgical exploration with the intention of possible nerve repair is warranted. This is paramount in proximal lesions, in which a prolonged waiting period for possible recovery cannot be afforded.

Fowler and Ochoa[16] have documented the relative resistance of unmyelinated nerve fibers to compressive injury. A nerve injury that results in loss of function subserved by unmyelinated fibers (autonomic function) is presumptive evidence for an insult severe enough to justify early surgical exploration.[23] However, severe axonotmesis may also present this way, particularly with high-velocity missile penetration of tissue contiguous with nerves. This has the effect of transmitting the energy of the projectile to surrounding tissue and may result in complete disintegration of all axons over a short segment in a nerve trunk.[7, 74] In such cases, surgical inspection of the nerves is the only available means of ensuring the anatomic continuity necessary for functional regeneration.

ACUTE COMPRESSIVE NERVE LESIONS

The Role of Ischemia in Producing Nerve Dysfunction

Short-term compression of a peripheral nerve above systolic pressure results in *rapidly reversible physiologic block* of nerve conduction, which is due to ischemia of the compressed nerve and not to the direct effects of pressure itself. Lewis, Pickering, and Rothchild[41] demonstrated this elegantly in experiments conducted on themselves in the early 1930s. Additionally, they established the sequence of sensory modality loss during nerve compression and accurately described the paresthesiae perceived during recovery from the ischemic insult. Their findings, detailed below, are important to recall when assessing possible ischemic nerve dysfunction in a patient experiencing sensory disturbances of a limb.

A pneumatic tourniquet is placed proximally on an arm at suprasystolic pressures (250 to 300 mm Hg). By the end of 13 to 15 minutes, numbness is detected in the tips of the fingers. Most commonly, it begins in the index or middle finger, spreads slowly to other fingers, and then moves proximally to include the bases of all fingers by the end of 16 to 17 minutes. At this time, light touch, as tested with cotton wool or Frey's hair, is lost at the finger tips. Subjective numbness and anesthesia to light touch and pressure continue to spread centripetally at about 3 to 4 cm/minute until all the skin below the tourniquet is affected. Joint position sense becomes impaired more or less in parallel with touch. Diminution of pain sense lags behind diminished touch by 15 to 20 cm, with absolute analgesia never obtained during a 40-minute arrest of arm circulation. The perception of "thermal sense" is delayed and distorted in quality but is not actually blunted at the time of total anesthesia to touch and pressure. Autonomic function (pilomotor and vasomotor), such as pain, cold, or warm modalities, remains relatively spared by the end of 30 to 40 minutes. Motor paralysis would also start distally and spread proximally, lagging behind the spread of anesthesia, with complete paralysis occurring by 35 minutes of arrested circulation. If the tourniquet is removed at the time of total arm paralysis, functional recovery occurs in the exact reverse of its loss. Sensation is fully restored in approximately 30 seconds and full muscle power at some time after 10 minutes.

If limb compression lasts 10 minutes or more, recovery is always accompanied by tingling paresthesiae. This "pins and needles" sensation begins 45 to 70 seconds after release of compression, becomes unusually intense if the fingers are manipulated, and subsides after 4 to 6 minutes. Although post-ischemic paresthesiae may be intense and uncomfortable, they are rarely painful.

This sequence of sensorimotor nerve disturbance in tourniquet limb compression experiments is well known to the layman and is often described as an arm or leg having "gone to sleep." But are these symptoms of nerve dysfunction attributable to nerve ischemia or to the direct effects of pressure on the nerve? Lewis et al.[41] clarified this by placing a second pressure cuff on the extremity, proximal to the first, at the time when total anesthesia is achieved (approximately 15 minutes). Release of the lower cuff, and hence release of local nerve compression without restoration of nerve blood supply, failed to result in nerve recovery. Instead, anesthesia and paralysis progressed; thus, these findings argue heavily in favor of an ischemic etiology for nerve dysfunction.

The stereotyped sequence of sensory modality loss and motor paralysis is remarkable. It suggested to Lewis et al. that different caliber nerve fibers have different tolerances to ischemia, the most vulnerable of these being large myelinated fibers. Electrophysiologic studies have documented, in animal experiments, that the nerve conduction defect occurs distal to the cuff as well as under it.[3, 8, 21, 35, 37] This has more recently been corroborated in humans, although the order of block in myelinated fibers of various caliber is yet to be established.[2, 8, 9, 54] Human and animal unmyelinated nerve fibers are clearly more resistant to anoxia-induced conduction block than are myelinated fibers.[17, 27, 29, 59, 80] The precise mechanism by which anoxia blocks excitability of nerves is currently unknown. Potential clamp analysis of single myelinated fibers from rats would suggest, however, that anoxia blocks impulse generation after 15 minutes by a decrease in the maximum peak of sodium permeability (PNa) combined with an increase in PNa inactivation.[6]

Our understanding of the pathology of ischemic injury has been limited in the past by an inability to produce sufficient local nerve ischemia in experimental animals without also producing nerve compression.[23] In reversible physiologic block, there is no demonstrable microscopic pathology, although the character of excitable nerve membranes must be deranged in some unknown way to account for the temporary conduction block.[58] Reproducible experimental infarction of nerves is difficult to achieve owing to the elaborate system of longitudinal blood vessels in epineurium, perineurium, and endoneurium, which is sustained by multiple regional vessels entering at intervals along its course. Korthals and Wisniewski[34] have developed a reliable method of producing experimental nerve ischemia in animal models. In a modification of this technique, Hess et al.[31] demonstrated that nerve infarction resulted in degeneration of all myelinated fibers of a fascicle, with sparing of unmyelinated fibers. In contrast to these results, when focal nerve infarcts were created by infusion of arachidonic acid into femoral arteries of rats, small myelinated and unmyelinated fibers appeared most vulnerable to ischemia.[68] In humans, overt pathologic changes have been described in nerve specimens obtained from lower limbs of patients suffering from chronic obstructive arterial disease.[13, 20, 56] Such changes involve both segmental demyelination and remyelination and Wallerian (axonal) degeneration and regeneration.

Spontaneous impulse generation has been confirmed as the basis for post-ischemic paresthesiae. Indeed, it is consistently possible to record early and progressive spontaneous muscle action potentials in normal individuals subjected to proximal limb compression at suprasystolic pressures. Since these discharges resemble motor unit rather than single muscle fiber potentials, it follows that spontaneous activity is likely initiated in the motor nerve fiber.[36, 38] Kugelberg and Cobb[38] concluded that motor and sensory nerve fibers at proximal levels behave as pacemakers in response to an inappropriate microenvironment.

Torebjörk et al.[81] and Ochoa and Torebjörk[65] obtained intraneural microelectrode recordings from sensory fascicles in individuals experiencing post-ischemic paresthesiae. Distal local anesthetic blocks, which failed to eliminate the paresthesiae or single unit discharge, indicated that impulses were generated ectopically along nerve fibers and not primarily from skin receptors. The subjective quality of various paresthesiae, which lacked pain or thermal modalities, and the failure to record ectopic discharges in unmyelinated fibers suggested that myelinated fibers were the likely source of paroxysmal events.

Why paresthesiae should surge during the post-ischemic state, after recovery from numbness, is rather disturbing, since spontaneous activity is unlikely to be confined to the recovery phase judging from what we know about sustained ischemic discharges of early onset in *motor* nerves. It is conceivable that spontaneous discharges in *sensory* fibers starting early after placement of the cuff are also sustained, but the impulses are blocked under the site of compression and, hence, never reach conscious levels.[9] Indeed, Weddell and Sinclair[84] in 1947 were surprised that Lewis et al. never mentioned early paresthesia "tingling" occurring a few minutes after inflation of the pneumatic cuff. Weddell and Sinclair distinguished this "tingling" from post-ischemic "pricking" sensations and believed that tingling specifically originated in sensory nerve endings. Others have also documented early paresthesiae in cuff experiments and have provided indirect evidence in favor of nerve fiber as the source of origin.[38, 51, 64]

Neurapraxia

Erb,[14] as early as 1876, defined electrophysiologically a type of nerve dysfunction that was more prolonged than the typical reversible physiologic block, yet less severe than that resulting from transection of a nerve. Seddon[74] emphasized that patients with this type of nerve dysfunction, although developing paralysis and sensory loss in a limb, did not develop muscle atrophy and their sensory functions were peculiarly dissociated: pain and temperature modalities were relatively preserved. Seddon called this *neurapraxia* ("Saturday night paralysis," "tourniquet paralysis") and noted that full recovery could occur after as long as 3 months. Denny-Brown and Brenner[11, 12] demonstrated that neurapraxia could be produced in experimental animals with the use of a high-pressure tourniquet and spring clip and was the result of segmental demyelination of the nerve. They erroneously concluded, however, that this lesion was ischemic in nature and a complication of the immediately reversible ischemic nerve block so elegantly described by Lewis, Pickering, and Rothchild.

If a pneumatic cuff is used to produce this kind of nerve dysfunction, the pressure needed is much higher than that required to occlude blood vessels. Figure 2–1 shows this experiment in the limb of a baboon. A pneumatic cuff is inflated to 10 pounds/sq. inch or approximately 1000 mm Hg for 90 to 120 minutes. One day later, motor conduction studies of the posterior tibial nerve show normal conduction below the lesion and failure to conduct through it.[15] Electrophysiologic and functional nerve recovery proceeds gradually over the next 3 months. Gilliatt[22] has summed up this situation succinctly:

From experiments of this kind, we are able to determine the pressure required to produce neurapraxia or demyelinating block. If a standard two hour period of compression is used, 1000 mm Hg regularly produces demyelination, 500 mm Hg produces some demyelination with conduction block and 250 mm Hg produces only rapidly reversible physiologic block. Since the systolic pressure of the anesthetized baboon is about 120 mm Hg, all of the pressures are sufficient to arrest circulation in the limb yet only the higher pressures produce demyelination.

More evidence against an ischemic etiology of demyelination was gleaned by serial sections of the nerve in the area of the limb where the cuff had been placed. The affected parts of the nerve corresponded only to the edges of the cuff, where pressure is changing, rather than to the center of the cuff, where ischemia is maximal.[24]

The mechanical nature of the primary structural lesion was elucidated by Ochoa and collaborators[60, 61] and is shown in Figures 2–2 and 2–3. Under the edges of the compressed region, there is evidence of displaced axoplasm and myelin in opposite directions, away from compression, invaginating the nodes of Ranvier of large myelinated fibers. The node of Ranvier is prolapsed into the paranodal area, moving a considerable distance away from its original position. Since the axoplasmic movement is away from the edges of the cuff, the driving force for this axoplasmic displacement is likely the pressure difference between compressed and uncompressed portions of the nerve.[60, 61] Myelin, which appears to be relatively firmly attached to the axonal membrane, is pas-

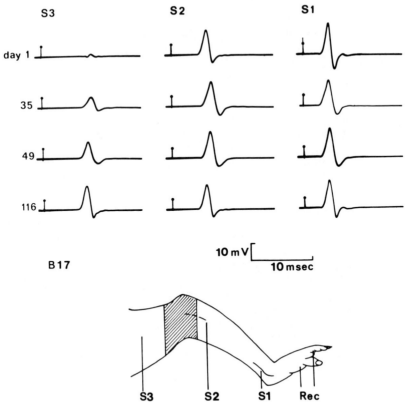

Figure 2–1. Evoked muscle action potentials from abductor hallucis muscle at different intervals after a cuff is inflated to 1000 mm Hg around the knee for 95 minutes. Sites of stimulation and recording electrodes are shown below. (From Fowler, T. J., Danta, G., and Gilliatt, R. W.: J. Neurol. Neurosurg. Psychiatry, *35*:638, 1972.)

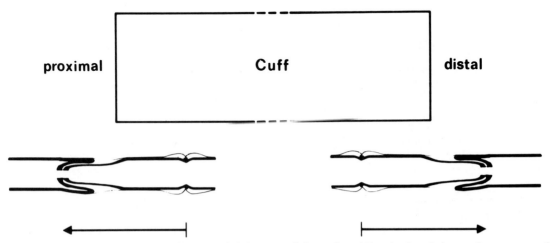

Figure 2–2. Diagram describing the direction of dislocation of the nodes of Ranvier in relation to the compressed zone. (From Ochoa, J., Fowler, T. J., and Gilliatt, R. W.: J. Anat., *113*:433, 1972.)

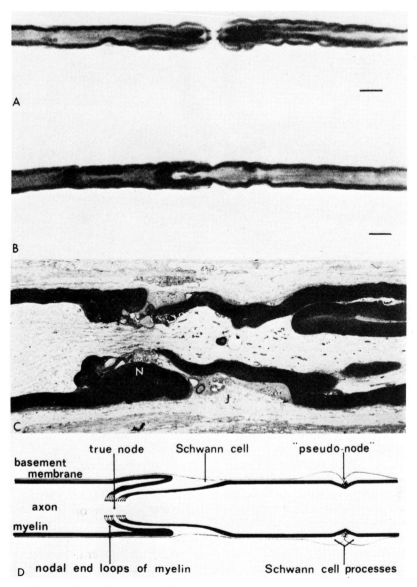

Figure 2–3. *A,* Normal microdissected myelinated fiber showing node of Ranvier. Baboon tibial nerve (bar = 10 μm). *B,* Abnormal fiber, early after acute compression. The nodal gap is occluded owing to intussusception from right to left. An indentation (pseudo-node) marks the original site of the node (bar = 10 μm). *C,* Low-power electron micrograph of abnormal myelinated fiber, cut longitudinally after microdissection. Note indentation at Schwann cell junction (J) and new position of the node (N) under infolded myelin. (From Rudge, P., Ochoa, J., and Gilliatt, R. W.: J. Neurol. Sci., 23:403, 1974). *D,* Diagram of affected fiber showing invagination of one paranode by the adjacent one, movement occurring from right to left. (From Ochoa, J., Fowler, T. J., and Gilliatt, R. W.: *In* Desmedt, J. E. (ed.): New Developments in Electromyography and Clinical Neurophysiology, Vol. 2, Basel, Karger, 1973, pp. 166–173.)

sively dragged along with the prolapsed axon, rather than becoming sheared off at the node. The Schwann cell junction remains fixed to the endoneurium and provides a useful reference point for the extent of axonal dislocation.[61, 72] This behavior of Schwann cells, that of dissociating from myelin rather than from their basal lamina and surrounding collagen, probably reflects a stronger attach-ment to the latter structures.[56] This type of specific large myelinated fiber injury also explains the clinical observation that pain, temperature sensation, and autonomic func-tions tend to be preserved in neurapraxic lesions. The reason for sparing small myeli-nated fibers is less obvious. It may simply be that greater pressure is needed to displace the viscous contents of smaller diameter

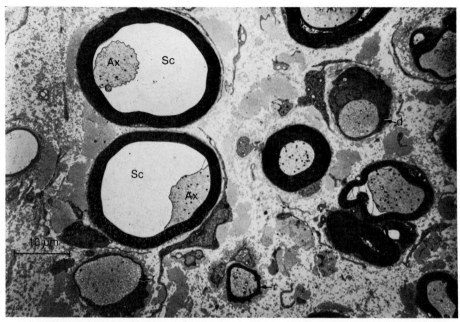

Figure 2–4. Low-power electron micrograph of transverse section of peripheral nerve obtained from a baboon 6 weeks after severe local compression of the limb with a pneumatic cuff, causing prolonged local conduction block. The striking feature is the presence of demyelinated (d) and remyelinated (r) fibers coexisting with abnormal ballooned myelinated fibers. The latter result from distention of the myelin sheaths due to edema of the ad-axonal Schwann cell tongue (Sc). Note shrunken axons (Ax).

tubes and that axons are likely physically crushed and develop Wallerian degeneration before this pressure is attained.[58]

During recovery, paranodal regions of invaginated myelin disintegrate, but demyelination of complete segments is unusual. Schwann cells proliferate and are intercalated into the injured zones, investing the naked axons with new myelin. Functional recovery of the limb parallels recovery of nerve conduction and remyelination. In experimental baboon studies, the fastest rates of recovery take place within 3 to 6 weeks.[15] But recovery may be protracted over 3 to 4 months in some cases of neurapraxia due to severe compression. In these circumstances, the development of intramyelin and periaxonal edema, perhaps due to anoxia, delays repair owing to late scavenging of the myelin defect, a prerequisite for myelination[61] (Fig. 2–4).

CHRONIC NERVE COMPRESSION

Thus far, we have described morphologic and physiologic reactions of peripheral nerves to sudden compressive injury. If a nerve fiber is chronically constricted, compressed, or entrapped, it may also cease to function properly. In particular, there may be slowing or block of conduction through the area of compression and histologic evidence of focal demyelination. Is nerve dysfunction a result of cumulative subclinical acute injuries, chronic vascular compromise, or some entirely novel form of mechanical insult? The answer lies in the histopathology of the single nerve fiber histopathology in chronic compressive nerve injury, which convincingly argues in favor of a peculiar mechanical distortion of normal fiber architecture quite unlike that seen in acute injuries.

Using vintage myelin stains of 1913, Pierre-Marie and Foix[49] discovered that a cause for some forms of thenar muscle wasting was a lesion of the median nerve at the level of the carpal tunnel in the wrist. They did not pursue histological evaluation of the nerve distal to the wrist, however. This was not reexamined until 50 years later, when in 1963 Thomas and Fullerton[79] demonstrated that local slowing of conduction in a case of proven carpal tunnel syndrome was due to a focal demyelination of the nerve seen on histologic section. A naturally occurring animal model for the chronic compressive nerve lesion was identified in the 1960s by Fullerton and Gilliatt.[18, 19] They found that elderly guinea pigs had a high incidence of "carpal tunnel syndrome" and described a peculiar form of demyelination of nerve proximal to the wrist in these animals. In working with this animal model, it was soon found that the severity of the entrapment could be predicted from the results of nerve conduction studies. Conduction delay and eventually conduction block were associated with progressively severe focal demyelinating lesions of nerve extending 2 to 3 mm in length under the carpal band.[22] In severe cases, there was gross narrowing of the entire nerve trunk and its constituent fascicles with evidence of Wallerian degeneration of myelinated fibers at the level of compression.

In 1973, Ochoa and Marotte,[63] who were interested in the mechanism of production of these lesions, studied guinea pigs during very early stages of nerve entrapment. Animals were selected at a time before gross demyelination had occurred and when nerve fiber conduction studies were still normal. The authors demonstrated that along stretches of 20 mm or more proximal or distal to the entrapment, myelin internodes were distorted into tapered spermlike segments with bulbous ends polarized away from the site of compression (Fig. 2–5). Figure 2–6 is a schematic illustration of how chronic compression might appear at different stages of its development. With older animals and more prolonged nerve injury, demyelination under the tunnel is associated with abnormal segments leading away from the entrapment

site (Fig. 2–6B). In severe lesions, Wallerian degeneration and regeneration are identified (Fig. 2–6C).

Examining abnormal myelin segments of the early stage lesions by electron microscopy revealed the pathogenesis and its likely mechanical origin. The internal myelin lamella, which should have attached to the axon membrane at the node of Ranvier, had retracted at the tapered ends and drifted along the fiber, resulting in "buckling" of redundant myelin at bulbous ends (Fig. 2–7). This initiated the sequence of demyelination with progressive retraction of unattached myelin, followed by complete exposure of the axon at one end of the internode.[53] Figure 2–8A shows the myelin tapering and bulb formation in a single myelinated fiber taken from a human biopsy specimen of the superficial radial nerve at the wrist. The electron micrograph in Figure 2–8B shows a single representative human myelinated fiber from chronic median nerve entrapment at the wrist. There is stepwise tapering of myelin on the left (not an intercalated segment) and redundant folds of telescoped myelin at the bulb on the right of the node of Ranvier. J. Ochoa has suggested that detachment of terminal loops and subsequent myelin deformation may be due to repeated longitudinal stretching of friction against flexor tendon, producing pressure waves that propagate away from the entrapment (Fig. 2–9).

In 1978, Sunderland[78] suggested that nerve

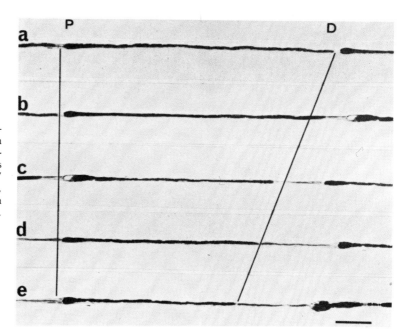

Figure 2–5. Five consecutive internodes, a to e, taken from above the wrist, displayed to emphasize asymmetry of internodes and progressive "demyelination" of tapered ends. P, Proximal; D, distal. Bar = 100 μm. (From Ochoa, J., and Marotte, L. R.: J. Neurol. Sci., 19:491, 1973.)

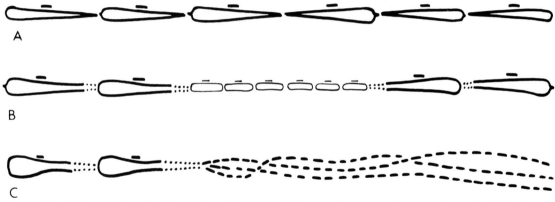

A

B

C

Figure 2–6. *A,* Diagram showing distorted myelin segments from median nerve of young guinea pig. Note reversal of polarity at the wrist. *B,* Further distortion and exposure of the axon proximal and distal to the site of entrapment. The median nerve under the carpal tunnel has lost its original myelin segments. Multiple, short, remyelinated internodes repair the lesion. *C,* Advanced lesion with massive bulbs and axonal Wallerian degeneration and regeneration. (From Ochoa, J.: *In* Omer, G. E., and Spinner, M. (eds.): Management of Peripheral Nerve Problems. Philadelphia, W. B. Saunders Co., 1980, pp. 482–499.)

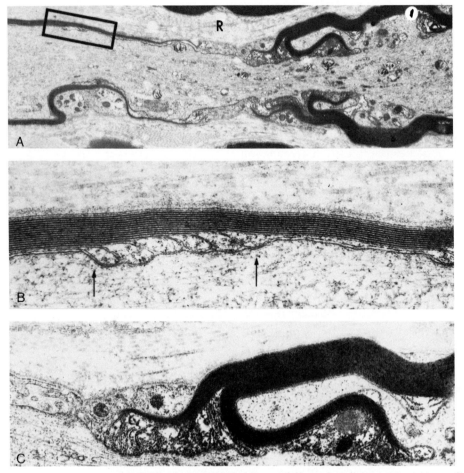

Figure 2–7. Low-power electron micrograph of a moderately abnormal fiber taken from a guinea pig median nerve above the wrist. The paranode on the left is tapered. The bulbous paranode on the right shows inturning of a group of inner lamella (R = node of Ranvier) (× 7000). *B,* Enlargement of the area enclosed in the rectangle in *A.* Six myelin, lamellae end in cytoplasmic loops between arrows (× 48,000). *C,* Detail of the bulbous paranode (× 20,000). (From Ochoa, J., and Marotte, L. R.: J. Neurol. Sci., *19*:491, 1973.)

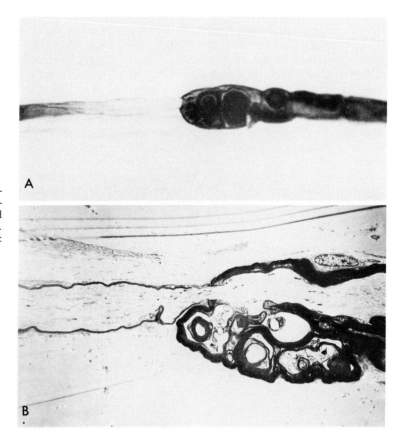

Figure 2–8. *A,* Single distorted fiber (× 500). *B,* Low-power electron micrograph of single distorted fiber cut longitudinally (× 1400). (From Ochoa, J., and Neary, D.: Lancet *1:*7907, 1975.)

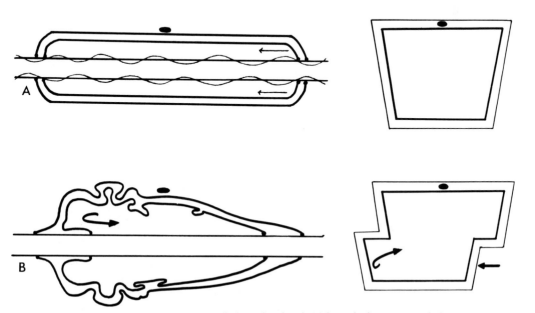

Figure 2–9. *A,* Normal myelin segment and unrolled myelin sheath (*right*), which is trapezoid shaped. Hypothetical pressure waves are shown in the direction of the arrows along the axon. *B,* Distorted segment with tapered end caused by myelin slippage and bulbous end containing inturned redundant myelin lamellae. If myelin were unrolled, it would be altered as indicated (*right*). (From Ochoa, J.: *In* Omer, G. E., and Spinner, M. (eds.): Management of Peripheral Nerve Problems. Philadelphia, W. B. Saunders Co., 1980, pp. 487–501.)

fiber damage is due to ischemia caused by local obstruction of venous return and subsequent increased pressure under the site of entrapment. More recent techniques of endoneurial fluid pressure recordings, using experimental models of chronic neuropathy, have not demonstrated elevated pressures sufficient to collapse endoneurial and perineurial capillaries anticipated in the Sunderland hypothesis.[42, 43]

What role, then, does ischemia play in chronic compressive lesions? The answer is still uncertain, but it seems unlikely that ischemia is responsible for the primary pathology described for myelinated fibers. On the other hand, episodic symptomatology, in particular positive sensory manifestations such as paresthesiae and even pain, may well be due to nerve fiber dysfunction induced by ischemia, which in turn may be due to direct compression of the nerve trunk and its vasculature.[25, 59, 64] Such manifestations are identical to those described in the classic experiment of Lewis, Pickering, and Rothchild.

TRAUMATIC LESIONS CAUSING PAIN

While we now know a great deal about the pathophysiology of local nerve lesions, we know very little about the anatomic substrates and mechanisms that cause pain in these patients. Noordenboos[55] has suggested that selective loss of large-diameter fast-conducting afferents disinhibits the pain-transmitting small fibers, which are more resistant to compression injuries. This "fiber dissociation" theory was based on clinical observations of post-herpetic neuralgia, which showed predominantly large myelinated fiber drop-out in intercostal nerves supplying painful dermatomes. This theory was inspired by Henry Head's concept of two conflicting peripheral sensory systems and is in harmony with the "gate control" theory of pain.[50]

Another theory used to explain the occurrence of pain with local nerve lesions is that of ephaptic transmission, in which an "artificial synapse" or "short circuit" created at the site of the lesion is thought to allow normal ascending or descending impulses to cross-excite the afferent pain pathways. Ephaptic excitation has been shown to occur transiently following acute local nerve injury in animals[26] and as a more stable phenome-

non in experimental neuroma.[76] Rasminsky[71] has elegantly shown that "cross-talk" may occur between contiguous single fibers of dysmyelinated spinal roots of dystrophic mice. In this animal model, lumbosacral spinal roots of the mutant mouse dystrophia muscularis are often thinly myelinated or without any Schwann cell investment at all. Nerve impulse conduction is slowed in the abnormal spinal roots and is continuous rather than saltatory. Ephaptic transmission can be demonstrated by selecting contiguous ventral root fiber and monitoring the response of one fiber with electrical activity incited in its neighbor (Fig. 2–10).[70]

A third explanation proposes that nerve injury results in spontaneous electrical discharges generated in abnormal nerve fibers. In 1974, Wall and Gutnick[83] used animal models to demonstrate that spontaneous impulse generation in experimental neuromas may arise from axon sprouts of small-diameter afferents. Similarly, Rasminsky,[71] in 1980, showed spontaneous ectopic impulse generation in single dysmyelinated spinal root axons. Presently, there is an emerging body of evidence incriminating ectopic impulse generators in abnormal axons as the basis for positive sensorimotor phenomena.[10]

There are no structural correlates in humans that are likely to identify the "artificial synapse" or the "spontaneous ectopic generators" that cause neuralgia. Quantitative studies from human painful neuromas in continuity are revealing. These show increased total numbers of fibers, many of them immature, at the level of the lesion compared with areas proximal and distal to it. The excess of immature fibers suggests that axon sprouts fail to mature as a consequence of the regenerating fiber's inability to reach *peripheral targets* (Fig. 2–11).

CONCLUSION

In summary, we have examined the histopathology of acute and chronic mechanical nerve lesions and discussed possible mechanisms of causation and factors responsible for symptoms of pain, paresthesiae, and weakness in these nerve injuries. Acute compression may cause transient physiologic block, i.e., an ischemic interruption of nerve conduction associated with no specific nerve pathology. Neurapraxia consists of intussusception of axon and myelin through the

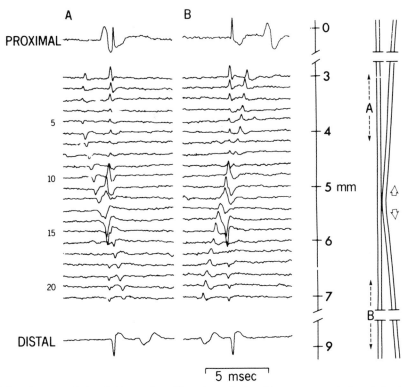

Figure 2–10. Ephaptic transmission between two fibers in a dystrophic mouse ventral root for two directions of propagation in the exciting fiber. Simultaneous recordings were made from proximal and distal electrode pairs, separated by almost 9 mm, which remained fixed throughout and from a third pair of mobile electrodes (records 1–21), which were moved in steps of 200 μm. Note that downgoing and upgoing spikes reflect impulses propagating away from and toward the spinal cord, respectively. The trigger spike for all records was the large amplitude downward spike at the distal electrodes (see Rasminsky[71] for details of recording technique). Sequence A was generated for single sweeps in which the large-amplitude downward spike at the distal electrodes was followed by a smaller amplitude downward spike. In this sequence an impulse arises ectopically in the exciting fiber at recording site 4 and is propagated toward the spinal cord (records 3–1 and PROXIMAL) and toward the periphery (records 5–21 and DISTAL). A second fiber is ephaptically excited between recording sites 12 and 13, and the impulse in this fiber is propagated toward the spinal cord (records 12–1 and PROXIMAL) and toward the periphery (records 13–21 and DISTAL). Sequence B was generated for single sweeps in which the large-amplitude downward spike at the distal electrodes was preceded by a smaller amplitude downward spike. In this sequence an impulse arises ectopically in the exciting fiber between recording site 21 and the DISTAL electrodes and is propagated toward the spinal cord (records 21–1). (From Rasminsky, M.: *In* Culp, W., and Ochoa, J. (eds.): Abnormal Nerves and Muscles as Impulse Generators. New York, Oxford University Press, 1982.)

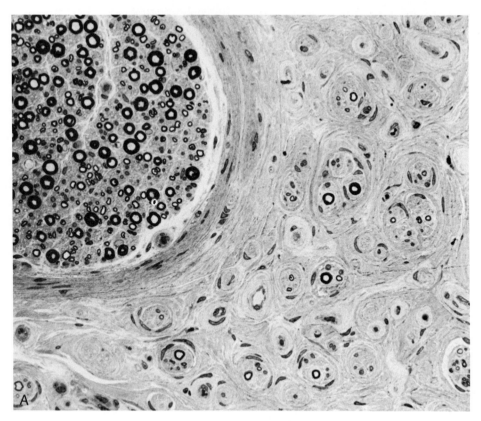

MYELINATED FIBERS

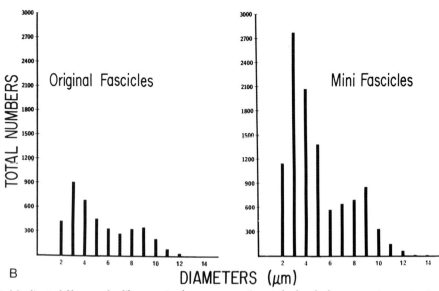

Figure 2–11. Myelinated fibers and caliber spectra from cross section at the level of neuroma-in-continuity. *A*, Original fascicle defined by perineurium (*left*) surrounded by newly formed minifascicles (light micrograph, × 390). *B*, Caliber spectra of all myelinated fibers; (*left*) from within original fascicles (*right*) within minifascicles where immature fibers predominate. (From Ochoa, J.: *In* Culp, W., and Ochoa, J. (eds.): Abnormal Nerves and Muscles as Impulse Generators. New York, Oxford University Press, 1982.)

nodes of Ranvier, resulting in prolonged nerve conduction block. Axonotmesis and neurotmesis describe more severe disruptions of nerve fiber architecture, are difficult to distinguish electrophysiologically, and have poorer prognoses for functional regenerative repair.

Chronic entrapment lesions consist of telescoping myelin internodes and tapering of the sheaths with bulbous polarization of internodes away from the site of injury. Both acute and chronic lesions chiefly involve large myelinated fibers and both may create neuralgia, although the mechanism by which this occurs is poorly understood. Presently, increasing evidence suggests that ectopic impulse generators and ephaptic transmission may be responsible for sensorimotor phenomena in these lesions.

References

1. Adams, W. E.: The blood supply of nerves. I. Historical review. J. Anat., 76:323, 1942.
2. Behse, F., and Buchthal, F.: Slowing in maximum nerve conduction velocity during acute hypoxia due to block of large fibers or to slowing along all fibers. Presented at the 21st Scandinavian Congress of Neurology, Stockholm, June, 1975.
3. Bently, F. H., and Schlapp, W.: Experiments on the blood supply of nerves. J. Physiol. (Lond.), 102:62, 1943.
4. Berthold, C. H.: Ultrastructure of postnatally developing feline peripheral nodes of Ranvier. Acta Soc. Med. Upsal., 73:145, 1968.
5. Bischoff, A., and Thomas, P. K.: Microscopic anatomy of myelinated nerve fibers. In Dyck, P. J., Thomas, P. K., and Lambert, E. H. (eds.): Peripheral Neuropathy, Vol. 1. Philadelphia, W. B. Saunders Company, 1978.
6. Brismar, T.: Potential clamp analysis of the effect of anoxia on the nodal function of rat peripheral nerve fibers. Acta Physiol. Scand., 112:495, 1981.
7. Bristaw, W. R.: Injuries of peripheral nerves in two world wars. Br. J. Surg., 34:333, 1947.
8. Caruso, G., Labianca, O., and Ferrannini, E.: Effects of ischemia on sensory potential of normal subjects of different ages. J. Neurol. Neurosurg. Psychiatry, 36:455, 1973.
9. Caruso, G., Santori, L., Perretti, A., and Amantea, B.: Recovery of sensory potentials after ischaemic block by pneumatic compression of varying duration. Proceedings of the International Symposium on Peripheral Neuropathies, Milan, June, 1978.
10. Culp, W., and Ochoa, J. (eds.): Abnormal nerves and muscles as impulse generators. London, Oxford University Press, 1982.
11. Denny-Brown, D., and Brenner, C.: Lesion in peripheral nerve resulting from compression by spring clip. Arch. Neurol. Psychiatry, 52:1, 1944.
12. Denny-Brown, D., and Brenner, C.: Paralysis of nerve induced by direct pressure and by tourniquet. Arch. Neurol. Psychiatry, 51:1, 1944.
13. Eames, R. A., and Lange, L. S.: Clinical and pathological study of ischemic neuropathy. J. Neurol. Neurosurg. Psychiatry, 30:215, 1967.
14. Erb, W.: Diseases of the peripheral cerebrospinal nerves. In Ziemssen, H. von: Cyclopedia of the Practice of Medicine, Vol. XI. London, Samson, Low, Marston, Searle, and Rivington, 1876.
15. Fowler, T. J., Danta, G., and Gilliatt, R. W.: Recovery of nerve conduction after pneumatic tourniquet: observation on the hind-limb of the baboon. J. Neurol. Neurosurg. Psychiatry, 35:638, 1972.
16. Fowler, T. J., and Ochoa, J.: Unmyelinated fibers in normal and compressed peripheral nerves of the baboon: a quantitative electron microscope study. Neuropathol. Appl. Neurobiol., 1:247, 1975.
17. Fox, J. D., and Kenmore, P.: The effect of ischemia on nerve conduction. Exp. Neurol., 17:403, 1967.
18. Fullerton, P. M.: The effect of ischemia on nerve conduction in carpal tunnel syndrome. J. Neurol. Neurosurg. Psychiatry, 26:385, 1963.
19. Fullerton, P. M., and Gilliatt, R. W.: Median and ulnar neuropathy in the guinea pig. J. Neurol. Neurosurg. Psychiatry, 30:393, 1967.
20. Gairns, F. W., Garven, H. S. D., and Smith, G.: The digital nerves and the nerve endings in progressive obliterative vascular disease of the leg. Scot. Med. J., 5:382, 1960.
21. Gilliatt, R. W.: Nerve conduction in human and experimental neuropathies. Proc. Roy. Soc. Med., 59:989, 1966.
22. Gilliatt, R. W.: Peripheral nerve compression and entrapment. The Oliver Sharpey Lecture. In Lant, A. F. (ed.): Eleventh Symposium on Advanced Medicine. New York, Pitman Medical Publishing, 1975, p. 114.
23. Gilliatt, R. W.: Physical injury to peripheral nerves. Physiologic and electrodiagnostic aspects. Mayo Clin. Proc., 56:361, 1981.
24. Gilliatt, R. W., McDonald, W. I., and Rudge, P.: The site of conduction block in peripheral nerves compressed by a pneumatic tourniquet. J. Physiol. (Lond.), 238:31, 1974.
25. Gilliatt, R. W., and Wilson, T. G.: Ischemic sensory loss in patients with peripheral nerve lesions. J. Neurol. Neurosurg. Psychiatry, 17:104, 1954.
26. Granit, R., and Skoglund, C. R.: Facilitation, inhibition and depression at the artificial synapse formed by the cut end of a mammalian nerve. J. Physiol., 101:489, 1943.
27. Grundfest, H.: Properties of mammalian B fibers. Am. J. Physiol., 127:252, 1939.
28. Gutrecht, J. A., and Dyck, P. J.: Quantitative teased fiber and histologic studies of human sural nerve during postnatal development. J. Comp. Neurol., 138:117, 1970.
29. Heinbecker, D.: Effect of anoxemia, carbon dioxide and lactic acid on electrical phenomena of myelinated fibers of the peripheral nervous system. Am. J. Physiol., 89:58, 1929.
30. Hess, A., and Young, J. Z.: The nodes of Ranvier. Proc. Roy. Soc. Lond. (Biol.), 140:301, 1952.
31. Hess, K., Eames, R. A., Darveniza, P., and Gilliatt, R. W.: Acute ischemic neuropathy in the rabbit. J. Neurol. Sci., 44:19, 1979.
32. Hiscoe, H. B.: Distribution of nodes and incisures in normal and regenerated nerve fibers. Anat. Rec., 99:447, 1947.
33. Horch, K. W., and Lisney, S. J. W.: On the number and nature of regenerating myelinated axons after

lesions of cutaneous nerves in the cat. J. Physiol., 313:275, 1981.

34. Korthals, J. K., and Wisniewski, H. M.: Peripheral nerve ischemia. Part 1: Experimental model. J. Neurol. Sci., 24:65, 1975.
35. Kugelberg, E.: Accommodation in human nerves. Acta Physiol. Scand., 8(Suppl. 24):105, 1944.
36. Kugelberg, E.: Activation of human nerves by ischemia. Arch. Neurol. Psychiatry, 60:140, 1948.
37. Kugelberg, E.: Injury activity and trigger zones in human nerves. Brain, 69:310, 1946.
38. Kugelberg, E., and Cobb, W.: Repetitive discharges in human motor nerve fibers during the postischemic state. J. Neurol. Neurosurg. Psychiatry, 14:88, 1951.
39. Landon, D. N., and Langley, O. K.: The local chemical environment of nodes of Ranvier: a study of cation binding. J. Anat., 108:419, 1971.
40. Landon, D. N., and Williams, P. M.: The ultrastructure of the node of Ranvier. Nature (Lond.), 199:575, 1963.
41. Lewis, T., Pickering, G. W., and Rothchild, P.: Centripetal paralysis arising out of arrersted blood-flow to the limb including notes on a form of tingling. Heart, 16:1, 1931.
42. Low, P. A., and Dyck, P. J.: Increased endoneurial fluid pressure in experimental lead neuropathy. Nature, 269:427, 1977.
43. Low, P. A., Dyck, P. J., and Schmelger, J. D.: Chronic elevation of endoneurial fluid pressure is associated with low-grade fiber pathology. Muscle Nerve, 5:162, 1982.
44. Low, P., Marchard, P., Knox, F., and Dyck, P. J.: Recorded endoneurial fluid pressure by means of small polyethylene matrix capsules. Brain Res., 122:373, 1977.
45. Lubinska, L.: Axoplasmic streaming in regenerating and in normal nerve fibers. In Singer, M., and Schadé, J. P. (eds.): Progress in Brain Research, Vol. 13, Mechanisms of Neural Regeneration. Amsterdam, Elsevier Publishing Company, 1964, pp. 1–71.
46. Lubinska, L.: Demyelination and remyelination in the proximal parts of regenerated nerve fiber. J. Comp. Neurol., 117:275, 1961.
47. Lubinska, L.: Region of transition between preserved and regenerating parts of myelinated nerve fibers. J. Comp. Neurol., 113:315, 1959.
48. Lubinska, L., and Lukaszewska, I.: Shape of myelinated nerve fibers and proximodistal flow of axoplasm. Acta Biol. Exp. Vars., 17:115, 1956.
49. Marie, P., and Foix, C.: Atrophie isolée de l'éminence thenar d'origin neuritique. Rôle du ligament annulaire antérieur du carpe dans la pathogénie de la lésion. Rev. Neurol., 26:647, 1913.
50. Melzack, R., and Wall, P. D.: Pain mechanisms: a new theory. Science, 150:971, 1965.
51. Merrington, W. R., and Nathan, P. W.: A study of postischemic paresthesiae. J. Neurol. Neurosurg. Psychiatry, 12:1, 1949.
52. Nathaniel, E. J. H., and Pease, D. C.: Collagen and basement membrane formation by Schwann cells during nerve regeneration. J. Ultrastruct. Res., 9:550, 1963.
53. Neary, D., Ochoa, J., and Gilliatt, R. W.: Sub-clinical entrapment neuropathy in man. J. Neurol. Sci., 24:283, 1975.
54. Nielsen, V. K., and Kardel, T.: Decremental conduction in normal human nerves subject to ischemia. Acta Physiol. Scand., 92:249, 1974.
55. Nordenboos, W.: Pain. Amsterdam, Elsevier Publishing Company, 1959.
56. Ochoa, J.: Histopathology of common mononeuropathies. In Jewett, D. L., and McCarroll, J. R. (eds.): Nerve Repair: Its Clinical and Experimental Basis. St. Louis, C. V. Mosby Company, 1980.
57. Ochoa, J.: Microscopic anatomy of unmyelinated nerve fibers. In Dyck, P. J., Thomas, P. K., and Lambert, E. H. (eds.): Peripheral Neuropathy, Vol. 1. Philadelphia, W. B. Saunders Company, 1975, p. 131.
58. Ochoa, J.: Nerve fiber pathology in acute and chronic compression. In Omer, G. E., and Spinner, M. (eds.): Management of Peripheral Nerve Problems. Philadelphia, W. B. Saunders Company, 1980, p. 487.
59. Ochoa, J.: Pain in local nerve lesions. In Culp, W., and Ochoa, J. (eds.): Abnormal Nerves and Muscles as Impulse Generators. London, Oxford University Press, 1982.
60. Ochoa, J., Danta, G., Fowler, T. J., and Gilliatt, R. W.: Nature of the nerve lesion caused by pneumatic tourniquet. Nature, 233:265, 1971.
61. Ochoa, J., Fowler, T. J., and Gilliatt, R. W.: Anatomical changes in peripheral nerves compressed by a pneumatic tourniquet. J. Anat., 133:433, 1972.
62. Ochoa, J., and Mair, W. G.: The normal sural nerve in man: ultrastructure and numbers of fibers and cells. Acta Neuropath. Berl., 13:197, 1969.
63. Ochoa, J., and Marotte, L.: Nature of the nerve lesion underlying chronic entrapment. J. Neurol. Sci., 19:49, 1973.
64. Ochoa, J., and Noordenbos, W.: Pathology and disordered sensation in local nerve lesions: an attempt at correlation. In Bonica, J. J., et al. (eds.): Advances in Pain Research and Therapy, Vol. 3. New York, Raven Press, 1979.
65. Ochoa, J. L., and Torebjörk, H. E.: Paresthesiae from ectopic impulse generation in human sensory nerves. Brain, 103:835, 1980.
66. Ochs, J., and Hollingsworth, D.: Dependence of fast axoplasmic transport in nerve on oxidative metabolism. J. Neurochem., 18:107, 1971.
67. Olsson, Y., and Kristensson, K.: The perineurium as a diffusion barrier to protein tracers following trauma to nerves. Acta Neuropath. Berl., 23:105, 1973.
68. Parry, G. J., and Brown, M. J.: Selective fiber vulnerability in acute ischemic neuropathy. Ann. Neurol., 11:147, 1982.
69. Ramón y Cajal S: Degeneration and Regeneration of the Nervous System. Vol. 1. London, Oxford University Press, 1928.
70. Rasminsky, M.: Ectopic excitation, ephaptic excitation and autoexcitation in peripheral nerve fibers of mutant mice. In Culp, W., and Ochoa, J. (eds.): Abnormal Nerves and Muscles as Impulse Generators. London, University Press, 1982.
71. Rasminsky, M.: Ephaptic transmission between single nerve fibers in the spinal nerve roots of dystrophic mice. J. Physiol., 350:151, 1980.
72. Rudge, P., Ochoa, J., and Gilliatt, R. W.: Acute peripheral nerve compression in the baboon. J. Neurol. Sci., 23:403, 1974.
73. Schlaepfer, W. W., and Myers, F . K.: Relationships

of myelin internode elongation and growth in the rat sural nerve. J. Comp. Neurol., *147*:255, 1973.

74. Seddon, H. J.: Peripheral nerve injuries in Great Britain during World War II: a review. Arch. Neurol. Psychiatry, *63*:171, 1950.

75. Seddon, H. J.: Three types of nerve injury. Brain, *66*:237, 1943.

76. Seltzer, C. A., and Devor, M.: Ephaptic transmission in chronically damaged peripheral nerves. Neurology, *29*:1061, 1979.

77. Spinner, M., and Spencer, P. S.: Nerve compression lesions of the upper extremity. Clin. Orthop., 104:46, 1974.

78. Sunderland, S.: Nerve and Nerve Injuries. London, Churchill Livingstone, 1978.

79. Thomas, P. K., and Fullerton, P. M.: Nerve fiber size in the carpal tunnel syndrome. J. Neurol. Neurosurg. Psychiatry, *26*:520, 1963.

80. Torebjörk, H. E., and Hallin, R. G.: Responses in human A and C fibers to repeated electrical intra-dermal stimulation. J. Neurol. Neurosurg. Psychiatry, *37*:653, 1974.

81. Torebjörk, H. E., Ochoa, J. L., and McCann, F. V.: Paresthesiae: abnormal impulse generation in sensory nerve fibers in man. Acta Physiol. Scand., 105:518, 1979.

82. Vizoso, A. D., and Young, J. Z.: Internode length and fiber diameter in developing and regenerating nerves. J. Anat., *82*:110, 1948.

83. Wall, P. D., and Gutnick, M.: Properties of afferent nerve impulses originating from a neuroma. Nature, *248*:740, 1974.

84. Weddell, G., and Sinclair, D. C.: "Pins and Needles": observations on some of the sensations aroused in a limb by the application of pressure. J. Neurol. Neurosurg. Psychiatry, *10*:24, 1947.

85. Williams, P. L. and Hall, S. M.: Prolonged in vivo observation of normal peripheral nerve fibers and their acute reactions to crush and deliberate trauma. J. Anat., *108*:397, 1971.

3

Current Models for Nerve Research

■

A. Lee Dellon, M.D.
Susan E. Mackinnon, M.D.

Advancement of our understanding of the pathophysiology of human peripheral neuropathy is limited, primarily because of lack of availability of neural tissue to investigate. People are understandably hesitant to give up their compressed median nerve for study! They are also hesitant to undergo surgery, e.g., to have a microsurgical internal neurolysis on their left median nerve and carpal tunnel decompression with or without local steroid instillation on their right. The development of new models for nerve research and the refinement of older models thus become the cornerstone upon which future neural investigations can build. Frequently, further insight is gained by applying a new assay technique to an existing model or previously studied problem, e.g., the histochemical horseradish peroxidase reaction to the "fascicular versus epineurial repair" controversy.[17] This chapter, however, details the current status of research models that will permit present and future assay techniques to investigate, at a basic level, the equivalents of clinical compression neuropathy, neuroma formation, and neural regeneration across a gap.

PERIPHERAL COMPRESSION NEUROPATHY

The apparent epidemic of peripheral compression neuropathy is due to a combination of (1) increased clinical awareness that spe-

cific peripheral nerves can become compressed and (2) increased recreational and occupational stress upon those nerves at specific sites. The first carpal tunnel releases were done about 1940,[22, 124] the first submuscular anterior transposition of the ulnar nerve performed in 1942,[58] the cubital tunnel syndrome described in 1957 and 1958,[37, 91] the tarsal tunnel syndrome described in 1962,[55] and the "double crush syndrome" hypothesized in 1972.[116] Contemporaneously, assembly-line work, hair styling, computer programming, word processing, desk work, increased telephone use, etc., in addition to entrance of women into the labor force, have combined to create a group of people with flexed wrists and elbows and vibrating, supinating, and pronating forearms that place the peripheral nerves at increased pressure in sites of anatomic tightness. Environmental toxins, such as lead, alcohol, and sorbitol, and systemic illnesses, such as diabetes, arthritis, and thyroid dysfunction, further increase the likelihood for compression neuropathy.

Yet, a good experimental model for *chronic* peripheral nerve compression neuropathy does not exist. In the absence of such a model, there is no experimental basis for any of our current treatment modalities for these problems.

A valid experimental model of peripheral nerve compression must produce pathophysiologic changes that reflect what is known to occur in human peripheral compression neuropathy. Such information is available by means of postmortem material. For an understanding of "severe compression," two median nerves,[75, 113] one ulnar nerve,[84] and one posterior tibial nerve[69] have been studied. For less severe, or "subclinical," nerve compression, twelve median and ulnar nerves[85] and ten lateral femoral cutaneous nerves[54] have been studied. Our interpretation of these human studies suggests a sequential change that begins with intraneural edema proximal to the constriction and proceeds to epifascicular and interfascicular epineurial fibrosis, perineurial thickening, and then to endoneurial fibrosis. Associated with these connective tissue changes is "drop out" of large myelinated axons beneath the site of constriction, with a shift in the fiber histogram to a lower mean fiber diameter. In these relatively less severe cases, the fiber histogram becomes bimodal again distal to the constriction, and electron microscopy suggests that the "large fiber drop out" is due to loss of myelin rather than to axonal degeneration. In more severe compression, there is abnormal distal motor latency and loss of large myelinated fibers associated with Wallerian degeneration. Remyelination and regenerating axon clusters are found distal to the compression.

The experimental models that have been utilized in the past have been able to produce pathophysiologic changes compatible with the above changes noted in human material, but each technique or study either has a major disadvantage or was not studied sufficiently long enough to be a suitable model for chronic peripheral nerve compression. The earliest studies employed wrapping an arterial cuff about a nerve repair[121] or tying thin threads about a nerve[36] and were more models of nerve degeneration and regeneration rather than of chronic compression. The best potential model was that described by Osborne,[120] in which he doubled a Silastic tube wrapping about a nerve. The two criticisms of his study are that he produced up to 50 per cent constriction of the rat sciatic nerve and followed the animals only up to 5 weeks. This model, however, demonstrated the relative increased "drop out" of large myelinated fibers from the periphery of the fascicle versus the center and the presence of proximal edema, epineurial fibrosis, and neovascularization in the epineurium. Extensive electrodiagnostic studies have been done with the "naturally occurring" guinea pig

model, which does demonstrate chronic pathophysiologic changes in adult guinea pigs that are housed in wire cages.[40–42] We believe the drawbacks to this model are that the carpal tunnel in guinea pigs contains a large median artery and a fibrocartilaginous bar that ossifies with time and the tarsal tunnel model occurs without predictability in these animals. From a practical standpoint, it is difficult to obtain "old" breeder guinea pigs. At a more fundamental level, this is a "developmental model" that we believe is invalid because of the possibility of adaptive central peripheral mechanisms. For example, with progressive loss of median nerve function during growth and maturation, does a different portion of the somatosensory cortex take over previous thumb–index finger territory, and do ulnar and radial nerves from adjacent peripheral territories extend into the former median-innervated area? The same type of criticism is directed at the Silastic band model, which, although sufficiently chronic, relied upon nerve fiber maturation from the neonatal period to adulthood to supply the compressive force.[1]

The ideal model for chronic peripheral nerve compression must demonstrate sequential changes that correspond to what is known of human pathophysiology and should occur in an adult animal. The degree of compression must not be so severe initially that the first pathophysiologic changes include Wallerian degeneration. The area of the nerve over which compression occurs should be broad relative to the nerve, and not a narrow constriction, as human peripheral compression neuropathy typically occurs beneath a band 1 to 2 cm in length. The model should be predictable in terms of its time-course to permit investigation of therapeutic modalities at appropriate points in the "natural history" of the problem. The placement of a band about the sciatic nerve of the rat has now been evaluated sufficiently to suggest that this may be the ideal model.[71]

In the rat sciatic nerve model for peripheral compression neuropathy, 250-gm Sprague-Dawley rats (adult) are utilized. Their sciatic nerve is 1.2 mm in diameter. A series of 1-cm-long tubes (0.6-mm and 0.9-mm internal diameter Silastic and 1.5-mm internal diameter polyvinyl) were investigated to determine the degree of constriction necessary to produce chronic compression (Fig. 3–1). The sciatic nerve is exposed and dissected from surrounding tissue, the band is slit longitudinally, and the nerve is unsheathed. Three sutures of 10–0 nylon are placed to close the tube. With a single stitch, the muscle layer is closed over the tube and the skin is sutured.

Evaluation of the effects of compression were done at intervals by reopening the wounds and recording the distal motor latency. At appropriate intervals, sciatic nerves were taken for light and electron microscopy studies. The results demonstrated that the smaller diameter tubes (0.6 mm and 0.9 mm) created sufficient compression to produce prolonged latency and Wallerian degeneration within 1 to 2 months (Fig. 3–2).

The 1.5-mm band, with an internal diameter only slightly larger than the diameter of the sciatic nerve, did not cause a change in the electrodiagnostic studies by 4 months of compression. Grossly, the nerves appeared swollen proximal to the band. With the bands removed, increased vascularity was noted along the length of the compressed nerve (Fig. 3–3). After 4 months of compression at this minimal degree of banding (1.5 mm), there were morphologic changes in connective and neural tissue, i.e., epineurial fibrosis and perineurial thickening and a greater "drop out" of large myelinated fibers from the periphery than from the center of the fascicle (Fig. 3–4). With compression for longer periods of time, there was progressive interfascicular epineurial fibrosis, perineurial thickening, and the development of endoneurial fibrosis. There was also corresponding decrease in amplitude of the compound action potential and prolongation of latency.

After 6 months of compression, Wallerian degeneration was evident. With further time, regeneration clusters occurred distally. Quantitatively, there was a decrease in the percentage of neural tissue with increased duration of compression; this occurred not only from the periphery versus the center of the fascicle but from a region distal to the band of compression versus a region beneath the band (Fig. 3–5). The earliest pathophysiologic alteration was a loss of the blood-nerve barrier, as demonstrated by leakage of Evans blue albumin from the endoneurial capillaries and from outside to within the perineurium. This change occurred by 4 months of compression and was noted as early as 2 months. The electron microscopic evaluation demonstrated changes by 4 months consistent with Ochoa's concept of the pathophysiology of chronic nerve compression,[86] such as paranodal myelin swelling, demyelination, and finally segmental demyelination. The model has been followed for 1 year.

This model for chronic peripheral nerve compression has been extended to the primate.[72a] Silastic tubing of the same internal diameter as the median nerve external diameter (2.5 mm) in the adult cynomolgus monkey was slit longitudinally and placed about the median nerve in the carpal tunnel (Fig. 3–6). The deep transverse carpal ligament was sutured with a single 5–0 nylon stitch before closing the skin. By 4 months of compression, a histologic picture similar to that reported for compressed human peripheral nerves[69, 84, 113] had developed, with

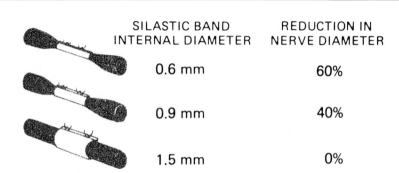

RAT MODEL:
CHRONIC NERVE COMPRESSION

	SILASTIC BAND INTERNAL DIAMETER	REDUCTION IN NERVE DIAMETER
	0.6 mm	60%
	0.9 mm	40%
	1.5 mm	0%

Figure 3–1. Schematic diagram of different degrees of nerve compression achieved by applying cuffs of different internal diameters to adult rat sciatic nerve. (From Mackinnon, S. E. et al.: Ann. Plast. Surg., *13*:112–120, 1984.)

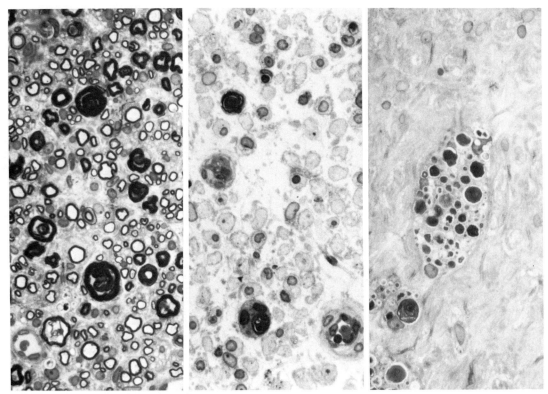

Figure 3–2. Composite photomicrograph of adult rat sciatic nerve banded with a 0.6-mm internal diameter cuff evaluated after 1 month of compression (*left*). Proximal to cuff, edematous normal nerve (*center*) beneath cuff, loss of myelinated axons (*right*) distal to cuff, and early regenerating nerve clusters are seen. This demonstrates a model of acute compression, degeneration, and regeneration rather than chronic compression. (From Mackinnon, S. E. et al.: Ann. Plast. Surg., *13*:112–120, 1984.)

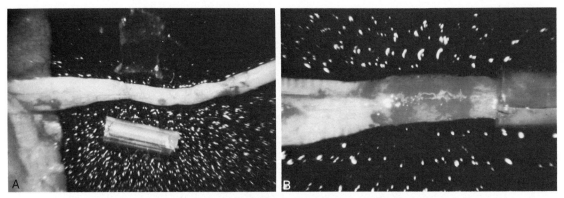

Figure 3–3. *A*, With the cuff removed, proximal swelling of the nerve is apparent (to the left). Note the removed pseudosheath lying above the nerve and the cuff lying below the nerve. *B*, With half the tube removed, the underlying vascularity in the compressed nerve is noted. (From Mackinnon, S. E. et al.: Ann. Plast. Surg., *13*:112–120, 1984.)

significant epineurial fibrosis, interfascicular fibrosis, perineurial thickening, and beginning endoneurial fibrosis (Fig. 3–7). There was a relatively increased "drop out" of large myelinated fibers in fascicles located at the periphery of the median nerve versus those located within the center of the nerve. No significant changes occurred in distal motor latency throughout the course of this study in which the model was followed for 1 year.

We believe that this model for peripheral compression neuropathy is valid and reproducible. As such, alterations in the model may now be introduced to produce models for other clinical situations and to simulate clinical therapeutic interventions. For example, preliminary obsevations[103] demonstrate that by placing a second Silastic band about the tibial nerve in the rat model, a model for the double crush syndrome can be produced. This suggests that these models can be utilized to evaluate the effects of subclinical nerve entrapment at one level on a second level of entrapment, either proximal or distal. Such susceptibility[114] of a peripheral nerve to compression may now be evaluated in this model for systemic conditions such as alcoholism and diabetes, in addition to a second

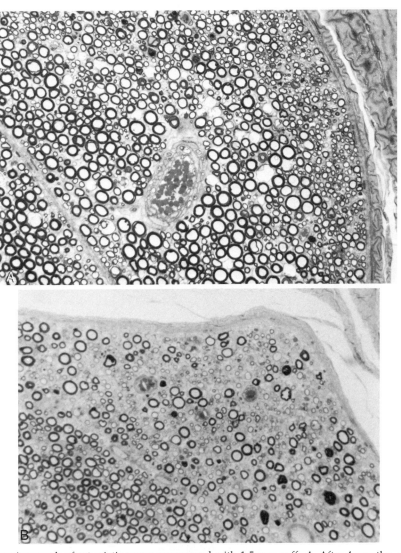

Figure 3–4. Photomicrograph of rat sciatic nerve compressed with 1.5-mm cuff. *A,* After 4 months, a "drop out" of large myelinated fibers at the periphery of the fascicle versus the center of the fascicle is noted. *B,* After 6 months of compression, further "drop out" of large myelinated fibers at the periphery of the fascicle is seen (toluidine blue, × 25). (From Mackinnon, S. E. et al.: Ann. Plast. Surg., *13:*112–120, 1984.)

Percentage Neural Tissue

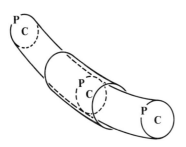

month compression	Proximal		Cuff		Distal	
	P	C	P	C	P	C
2	51	51	48	48	50	50
4	35	60	30	45	35	48
6	20	45	30	40	15	20

Figure 3–5. Schematic demonstration of change in percentage of neural tissue present proximal, beneath, and distal (to the right) of the cuff after varying periods of nerve compression. Note change in the percentage of neural tissue at the periphery (P) versus the center (C) of fascicle at each location along the nerve. (From Mackinnon, S. E. et al.: Ann. Plast. Surg., 13:112–120, 1984.)

localized site of compression. Since significant divergence of opinion exists as to whether the intraneural fibrosis of prolonged compression persists following simple decompression, thus requiring an internal neurolysis,[24] whether this fibrosis will resolve with time,[90] or whether intraneural dissection increases fibrosis,[101] this model may be utilized to resolve these questions. The model may also be used to study the pharmacologic effects of drugs, such as steroids, upon the development and treatment of intraneural fibrosis. Since discrepancies remain between detailed evaluations of sensibility and electrodiagnostic studies,[107] this model may prove useful by allowing removal of the Silastic band and subjecting the compressed area of nerve to teased-fiber preparations. Then single-unit electrical recordings can be employed to study the pathophysiology of these syndromes and correlate the abnormal electrodiagnostic studies with the abnormal morphology. Using this technique it would also be possible to investigate the suggestion that

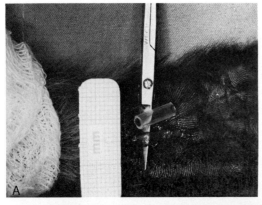

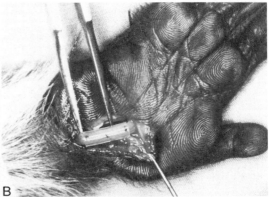

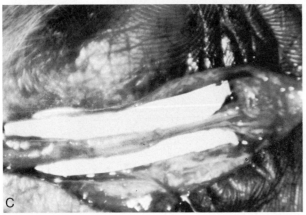

Figure 3–6. Nerve compression model in primate (cynomolgus monkey) carpal tunnel. *A*, Cuff prior to placement about median nerve in carpal tunnel. *B*, Cuff in place. *C*, Median nerve with cuff removed after 4 months of compression distal to right. Note large proximal swelling of the median nerve and relative narrowing in the area of banding. (From Mackinnon, S. E. et al.: Reconstr. Microsurg., 1:185–194, 1985.)

the earliest perception of nerve compression is one of heightened sensitivity[28, 29] and possibly to correlate an early increase in the compound action potential[33, 63] and alteration of its wave form with mechanisms involved in states of hypersensitivity (hyperalgesia), such as causalgia.[82]

NEUROMA FORMATION

The occurrence of painful neuromas is so prevalent that clinicians accept neuroma formation as the inevitable result of nerve injury. Nevertheless, for at least 65 years attention, both clinically and in the laboratory, has been directed to techniques that attempt to "prevent" neuroma formation[81] or at least relocate the neuroma into "quiet" areas.[50, 57, 115] Experimentally, neuromas have been induced by crushing the nerve (incontinuity neuroma) or dividing the nerve and mechanically or chemically treating the proximal end of the divided nerve in models that have included rats, cats, horses, and subhuman and human primates.[6, 10, 16, 39, 48, 52, 60, 83, 93–95, 105,]

[109, 111] Generalizations that may be concluded from these studies are:

1. Disruption of continuity of the nerve fiber results in neural regeneration, which, if prevented from reaching an appropriate sensory or motor end-organ, will form a disorganized mass of collagen and randomly-oriented small neural fascicles, i.e., a classic neuroma (Fig. 3–8).

2. Not all neuromas are symptomatic.

3. A painful classic neuroma cannot be distinguished morphologically from a classic neuroma that is not painful.

4. Approximately 70 per cent of patients achieve relief of pain after treatment of a painful neuroma regardless of technique used, but successive attempts to treat patients in this group who failed to achieve relief initially are less and less successful regardless of technique.

5. Some nerves are more "resistant" to treatment than others, e.g., the radial sensory nerve.

6. No single treatment technique has been uniformly successful.

7. Amputation neuromas with phantom

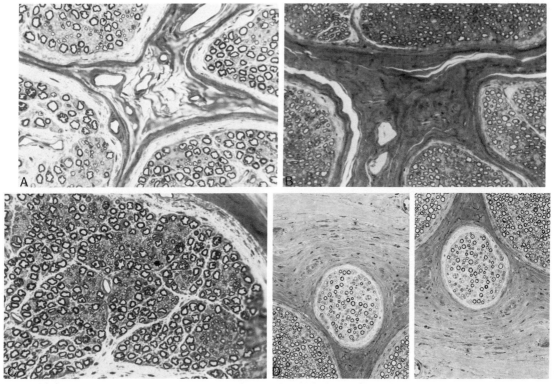

Figure 3–7. Photomicrograph of monkey median nerve from within carpal tunnel. *A,* Normal. *B,* After 4 months of compression. *C,* Outer fascicle: Note increased epifascicular epineurium and "drop out" of large myelinated fibers after 4 months of compression. *D,* Central fascicle: Note connective tissue changes of interfascicular epineurial fibrosis and perineurial thickening with minimal change as of yet in myelinated fiber population (toluidine blue, × 100, × 64, × 100). (From Mackinnon, S. E. et al.: J. Reconstr. Microsurg., 1:185–194, 1985.)

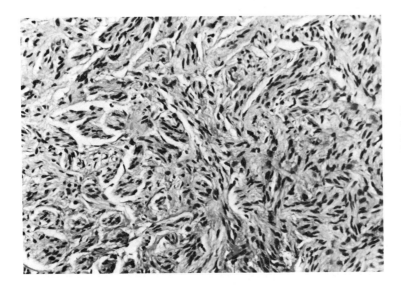

Figure 3–8. Photomicrograph of classic neuroma from radial sensory nerve in man (hematoxylin and eosin, × 240). (From Dellon, A. L. et al.: J. Hand Surg., in press, 1986.)

limb pain may involve a different pathophysiology than incontinuity or non-amputation end-bulb neuromas.

8. The pathophysiology of neuroma pain is not understood.

With this background, it is clear that a productive approach to neuroma investigation must consider that etiology of the painful neuroma is multifactorial and must employ a neuroma model that can isolate different etiologic variables. Because of significant species variability in neural regenerative capacity, it is best to utilize a primate model. It is also clear that an experimental model cannot give information about a subjective variable such as pain and that the observations made in the laboratory would have to be confirmed in patients with long-term follow-up. Within this framework, two different avenues of neuroma investigation can be utilized, neurophysiologic and morphometric.

The technique for producing a neuroma must be one that predictably results in the formation of a classic neuroma. Previously, there were no primate models to follow, and thus we began with a technique planned to maximize neuroma formation. In the baboon, the radial sensory nerve was transected at the wrist level, and the proximal end was crushed between the serrated jaws of a hemostat for 30 seconds. Two centimeters of the distal nerve were excised. The crushed end was left in the subcutaneous tissue at the wrist level. The extremity was not splinted. This technique reproducibly resulted in 1-cm masses that were palpable subcutaneously by 2 months postoperatively. At exploration between 4 and 6 months post-

operatively, these neuromas were found to be adherent to overlying skin and subjacent structures, with sprouts having regenerated from the neuroma distally into the skin (Fig. 3–9). In subsequent work, in an attempt to produce a neuroma in a manner more analogous to the clinical situation, we simply transected the nerve and resected 2 cm from the distal end. Even without crushing, we found in the baboon and then in the cynomolgus monkey that not only the radial sensory nerve (RSN) but also the palmar cutaneous branch of the median nerve (PCM) and the dorsal cutaneous branch of the ulnar nerve (DCU) predictably formed classic end-bulb neuromas (Fig. 3–10).

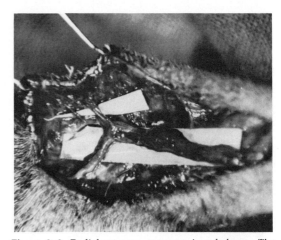

Figure 3–9. Radial sensory neuroma in a baboon. The neuroma was formed by nerve transection followed by nerve crush. Distal regeneration of the nerve from the neuroma into skin is demonstrated. (From Meyer, R. A. et al.: Proc. Soc. Neurosci., *8*:855, 1982.)

The neurophysiologic investigation of a neuroma may seek to answer questions such as:

1. What type of neural activity may be recorded proximal to the neuroma?

2. Is the neural activity spontaneous in origin?

3. What type of neural activity results from chemical, mechanical, or thermal stimulation of the neuroma or stimulation of its overlying or reinnervated distal skin?

4. Is there evidence of ephaptic transmission?

5. What subpopulations of nerve fibers are involved in any of this neural activity, etc.?

Pioneering work with these techniques has come from Wall's[119] and Devor's[104] groups, and this work continues to be extended.[9, 61] These groups utilized end-bulb neuromas formed by transection of the nerve and then ligation of its distal end ("to prevent regeneration")[9, 61, 104, 109] and by nerve transection but leaving the ends left in continuity to form a non-crushed incontinuity neuroma[61] in rat or cat models. These investigators found spontaneous neural activity originating from the neuromas and transmitted via small myelinated and non-myelinated fibers. They also found one-way and two-way ephaptic conduction through the neuromas. Whether the mechanism was a true ephapse interaction between two nerve fibers or whether action potentials are propagated along retrograde sprouts remains to be determined, but these observations suggest that neural activity arising within the neuroma itself may serve as the basis for neuromatous pain.

The neurophysiologic implications just discussed suggest that spontaneous neural activity and ephaptic conduction are abnormal. Other (non-neuromatous) ectopic generator research has been reviewed more recently.[98] However, observations similar to these have been made, although rarely, in normal or control nerves.[15, 61, 96] If the degree or type (C-fiber to C-fiber, A-delta to A-delta, C-fiber to A-delta) of ephaptic transmission or spontaneous activity is significantly different in nerve fibers proximal to a neuroma, this suggests that the clinical method of neuroma treatment should be altered. For example, such neurophysiologic observations suggest the "old" or "mature" neuromas should be resected in the hope that the subsequent random intraneuroma formation will result in a different set, type, or proportion of ephapses.

The preliminary observations made in our primate model have demonstrated that spontaneous C-fiber activity, as well as ephaptic transmission, occurs in the radial sensory nerve of the baboon proximal to a transection/crush-induced neuroma and that the proportion of these activities alters as the neuroma "matures" from 1 to 6 months.[79] Similar observations have been noted, but to

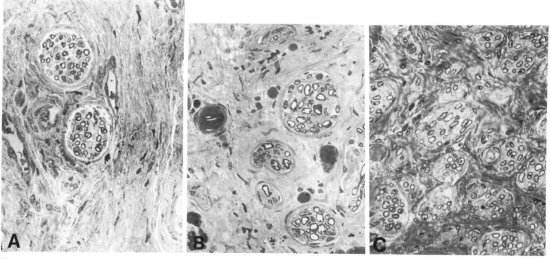

Figure 3–10. Comparison of percentage of neural tissue in neuroma groups in cynomolgus monkeys. *A*, Control group, 20%; *B*, "proximal resection group," 21%; *C*, muscle implantation group, 50%. The p value is <0.001 for the last group versus each of the other two groups. (From Mackinnon, S. E. et al.: Plast. Reconstr. Surg., 76:345–351, 1985.)

a lesser extent, in recordings from two normal baboon radial sensory nerves.[20] The definition of an ephapse, experimentally, is still evolving, however, and it is probably necessary to use a muscle-blocking agent in an intubated animal to be certain that afferent impulses being recorded are not from muscle spindles.[21] This blockade has not been utilized in previous model controls. Clearly, this avenue of investigation holds much future promise.

Morphometric analysis of the neuroma permits evaluation of the end result of various interventions in the natural course of neuroma formation. If we view the neuroma formation as multifactorial, we can then alter each factor to produce a microenvironment in which morphometric analysis may reveal an alteration in this process. Such an alteration, of course, does not necessarily imply altered pathophysiology. The factors that we considered are:

1. Location of the neuroma, i.e., a "quiet" area away from movement and new trauma.

2. Tension upon the neuroma, i.e., avoidance of proximal tethering or distal traction or overlying compression.

3. Absence of neuronotrophic factors, i.e., absence of denervated skin from the immediate environment.

4. Minimal surrounding scar tissue.

Our present model for morphometric analysis of neuroma formation comes from preliminary clinical observations and experimental observations in the baboon.[32] We observed that placement of the proximal end of the nerve into muscle after resection of the "mature" end-bulb neuroma appeared to alter classic neuroma formation. From theoretical considerations of the effect of proximal tethering and distal traction upon the susceptibility of the radial sensory nerve to form a painful neuroma,[30] the following protocol evolved for study in the cynomolgus monkey. In one upper extremity, the (control) neuroma was formed by division of the nerve and resection of its distal 2 cm; the transected proximal stump was left at the level of the wrist, thus maximizing proximity of the nerve end to scar tissue, joint movement, denervated skin, and daily trauma. In the contralateral limb of one group of monkeys, the "standard" clinical procedure, a "proximal level of resection," was done, in which the nerve was treated as just described, but its proximal end was resected proximally an additional 2 cm to permit the nerve end to

lie in non-scarred subcutaneous tissue and away from wrist joint movement and the denervated skin. In another group of monkeys, the contralateral hand was treated by implanting the proximal end of the transected nerve into muscle. A 2 cm tunnel was made from distal to proximal through the muscle, the transected end was brought into the tunnel and secured there with a proximal 6–0 nylon epineurial-epimyseal stitch, and the distal muscle tunnel opening was closed with a suture. In each animal, the RSN, DCU, and PCM were used. During muscle implantation, the RSN was placed into the brachioradialis, the DCU into the flexor carpi ulnaris, and the PCM into the sublimis muscle. In this group of animals, the limb with the muscle implantation was placed into a protective Orthoplast wrist splint for 6 weeks.[99] The neuromas were excised and evaluated 4 to 7 months postoperatively.

The results of the alteration of the microenvironment of transected cutaneous nerves in the cynomolgus monkeys[72] suggested that reducing tension, reducing local extrinsic scarring, and eliminating the presence of denervated skin all alter the formation of a classic end-bulb neuroma. The largest end-bulb neuromas were present grossly in all the control group limbs, whereas the "proximal resection" group had small end-bulb neuromas grossly, and the group with the nerve end implanted into muscle had little, if any, grossly palpable neuroma present. Histologic evaluation of the three groups demonstrated progressively less fascicular disorganization and less connective tissue present from the control group to the proximal resection group to the muscle implantation group. For example, using a particle analyzer, the percentage of neural tissue was found to be increased from 20 per cent in the control group to 59 per cent in the muscle implantation group ($p < 0.001$) (see Fig. 3–10). The "proximal resection" group was not distinguished histologically from the control group. The nerve/muscle interface showed an orderly setting of minifascicles and an absence of collagen whirls. A classic neuroma did not form in the muscle implantation group (Fig. 3–11).

Application of these observations to the clinical situation has begun. In 34 patients, 47 nerves were treated by neuroma resection and implantation of the proximal end into muscle.[68] Although 100 per cent follow-up is available thus far, the length of follow-up is short (4 to 22 months, mean 9 months) and the results are therefore considered preliminary. This was a group of "previous treatment failures," with 19 of the patients (56 per cent) having had at least one earlier procedure and 11 of the patients (32 per cent) having had three or more previous procedures. In 65 per cent of the patients, Workmen's Compensation was involved. Considering the entire group, 74 per cent had excellent and 14 per cent had good relief of pain postoperatively. If just the 16 patients with radial sensory neuromas are considered, 56 per cent had excellent and 18 per cent had good relief of pain. No one had increased pain. Just 6 per cent of the entire group and 13 per cent of the radial nerve group reported no improvement postoperatively. Among the 19 patients with other than radial sensory neuromas, 89 per cent had excellent and 11 per cent had good relief of pain postoperatively.

We are encouraged by these early results of nerve implantation into muscle and continue to do this procedure and follow these patients. Two important technical details should be noted. The muscle tunnel is now made from distal to proximal because in the monkeys we noted a tendency for an occasional axon sprout to grow distally along the myofascial or musculotendinous planes. Also, the recipient muscle must be one with minimal excursion, such as the brachioradialis. In four patients, the radial sensory neuroma was resected and the nerve implanted into the outcropping thumb extensor/abductor muscle group. Although the pain was relieved distally and good wrist function returned, there was pain with thumb abduction/extension! So far three patients have been re-operated upon,[68] the nerve relocated into the brachioradialis with good restoration of thumb function (Fig. 3–12).

In this model myofibroblasts (Fig. 3–13) have been observed to be present in the control and "proximal resection" groups but not in the muscle implantation group of neuromas.[72] The presence of myofibroblasts in these groups supports the concept that tension and motion are critical components of the microenvironment that are favorable to formation of classic end-bulb neuromas. This presence of myofibroblasts is not surprising considering their documented presence in contracting wounds,[43] tension-induced scar,[7] Dupuytren's contracture,[78] and the capsular

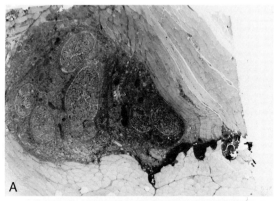

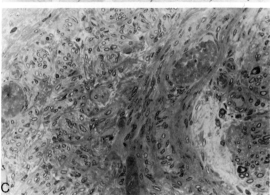

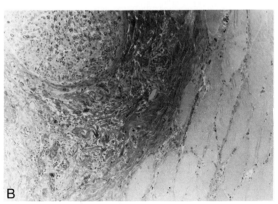

Figure 3–11. Nerve implanted into monkey muscle, 6-month specimens: *A,* Low-power view (× 20). Note preservation of large fascicles in nerve trunk surrounded by muscle. *B,* At end of nerve/muscle interface, multiple minifascicles occur between large fascicle and muscle (× 140). *C,* High-power view (× 200). Note orderly pattern of minifascicles (?axon sprouts) and absence of collagen whirls. (From Mackinnon, S. E. et al.: Ann. Plast. Reconstr. Surg., *76:*345–381, 1985.)

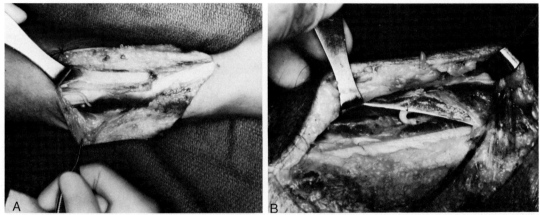

Figure 3–12. Clinical implantation of radial sensory nerve from proximal to distal into thumb abductor/extensor group. *A,* The "wrong technique." *B,* Current technique radial sensory nerve into brachioradialis muscle, from distal to proximal (see text for explanation). (From Dellon, A. L. et al.: Plast. Reconstr. Surg., in press, 1986.)

contracture about Silastic implants.[100] Perhaps the activity of these cells is related to neural discharge from the neuromas. The presence of myofibroblasts and their relationship to the maturity of the neuroma need to be evaluated.

Further applications of this model are apparent. The model so far has evaluated only the relationship of cutaneous nerves to muscle. What about the effect of implantation of a mixed nerve into muscle upon neuroma formation? What effect would denervation of the muscle have upon these relationships? This model might also be utilized to evaluate the effect of a proximal transection and repair upon an established neuroma.

Finally, this approach to neuroma investigation may be useful in evaluating the central nervous system component in patients with a painful neuroma. There is evidence that after a period of time, pain in some way becomes "fixed" in the central nervous system and will remain regardless of what peripheral treatment is given.[5, 123, 125] With increasing ability to utilize histochemistry and immunochemistry histologic and tracer techniques, "pain transmitters and/or receptors" (such as substance P) may be directly evaluated in these models.

NEURAL REGENERATION

Neural regeneration is generally considered to be the sequence of events occurring after nerve repair. Experimental models to study nerve regeneration have employed variations in the *technique* of nerve repair (i.e.,

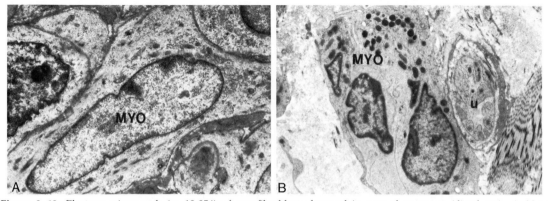

Figure 3–13. Electron micrograph ($\times$ 10,054) of myofibroblast observed in control neuroma (distal cut). *A,* Note unmyelinated fibers (u) between myofibroblast (MYO) and collagen bundles (*B*). (From Mackinnon, S. E. et al.: Plast. Reconstr. Surg., 76:345–351, 1985.)

epineurial versus perineurial,[11, 12, 17, 18, 46, 49, 53, 89, 108] tension-free repair [autograft] versus repair across a gap,[44, 80, 102, 112] autograft versus allograft[2, 73]) or the *timing* of nerve repair (i.e., primary versus secondary repair[45, 51]) or the *method* of repair (i.e., suture versus clot,[110] arterial cuff,[122] tubulation,[14, 56] or laser[4]). Thus, models to study nerve regeneration were concerned more with the mechanisms of nerve *repair*, how best to repair a nerve given different clinical situations. There has, however, been some investigation of the biology of nerve regeneration. The earlier studies described the biologic events preceding nerve regeneration (i.e., Wallerian degeneration of the nerve trunk[96, 97] and end-organ[26]), then described end-organ regeneration.[3, 25, 27, 88] More recently, the metabolism of neural regeneration and axoplasmic flow[31, 47, 81] has been investigated. As more about the biology of neural regeneration is learned, it becomes possible that clinical results will be improved in the future more by manipulating the microneural environment than by microneurosurgery. To this end, an experimental model other than a form of nerve repair is required.

To investigate the biologic capacity of nerve to regenerate requires permitting the nerve to attempt regeneration unencumbered by the investigator's concept of what is required for this biologic event to occur. The concept of trophic factors, neuronotropism, Schwann cell interactions, and effect of the presence of a distal nerve stump or denervated tissue or end-organs and vascularity upon this biologic capacity for neural regeneration,[34, 59, 62, 74, 117, 118]—all these can be investigated in a model that presents a transected nerve with a space into which to regenerate. The model, as perfected by Lundborg, has a "preformed tissue space" into which the proximal nerve may be inserted. The other end of the "preformed tissue space" may serve as a receptacle for the other end of the transected nerve, another nerve (sensory versus motor), or a nerve substitute (tendon).[106] The "preformed tissue space" may be either artificial, such as Silastic tubing,[67] or a mesothelial-lined sheath.[64, 65]

Lundborg's[62, 64, 65, 67] and Spencer's[106] groups have investigated these models in the rat over distances of less than 12 mm. Bora[13] has studied neural regeneration in a cat model over distances approaching 15 mm. However, Campbell et al.,[19] in 1957, reported regeneration of the cat sciatic nerve across a 25-mm Millipore filter gap. The only previous primate investigation of which we are aware is that of Matson et al.,[77] in 1948. These investigators demonstrated neural regeneration across a 10- to 14-mm tibial nerve gap. Because primates are generally considered to have a poorer capacity for neural regeneration than lower order animals, we have extended Lundborg's model, using the vascularized mesothelial-lined sheath, to the primate.[70]

In the primate model for neural regeneration, the mesothelial-lined sheath was created by implanting a 4-cm length of a No. 18 Fr Silastic Foley catheter into the subcutaneous tissue of the antecubital fossa of a baboon. The catheter had been first wrapped circumferentially with No. 26 stainless steel wire along its entire length. The baboon received intramuscular penicillin. The catheter and wire had been soaked in povidone-iodine (Betadine) solution for 5 minutes and had been pre-sterilized. Aseptic technique was used for the operation. This apparatus was left in place for 6 weeks, at which time the vascularization of the formed mesothelial sheath was maximum.[8] At that time, the wound was re-opened and extended, with the baboon again anesthetized with a combination of ketamine (Ketaset) and acepromazine. The ulnar nerve was transposed anteriorly. A tourniquet was not used. A 3-cm segment of the nerve was excised. The implanted apparatus was not dissected from the surrounding connective tissue but was left on a mesothelial stalk attached to its deep surface to maintain the vascularization of the new "preformed tissue space." The soft tissue about the end of the catheter was transected and discarded. The Silastic catheter was removed, leaving a mesothelial tube supported in the "open" position by its skeleton of coated wire. The proximal end of the ulnar nerve was drawn into the sheath by a horizontal mattress suture of 8–0 nylon. The distal end of the ulnar nerve was drawn into the distal end of the sheath by 8–0 nylon. The gap between the nerve ends was adjusted to be 3 cm. At this operation, the baboon received another injection of penicillin. The nerve in the mesothelial sheath was protected by placing the elbow at 120° of flexion and into an Orthoplast splint, which had been fabricated for the particular baboon's upper extremity prior to the operation.[99]

The splint left the wrist and finger free for use so that the operation could be done

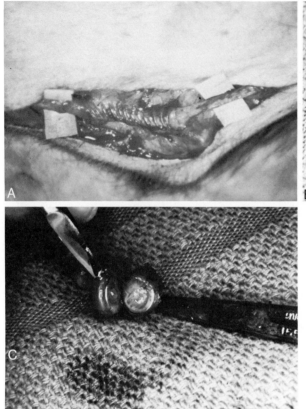
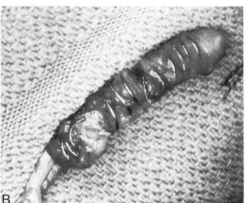

Figure 3–14. *A*, Ulnar nerve and sheath in situ. *B*, Excised ulnar nerve and sheath. *C*, Sheath transected with view of regenerated nerve within. (From Mackinnon, S. E. et al.: Plast. Reconstr. Surg., June, 1985.)

bilaterally and simultaneously and still permit the animal to feed if food was placed within the cage so that the baboon did not have to reach out between the bars. The extremities remained splinted for 6 months, unless the biopsy specimens were obtained earlier. This degree of splinting was thought to be required to prevent the nerves from pulling out of the pseudosheaths. Five baboons had both arms operated upon. Neural regeneration was evaluated at 1, 3, 7, and 9 months after implantation of the nerve into the sheath. At the time of re-exploration to harvest the nerve, one infection and one nerve that had pulled out the sheath were found. Thus, a total of eight specimens were available for evaluation by light and electron microscopy. Ability of the regenerated nerve to conduct an electrical impulse was evaluated at 3 months in two extremities and at 7 months in one extremity. For histologic evaluation, the specimen was resected from 2 cm proximal to 2 cm distal to the sheath (Fig. 3–14).

The investigation of neural regeneration in the baboon demonstrated that a multifascic-ular nerve would regenerate across a 3-cm vascularized preformed tissue space.[70] By 3 months after nerve implantation into the sheath, morphologic evaluation demonstrated individual minifascicles with groups of thinly myelinated and unmyelinated nerve fibers in a matrix of collagen (Fig. 3–15). By 9 months, the central portion of the sheath contained a well-organized multifascicular nerve. Each minifascicle was delineated by perineurium (Fig. 3–16). The fascicles were smaller than those in the proximal ulnar sections and at the mid-sheath level resembled the fascicular pattern of neither the proximal nor the distal ulnar nerve. The ulnar nerve proximal to the sheath was normal. At 3 months after neural regeneration the ulnar nerve sections distal to the sheath demonstrated Wallerian degeneration, but by 9 months the sections had the appearance of a nerve distal to the site of a good nerve repair.

The future investigations with this model have at least two divergent directions. Collection of the fluid within the sheath early in the course of neural regeneration can be assayed for neuronotrophic factors[66] and

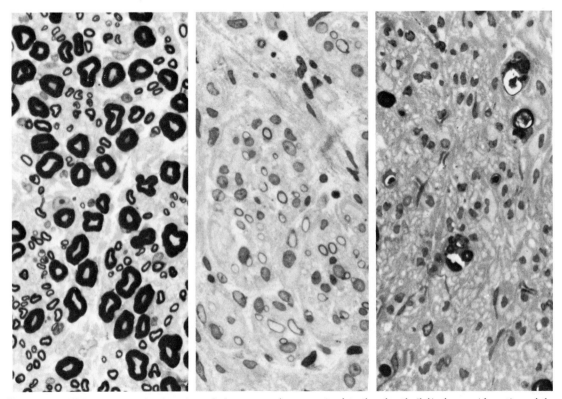

Figure 3–15. Photomicrograph of section of ulnar nerve from proximal to the sheath (*left*), from mid-portion of the sheath (*center*), and from the ulnar nerve distal to the sheath (*right*) (toluidine blue, × 100). This specimen was taken 3 months following implantation of the nerve into the pseudosheath. Note normal ulnar nerve proximal to the sheath, early minifascicle regeneration with thinly myelinated nerve fibers in matrix of collagen, and distal remnants of Wallerian degeneration. (From Mackinnon, S. E. et al.: Plast. Reconstr. Surg., June, 1985.)

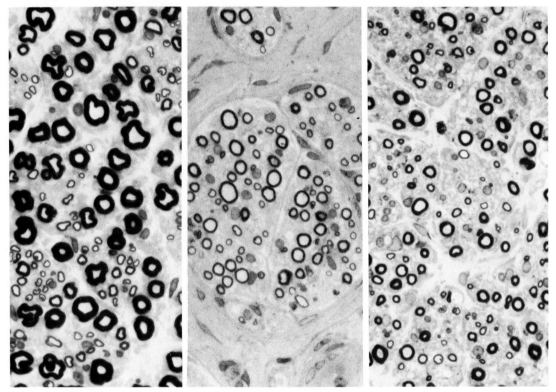

Figure 3–16. Specimen taken 9 months after implantation of nerve into pseudosheath, same arrangement of sections (left to right) as Figure 3–15. Note normal ulnar nerve proximal to sheath, well-developed multifascicular nerve with increasing myelination of fibers within minifascicles, and regeneration of ulnar nerve distal to sheath. (From Mackinnon, S. E. et al.: Plast. Reconstr. Surg., June, 1985.)

morphologic investigation early during regeneration can be done to determine the relative role of Schwann cell migration with respect to axonal sprouting, thereby continuing the research into the basic neurobiology of regeneration. The other avenue of investigation must lead to comparing the results of neural regeneration by means of preformed tissue spaces with the results of nerve grafting. For example, Chiu and Januka[23] have demonstrated comparable degrees of regeneration of sciatic nerve in the rat by an autogenous orthotopic graft and by neural regeneration using an autogenous vein. If, in the primate, the degree of regeneration in the distal nerve trunk and the degree of sensory and motor reinnervation that occurred after neural regeneration by means of a preformed tissue space were comparable to those obtained by means of a nerve graft, it would be conceivable to suggest an alternative to nerve grafting over at least short nerve gaps in human patients.

The demonstration that a primate peripheral nerve can regenerate a multifascicular nerve over distances greater than 15 mm supports the concept that given the appropriate microenvironment, which seems to require the presence of a non-scarred, well-vascularized, tension-free preformed tissue space, neural regeneration has a greater capacity than we had previously imagined. Although it is too soon to suggest that the outcome of these investigations may lead to use of an "off-the-shelf" preformed tissue space suitable for repair of 2-cm nerve gaps instead of nerve grafting, it is appropriate to raise again the possibility that locally acting biologic factors may yet prove more critical in producing better quality results in nerve repair than more precise microsurgical technique.

References

1. Aguayo, A., Nair, C. P. O., and Midgely, R.: Experimental progressive compression neuropathy in the rabbit. Arch. Neurol., 24:357–364, 1971.
2. Aguayo, A. J., and Bray, G. M.: Experimental nerve grafts. *In* Jewett, D. L., and McCarroll, H. R., Jr. (eds.): Nerve Repair and Regeneration. St. Louis, C. V. Mosby Company, 1980.
3. Aitken, S. T., Shorman, B., Young, J. Z.: Maturation of regenerating nerve fibers with various peripheral connections. J. Anat., 81:1–22, 1947.
4. Almquist, E. E.: Use of argon laser in peripheral nerve repair. Sunderland Society Meeting, May, 1983.
5. Battista, A. F.: Pain of peripheral nerve origin: Fascicle ligation for the prevention of painful neuroma. Adv. Pain Res. Ther., 3:167–172, 1979.
6. Battista, A. F., Cravioto, H. M., and Budzilovich, G. N.: Painful neuroma: Changes produced in peripheral nerve after fascicle ligation. Neurosurgery, 9:589–600, 1981.
7. Baur, P. S., Larson, D. L., and Stacey, T. R.: The observation of myofibroblasts in hypertrophic scars. Surg. Gynecol. Obstet., 141:22, 1975.
8. Berry, R. B., Ewart, W. R., Reeve, D. R. E., and Sommerlac, B. C.: Experimental observations of the behavior of nerve grafts in sheaths formed around silicone rods. Br. J. Plast. Surg., 33:324–339, 1980.
9. Blumberg, H., and Janig, W.: Activation of fibers via experimentally produced stump neuromas of skin nerves—Ephaptic transmission or retrograde sprouting. Exp. Neurol., 76:468–482, 1982.
10. Boldney, E.: Amputation neuroma in nerves implanted in bone. Ann. Surg., 118:1052–1057, 1943.
11. Bora, F. W.: Peripheral nerve repair in cats: The fascicular stitch. J. Bone Joint Surg., 49A:659–666, 1967.
12. Bora, F. W., Pleasure, D. E., and Didizian, N. A.: A study of nerve regeneration and neuroma formation after nerve suture by various techniques. J. Hand Surg., 1:138–143, 1976.
13. Bora, W. F., Unger, A. S., and Osterman, A. L.: The local inhibition of nerve scar by the biodegradable vehicle, alzamer, carrying *cis*-hydroxyproline. Presented at American Society of Surgery of the Hand Meeting, March, 1983.
14. Braun, R. M.: Comparative studies of neurorrhaphy and sutureless peripheral nerve repair. Surg. Gynecol. Obstet., 122:15, 1966.
15. Brennan, A., and Mathews, B.: Coupling between nerve fibers supplying normal and injured skin in the cat. J. Physiol., 334:70–71, 1983.
16. Brown, H., and Flynn, J. E.: Abdominal pedicle flap for hand neuromas and entrapped nerves. J. Bone Joint Surg., 55:575–578, 1973.
17. Brushart, T. M., Tarlov, E. C., and Mesulam, M. M.: Specificity of muscle reinnervation after epineurial and individual fascicular suture of the rat sciatic nerve. J. Hand Surg., 8:248–253, 1983.
18. Cabaud, H. E., Rodkey, W. G., McCarroll, H. R., Muty, S. B., and Niebauer, J. J.: Epineurial and perineurial fascicular nerve repairs: A critical comparison. J. Hand Surg., 1:131–137, 1976.
19. Campbell, J. B., Bassett, C. A., Gerado, J. M., Seymour, R. J., and Rossi, J. P.: Application of monomolecular filter tubes in bridging gaps in peripheral nerves and for prevention of neuroma formation. J. Neurosurg., 13:635–637, 1957.
20. Campbell, J. N., et al.: Unpublished observations, 1982.
21. Campbell, J. N.: Personal communication, 1983.
22. Cannon, B. W., and Love, J. G.: Tardy median palsy: median neuritis: median thenar neuritis amenable to surgery. Surgery, 20:210–216, 1946.
23. Chiu, D. T., Januka, I., Krizek, T. J., Wolff, M., and Lovelace, R. E.: Autogenous vein graft as a conduit for nerve regeneration. Surgery, 91:226–233, 1982.
24. Curtis, R. M., and Eversmann, W. W., Jr.: Internal neurolysis as an adjunct to the treatment of carpal tunnel syndrome. J. Bone Joint Surg., 55A:733–740, 1973.
25. Dellon, A. L.: Reinnervation of denervated Meissner corpuscles: A sequential histologic study in the

monkey following fascicular nerve repair. J. Hand Surg., 1:98–109, 1976.

26. Dellon, A. L.: Sensory corpuscles after nerve division. In Dellon, A. L. (ed.): Evaluation of Sensibility and Re-education of Sensation in the Hand. Baltimore, Williams & Wilkins Company, 1981, Chapter 4.

27. Dellon, A. L.: Sensory corpuscles after nerve repair. In Dellon, A. L. (ed.): Evaluation of Sensibility and Re-education of Sensation in the Hand. Baltimore, Williams & Wilkins Company, 1981, Chapter 5.

28. Dellon, A. L.: The clinical use of vibratory stimuli to evaluate peripheral nerve injury and compression neuropathy. Plast. Reconstr. Surg., 65:466–476, 1980.

29. Dellon, A. L.: The Vibrometer. Plast. Reconstr. Surg., 71:427–431, 1983.

30. Dellon, A. L., and Mackinnon, S. E.: Susceptibility of the superficial sensory branch of the radial nerve to form painful neuromas. J. Hand Surg. (Brit.) 1984.

31. Dellon, A. L., Mackinnon, S. E., Hudson, A., Hunter, D., and Seiler, W. A.: Primate model for median nerve compression in the carpal tunnel. Sunderland Society Meeting, May, 1983.

32. Dellon, A. L., Mackinnon, S. E., and Pestronk, A.: Implantation of sensory nerve into muscle. Preliminary clinical and experimental observations on neuroma formation. Ann. Plast. Surg., 12:30–40, 1984.

33. Dellon, A. L., Schneider, R., and Burke, R.: Effect of acute compartment pressure changes upon response to vibratory stimuli. Plast. Reconstr. Surg., 72:208–216, 1983.

34. Drachman, D. B. (ed.): Trophic Functions of the Neuron. New York, New York Academy of Science, 1974.

35. Ducker, T. B., Kempe, L. G., and Hayes, G. J.: The metabolic background for peripheral nerve surgery. J. Neurosurg., 30:270, 1969.

36. Duncan, D.: Alterations in the structure of nerves caused by restricting their growth with ligatures. J. Neuropathol. Exp. Neurol., 7:261–273, 1948.

37. Feindel, W., and Stratford, J.: Cubital tunnel compression in tardy ulnar palsy. Can. Med. Assn. J., 78:351–354, 1958.

38. Forman, D. S., and Berenberg, R. A.: Regeneration of motor axons in the rat sciatic nerve studied by labelling with axonally transported radioactive proteins. Brain Res., 156:213, 1978.

39. Frackelton, W. H., Teasley, J. L., and Tauras, A.: Neuromas in the hand treated by nerve transposition and silicone capping. J. Bone Joint Surg., 53A:813, 1971.

40. Fullerton, P. M., and Gilliattt, R. W.: Changes in nerve conduction in caged guinea-pigs. J. Physiol., 178:47–48, 1965.

41. Fullerton, P. M., and Gilliatt, R. W.: Median and ulnar neuropathy in the guinea-pig. J. Neurol. Neurosurg. Psychiatry, 30:393–402, 1967.

42. Fullerton, P. M., and Gilliatt, R. W.: Pressure neuropathy in the hind foot of the guinea-pig. J. Neurol. Neurosurg. Psychiatry, 30:18–25, 1967.

43. Gabbiani, G., Hirschel, J., Ryan, G. B., Statkov, P. R., and Majno, G.: Granulation tissue as a contractile organ: A study of structure and function. J. Exp. Med., 135:719, 1972.

44. Goto, Y.: Experimental study of nerve autografting by funicular suture. Arch. Japan Chir., 36:478–494, 1967.

45. Grabb, W. C.: Median and ulnar nerve suture: An experimental study comparing primary and secondary repair in monkeys. J. Bone Joint Surg., 50A:964, 1968.

46. Grabb, W. C., Spencer, L. B., Koepke, G. H., and Green, R. A.: Comparison of methods of peripheral nerve suturing in monkeys. Plast. Reconstr. Surg., 46:31–38, 1970.

47. Griffin, J. W., Price, D. B., and Drachman, B.: Fast axonal transport in motor nerve regeneration. J. Neurobiol., 7:355, 1976.

48. Guttman, L., and Medawar, P. B.: The chemical inhibition of fibre regeneration and neuroma formation in peripheral nerves. J. Neurol. Neurosurg. Psychiatry, 5:130–141, 1942.

49. Hakstian, R. W.: Funicular orientation by direct stimulation. J. Bone Joint Surg., 52A:1178–1186, 1968.

50. Herndon, J. H., Eaton, R. G., and Littler, J. W.: Management of painful neuromas in the hand. J. Bone Joint Surg., 58A:369–373, 1976.

51. Holmes, W., and Young, J. Z.: Nerve regeneration after immediate and delayed suture. J. Anat., 77:63, 1942.

52. Huber, G. C., and Lewis, D.: Amputation neuromas. Their development and prevention. Arch. Surg., 1:85–113, 1920.

53. Hudson, A., Hunter, D., Kline, D. G., and Bratton, B. R.: Histologic studies of experimental interfascicular graft repairs. J. Neurosurg., 51:333, 1979.

54. Jefferson, D., and Eames, R. A.: Subclinical entrapment of the lateral femoral cutaneous nerve: an autopsy study. Muscle Nerve 2:145–154, 1979.

55. Keck, C.: The tarsal-tunnel syndrome. Lancet 2:1354–1355, 1962.

56. Kline, D. G., and Hayes, G. J.: The use of resorbable wrapper for peripheral nerve repair. J. Neurosurg., 21:737, 1964.

57. Laborde, K. J., Kalisman, M., and Tsai, T.: Results of surgical treatment of painful neuromas of the hand. J. Hand Surg., 7:190–193, 1982.

58. Learmouth, J. R.: A technique for transplanting the ulnar nerve. Surg. Gynecol. Obstet., 75:792–793, 1942.

59. Levi–Montalcini, E.: The nerve growth factor. Its mode of action on sensory and sympathetic nerve cells. Harvey Lecture, 60:217–259, 1966.

60. Linscheid, R. L.: Injuries to radial nerve at wrist. Arch. Surg., 91:942–946, 1965.

61. Lisney, S. J. W., and Pover, C. M.: Coupling between fibres involved in sensory nerve neuromata in cats. J. Neurol. Sci., 59:255–264, 1983.

62. Lundborg, G., Dahlin, L., Danielsen, N., Hansson, H., Johannesson, A., Longo, F. M., Varon, S., and Engin, D.: Nerve regeneration across an extended gap: A neurobiologic view of nerve repair and the possible involvement of neuronotrophic factors. J. Hand Surg., 7:580–587, 1982.

63. Lundborg, G., Gelberman, R. H., Minteer-Convery, M., Lee, F. F., and Hargens, A. R.: Median nerve compression in the carpal tunnel—functional response to experimentally induced controlled pressure. J. Hand Surg., 7:252–259, 1982.

64. Lundborg, G., and Hanson, H. A.: Nerve regeneration through preformed pseudosynovial tubes. A preliminary report of a new experimental model for studying the regeneration and reorganization capacity of peripheral nerve tissue. J. Hand Surg., 5:35–38, 1980.

65. Lundborg, G., and Hanson, H. A.: Regeneration

of peripheral nerve through a preformed tissue space. Preliminary observations on the reorganization of regenerating nerve fibers and perineurium. Brain Res., 178:573–576, 1979.

66. Lundborg, G., Longo, F. M., and Varon, S.: Nerve regeneration: Its association with neuronotrophic factors. Presented at the American Society for Surgery of the Hand Meeting, March, 1983.

67. Lundborg, G., Longo, F. M., and Varon, S.: Nerve regeneration model and trophic factors in vivo. Brain Res., 232:157–161, 1982.

68. Mackinnon, S. E., and Dellon, A. L.: Treatment of painful neuroma by neuroma resection and muscle implantation. Plast. Reconstr. Surg., in press, 1986.

69. Mackinnon, S. E., Dellon, A. L., and Daneshvar, A.: Histopathology of the tarsal tunnel syndrome: examination of a human posterior tibial nerve. Contemp. Orthop., 9:43–48, 1984.

70. Mackinnon, S. E., Dellon, A. L., Hudson, A. B., and Hunter, D.: Regeneration of ulnar nerve through a mesothelial tube in the baboon. Plast. Reconstr. Surg., June, 1985.

71. Mackinnon, S. E., Dellon, A. L., Hudson, A., Hunter, D., and Seiler, W. A.: Chronic nerve compression: An experimental model in the rat. Arch. Plast. Surg., 13:112–120, 1984.

72. Mackinnon, S. E., Dellon, A. L., Hudson, A., Hunter, D., and Seiler, W.A.: Alteration of neuroma formation by manipulation of its microenvironment. Plast. Reconstr. Surg., 76:345–351, 1985.

72a. Mackinnon, S. E., Dellon, A. L., Hudson, A., Hunter, D., and Seiler, W. A.: Primate model for chronic nerve compression. J. Reconstr. Microsurg., 1:185–194, 1985.

73. Mackinnon, S. E., Hudson, A., Falk, R. E., and Hunter, D.: The peripheral nerve allograft: An immunological assessment of pretreatment methods. Plast. Surg. Forum 5:172–174, 1983.

74. Manthorpe, M., Varon, S., and Adler, R.: Neurite promoting factor (NPF) in conditioned medium from RNZZ schwannoma cultures: bioassay, fractionation and other properties. J. Neurochem., 37:759–767, 1981.

75. Marie, P., and Foix, C.: Atrophie isolée de l'éminence thénar d'origine névritique. Rôle du ligament annulaiare antérieur du carpe dans la pathogénie de la lésion. Rev. Neurol., 26:647–648, 1913.

76. Mathews, B.: Coupling between cutaneous nerves. J. Physiol., 254:37–38, 1976.

77. Matson, D. D., Alexander, E., Jr., and Weiss, P: Experiments on the bridging of gaps in severed peripheral nerves of monkeys. J. Neurosurg., 5:230–248, 1948.

78. McFarlane, R. M., and Chiu, H. F.: Pathogenesis of Dupuytren's contracture. J. Hand Surg., 3:1–10, 1978.

79. Meyer, R. A., Campbell, J. N., Raja, S. N., Mackinnon, S. E., Burke, R., and Dellon, A. L.: Neural activity originating from a neuroma in the baboon. Proc. Soc. Neurosci., 8:855, 1982.

80. Millesi, H., Meissl, G., and Berger, A.: Interfascicular nerve grafting of the median and ulnar nerves. J. Bone Joint Surg., 54A:727–750, 1972.

81. Moszkowicz, L.: Zur Behandlung der schmerzhaften Neurome. Zntrlbl. Chir., 45:547, 1918.

82. Mountcastle, V. B.: Personal communication, July, 1983.

83. Munro, D., and Mallory, G. K.: Elimination of the so-called amputation neuromas of divided peripheral nerves. N. Engl. J. Med., 260:358–361, 1959.

84. Neary, D., and Eames, R. A.: The pathology of ulnar nerve compression in man. Neuropathol. Appl. Neurobiol., 1:69–88, 1975.

85. Neary, D., Ochoa, J., and Gilliatt, R. W.: Subclinical entrapment neuropathy in man. J. Neurol. Sci., 24:283–298, 1975.

86. Ochoa, J., and Marotte, L.: Nature of the nerve lesion underlying chronic nerve entrapment. J. Neurol. Sci., 19:491, 1973.

87. Ochs, S., and Worth, R. M.: Calcium requirement for axoplasmic transport in mammalian nerve. Nature, 270:748, 1977.

88. Orgel, M., Aguayo, A., and Williams, H. B.: Sensory nerve regeneration: An experimental study of skin grafts in the rabbit. J. Anat., 111:121, 1972.

89. Orgel, M. G., and Terzis, J. K.: Epineurial versus perineurial repair: An ultrastructural and electrophysiological study of nerve regeneration. Plast. Reconstr. Surg., 60:80–90, 1977.

90. Osborne, G.: Compression neuritis of the ulnar nerve at the elbow. Hand, 2:10–13, 1970.

91. Osborne, G. V.: The surgical treatment of tardy ulnar neuritis. J. Bone Joint Surg., 39:782, 1957.

92. Parry, C. B. W.: Painful conditions of peripheral nerves. Aust. N. Z. J. Surg., 50:233–236, 1980.

93. Petropoulos, P. C., and Stefanko, S.: Experimental observations on the prevention of neuroma formations. J. Surg. Res., 1:241–248, 1961.

94. Petropoulos, P. C., and Stefanko, S.: Experimental studies of post-traumatic neuromas under various physiologic conditions. J. Surg. Res., 1:235–240, 1961.

95. Poth, E. J., Bravo-Fernandez, E., and Drager, G. A.: Prevention of formation of end-bulb neuromata. Proc. Soc. Exp. Biol. Med., 60:200–207, 1945.

96. Ramon y Cajal, S.: Degeneration and Regeneration of the Nervous System. Vol 1, English Ed. London, Oxford University Press, 1928.

97. Ranson, S. W.: Degeneration and regeneration of nerve fibers. J. Comp. Neurol., 22:487–546, 1912.

98. Rasminsky, M.: Ectopic generation of impulses in pathologic nerve fibres. In Jewett, D. L., and McCarroll, H. R., Jr. (eds.): Nerve Repair and Regeneration. St. Louis, C. V. Mosby Company, 1980, pp. 178–185.

99. Rose, B. W., Mackinnon, S. E., Dellon, A. L., and Snyder, R. A.: Design of a protective splint for the non-human primate extremity. Lab. Ani. Sci., 33:306–308, 1983.

100. Rudolph, R., Abraham, J., Vecchione, T., Guber, S., and Woodward, M.: Myofibroblasts and free silicone around breast implants. Plast. Reconstr. Surg., 62:185–190, 1978.

101. Rydevik, B., Lundborg, G., and Nordborg, C.: Intraneural tissue reactions induced by internal neurolysis. Scand. J. Plast. Reconstr. Surg., 10:3–8, 1976.

102. Seddon, H. J.: The use of autografts for repair of large gaps in peripheral nerves. Br. J. Surg., 35:151, 1947.

103. Seiler, W. A., Schlegel, R., Mackinnon, S. E., and Dellon, A. L.: The double crush syndrome: development of a model. Surg. Forum, 33:596–598, 1983.

104. Seltzer, Z., and Devor, M.: Ephaptic transmission in chronically damaged peripheral nerves. Neurology, 29:1061–1064, 1979.

105. Smith, J. R., and Gomez, N. H.: Local injection therapy of neuromata of the hand with triamcinolone acetonide. A preliminary study of twenty-two patients. J. Bone Joint Surg., 52A:71–83, 1970.

106. Spencer, P.: Sunderland Society Meeting, May, 1983.
107. Spindler, H. A., and Dellon, A. L.: Nerve conduction studies and sensibility testing in carpal tunnel syndrome. J. Hand Surg., 7:260–263, 1982.
108. Sunderland, S.: Funicular suture and funicular exclusion in the repair of severed nerves. Br. J. Surg., 40:580, 1953.
109. Swanson, A. B., Boeve, N. R., and Biddulph, S. L.: Silicone-rubber capping of amputation neuromas. Investigational and clinical experience. Interclin. Info. Bull., 11:1, 1972.
110. Tarlov, I. M.: Plasma clot suture of nerves. Surgery, 15:257, 1944.
111. Teneff, S.: Prevention of amputation neuroma. J. Int. Coll. Surg., 12:16, 1949.
112. Terzis, J. K., Faibisoff, B., and Williams, H. B.: The nerve gap: Suture under tension versus graft. Plast. Reconstr. Surg., 56:166–170, 1975.
113. Thomas, P. K., and Fullerton, P. M.: Nerve fiber size in the carpal tunnel syndrome. J. Neurol. Neurosurg. Psychiatry, 26:520–527, 1963.
114. Tsairis, P.: Differential diagnosis of peripheral neuropathies. *In* Omer, G. E., and Spinner, M. (eds.): Management of Peripheral Nerve Problems. Philadelphia, W. B. Saunders Company, 1980, pp. 712–726.
115. Tupper, J. W., and Booth, D. M.: Treatment of painful neuromas of sensory nerves in the hand: A comparison of traditional and newer methods. J. Hand Surg., 1:144–151, 1976.
116. Upton, A. R. M., and McComas, A. J.: The double crush in nerve entrapment syndromes. Lancet 2:359, 1972.
117. Varon, S.: Nerve growth factor and its mode of action. Exp. Neurol., 48:75–92, 1975.
118. Varon, S., and Adler, R.: Nerve growth factors and control of nerve growth. Curr. Topics Dev. Biol., 16:207–252, 1980.
119. Wall, P. D., and Gutnick, M.: Properties of afferent nerve impulses originating from a neuroma. Nature, 248:740–742, 1974.
120. Weisl, H., and Osborne, G. V.: The pathological changes in rats' nerves subject to moderate compression. J. Bone Joint Surg., 46B:297–306, 1964.
121. Weiss, P., and Hiscoe, H. B.: Experiments on the mechanism of nerve growth. J. Exp. Zool., 107:315–395, 1948.
122. Weiss, P. A., and Taylor, A. C.: Guides for nerve regeneration across gaps. J. Neurosurg., 3:400, 1946.
123. Wilson, P. R.: Neurological mechanisms of pain: Modifications by neural blockage. *In* Cousins, M. J., and Bridenbough, P. O. (eds.): Neural Blockade in Clinical Anesthesia and Management of Pain. Philadelphia, J. B. Lippincott Company, 1982, pp. 557–585.
124. Wolton, M. W. J.: Neuritis associated with acromegaly. Arch. Neurol. Psychiatry, 45:680–682, 1941.
125. Yaksh, T. L., and Hammond, D. L.: Peripheral and central substrates involved in the rostrad transmission of nociceptive information. Pain, 13:1–85, 1982.

4

Effects of Repeated Experimental Localized Freezings in the Distal Stump of Peripheral Nerves

■

Jean-Claude Mira, D.Sc.

The earliest observations on peripheral nerve regeneration after repeated injuries were made at the end of the last century by Mayer[16] and Vanlair.[40] From that time onward, relatively few studies have been devoted to this subject, and the morphologic and/or electrophysiologic results of these investigations have often been conflicting. Indeed, some results show that the neuronal regenerative power is lessened after repeated injuries,[33] whereas others indicate that it is unchanged,[4, 5, 7, 8, 10] and still others demonstrate that it is enhanced.[1, 3, 9]

Thus, Duncan and Jarvis,[4] when studying regeneration of the motor branches of the cat facial nerve, reported that recovery was apparently achieved about 1 month after each of five successive sections, eight successive crushes, and nine successive chemical treatments (e.g., destruction of nerve fibers with 10% benzyl alcohol in sweet almond oil). Moreover, 3 months after the last injury, the number of fibers peripheral to the site of lesion was greatly reduced in the sectioned nerves, slightly reduced in the crushed nerves, and definitely increased in chemically treated nerves. Duncan and Jarvis concluded that, using their methods, small motor nerves were capable of repeated regenerations without reducing the intensity of the

reaction and without demonstrable effects on parent neuronal cell bodies. Holmes and Young[10] considered that the capacity of a proximal stump to send out new fibers was not reduced if the stump was injured a second time, either within 1 week of the first injury or after an interval as long as 1 year. Gutmann[7, 8] found that repeated injuries to the same nerve did not affect the axonal regenerative capacity; thus, repeated crushes were often followed by functional recovery, the rate of regeneration remaining virtually unchanged even after the eighth crush. In contrast, Gutmann and Holubar[9] observed that "prophylactic" crushing of the proximal stump of a severed nerve stimulated the cell bodies and enhanced their metabolic activities, since the number of nerve fibers and the thickness of their myelin sheaths were greater in the proximal stump where the crush had been performed. Accordingly, the conduction velocity and the amplitude of the action potentials were greater on the injured side than on the control side. Ducker et al.[3] indicated that the axonal growth proceeded faster after the second injury than after the first if there was a 2- to 3-week interval between the lesions; however, in the spinal cord, the neuronal metabolic response was not as intense the second time. In the same way, Thomas[37, 38] observed a gradual increase in the number of nuclei ($\times 8$) and in nuclear density ($\times 4$) following the ninth crush of the rabbit peroneal nerve; there was an approximately linear relationship between the changes in the nuclear counts and the number of crushings. Proliferation was mainly observed in Schwann cells; moreover, following repeated Wallerian degeneration with intervening regeneration, nerve transverse sections showed extensive nerve fiber systems composed of groups of several myelinated and unmyelinated axons with associated Schwann cells and collagen fibrils. Each of these clusters was the product of a single Büngner band, which gradually grew larger and was subdivided by the repeated degeneration and regeneration of multiple axonal sprouts. These clusters resembled those sometimes observed in chronic neuropathies associated with repeated axonal degeneration and regeneration. Similar "hyperneurotization" of Büngner bands was also noted by Schröder[34] in sciatic nerves of rats with experimental isoniazid neuropathy.

More recent experimental works have established that the axonal regeneration following nerve section may be accelerated in neurons that have undergone previous axonal injury. Thus, a "conditioning" lesion performed before the "test" lesion may facilitate the response of some neurons. The results in this respect can be summed up as follows:

1. Regeneration of the motor axons[12, 36] and sensory axons[15] is accelerated, whereas that of the adrenergic axons is considerably slowed down.[14]

2. The initial delay (i.e., the time required for the neuron to recover and to enable regeneration to begin and for regenerating axons to cross the zone of traumatic degeneration) is decreased from 1.6 days to 0.9 day for sensory axons[6] and from 1.3 days to 0.6 day for adrenergic axons.[14]

3. The overall number of regenerated nerve fibers does not increase[13] and can even be reduced.[14] However, as will be described, the results are different after repeated localized freezings.

4. The axonal response is facilitated when the test lesion is performed at least 48 hours after the conditioning lesion; the response seems to be maximal between 7 and 14 days and regresses after 21 days.[35]

5. The return of motor function is accelerated, but only if the denervated muscle undergoes daily electrical stimulation[36]; this form of stimulation appears to prevent muscle atrophy resulting from denervation after creating the conditioning lesion.

These divergent findings prompted us to undertake a study of peripheral nerve regeneration and muscle reinnervation following repeated nerve injury. For this purpose, the present author has chosen the freezing procedure, since results of this technique have always shown that anatomic and electrophysiologic recovery is faster and more complete than after crushing or section.[11, 19, 20, 23, 26, 28, 31] In addition, this experimental procedure is very easy to perform and is perfectly controllable and perfectly reproducible, which is not the case even for localized crushing. Consequently, all results of freezing are more constant than those of any type of experimental peripheral nerve injury.[11, 23, 28] This technique consists of localized freezing of the nerve, performed *in situ*, using a liquid nitrogen cryode.[23, 26] The active point of this probe is quickly brought to a temperature of about $-180°$ C. To perform the freezing, the cryode is directly applied to the rat sciatic nerve at three points of the same nerve circumference; the near circle formed by these points is indicated by a suture of nonresorbable Flexilon thread placed in the perineurium and marking the approximate center of the frozen area. Under the usual conditions, the total duration of freezing and thawing never exceeds 30 to 40 seconds and the frozen area is 2 to 3 mm long.

All the axons and their myelin sheaths undergo irreversible changes and degenerate, whereas the general organization of the connective tissue sheaths (epineurium, perineurium, and endoneurium) and the blood vessels supplying them does not appear to be affected by the cold injury. Moreover, the basal laminae surrounding the nerve fibers, both myelinated and unmyelinated, remain intact throughout the frozen segment and into the distal stump.[2, 17, 41] This technique therefore enabled me to study nerve regeneration under extremely favorable conditions.

ULTRASTRUCTURAL ASPECTS OF MYELINATED NERVE FIBER REGENERATION

Axonal regeneration began at the upper limit of the necrosed zone, i.e., the proximal part of the frozen area and the proximal segment affected by traumatic degeneration. Within hours of the cold injury, small axoplasmic outgrowths extended from the fiber extremity, which remained continuous with the neuronal cell body. However, these first axonal sprouts degenerated, since the final sprouting occurred only after 24 hours and developed within the basal lamina tube, which had remained intact and continuous after the freezing injury.

In the proximal stump, axonal regeneration could be detected electrophysiologically within 24 to 36 hours of the injury[29] and was noted histologically by the second day at the most distal node of Ranvier, which had remained undamaged.[28] This was, in fact, a half-node, since the proximal part of the axon was ensheathed by normal myelin, whereas the distal part was not yet myelinated (Fig. 4–1a). Myelination of the regenerating axon began toward the end of the first week. By this time, a thin sheath consisting of a few lamellae was forming around the distal part, whereas the proximal part still preserved its normal sheath (Fig. 4–1b).

During the first 2 weeks, there was a phase of active axonal sprouting in the necrosed zone and distal stump. Whereas in the normal nerve each myelinated fiber basically consists of a single axon, in the regenerating nerve two myelinated structures were found: "simple" fibers with a single axon, as in the intact nerve (Fig. 4–1c), and "compound" fibers containing at least two myelinated and numerous unmyelinated axons (Fig. 4–2c). I have kept the term *faisceaux de régénération*, which Nageotte[32] used to describe the somewhat unusual structures formed in the early stages of peripheral nerve regeneration.[18] Similar structures seen by different authors have been called "clusters," "Schwann cell families," or "regenerating units." It is generally assumed that these compound fibers result from the sprouting of a single initial fiber, an assumption now confirmed by electron microscopic examination of semi-serial transverse and longitudinal sections made after localized freezing.[18, 20, 28]

At the upper limit of the necrosed area, from the second day onward, some fibers began to ramify actively within a common basal lamina, the same structure that surrounded the fiber in the intact nerve. This "old" tube was still present and continuous after freezing, but appeared in the form of folds of varying depth running parallel to the fiber axis (Fig. 4–1c). The Schwann cell plasma membrane was therefore no longer in close apposition to the base of the deepest gutters. One terminal sprout (Fig. 4–1a to c) or several terminal sprouts of various sizes (Fig. 4–2a) were seen to extend from the axonal tip; more distally, collaterals protruded in the entire regenerated segment, but only at the site of a node (Fig. 4–2b). All these sprouts developed within the old basal lamina and formed a *faisceau de régénération*.

The bare peripheral axons were progressively wrapped in cytoplasmic expansions from the Schwann cells and thus acquired their individual Schwann cell sheath. By the fifth postoperative day, short segments of new basal laminae with free extremities appeared close to the areas of the Schwann cell plasma membrane not covered by the original tube. By the sixth day, these new segments linked up with the old ones in such a way that the Schwann cell was now covered by a continuous basal lamina closely enveloping its plasma membrane. Consequently, each Schwann cell that still contained one or several axons was isolated from its neighbors by its own basal lamina; however, the outermost fibers were surrounded by a tube made up partly of segments of the old basal lamina and partly of newly formed segments, whereas the innermost fibers were covered by an entirely new tube. Moreover, the lumen of the initial tube was partitioned by these basal laminae, and longitudinal collagen fibrils then appeared in the extracellular spaces thus created. By now, the small bunch of initial axonal sprouts had become a *faisceau de régénération*. Myelination of some axons began by the end of the first week (Fig. 4–2c). By the fourth week, the old basal lamina, which still enclosed all the fibers of each *faisceau de régénération*, disintegrated and allowed the release of new fibers in the endoneurial spaces. However, these fibers were not all myelinated, and those that were unmyelinated quickly degenerated. Accordingly, while the number of axonal sprouts was about 6 to 7 times greater than that in the normal nerve, the possible number of regenerated and fully myelinated fibers was only 1.2 to 2.0 times the original number, as will be described.

Axonal sprouting was not restricted to the regenerating parts. At the beginning of the second postoperative week, fine new collaterals could be seen originating in the proximal stump in a zone that had apparently remained normal and was located about 3 to 4 mm proximal to the upper limit of the necrosis.[20, 28] These small sprouts, which originated within the basal lamina tube of the parent fiber, developed proximodistally, joined the more distal sprouts, and helped to form a *faisceau de régénération*.

The evolution of the Schwann cell basal laminae, as observed in time and space on semi-serial ultrathin sections, led to the conclusion that each *faisceau de régénération* is a morphologic entity including all the preterminal, terminal, and collateral sprouts originating from a single myelinated fiber and confined for 3 or 4 weeks within a common basal lamina; it is this old tube that, in the intact nerve, originally covered the myelinated fiber, giving rise to all the sprouts.

In addition, the formation and evolution of the *faisceaux de régénération* explain the increase in the number of myelinated fibers in regenerating peripheral nerves.

QUANTITATIVE ASPECTS OF MYELINATED NERVE FIBER REGENERATION

Quantitative studies involving different populations of nerve fibers require the determination of their number and the measurement of their size. This can be performed in the living animal as well as in teased preparations or can be carried out in the whole nerve after fixation and staining. The diameter can be measured at different points along the teased fibers or, more often, in enlarged photographic prints of transverse sections of the nerve trunk. Numerical data obtained by various methods concern the total, maximal, or minimal diameter of each fiber, the mean diameter of all the fibers, etc.

Measurement of the total diameter (axon + myelin) of each myelinated fiber allows the construction of a histogram and the study of fiber size distribution. Histograms have often been used as an anatomic basis for electrophysiologic studies (reconstruction of compound action potentials, relationship between diameter and conduction velocity, etc.), as well as for anatomic studies. However, it should be emphasized that the histogram made from such measurements is definitely subjective. If each fiber were to have a constant diameter throughout its length and no artifacts were introduced by histologic treatment, the histogram drawn up on the basis of a single transverse section could be considered a good representation of fiber distribution in a particular nerve. However, since fiber diameter varies with the age (or weight) and sex of the rats,[21] the histogram can never be characteristic of a fiber population as a whole, nor can it be considered as anything other than one sample of diameters in the nerve.

The size distribution of myelinated fibers has also been used as a criterion in numerous studies of peripheral nerve regeneration. Thus, some authors have used the contralateral nerve as a control, whereas others have preferred to obtain their reference material from both sides of the lesion. I have used the first method, since it obviates the need to count and calibrate an excessively large number of fibers (the rat sciatic nerve contains approximately 15,000 myelinated fibers at the site of localized freezing) and hence avoids a high degree of error in measurements, allows a large number of animals to be tested, and eliminates individual variations due to the age, weight, or sex of the rats. However, it should be noted that variations in the number and size of myelinated fibers, which are often quite marked, can be recorded in the contralateral nerve after creation of all types of lesions.[26]

Figure 4–1. Regenerating rat sciatic nerve: "simple" myelinated fibers. *a*, 5 days after freezing. Longitudinal section at the upper limit of the necrosed area. The proximal part of an axon was seen to be ensheathed by normal myelin, while its distal part was not myelinated. This was a half-node of Ranvier (× 9500). *b*, 9 days after freezing. Longitudinal section at the upper limit of the necrosed area. When myelination had started, the newly restored node was formed by two distinct half-nodes: the more proximal was normal and complex, the more distal was more simple. The proximal part of the axon had always preserved its normal sheath, while a thin sheath was forming on distal side. Note the presence of two distinct basal laminae (× 9400). *c*, 9 days after freezing. Transverse section of a regenerating fiber with very marked folding of its old basal lamina, while the new one was molded to the contour of the Schwann cell. Note the junctions between the two basal laminae (*arrows*) and the presence of rare longitudinal collagen fibrils in the extracellular spaces formed between the two basal laminae (*arrowhead*) (× 8800). D = distal part of nerve fiber; EC = endoneurial collagen; NBL = new basal lamina; NR = node of Ranvier; ½NR = half node of Ranvier; OBL = old basal lamina; P = proximal part of nerve fiber. (From Mira, J.-C.: Clin. Plast. Surg., *11*:18, 1984.)

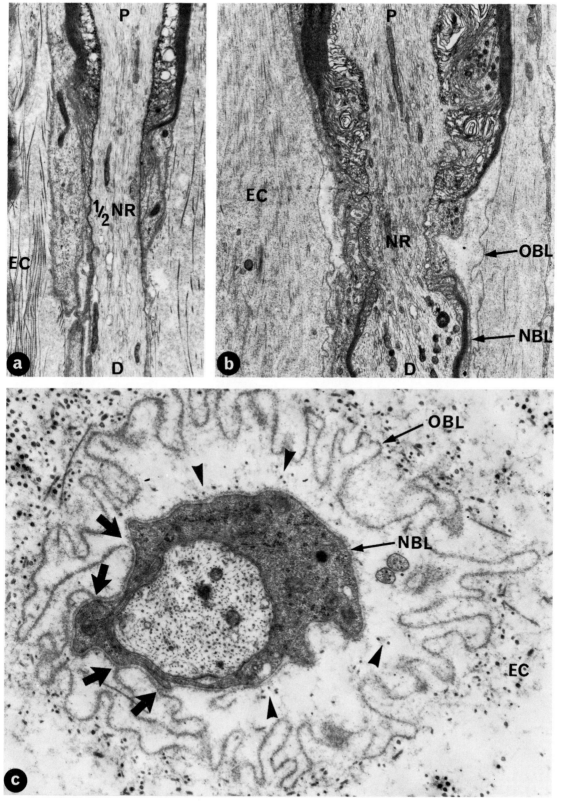

Figure 4–1. *See legend on opposite page.*

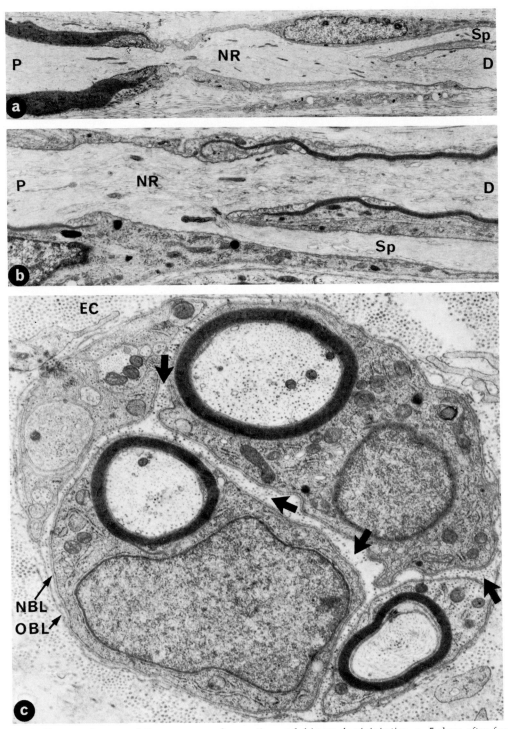

Figure 4–2. Regenerating rat sciatic nerve: axonal sprouting and *faisceau de régénération. a,* 5 days after freezing. Longitudinal section at the upper limit of necrosis, passing through a newly restored node and showing terminal sprouting. The sprout was much finer than the main axon, still unmyelinated and confined within the Schwann cell cytoplasm of the parent fiber. The proximal part of the main axon was ensheathed by normal myelin, the distal part by a thin sheath (× 3100). *b,* 13 days after freezing. Longitudinal section. Example of collateral sprouting at a node, in the distal part of the frozen area (× 9000). *c,* 11½ days after freezing. Transverse section. This *faisceau de régénération* contained 12 axons, only 3 of which were myelinated. In one fiber, several nonmyelinated axons were seen in the same Schwann cell. Note that the whole cluster was surrounded by a common basal lamina. In addition, each fiber had its own basal lamina formed partly by the old one and partly by the new one. Note also the presence of fine longitudinal collagen fibrils (*arrows*) in the extracellular spaces between the two basal laminae (× 20,000). D = distal part of nerve fiber; EC = endoneurial collagen; NBL = new basal lamina; NR = node of Ranvier; OBL = old basal lamina; P = proximal part of nerve fiber; Sp = axonal sprout. (From Mira, J.-C.: Clin Plast. Surg., *11*:20, 1984.)

The literature contains numerous studies of the peripheral nerves of humans and various animals. However, since such studies have not been performed on the same nerves and since various histologic techniques have been used, the results are not always comparable and may even be conflicting. For instance, although the number and size of myelinated fibers generally appear to be restored after crushing, the data are highly variable and even contradictory after nerve section.[22] Thus, it is obvious that the type of nerve, the level at which injury and sampling are performed, and the histologic technique used are of primary importance and may, at least partially, explain the conflicting published results.

However, the standardization of all stages (material used, operation, samplings performed, histology, photography, and measurements) in the current methods should enable data to be obtained for an acceptable comparison of certain parameters, particularly the total diameter (axon + myelin), which is often used to identify different populations of myelinated fibers.[39]

I have attempted to achieve this in my studies. Animals were always albino rats, about 6 weeks old and weighing from 160 to 180 gm at the time of operation. Injury (section, crushing, single or repeated localized freezings) was always performed at roughly the same site on the left sciatic nerve shortly after its entry into the sciatic fossa. Samplings and controls were performed at standardized levels using the nerve to the medial head of the left and right gastrocnemius muscles; this small nerve branches off from the tibial nerve 30 to 40 mm below the point where the injury is produced in the sciatic nerve. After fixation with glutaraldehyde, post-fixation with osmium tetroxide, and embedding in an epoxy resin (Araldite), 30 to 40 serial semi-thin transverse sections of the same nerve were stained with toluidine blue. Only perfect sections of each nerve were selected and photographed. Myelinated fiber counts and measurements were made on the two to three best photographic prints at a final magnification of ×1000. Under an oil-immersion objective, each fiber was simultaneously identified in the corresponding and adjacent transverse sections, with special attention being paid to the finest fibers. The total diameter of each fiber was measured over the contour of its myelin sheath, using a series of graduated circles printed on rhodoid. These measurements allowed the study of fiber size distribution for each nerve. The mean diameter of all the myelinated fibers was also calculated.

Unoperated Animals[21, 27]

Number of Fibers. Myelinated fibers were systematically counted at standardized levels in the nerve to the medial head of the left and right gastrocnemius muscles (LGM and RGM nerves). Twenty-four rats were used, 11 males weighing between 150 and 450 gm, and 13 females weighing between 110 and 480 gm.

When neither the weight nor sex of the rats was taken into account, RGM nerve was found to contain an average of 271 ± 5 myelinated fibers and LGM nerve, 272 ± 4 myelinated fibers. Slight variations were recorded when weight and sex were considered. However, for a given animal, differences between the two nerves were not significant and thus could be disregarded.

Fiber Size Distribution. In both LGM and RGM nerves of unoperated rats, the size distribution of myelinated fibers was always bimodal, since two different fiber populations were constantly detected and characterized by their respective peaks (i.e., maximal concentration). The peak of the small fibers was usually located at 2 to 4 μm and that of the large ones at 10 to 12 μm. The finest fibers had a diameter of 2 μm, and the thickest seldom exceeded 14 to 15 μm. The lower limit of the large fiber population clearly overlapped the upper limit of the small fibers; the intersection was probably not located where the fiber concentration was lowest (generally between 6 and 8 μm). The exact site of this intersection has not been determined. However, since all the numerical data varied only slightly, both from one animal to another and within the symmetrical nerves of the same rat, the mean diameter of all the myelinated fibers has been used to distinguish between the two populations in a given nerve. Like many other authors, I have arbitrarily classified as large fibers all those whose diameter equals or exceeds this mean value. According to this criterion, the average number of myelinated fibers in each population for most of the rats studied was noticeably similar for both nerves (40% for small and 60% for large fibers), and, with very few exceptions, histograms for RGM and LGM nerves of the same animal were superimposable.

Mean Diameter. The mean diameter of all the myelinated fibers in RGM nerve was 8.1 ± 0.1 μm and in LGM nerve, 8.0 ± 0.1 μm. Here again, there were certain variations according to weight and sex, but for a given animal these were minor and could be disregarded.

Single Localized Freezing[19, 23, 28]

Measurements were made in the RGM and LGM nerves of 45 rats between 10 and 720 days after freezing their left sciatic nerve.

Number of Fibers. The first myelinated fibers appeared between 12 and 15 days, and their number subsequently increased progressively, exceeding that of the opposite side at the end of the first month. From this time onward, all the regenerating nerves contained a larger number of fibers than the contralateral nerves used as a control; there was virtually no increase in number, and variations remained within relatively narrow limits (from 121 to 131%), with a general mean slightly above 124 ± 7%. This value was still found 2 years after the cold injury (Fig. 4–3).

Fiber Size Distribution. Fiber diameter regularly increased, and restoration was apparently complete at the beginning of the second postoperative year (Fig. 4–3). The first large fibers appeared at the end of the first month, and their number became almost normal at about 18 months.

At the beginning of the second month, bimodal distribution was detectable in all the regenerating nerves and was obvious from 75 days onward (Fig. 4–4b). However, it was necessary to wait until the end of the first year before the regenerated nerve histogram became superimposable with that of the contralateral nerve (Fig. 4–4d).

Repeated Localized Freezings[24, 25, 28, 30]

To determine the optimal period between two successive cold injuries, a single localized freezing was performed on the sciatic nerve of eight rats. Using Bielschowsky-Gros silver impregnation, the first regenerating nerve endings were detected in the middle part of the gastrocnemius and soleus muscles 11 to 12 days after freezing. Consequently, it was decided to freeze at intervals of 3 weeks, so that muscle reinnervation occurred before the nerve was once again damaged.

Repeated localized freezings were performed using the same experimental procedure as for single freezing, but were done in two different ways:

1. In a first series (group I), the left sciatic nerve of 12 rats was frozen 2 to 5 times at 23- to 25-day intervals. For each animal, results were investigated in the RGM and LGM nerves about 1 month after the final freezing.

2. In a second series (group II), based upon the results of the first group, the left sciatic nerve of 15 rats underwent three successive localized freezings and results were recorded from 1 to 18 months later.

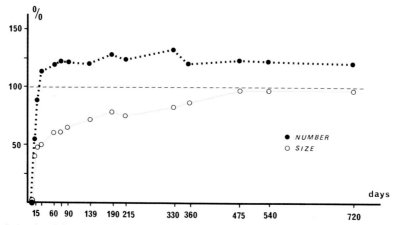

Figure 4–3. Single localized freezing. Mean values are of the number and size of regenerated myelinated fibers, as a function of the contralateral nerve values and the time elapsing since injury. (From Mira, J.-C.: Clin. Plast. Surg., 11:21, 1984.)

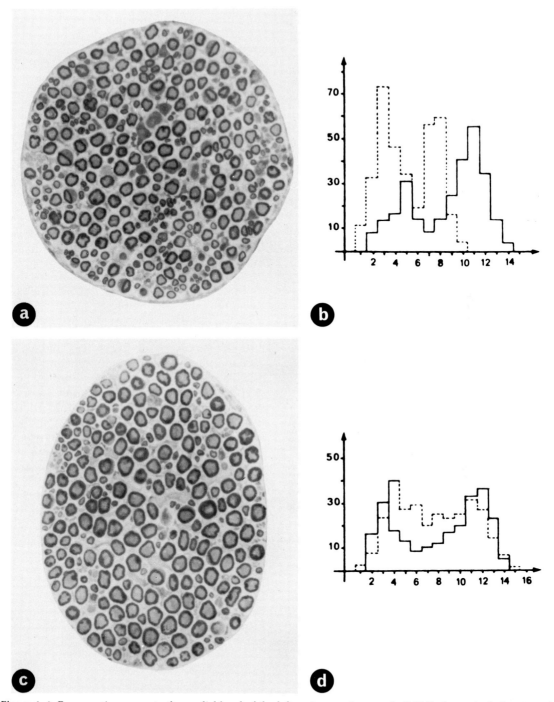

Figure 4–4. Regenerating nerve to the medial head of the left gastrocnemius muscle (LGM) after a single freezing of the left sciatic nerve. The contralateral nerve (RGM) was used as a control. *a,* 75 postoperative days. Semi-thin transverse section of the LGM nerve stained with toluidine blue. There were 283 myelinated fibers in RGM and 357 (i.e., 126.2%) in LGM. Mean diameters were 8.8 and 5.3 μm, respectively (i.e., 60.2%) (× 400). *b,* Histogram of the same nerve (*solid lines* = RGM nerve; *dotted lines* = LGM nerve). The number of myelinated fibers is plotted on the ordinate and their size (in μm) on the abscissa. *c,* 376 postoperative days. Semi-thin transverse section of the LGM nerve stained with toluidine blue. There were 245 myelinated fibers in RGM and 304 (i.e., 124.1%) in LGM. Mean diameters were 8.5 and 7.7 μm, respectively (i.e., 90.6%) (× 400). *d,* Histogram of the same nerve. (From Mira, J.-C.: Clin. Plast. Surg., *11:*22, 1984.)

Group I (Fig. 4–5)

Number of Fibers. One month after a single localized freezing, the number of regenerating and myelinated fibers reached a mean value of 117% (see Fig. 4–3), i.e., the regenerating LGM nerve contained 17% more myelinated fibers than the contralateral RGM nerve used as a control.

About 1 month after the last of the repeated localized freezings, all the regenerating nerves contained a larger number of myelinated fibers than did control nerves. An average of 154% fibers was found 28 days after the second freezing, 212% 30 days after the third freezing, and about 218% 28 days and 34 days after the fourth and fifth freezings, respectively (Fig. 4–6). The number of myelinated fibers in the LGM nerve gradually increased after the first three freezings of the sciatic nerve, but the two final injuries did not seem to bring about noticeable changes, since the fiber number remained close to 220% of the control value determined in the contralateral RGM nerve.

Fiber Size Distribution. In the RGM and LGM nerves of unoperated rats, size distribution of myelinated fibers was always bimodal and averaged 40% for small and 60% for large fibers. In the uninjured RGM nerve of the operated rats, fiber size distribution was again always bimodal and averaged 37.5% for small and 62.5% for large fibers. In all the regenerating LGM nerves, myelinated fibers were very small, and their size distribution was always unimodal 1 month after the last freezing of the left sciatic nerve. Only one fiber population was found in which the diameter of most fibers ranged from 2 to 5 μm; there were no large fibers (see Fig. 4–5b to d).

Mean Diameter. In the RGM nerve of the unoperated rats, the mean diameter for all the myelinated fibers was 8.1 μm. One month after a single localized freezing, regenerating myelinated fibers had already grown to half their normal size. One month after the last of the repeated cold injuries, a gradual reduction in fiber size was recorded, i.e., to 50%, 46%, 41%, 37%, and 36% after one, two, three, four, and five freezings, respectively (Fig. 4–6). There were no large fibers.

Group II (Fig. 4–7)

Number of Fibers. One month after the third localized freezing, the number of regenerating and myelinated fibers reached 212% of the control value (Fig. 4–6). At the beginning of the second month after a third and final cold injury, myelinated fibers decreased in number by about 30% and from then on no further variations occurred, with their number remaining close to 190% of the contralateral value (Fig. 4–8).

Fiber Size Distribution. In the uninjured RGM nerve of operated rats, the size distribution of myelinated fibers was always bimodal and averaged 39% for small and 61% for large fibers. In the regenerating LGM nerves, the fiber size distribution and number of large fibers varied as the time interval increased following the third and final localized freezing of the left sciatic nerve. One month later, the size distribution was unimodal with a single peak at 3 μm; there were no large fibers. From the third month onward, the fiber size became bimodal and the large fibers appeared. However, even at the eighteenth month, which was the longest period of regeneration allowed in these experiments, peaks did not have the same location on both sides (4 and 14 μm in the RGM nerve, 3 to 5 and 12 to 13 μm in the LGM nerve), although size distribution was comparable in the two nerves. In addition, histograms of RGM and LGM nerves were not superimposable.

Figure 4–5. Regenerating nerve to the medial head of the left gastrocnemius muscle (LGM) after repeated freezings of the left sciatic nerve. The contralateral nerve (RGM) was used as a control. *a,* 31 days after three freezings. Semi-thin transverse section of the LGM nerve stained with toluidine blue. There were 262 myelinated fibers in RGM and 517 (i.e., 197.3%) in LGM. Mean diameters were 8.3 and 3.2 μm, respectively (i.e., 38.6%) (× 400). *b,* Histogram of the same nerve (*solid lines* = RGM nerve; *dotted lines* = LGM nerve). The number of myelinated fibers is plotted on the ordinate and their size (in μm) in the abscissa. *c,* 28 days after four freezings. Semi-thin transverse section of the LGM nerve stained with toluidine blue. There were 262 myelinated fibers in RGM and 543 (i.e., 207.3%) in LGM. Mean diameters were 9.5 and 3.1 μm, respectively (i.e., 32.6%) (× 400). *d,* Histogram of the same nerve. (From Mira, J.-C.: Clin. Plast. Surg., *11*:24, 1984.)

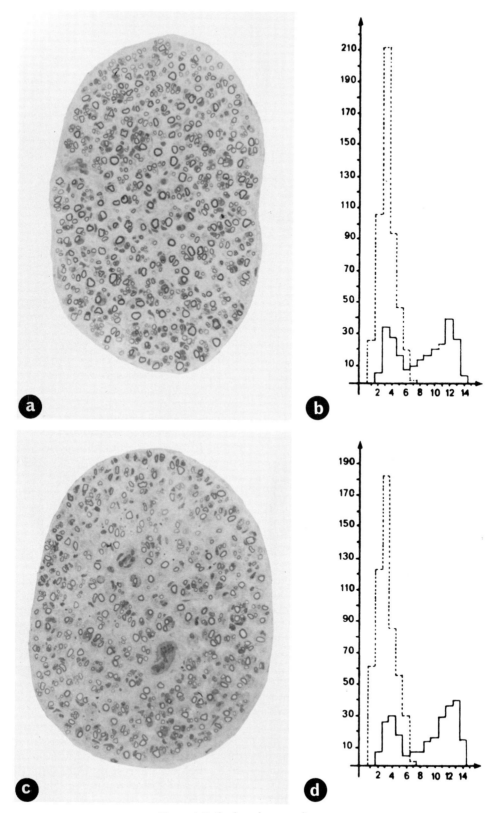

Figure 4–5. *See legend on opposite page.*

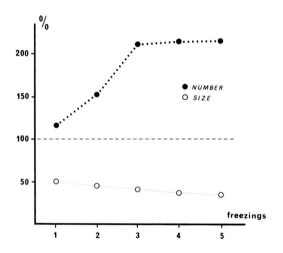

Figure 4–6. Repeated localized freezings. Shown are mean values of the number and size of regenerating myelinated fibers, as a function of the contralateral nerve values and the number of injuries. (From Mira, J.-C.: Clin. Plast. Surg., *11*:23, 1984.)

Mean Diameter. A regular increase in fiber size was observed in the LGM nerve between the first and eighteenth month after the third and final freezing of the left sciatic nerve. The mean diameter increased from 41% after 1 month to 52% after 3 months, 62% after 6 months, 67% after 12 months, and 70% after 18 months (Fig. 4–8). In the final stage of the study, the mean diameter of all the myelinated fibers remained very much below the control value.

CONCLUSIONS

Conclusions concerning the ultrastructural and quantitative aspects of peripheral nerve regeneration after localized freezing(s) of the rat sciatic nerve may be summarized as follows:

1. The maintenance of the continuity of connective tissue sheaths, particularly of basal lamina, is of fundamental importance in regeneration, since these tubes ensure that axonal sprouts are guided toward the periphery without encountering any obstruction. Consequently, regenerating axons are directed to the end-organs with which the normal fibers were initially connected. In this respect, the localized freezing procedure provides very favorable conditions for peripheral nerve regeneration and its experimental study.

2. The evolution of the Schwann cell basal laminae, as observed in time and space on semi-serial ultrathin sections, indicates that each *faisceau de régénération* is a morphologic entity consisting of all the axonal sprouts belonging to a given fiber and temporarily confined within a common basal lamina; this latter is the old or initial tube that in the intact nerve covered the parent myelinated fiber that gave rise to these sprouts.

3. The formation and evolution of the *faisceaux de régénération* explain the increase in the number of myelinated fibers in regenerating peripheral nerves.

4. After a single localized freezing, anatomic recovery is more complete and more constant than after any type of experimental nerve injury.

5. After repeated localized freezings, results may be divided into two different categories: (a) when measurements are made 1 month after the last of two to five injuries, the number of myelinated fibers increases considerably after the first three operations, reaching about 220% of the control value, but shows little variation after four or five freezings, and (b) when measurements are made between 1 and 18 months after a third and final cold injury, about 220% of the myelinated fibers are found in the regenerating nerves at the end of the first month; only 190% are recorded thereafter.

These observations show that repetition of an experimental nerve injury induces a large and lasting increase in the number of myelinated fibers, but with an accompanying reduction in their size. These findings may also be of medical interest by indicating possible uses for facilitating reinnervation of muscles that have been partially or totally deprived of their motor supply.

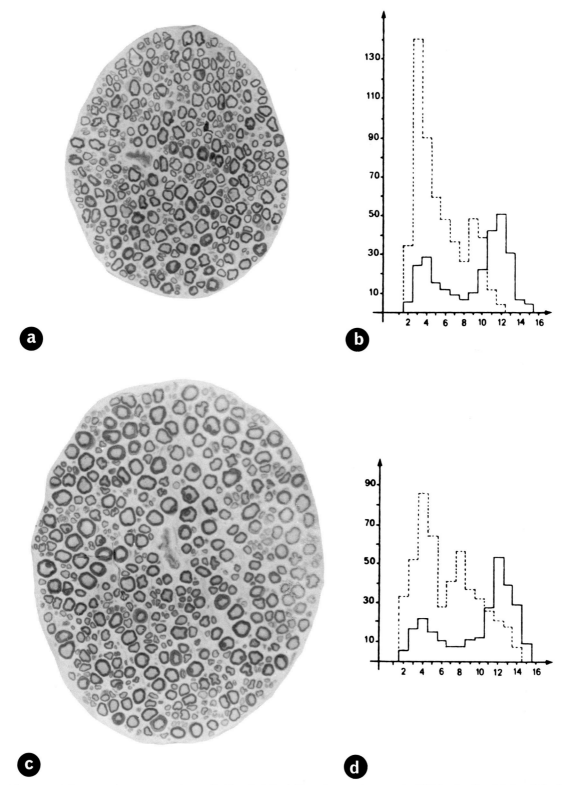

Figure 4–7. Regenerating nerve to the medial head of the left gastrocnemius muscle (LGM) after the third and final freezing of the left sciatic nerve. The contralateral nerve (RGM) was used as a control. *a,* 6 postoperative months. Semi-thin transverse section of the LGM nerve stained with toluidine blue. There were 267 myelinated fibers in RGM and 536 (i.e., 200.8%) in LGM. Mean diameters were 9.0 and 5.4 μm, respectively (i.e., 60.0%) (× 340). *b,* Histogram of the same nerve (*solid lines* = RGM nerve; *dotted lines* = LGM nerve). The number of myelinated fibers is plotted in the ordinate and their size (in μm) in the abscissa. *c,* 12 postoperative months. Semi-thin transverse section of the LGM nerve stained with toluidine blue. There were 266 myelinated fibers in RGM and 501 (i.e., 188.4%) in LGM. Mean diameters were 9.8 and 6.6 μm, respectively (i.e., 67.4%) (× 340). *d,* Histogram of the same nerve.

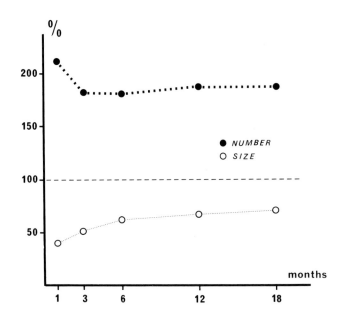

Figure 4–8. Repeated localized freezings. Shown are values of the number and size of regenerated myelinated fibers, as a function of the contralateral nerve values and the time elapsing since the third and final cold injury.

References

1. Abercrombie, M., and Santler, J. E.: An analysis of growth in nuclear population during Wallerian degeneration. J. Cell Comp. Physiol., *50:*429, 1957.
2. Basbum, C. B.: Induced hypothermia in peripheral nerve: electron microscopical and electrophysiological observations. J. Neurocytol., *2:*171, 1973.
3. Ducker, T. B., Kempe, L. G., and Hayes, G. J.: The metabolic background for peripheral nerve surgery. J. Neurosurg., *30:*270, 1969.
4. Duncan, D., and Jarvis, W. H.: Observations on repeated regeneration of facial nerve in cats. J. Comp. Neurol., *79:*315, 1943.
5. Falin, L. I.: Regeneration of nerve fibers after repeated injuries of the nerve trunk (in Russian). Voprosy Nejrokhirurgii, *25:*5, 1961.
6. Forman, D. S., McQuarrie, I. G., Labore, F. W., Wood, D. K., Stone, L. S., Braddock, C. H., and Fuchs, D. A.: Time course of the conditioning lesion effect on axonal regeneration. Brain Res., *156:*213, 1980.
7. Gutmann, E.: Factors affecting recovery of motor function after nerve lesions. J. Neurol. Neurosurg. Psychiatry, *5:*81, 1942.
8. Gutmann, E.: Effect of delay of innervation on recovery of muscle after nerve lesions. J. Neurophysiol., *11:*279, 1948.
9. Gutmann, E., and Holubar, J.: Atrophy of fibres in the central stump following nerve section and the possibilities of its prevention. Arch. Intern. Stud. Neurol., *1:*314, 1951.
10. Holmes, W., and Young, J. Z.: Nerve regeneration after immediate and delayed sutures. J. Anat. (Lond.), *77:*63, 1942.
11. Legrain, Y.: Méthode de comparaison de la vitesse de régénération des fibres du nerf sciatique de rat. J. Physiol. (Paris), *73:*13, 1977.
12. McQuarrie, I. G.: The effect of a conditioning lesion on the regeneration of motor axons. Brain Res., *152:*597, 1978.
13. McQuarrie, I. G.: Accelerated axonal sprouting after nerve transection. Brain Res., *167:*185, 1979.
14. McQuarrie, I. G., Grafstein, B., Dreyfus, C. F., and Gershon, M. D.: Regeneration of adrenergic axons in rat sciatic nerve: effect of a conditioning lesion. Brain Res., *141:*21, 1978.
15. McQuarrie, I. G., Grafstein, B., and Gershon, M. D.: Axonal regeneration in the rat sciatic nerve: effect of a conditioning lesion and dbc-AMP. Brain Res., *132:*443, 1977.
16. Mayer, S.: Über Vorgänge der Degeneration und Regeneration in unversehrten peripherischen Nervensystem. Eine biologische Studie. Z. Heilkunde, *2:*154, 1881.
17. Mira, J. C.: Maintien de la continuité de la lame basale des fibres nerveuses myélinisées après une congélation localisée. C.R. Acad. Sci. Paris, Série D, *273:*1836, 1971.
18. Mira, J. C.: Effets d'une congélation localisée sur la structure des fibres myélinisées et leur régénération. J. Micr. (Paris), *14:*155, 1972.
19. Mira, J. C.: Variations du nombre et du calibre des fibres nerveuses myélinisées après une "section" des axones par congélation localisée. C.R. Acad. Sci. Paris, Série D, *275:*979, 1972.
20. Mira, J. C.: Observations histophysiologiques sur la dégénérescence et la régénération des fibres nerveuses périphériques à la suite d'une congélation localisée. In Guiraud, B., and Mansat, M. (eds.): Pathologie du Nerf Périphérique. Paris, Editions Médicales Pierre Fabre, 1976, pp. 9–23.
21. Mira, J.C.: Etudes quantitatives sur la régénération des fibres nerveuses myélinisées. I. Variations du nombre et du calibre des fibres myélinisées dans les nerfs de rats normaux. Arch. Anat. Micr. Morphol. Exp., *65:*209, 1976.
22. Mira, J. C.: Etudes quantitatives sur la régénération des fibres nerveuses myélinisées. II. Variations du nombre et du calibre des fibres régénérées après un écrasement localisé ou une section totale. Arch. Anat. Micr. Morphol. Exp., *65:*255, 1976.
23. Mira, J. C.: Etudes quantitatives sur la régénération des fibres nerveuses myélinisées. III. Variations du nombre et du calibre des fibres régénérées après une congélation localisée. Arch. Anat. Micr. Morphol. Exp., *66:*1, 1977.

24. Mira, J. C.: Variations du nombre et du calibre des fibres nerveuses myélinisées régénérées après des congélations localisées itératives du nerf sciatique de rat. C.R. Acad. Sci. Paris, série D, *284*:2357, 1977.

25. Mira, J. C.: Quantitative studies of the regeneration of rat myelinated fibres: variations in the number and size of regenerating nerve fibres after repeated localized freezings. J. Anat. (Lond.), *129*:77, 1979.

26. Mira, J. C.: Contribution à l'Etude de la Régénération du Nerf Périphérique et des Changements du Muscle Squelettique Strié au cours de sa Réinnervation. Thèse de Doctorat d'Etat, Paris, Université Pierre et Marie Curie, 1980.

27. Mira, J. C.: The normal peripheral nerve. Intern. J. Microsurg., *3*:77, 1981.

28. Mira, J. C.: Degeneration and regeneration of peripheral nerves: ultrastructural and electrophysiological observations, quantitative aspects and muscle changes during reinnervation. Intern. J. Microsurg., *3*:102, 1981.

29. Mira, J. C., and Bondoux-Jahan, M.: Unpublished observations, 1979.

30. Mira, J. C., and Fardeau, M.: Nerve and muscle changes induced by repeated localized freezings of the sciatic nerve in the rat. In Canal, N., and Pozza, G. (eds.): Peripheral Neuropathies. Amsterdam, Elsevier, 1978, pp. 83–90.

31. Mira, J. C., and Pécot-Dechavassine, M.: Effets d'une congélation localisée d'un nerf périphérique sur la conduction de l'influx nerveux, au cours de la dégénérescence et de la régénération. Pflüger's Archiv, *330*:5, 1971.

32. Nageotte, J.: L'Organisation de la Matière Vivante dans ses Rapports avec la Vie. Etudes d'Anatomie Générale et de Morphologie Expérimentale sur le Tissu Conjonctif et le Nerf. Paris, Librairie Alcan, 1922.

33. Sabaino, D., and Solerio, L.: Sul comportamento numerico delle fibre rigenerate in tronchi nervosi sottoposti a ripetute neurotomie. Richerche sperimentali. Arch. Sci. Med., *93*:463, 1952.

34. Schröder, J.M.: Die Hyperneurotisation Büngnerscher Bänder bei der experimentelle Izoniazid-Neuropathie: Phasenkontrast- und electronenmikroskopische Untersuchungen. Virchou's Archiv, Abt. B, Zellpathol., *1*:131, 1968.

35. Sebille, A.: Personal communication, 1981.

36. Sebille, A., and Bondoux-Jahan, M.: Effects of electric stimulation and previous nerve injury on motor function recovery in rats. Brain Res., *193*: 562, 1980.

37. Thomas, P. K.: The effects of repeated regenerative activity on the structure of peripheral nerve. In Research in Muscular Dystrophy. London, Pitman, 1968, pp. 413–419.

38. Thomas, P. K.: The cellular response to nerve injury. 3. The effects of repeated crush injuries. J. Anat. (Lond.), *106*:463, 1970.

39. Tomé, F. M. S., and Mira, J.C.: Contribution of the morphological techniques to the study of peripheral nerve lesions in man and experimental animals. Intern. J. Microsurg., *3*:152, 1981.

40. Vanlair, C.: Sur la persistence de l'aptitude régénérative des nerfs. Bull. Acad. Roy. Sci. Belges, *16*:93, 1888.

41. Whittaker, D. K.: Degeneration and regeneration of nerves following cryosurgery. Br. J. Exp. Pathol., *55*:595, 1974.

5

Effects of Repeated Denervation on Muscle Reinnervation

■

Jean-Claude Mira, D.Sc.

Although numerous studies have been devoted to peripheral nerve regeneration, muscle changes during reinnervation, and the properties of reinnervation itself, no attempts have yet been made to collect and correlate these observations. For this reason, and in collaboration with Michel Fardeau and Monique Pécot-Dechavassine, I have tried to correlate changes in histologic and histochemical characteristics of muscle fibers, electrophysiologic events that occur at the motor end-plates during reinnervation, and morphologic and quantitative aspects of myelinated nerve fiber regeneration.

Refined techniques now available allow the follow-up of modifications in extrafusal muscle fibers after injury to their innervation. Thus, it is possible to study the arrangement and structure of the motor nerve endings in experimental muscles and in human histopathologic biopsy specimens.[6, 13] In the same materials, cytochemical techniques can be used to individualize different types of muscle fibers, e.g., an examination of myofibrillar adenosine triphosphatase (ATPase) activity reveals the presence of three principal fiber types in adult muscles.[2] Moreover, experiments using cross-innervation have shown that the muscle fiber type depends on its innervation[23] or on the rhythm of nerve stimulation.[40, 41] Finally, muscle fibers that are dependent on the same motor unit are known to have similar cytochemical characteristics[5, 12] and to retain their native

myosin-ATPase activity during the atrophy that follows denervation.[19] Consequently, by study of the cytochemical properties of muscle fibers, eventual topographic modifications of the different motor units may be followed at the periphery.

Thus, after a nerve injury that disrupts the continuity of all the axons, muscle fibers exhibit an evident atrophy that, as will be described, is independent of the nature and degree of the nerve lesion and is related solely to the cytochemical fiber type. However, during this period, there are no changes in the topographic distribution of muscle fiber types. When the first regenerated axons reach the muscle, reinnervation of the old motor end-plates (among other effects) induces an interruption in the atrophy process and a rather rapid return of muscle fibers to their initial volume. Moreover, reinnervation of some contiguous muscle fibers by collateral sprouts from the first regenerated axons induces topographic redistribution of the different muscle fiber types. Instead of distribution at random in a "mosaic" pattern, formation of small clusters consisting of contiguous fibers of the same cytochemical type is observed. Occasionally, clusters are even made up of a type unusual for the muscle being considered, such as type IIB in the rat soleus muscle.[3, 29, 30] This is a further demonstration of the subordination of the muscle fiber type to its innervation.

These data have been known for several

years[22, 24, 36] and, for the mammalian muscles studied, involve several corollaries that are explicit or implicit, depending on the different investigators: (1) the nerve fiber that reinnervates an end-plate is, and remains, single, (2) this reinnervation is stable, and (3) it induces the reversibility of structural changes created in muscle fibers by denervation.

To test these assumptions, I, along with Michel Fardeau and Monique Pécot-Dechavassine, have undertaken a study of muscle changes observed at different time intervals after a nerve injury, as well as a comparison of the effects of single and repeated injuries; controls have been performed at standardized levels in the gastrocnemius and soleus muscles. Nerve regeneration had previously been studied and quantified in the nerve to the medial head of the gastrocnemius muscle. Different aspects of our work have already been published elsewhere.[15, 27, 28, 30–35, 37]

TECHNIQUES

In our experimental studies, we used histochemical and histologic techniques to plot the time-course of the muscle changes over a long period, starting from the beginning of reinnervation. Parallel to this, we used electrophysiologic techniques to study the properties of the reinnervated synapses. These investigations were carried out principally on the medial head of the rat gastrocnemius muscle, which was dissected out after single or repeated localized freezings of the sciatic nerve.

Nerve Injury

One or several successive localized freezings were performed in situ on the left sciatic nerve of albino rats, according to the procedure described in Chapter 4.

The technique of localized freezing was chosen for investigating cytochemical and electrophysiologic changes in the skeletal muscles of the adult rat during reinnervation because all its results are perfectly reproducible. This method also has the advantage of focally destroying all the axons, while maintaining the anatomic continuity of the nerve trunk and preserving the basal laminae.[25, 27, 30]

Results following a single cold injury were recorded between 15 and 360 days after in-

jury. Repeated freezings were done in two different ways: in group I, the sciatic nerve was frozen 2 to 5 times and the results were recorded 1 month after the last injury; in group II, the test period lasted for several months after the third and final freezing.

Morphologic Techniques

In the gastrocnemius and soleus muscles of the operated rats, the changes induced by one or several successive localized freezings of the left sciatic nerve were determined by comparison with the contralateral muscle. These morphologic studies were conducted in cooperation with Michel Fardeau.[15, 29–33]

Muscle changes were investigated on cryostat serial transverse sections, using different histologic and histochemical techniques, depending on the information sought:

1. Observation of terminal motor innervation of muscle fibers by silver impregnation, according to the technique proposed by Bielschowsky and modified by Gros-Schultze.

2. Identification of muscle fiber types by their myosin-ATPase activity at three different pH values, according to the classification proposed by Brooke and Kaiser[2] and Fardeau.[14] Thus, at pH 9.4, rat fibers could be classified into two groups: the most numerous fibers were type II (dark), the least numerous, type I (light). After pre-incubation at pH 4.53, type I fibers became dark, whereas type II fibers divided into types IIA (slightly stained) and IIB (intermediate tint). After pre-incubation at pH 4.35, type I fibers were black and type IIA and most of type IIB fibers were colorless. Among type II fibers, however, some of them (type IIC) retained slight staining; they were absent from the normal muscle of adult rat, with the exception of the soleus muscle.

Electrophysiologic Techniques

The process of recovery was also studied electrophysiologically in the medial head of the gastrocnemius muscle. These studies were performed in cooperation with Monique Pécot-Dechavassine.[34, 35, 37] At varying times after sciatic nerve freezing, the nerve muscle preparation (sciatic nerve, nerve to the medial head of the gastrocnemius muscle, and gastrocnemius muscle itself) was rapidly removed from each anesthetized animal.

The preparation was then transferred to a recording chamber with two compartments—the first for the nerve, which was placed on two platinum electrodes in Vaseline oil at about 30 mm from the point of nerve entry into the muscle, and the second for pinning the muscle to a transparent rhodorsil base and bathing it in oxygenated physiologic liquid (Liley's solution) permanently perfused through the chamber. D-Tubocurarine ($1–3.10^{-7}M$) was added to the bathing solution when the end-plate potentials (EPPs) reached overthreshold and were able to induce muscle contraction.

Only the superficial fibers of the inner side of the gastrocnemius muscle were impaled; moreover, for the following reasons exploration was restricted to the "white" area of the muscle and to some fibers of the "red" area close to the limit between the two zones:

1. In the reinnervated muscle, the white zone has been observed to contain mainly acid-resistant ATPase fibers, which are distinguishable on serial sections as type I and especially type IIC fibers,[29, 30, 32, 33] whereas the latter fibers are virtually absent from the normal adult muscle.

2. The slight thickness of the muscle at this level and the almost complete absence of connective tissue allow easier identification of the reinnervated zones and the use of glass microelectrodes, without breaking them and without injury to muscle fibers.

The red area was excluded from our present investigations because of its excessively great thickness and the presence of highly developed aponeurosis. In order to explore the superficial fibers of the white portion, the nerve was placed on the red portion; moreover, the light microscopic examination of the extended muscle was used to identify the zones of motor innervation.

The nerve was stimulated by pulses of 0.1 msec duration at 0.5 Hz. Since the regenerating axons were less excitable and required higher currents, stimulation was gradually intensified so as to "mobilize" an increasing number of nerve endings. Evoked EPPs were recorded intracellularly by impaling muscle fibers with conventional glass microelectrodes filled with potassium chloride (3 M) and having a resistance ranging from 10 to 20 MΩ.

NORMAL MUSCLES OF THE ADULT RAT

Gastrocnemius Muscle

Macroscopically, two well-defined zones were consistently visualized in the transverse sections of the medial head of the adult rat gastrocnemius muscle (Fig. 5–1a): a crescent-shaped "white" area surrounding most of a "red" area in contact with an aponeurosis. At the junction of the two zones, a pedicle composed of vessels and nerves was often present.

In cryostat serial transverse sections, the study of myosin-ATPase activity was used to individualize three principal types of muscle fibers (types I, IIA, and IIB):

1. Type I fibers, slightly stained at pH 9.4, were considered as acid-resistant fibers, since they became black after pre-incubation at pH 4.53 and 4.35.

Type IIA fibers, markedly stained at pH 9.4, were considered as acid-sensitive fibers, since their ATPase activity was completely inhibited after pre-incubation at pH 4.53 and 4.35.

3. Type IIB fibers were as dark as type IIA fibers at pH 9.4; however, if their ATPase activity was also completely inhibited after pre-incubation at pH 4.35, they were still stained after pre-incubation at pH 4.53.

These various fiber types were not equally distributed throughout the muscle transverse sections, and the cytochemical preparations had a "mosaic" appearance with three tints. The red zone contained all the type I fibers, isolated from each other and randomly distributed among mostly type IIB fibers. The white zone contained only randomly distributed type IIA and IIB fibers.

Soleus Muscle

Macroscopically, the adult rat soleus muscle appeared "red" and homogeneous on cryostat transverse sections (Fig. 5–1b). The study of myosin-ATPase activities revealed that the preparations contained three types of muscle fibers (types I, IIA, and IIC):

1. Type I and IIA fibers displayed the same characteristics as those of the gastrocnemius muscle.

2. Type IIC fibers were peculiar to the

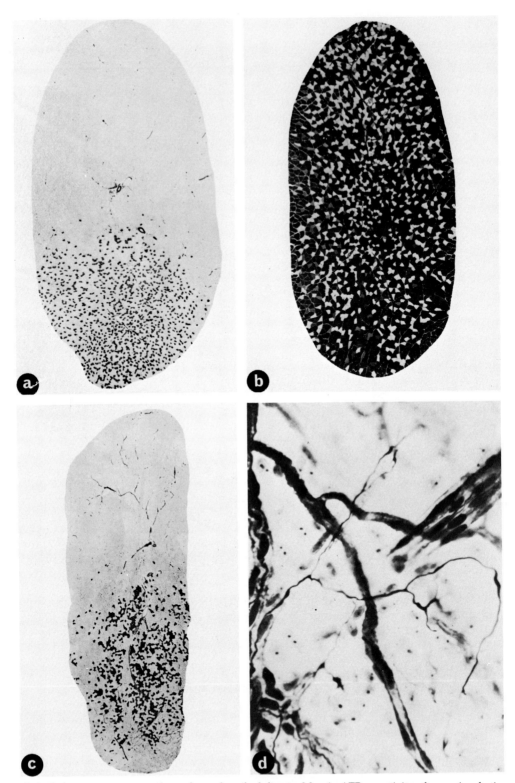

Figure 5–1. Cryostat transverse sections of muscles of adult rats. Myosin-ATPase activity after preincubation at pH 4.35 (*a*, *b*, *c*) and motor terminal innervation after silver impregnation (*d*). *a*, Normal rat; medial head of the left gastrocnemius muscle (× 10.3). *b*, Normal rat; right soleus muscle (× 23.2). *c*, 360 days after a single localized freezing of the left sciatic nerve. Left gastrocnemius muscle. There was limited type-grouping of fibers of the same histochemical type (× 10). *d*, 20 days after a single freezing of the sciatic nerve. Gastrocnemius muscle. A single axon innervated several contiguous muscle fibers (preterminal sprouting) (× 480). (From Mira, J.-C.: Clin. Plast. Surg., *11*:33, 1984.)

soleus muscle of the adult rat. They were markedly stained at pH 9.4, similar to acid-sensitive ATPase or type II fibers. However, they became partly negative after pre-incubation at pH 4.53 and 4.35, almost like acid-resistant ATPase or type I fibers. Because of these special characteristics, type IIC fibers were called "superfibers" by Brooke.[2]

Depending on the individual animals, there were great variations in the numerical proportions of type I and II(A and C) fibers. In some rats, one of the two soleus muscles was homogeneous for type I. However, in most animals, although type I fibers were always much more numerous than type II fibers, the latter were almost equally divided between types IIA and IIC.

Motor Innervation

The general scheme of the motor end-plate structure and innervation has become classic since the studies of René Couteaux.[7-9] Silver impregnation using the Bielschowsky-Gros technique showed that nerve endings were single. Each motor axon, when it came into close contact with the muscle fiber, divided into two or three fine terminal branches. This terminal branching was surrounded by a crown of vesicular muscle nuclei with several prominent nucleoli.

Electrophysiologic Recordings at End-Plates

In the normal gastrocnemius muscle of adult rat, all the recorded EPPs had a single peak and muscle fibers exhibited superimposed and similarly delayed EPPS, whatever the intensity of stimulation (see Fig. 5–3d). This clearly indicates that each muscle fiber is innervated by a single motor axon.

CHANGES INDUCED BY A SINGLE NERVE INJURY

In the gastrocnemius and soleus muscles of the operated rats, changes induced by a single localized freezing of the left sciatic nerve were determined by comparison with the contralateral muscle. Only changes in extrafusal muscle fibers were taken into account.

In order to include all results, three param-

eters must always be considered: the type of nerve injury (localized freezing, crush, or section), the muscle studied (gastrocnemius or soleus), and the time elapsed between nerve injury and muscle examination. However, the present study presents only the effects of a single localized freezing of the sciatic nerve in the gastrocnemius muscle, with results recorded 15 to 360 days later (for results of investigations in gastrocnemius and soleus muscles after crush and section injuries, see references 29 and 30).

Atrophy

By the fifteenth postoperative day, atrophy was evident as a decrease in the total weight of the gatrocnemius and soleus muscles and a reduction in the cross-sectional area of the muscle fibers. Atrophy of denervated muscle may have been due to both the disuse caused by muscle paralysis and the loss of special neurotrophic substances normally secreted by intact motoneurons.[10, 11, 39, 44]

Atrophy was independent of the nature and degree of the nerve injury; it was solely related to the cytochemical fiber type and, for a given fiber type, to the specific muscle studied. Thus, in the gastrocnemius muscle of the rat, type I fibers atrophied more slowly than type IIA and IIB fibers, whereas in the soleus muscle, type I fibers atrophied faster than type IIA and IIC fibers.

Topographic Distribution

In the gastrocnemius muscle, the topographic distribution of the different fiber types did not appear to be significantly modified 15 and 31 days after the sciatic nerve freezing. Type I fibers were always randomly distributed throughout the red area, and most of type I and II (A and B) fibers retained their native cytochemical characteristics.

From 75 days onward, limited redistribution was observed. Although type I fibers remained confined to a relatively well-defined zone comparable to, but slightly larger than, the red zone of the normal muscle, they were no longer isolated from each other and formed small clusters of 5 to 20 contiguous fibers. In the white zone, regrouping of type IIA and IIB fibers also occurred. The intensity of this phenomenon, known as "type-grouping," did not appear to be significantly different in muscles observed at 137, 190, and 360 days after nerve injury (Fig. 5–1c).

It must be noted that a number of type IIC fibers were detected 31 and 75 days after nerve freezing. When present, these fibers were in close contact with type I fibers and, as already mentioned, their myosin-ATPase activity was intermediate between type I (acid-resistant) and type II (acid-sensitive) ATPase fibers.

Motor Innervation

Modifications in terminal motor innervation of adult rat gastrocnemius muscle fibers were not systematically studied, since muscles of operated animals were preferentially used for electrophysiologic and histochemical investigations. However, this innervation has been observed at certain postoperative stages.

After silver impregnation, it was often possible to demonstrate collateral sprouting of the motor axons and innervation of several contiguous muscle fibers by the same nerve ending (Fig. 5–1d). These phenomena explain the topographic changes and appearance of the unusual fiber type (IIC) described earlier.

Electrophysiologic Events at the Motor End-Plates

Electrophysiologic changes were investigated in the left gastrocnemius muscle of rats whose sciatic nerve had been focally frozen 9 to 54 days previously. The first sign of muscle innervation could be detected between 10 and 11 postoperative days. At that time, it consisted of a subthreshold EPP with an amplitude of several millivolts; moreover, all the EPPs recorded displayed a single peak for all degrees of stimulation, as in normal muscle. Between 12 to 13 and 43 days, 3 to 22% (mean value, 14%) of EPPs exhibited two components of different latencies after a single stimulus, and in a few rare cases three or four components were detected. After 43 days, all the EPPs reverted to the simple form, as in control muscle.

Based on these results, which will be discussed later, it may be assumed that reinnervation of the gastrocnemius muscle of adult rat is completed in three successive stages:

1. Between 10 and 12 days after freezing of the sciatic nerve, all the EPPs recorded are simple, whatever the intensity of stimulation. This leads to the conclusion that, as in normal muscle, each muscle fiber is innervated by a single motor axon.

2. Between 12 to 13 and 43 days, a mean of 14% of fibers in each muscle exhibit compound EPPs after a single stimulus, indicating that they are innervated by more than one axon.

3. After 43 days, all the EPPs recorded are again simple, as in control muscle, indicating that each muscle fiber is innervated by a single axon.

CHANGES INDUCED BY REPEATED NERVE INJURIES

Investigations were carried out on the medial head of the gastrocnemius muscle, which had been dissected out after repeated localized freezings of the sciatic nerve. This model was especially suitable for our purpose (i.e., to correlate morphologic and electrophysiologic changes in the nerve and the muscle that it innervates), since I had previously shown that the number of myelinated nerve fibers was much higher after repeated freezings than after a single one (see Chapter 4). These results led us to believe that repeated cold injuries might also induce significant changes in muscle during reinnervation. Indeed, repetition of nerve injury every 3 weeks induced extensive changes, as detailed earlier. Two series (described under "Techniques") have been examined.

Morphologic Changes

Group I. In this group, the sciatic nerve was focally frozen from one to five times, at 3-week intervals, and results were recorded 1 month after the last injury.

One month after the first localized freezing, the gastrocnemius muscle exhibited a very limited grouping of fibers of the same histochemical type (Fig. 5–2a). Moreover, a number of type IIC fibers, absent in normal muscle, could be observed in contact with type I fibers. One month after two to five localized freezings, changes were more pronounced (Fig. 5–2b to d). There was a gradual but very marked extension of the area occupied by acid-resistant ATPase type I and IIC

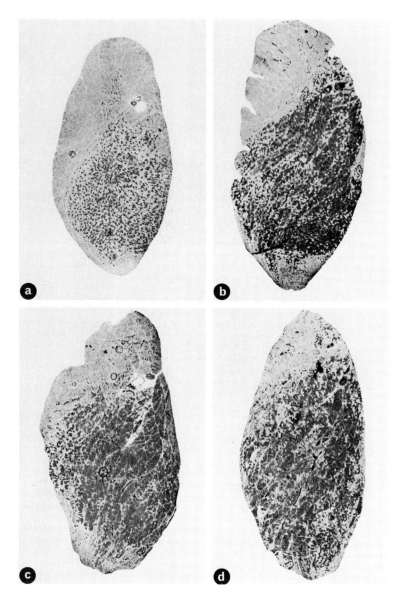

Figure 5–2. Medial head of the left gastrocnemius muscle of adult rats. Cryostat transverse sections after one to four localized freezings of the left sciatic nerve. Myosin-ATPase activity after preincubation at pH 4.35 (*a, b, c*) and 4.53 (*d*) (× 15.5), *a,* 28 days after a single freezing. There was limited type-grouping of fibers of the same histochemical type. Some type IIC fibers, absent from the normal muscle, were observed close to type I fibers. *b, c, d,* 30, 28, and 30 days after two, three, and four freezings. Repetition of nerve injury caused a gradual but very marked increase in the area occupied by type I and more especially type IIC fibers. The "white" area occupied by type IIA and IIB fibers was progressively reduced to a thin peripheral crescent. (From Mira, J.-C.: Clin. Plast. Surg., *11*:34, 1984.)

fibers. Examination of cryostat serial transverse sections (Fig. 5–3) showed that they were mainly of type IIC. In addition, their diameter did not significantly differ from that of control fibers. Concomitantly, type IIA and IIB fibers were detected only in a small crescent-shaped area at the muscle periphery (see Fig. 5–2*d*) and remained markedly atrophic longer than the acid-resistant ATPase fibers. Furthermore, type IIA and IIB fibers retained their original cytochemical characteristics, similar to type I fibers.

Group II. In this group, study of which was based on the results of the first group, the sciatic nerve was focally frozen three

times, always at 3-week intervals, and results were recorded 1 to 18 months later.

One month after the third and final freezing, most of the muscle transverse section was occupied by acid-resistant ATPase fibers belonging to type I and especially to type IIC fibers (see Fig. 5–2*c*). During the second postoperative month, the number of acid-resistant ATPase fibers considerably decreased, type IIC fibers entirely disappeared, and the diameters of type IIA and IIB fibers returned to subnormal values.

From this time onward, only a restricted grouping of the different fiber types (I, IIA, and IIB) persisted, and the muscle histo-

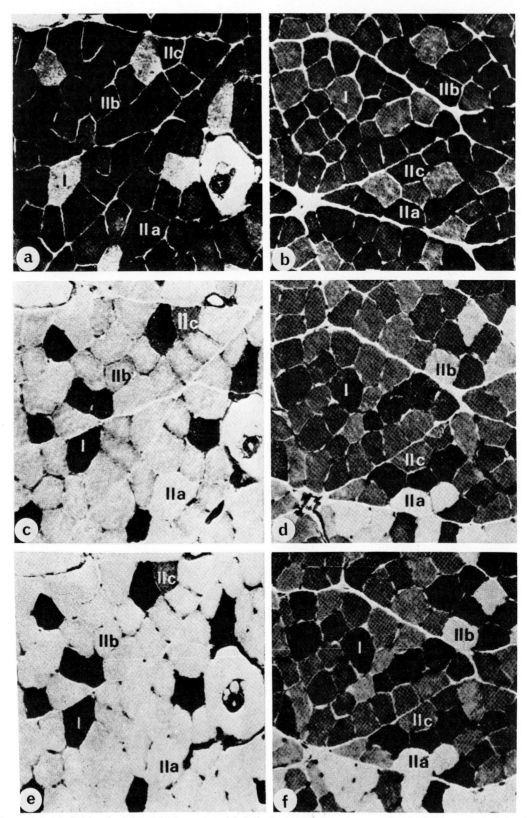

Figure 5–3. Medial head of the right (*a, c, e*) and left (*b, d, e*) gastrocnemius muscle of adult rat whose left sciatic nerve had undergone two successive localized freezings 1 month previously. Cryostat serial transverse sections (*f*). Numerous type IIC fibers are demonstrated (× 190). *a, b*: Myosin-ATPase activity at pH 9.4; *c, d*: myosin-ATPase activity after preincubation at pH 4.53; *e, f*: myosin-ATPase activity after preincubation at pH 4.35.

chemical pattern did not differ schematically, from that observed after a single nerve injury (see Fig. 5–1c). This appearance was the same at 3 months (Fig. 5–4a) and at 6, 12, and 18 months (Fig. 5–4b) later.

Electrophysiologic Changes at Motor End-Plates

After repeated nerve freezings, investigations were restricted to rats whose sciatic nerve had undergone three successive injuries (group II), since nerve and muscle changes had been noted to increase gradually in amplitude between the first and third freezing and to remain unchanged after further nerve injuries (see earlier discussion and Chapter 4).

The first signs of muscle reinnervation could be detected between 16 and 18 days after the third and final freezing of the sciatic nerve. Until the twentieth day, all the EPPs recorded displayed a single peak for all degrees of stimulation, as in control muscle (Fig. 5–4d). Between 20 and 35 days, 16 to 35% (mean value, 23%) of fibers had two components of different latencies after a single nerve stimulation (Fig. 5–4e). In rare cases, EPPs were composed of three or four components. After 35 days, all EPPs were again simple, as in control muscles.

As in the case of a single nerve freezing, reinnervation of the gastrocnemius muscle of the adult rat was completed in three principal stages:

1. A "simple innervation" stage, starting about the sixteenth postoperative day. During 3 or 4 days, all the EPPs recorded display a single peak, as in control muscles; therefore, muscle fibers are innervated by a single motor axon.

2. A "multiple innervation" stage (days 20 to 35) during which a mean of 23% of fibers in each muscle exhibit compound EPPs, indicating that certain fibers are innervated by more than one axon. Such multiple innervation is all the more evident, since each EPP component usually exhibits a different delay. Moreover, the rise-time is usually similar for compound EPPs recorded from the same fiber, suggesting that they result from the activity of several motor axons contacting the fiber in close proximity. This assumption is strengthened by the observation of several axons converging on the same end-plate after silver impregnation (Fig. 5–4c). The different delays for each EPP component suggest that the axons had different conduction velocities; this may be because they were at various stages of maturation related to different rates of regeneration, since the differences in delay appeared to decrease with time.

3. A final stage of "simple innervation" after 35 days, when all EPPs revert to the simple form, as in control muscles, indicating that muscle fibers are again definitively innervated by a single motor axon.

COMMENTS

In the muscle of adult rat, morphologic and electrophysiologic changes are much more pronounced after several localized freezings repeated every 3 weeks than after a single freezing.

The considerable cytochemical and topographic changes that we observed led to questioning the mechanism governing the gradual invasion of almost the entire muscle by a majority of type IIC fibers, which are absent from all normal muscles (except the soleus muscle) of the adult rat. Based on the works of Brooke et al.,[3] type IIC fibers are classically considered to correspond to an undefined ATPase type, observed during fetal development before the appearance of Type II(A and B) fibers and during reinnervation of adult muscle fibers. Type IIC fibers are therefore usually considered a transitional stage during conversion of one type of fiber into another, the "flip-flop" stage between type II(A and B) and type I fibers.[3]

In our experimental model, the fast recovery of subnormal volume by type I fibers and the persistence of atrophy for type IIA and IIB fibers (which also retain their native cytochemical characteristics) suggest a faster regeneration for axons belonging to type I motoneurons (type I axons) that normally innervate type I muscle fibers, with the entire system forming a type I motor unit. Since the muscle fibers of the same motor unit are known to have similar cytochemical properties[5, 12] and to retain their native myosin-ATPase activities during denervation atrophy,[19] any change in their innervation must alter their enzymologic properties. In addition, a new topographic distribution of the different fiber types, and even the appearance of new types, has been observed in adult muscles after reinnervation. These changes have been interpreted as resulting

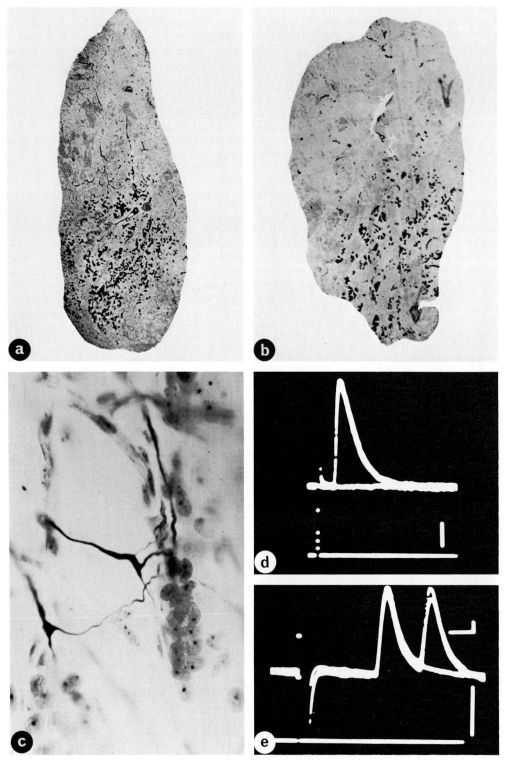

Figure 5–4. *See legend on opposite page.*

from the reinnervation of vacant end-plates by collateral sprouting of the first regenerated axons.[3, 22]

If this is so, then in our model, type I axons had to have reinnervated not only their original type I muscle fibers but also some contiguous type IIA and IIB fibers by collateral sprouting. Three of our observations support this assumption: (1) After nerve freezing(s), type I muscle fibers are no longer randomly distributed, but are regrouped in small clusters; (2) type IIC muscle fibers are always located close to type I fibers; and (3) after silver impregnation, reinnervation of several contiguous muscle fibers by the same axon is often observed (see Fig. 5–1d).

Additional questions concern the fate of the very numerous type IIC fibers, which are absent in the normal adult muscle. If the hypothesis for the stability of reinnervation is correct, the muscle transformation achieved after repeated nerve injuries must be stable. In other words, using the concept that type IIC fibers represent a transitional stage during conversion of one cytochemical type into another, it was expected, in our model, that they would be gradually transformed into type I fibers. Therefore, in a second experimental series, we studied muscles that had undergone three complete denervations followed by reinnervation, results being recorded from 1 to 18 months later. Much to our surprise, results were contrary to those expected, i.e., the muscle transformation is not stable; during the second postoperative month, all type IIC fibers have disappeared, and from then on the histochemical muscle pattern does not differ from that observed after a single cold injury.

Two hypotheses were initially advanced to explain this contradiction:

1. A correlation exists between the cytochemical type of muscle fibers and the diameter of afferent nerve fibers. Indeed, during the first months of regeneration, the size of myelinated nerve fibers is greatly reduced compared with controls, and there is a disappearance of the normal bimodal fiber size distribution.[28] However, the return of nerve fibers to normal size and distribution is much slower than the disappearance of type IIC muscle fibers.

2. A multiple innervation stage occurs, with a muscle fiber thus being transiently reinnervated by axons belonging to different motoneurons and taking on the characteristics of the undetermined type IIC fibers. In other words, some type IIA and IIB muscle fibers are reinnervated by type I axons (collateral sprouting) and then are temporarily converted into type IIC fibers before being "recaptured" by their native type II axons. This assumption is supported by the observation, after silver impregnation, of several axonal sprouts converging on the same endplate (Fig. 5–4c). These features disappear by the fortieth day after the last nerve injury.

This second hypothesis thus implies multiple and polyneuronal innervation of type IIC muscle fibers. However, although all our morphologic data pointed in this direction, they were insufficient for reaching a conclusion favoring this mode of innervation, and it was necessary to perform intracellular recordings of compound EPPs in order to clearly demonstrate its existence. These recordings were carried out 12 to 43 days after a single localized freezing of the sciatic nerve and 20 to 35 days after three freezings.

In summary, our histologic,[*] cytochemical,[†] and electrophysiologic[‡] observations can be explained by the transitory nature of the type IIC muscle fibers and their multiple innervation. These overall data lead to the conclusion that muscle reinnervation in the adult rat is completed in three principal stages, as illustrated in Figure 5–5 and summarized as follows:

---

*Electron microscopic observations of nerve fiber degeneration and regeneration, counts of myelinated nerve fibers (see Chapter 4), and silver impregnation of muscle sections.

†Analysis of muscle fiber types and changes in type grouping.

‡Intracellular recordings of evoked EPPs.

Figure 5–4. Medial head of the left gastrocnemius muscle of adult rats after three localized freezings of the left sciatic nerve. *a*, 3 months postoperatively. Transverse section. Myosin-ATPase activity after preincubation at pH 4.53. Type HC fibers have disappeared and the muscle histochemical pattern did not differ from that observed after a single freezing. There was only restricted type-grouping of fibers of the same cytochemical type (× 10.2). *b*, 12 months postoperatively. Transverse section. Myosin-ATPase activity after preincubation at pH 4.53 (× 10.2). *c*, 25 days postoperatively. Silver impregnation. Double innervation of the same motor endplate (× 570). *d* and *e*, Intracellular recordings of endplate potentials in the medial head of adult rat gastrocnemius muscle after three localized freezings of the sciatic nerve. (D-tubocurarine: $1–3.10^{-7}$ M. Calibrations: depolarization: 1 mV; stimulus: 2 volts; time: 5 msec). *d*, 18 days postoperatively. Simple innervation, as in control muscle. *e*, 19 days postoperatively. Double innervation. (From Mira, J.-C.: Clin. Plast. Surg., *11*:33, 1984.)

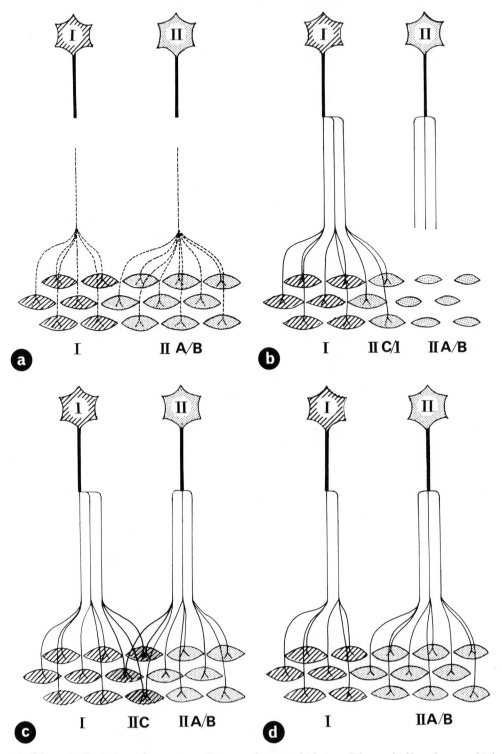

Figure 5–5. Schematic illustration of our assumption according to which type IIC muscle fibers have multiple and polyneuronal innervation. (From Mira, J.-C.: Clin. Plast. Surg., *11*:36, 1984.)

1. Initially, type I axons are the first to regenerate in their own basal laminae, which are not destroyed by the cold injury, and therefore reinnervate their native type I muscle fibers; the latter then recover their normal volume and retain their original cytochemical characteristics. At the muscle periphery, type IIA and IIB fibers, not yet reinnervated, remain atrophic, but retain their normal cytochemical properties (Fig. 5–5*a*). In contrast, in the rest of the muscle, a number of type II(A and B) fibers are reinnervated by collateral sprouts from foreign type I axons and thus assume the intermediate cytochemical characteristics of type IIC fibers (Fig. 5–5*b*).

2. Shortly thereafter, type II axons reach the muscle and reinnervate their type II(A and B) muscle fibers through maintenance of basal lamina continuity. The atrophic type II fibers, previously located at the muscle periphery, then recover a normal volume. In contrast, type IIC fibers, which remain innervated by foreign type I axons, are also reinnervated by their initial type II axons. Thus, they now have multiple and polyneuronal innervation (Fig. 5–5*c*).

3. Finally, the competition developing between foreign and original axons ends in favor of the latter (possibly shown by the 30% decrease in the number of myelinated nerve fibers, as described in Chapter 4). Type IIC muscle fibers are then innervated only by type II axons and progressively recover their initial cytochemical characteristics, i.e., those of type IIA or IIB fibers (Fig. 5–5*d*). This multiple innervation therefore appears to undergo the same reversibility that occurs in newborn mammals.[21, 38, 45]

Our results of studies of multiple innervation agree with the electrophysiologic data obtained by others after partial or total denervation of adult muscles of several species, including mammals[1, 4, 16–18, 20, 25, 40] However, our combined cytologic, cytochemical, and electrophysiologic data provide evidence for the polyneuronal character of this mode of innervation.

In conclusion, this experimental study of muscle reinnervation in adult rat should help to clarify events sometimes observed in human neuropathies, in which muscles are subjected to a series of denervation-reinnervation processes (inflammatory polyneuropathies, spinal amyotrophies, Charcot-Marie-Tooth amyotrophy). In all these diseases, a study of muscle biopsies shows (1) a type grouping for fibers of the same cytochemical characteristics, (2) a prevalence of type I muscle fibers, (3) a marked increase in the terminal innervation ratio,[6] and (4) the presence of type IIC fibers.[15, 42]

References

1. Benoit, P., and Changeux, J. P.: Consequences of blocking the nerve with local anaesthetic on the evolution of multiinnervation of the regenerating neuromuscular junction of the rat. Brain Res., *149*:89, 1978.
2. Brooke, M. H., and Kaiser, K. K.: Muscle fiber types: how many and what kind? Arch. Neurol., *23*:369, 1970.
3. Brooke, M. H., Williamson, E., and Kaiser, K. K.: The behavior of four fiber types in developing and reinnervated muscles. Arch. Neurol., *25*:360, 1971.
4. Brown, M. C., and Ironton, R.: Sprouting and regression of neuromuscular synapses in partially denervated mammalian muscles. J. Physiol. (Lond.), *278*:325, 1978.
5. Burke, R. E., Levine, D. N., Zajac, F. E., Tsairis, P., and Engel, W. K.: Mammalian motor units: physiological-cytochemical correlation in three types in cat gastrocnemius. Science, *174*:709, 1971.
6. Coërs, C., and Woolf, A. L.: The Innervation of Muscle. A Biopsy Study. Oxford, Blackwell Scientific Publishers, 1959.
7. Couteaux, R.: Contribution à l'étude de la synapse myoneurale. Rev. Can. Biol., *6*:563, 1947.
8. Couteaux, R.: Morphological and cytochemical observations on the post-synaptic membrane at motor endplate and ganglionic synapses. Exp. Cell Res., Suppl. 5, *294*, 1958.
9. Couteaux, R.: Motor endplate structure. *In* Bourne, G.H. (ed.): Structure and Function of Muscle, Vol. 1, New York, Academic Press, 1960, pp. 337–380.
10. Davis, H. L., and Kiernan, J. A.: Neurotrophic effects of sciatic nerve extract on denervated extensor digitorum longus muscle in the rat. Exp. Neurol., *69*:124, 1980.
11. Davis, H. L., and Kiernan, J. A.: Effect of nerve extract on atrophy of denervated or immobilized muscles. Exp. Neurol., *72*:582, 1981.
12. Edstrom, L., and Kugelberg, E.: Histochemical composition, distribution of fibres, and fatigability of single motor unit. Anterior tibial muscle of the rat. J. Neurol. Neurosurg. Psychiatry, *31*:424, 1968.
13. Fardeau, M.: Technique et résultats de l'étude des plaques motrices dans la pathologie du muscle squelettique. Rev. Neurol., *103*:30, 1960.
14. Fardeau, M.: Caractéristiques cytochimiques et ultrastructurales des différents types de fibres musculaires squelettiques extrafusales (chez l'homme et quelques mammifères). Ann. Anat. Pathol., *18*:7, 1973.
15. Fardeau, M., Godet-Guillain, J., Mira, J. C., and Tomé, F. M. S.: Dénervation et réinnervation du muscle squelettique. Comparaison des données expérimentales et des observations faites en pathologie humaine. *In* Singer-Polignac Foundation (ed.): La Transmission Neuromusculaire. Les Médiateurs et le Milieu Intérieur. Paris, Masson, 1980, p. 153.
16. Gorio, A., Carmignoto, G., Facci, L., and Finesso, M.: Motor nerve sprouting induced by ganglioside treatment. Possible implications for gangliosides on neuronal growth. Brain Res., *197*:236, 1980.

17. Gorio, A., Carmignoto, G., and Ferrari, G.: Axon sprouting stimulated by gangliosides: a new model for elongation and sprouting. *In* Rapport, M.M., and Gorio, A. (eds.): Gangliosides in Neurological and Neuromuscular Function. Development and Repair. New York, Raven Press, 1981, pp. 177–195.
18. Haimann, C., Mallart, A., and Zilber-Gachelin, N. F.: Competition between motor nerves in the establishment of neuromuscular junctions in striated muscles of Xenopus laevis. Neurosci. Letters, *3*:15, 1976.
19. Hogenhuils, L. A. H., and Engel, W. K.: Histochemistry and cytochemistry of experimentally denervated guinea-pig muscle. I: Histochemistry. Acta Anat., *60*:39, 1965.
20. Jansen, J. K. S., and Van Essen, D. C.: Reinnervation of rat skeletal muscle in the presence of α-bungarotoxin. J. Physiol. (Lond.), *250*:651, 1975.
21. Jansen, J. K. S., Thompson, W., and Kuffler, D. P.: The formation and maintenance of synaptic connections as illustrated by studies of the neuromuscular junctions. *In* Corner, M.A. et al. (eds.): Progress in Brain Research. Amsterdam, Elsevier, 1978, pp. 3–18.
22. Karpati, G., and Engel, W. K.: "Type-grouping" in skeletal muscles after experimental reinnervation. Neurology, *18*:447, 1968.
23. Koenig, J., and Fardeau, M.: Etude histochimique des muscles grands dorsaux antérieurs et postérieurs du poulet et des modifications observées après dénervation et réinnervation homologue et croisée. Arch. Anat. Micr. Morphol. Exp., *62*:249, 1973.
24. Kugelberg, E., Edström, L., and Abbruzesse, M.: Mapping of motor units in experimentally reinnervated rat muscles. J. Neurol. Neurosurg. Psychiatry, *33*:319, 1970.
25. McArdle, J. J.: Complex endplate potentials at the regenerating neuromuscular junction of the rat. Exp. Neurol., *49*:629, 1975.
26. Mira, J. C.: Maintien de la continuité de la lame basale des fibres nerveuses périphériques après "section" des axones par congélation localisée. C.R. Acad. Sci. Paris, Série D, *273*:1836, 1971.
27. Mira, J. C.: Etude quantitative sur la régénération des fibres nerveuses myélinisées. III: Variations du nombre et du calibre des fibres régénérées après une congélation localisée. Arch. Anat. Micr. Morphol. Exp., *66*:1, 1977.
28. Mira, J. C.: Quantitative studies of the regeneration of rat myelinated fibres: variations in the number and size of regenerating nerve fibres after repeated localized freezings. J. Anat. (Lond.), *129*:77, 1979.
29. Mira, J. C.: Contribution à l'Etude de la Régénération du Nerf Périphérique et des Changements du Muscle Squelettique Strié au cours de sa Réinnervation. Thèse de Doctorat d'Etat, Paris, Université Pierre et Marie Curie, 1980.
30. Mira, J. C.: Degeneration and regeneration of peripheral nerves: ultrastructural and electrophysiological observations, quantitative aspects, and muscle changes during reinnervation. Intern. J. Microsurg., *3*:102, 1981.
31. Mira, J. C.: Muscle changes during reinnervation after repeated nerve injuries. Reprod. Nutr. Dévelop., *22*:251, 1982.
32. Mira, J. C., and Fardeau, M.: Modifications dans la distribution des types de fibres musculaires provoquées par des congélations localisées itératives du nerf sciatique de rat. C.R. Acad. Sci. Paris, Série D, *286*:1367, 1978.
33. Mira, J. C., and Fardeau, M.: Nerve and muscle changes induced by repeated localized freezings of the sciatic nerve in the rat. *In* Canal, N., and Pozza, G. (eds.): Peripheral Neuropathies. Amsterdam, Elsevier, 1978, pp. 83–90.
34. Mira, J. C., and Pécot-Dechavassine, M.: Mise en évidence d'une innervation multiple des fibres musculaires squelettiques de rat à la suite de congélations localisées itératives du nerf sciatique. C.R. Soc. Biol., *172*:1063, 1978.
35. Mira, J. C., and Pécot-Dechavassine, M.: Induction of multiple and polyneuronal innervation in skeletal muscle fibres after repeated localized freezings of the adult rat sciatic nerve. Cryoletters, *1*:5, 1979.
36. Morris, C. J.: Human skeletal muscle fibre type grouping and collateral reinnervation. J. Neurol. Neurosurg. Psychiatry, *32*:440, 1979.
37. Pécot-Dechavassine, M., Fardeau, M., and Mira, J. C.: Effects of repeated nerve injuries on muscle histochemistry and reinnervation in the adult rat. *In* Gorio, A., Millesi, H., and Minigrino, S. (eds.): Post-Traumatic Peripheral Nerve Regeneration. Experimental Basis and Clinical Implications. New York, Raven Press, 1981, pp. 507–515.
38. Riley, D. A.: Multiple innervation of fiber types in the soleus muscle of postnatal rats. Exp. Neurol., *56*:400, 1977.
39. Riley, D. A., and Allin, E. F.: The effects of inactivity, programmed stimulation, and denervation on the histochemistry of skeletal muscle fiber types. Exp. Neurol., *40*:391, 1973.
40. Streter, F. A., Gergely, J., Salmons, A., and Romanul, F. C. A.: Synthesis by fast muscle of myosin light chains characteristic of slow muscle in response to long-term stimulation. Nature New Biol., *241*:17, 1973.
41. Streter, F. A., Pinter, K., Jolesz, F., and Mabuchi, K.: Fast to slow transformation of fast muscles in response to long-term phasic stimulation. Exp. Neurol., *75*:95, 1982.
42. Telerman-Toppet, N., and Coërs, C.: A third muscle fibre type related to collateral reinnervation in motor neuron and peripheral nerve diseases. Pathol. Eur., *6*:50, 1971.
43. Thompson, W.: Reinnervation of partially denervated rat soleus muscle. Acta Physiol. Scand., *103*:81, 1978.
44. Tomanek, R. J., and Lund, R. D.: Degeneration of different types of skeletal muscle fibers. II: Immobilization. J. Anat. (Lond.), *118*:531, 1974.
45. Tweedle, C. D., and Stephens, K. E.: Development of complexity in motor nerve endings at the rat neuromuscular junction. Neuroscience, *6*:1657, 1981.

6

Physiologic Assessment of Nerve Injuries

■

Nelson G. Publicover, Ph.D.
Julia K. Terzis, M.D., Ph.D.

The two major functions of the peripheral nervous system are (1) to serve as a *transducer* to encode information from the outside world into a form that can be manipulated internally and (2) to *transport* information from one portion of the body to another (possibly involving a limited amount of processing). The consequences of interrupting or even slowing this flow of information are devastating. In order to assist the body's inherent ability to regenerate these pathways, surgical techniques must be devised to (1) spatially localize regions of abnormal transmission and (2) assess the degree of the injury.

This chapter is devoted to providing the scientific basis for the rational use of electrophysiologic recordings as a tool to localize sites of neural injury accurately during invasive surgery. Knowledge of the exact locations of abnormal conduction minimizes the amount of neural repair that should be attempted and delineates those fascicles or bundles that do conduct, so that any function already present in the affected nerve will not be compromised. This type of electrophysiologic recording differs somewhat from electroencephalograms and electromyelograms[1, 16, 17] because synaptic junctions (including neuromuscular junctions) are *not* involved and because of the degree of localization that can be attained.

Neural propagation is governed by the properties of the axons of individual nerve cells. Therefore, this chapter contains a description of the basic mechanisms thought to regulate conduction at the axonal level. An understanding of these mechanisms is imperative if meaningful nerve conduction techniques are to be applied to intraoperative clinical diagnosis.

Man's first experiments with the nervous system were largely introspective.[5, 16] As early as the second century AD, Galen reportedly divided nerves into sensory and motor types. Perhaps the most interesting calculation of the speed of neural conduction came from Albrecht von Haller[8] in 1762. By reading the *Aeneid* aloud, he determined that he could read 1500 letters per minute. If each letter required 10 contractions of the styloglossus muscle, then each contraction lasted approximately 2 milliseconds (msec). Von Haller guessed that it required the full 2 msec to travel the 10 cm between the muscle and the brain. Thus, he arrived at a conduction velocity of 50 meters per second (m/sec). Although this value agrees with the conduction velocity in the human median nerve determined by Hermann von Helmholtz[9] nearly a century later, the value is remarkable because of the fallacious reasoning by von Haller at almost every step.

In 1791 Galvani published his observations of the relationships between electricity and muscle contractions in the frog. A few years later, Humboldt observed that the nerve must be intact to stimulate contractions in his own shoulder muscles. In 1870, Engelmann described the relationship between the strength and duration of a stimulating current to elicit muscle contraction. Lapicque (1909) named the threshold of muscle excitation the "rheobase" (see Fig. 6–4) and defined the minimal stimulus duration to elicit a contraction at twice the rheobase strength as the "chronaxie." By the turn of the century, electrodiagnosis was being used clinically by Brenner (1882), Cluzet (1911), and others.

In 1924 Erlanger and Gasser[6] reported their landmark study of motor and sensory conduction in bullfrogs and dogs. They demonstrated the proportional relationship between conduction velocity and the diameter of peripheral nerves. Since that time, many advances have been made to improve the instrumentation used to measure nerve conduction, including coaxial needle electrodes (Adrian, 1929), differential amplification (Matthews, 1934), constant-current stimulators (Bauwens, 1941), and photographic superimposition of nerve action potentials (Dawson, 1950).

In 1944, Berry, Grundfest, and Hinsey observed a substantially reduced conduction velocity in regenerating fibers following nerve crush or suture. Nerve conduction has subsequently been used to diagnose peripheral nerve injuries (Hodes, Larrabee, and German, 1948) and carpal tunnel syndrome (Simpson, 1956) and to distinguish between neuropathies and myopathies (Eaton and Lambert, 1956).

More recently, Buchthal and Rosenfalck[3] have contributed an excellent review describing both clinical methodology and our present understanding of sensory nerve conduction. Invasive intraoperative diagnosis was used in 1972 by Kline and Nulsen[13] to record the compound action potential from lesions in continuity. Terzis et al.[20] expanded the use of intraoperative diagnosis by refining these techniques to assess functional transmission at the level of individual nerve fascicles. Furthermore, the clinical assessment of cutaneous sensory territories was achieved for the first time by Terzis,[21] which led to the use of free neurovascular sensory skin transfers in reconstructive microsurgery.

THE ACTION POTENTIAL

The unitary basis of the extracellularly recorded compound action potential (CAP) is the response from a single excitable cell known as the action potential (AP).[10] Throughout the life of a neuron (nerve cell), an electrochemical gradient is maintained between the interior of the cell and the extracellular fluid. Potassium (K^+) and large protein anions are in high concentration within the axoplasm, whereas sodium (Na^+) and chloride (Cl^-) dominate the exterior. The magnitude of the electrical gradient that results from this separation of ions can be estimated from the Goldman equation. The potential across the cellular membrane is about 70 to 90 millivolts (mV), inside negative.

If the membrane potential depolarizes (becomes more positive) above a threshold potential in the range from -30 to -50 mV, the permeability of the membrane to sodium ions suddenly increases. As described by the Goldman equation, the change in permeability causes a depolarization of the potential across the membrane. This, in turn, causes an increase in permeability to sodium, which further depolarizes the cell. The result is a self-reinforcing or positive-feedback loop. Once initiated, the AP is a stereotyped response that shows no dependence on the initial subthreshold depolarization. For this reason, individual APs are "all or none" events. An example of an intracellularly recorded AP is shown in Figure 6–1.

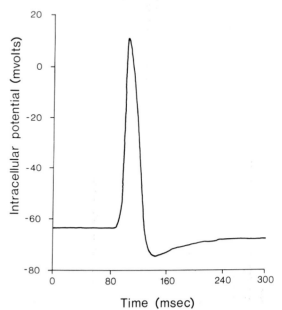

Figure 6–1. Intracellularly recorded action potential. A glass micropipette filled with 3M KCl has been used to record the potential from the interior of a salivary effector neuron in the invertebrate *Helisoma trivolvis*. Resting membrane potential is approximately -70 mV. The action potential propagates through the salivary nerves and results in the release of secretion from the salivary glands. (From Publicover, N., and Terzis, J. K.: Clin. Plast. Surg., *11*:40, 1984.)

The positive-going phase of the AP is dominated by the permeability increase to sodium. The membrane potential approaches the electrochemical gradient for sodium, which in nerve is about $+50$ mV. Thus, the total excursion of an individual AP is greater than 100 mV, i.e., from a resting level of -70 mV to $+50$ mV.

Shortly after the influx of a small number of sodium ions, the permeability of the membrane to potassium increases. The electrochemical gradient for potassium is in the opposite direction. This (along with the closing of the sodium channels) tends to repolarize the interior of the cell and hasten the recovery of the intracellular potential back to the resting level. The complete cycle of AP events may last less than 1 msec in mammalian neurons or extend to several tens of milliseconds in invertebrates.

THE COMPOUND ACTION POTENTIAL

The requirements for mechanical stability during intracellular recordings make the technique of recording from individual cells difficult to apply clinically. However, the electrical field generated by the flow of charge during an AP can also be sensed extracellularly[2] (Fig. 6–2). The magnitude of the extracellularly recorded signal depends on a number of factors, including (1) the distance between the neural membrane (axolemma) and the recording electrodes and (2) the electrical properties of the interposing non-neural tissue. In general, the signal from an *individual* axon is minute and can be recorded extracellularly only following special processing.

However, if all of the axons within a group are made to fire synchronously, the extracellularly recorded signal is the algebraic sum of the contributions from each fiber. In the case of the median nerve, which contains approximately 10,000 axons, the resultant signal from wire electrodes placed around the nerve is several millivolts in amplitude.

In contrast to individual APs, which are always the same amplitude, the magnitude of the CAP is a continuously variable or "graded" response. A "threshold" CAP (Fig. 6–3) is usually described as the smallest response that is clearly distinguishable from the noise without averaging. A "saturated" response is one in which all of the fibers within a nerve bundle have been activated. The amplitude of the CAP is dependent on a number of factors, including the total number of fibers that are synchronously active in the region near the recording electrode.

Eliciting a Compound Action Potential

To elicit a CAP,[3, 16, 17] a sufficient number of fibers must be synchronously depolarized above the AP threshold. In the case of intra-

Figure 6–2. Compound action potential (CAP). This figure shows a CAP recorded from the sciatic nerve of a frog using a monopolar recording setup. A large artifact caused by the application of the stimulus appears at the beginning of the trace. This is volume conducted through the tissues and is therefore synchronous with the stimulus application. The CAP itself appears to contain at least two "bumps" corresponding to populations of different fiber types contributing to the CAP. (From Publicover, N., and Terzis, J. K.: Clin. Plast. Surg., *11*:41, 1984.)

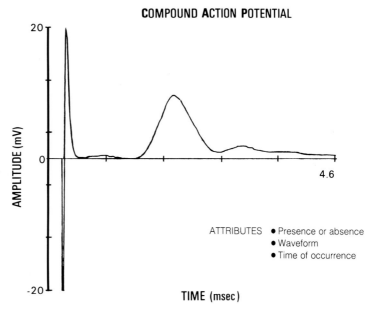

COMPOUND ACTION POTENTIAL

ATTRIBUTES • Presence or absence
• Waveform
• Time of occurrence

AMPLITUDE (mV)

TIME (msec)

THRESHOLD RESPONSE OF THE **CAP**

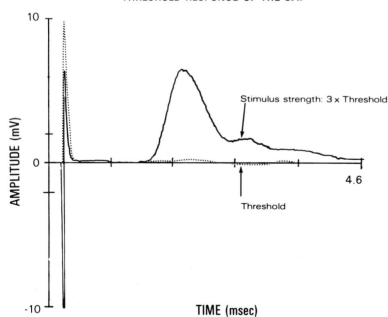

Figure 6–3. Threshold response of the CAP. The dotted line is just distinguishable from the baseline without averaging and is therefore considered to be a threshold response. The solid line shows the response following the application of three times the stimulus intensity used to obtain the threshold response. To offset the effects of a particular recording setup, stimulus intensities are often expressed in terms of the threshold intensity. (From Publicover, N., and Terzis, J. K.: Clin. Plast. Surg., *11*:41, 1984.)

operative recordings, this stimulus is usually delivered directly through a pair of metal (wire) electrodes.[4] An amount of charge must be delivered to the extracellular medium to cause the voltage across the axonal membranes to reach threshold. In the case of noninvasive evoked responses, receptors may be included in the conduction pathway. Flashes of light, clicks, and tactile applications are examples of common stimuli used to measure evoked responses. In addition, volume-conducted shocks and percutaneous needle electrodes can be used to stimulate nerve axons directly, bypassing the receptor. Direct neural stimulation can elicit APs in both sensory and motor nerves.

The amount of charge delivered to a neural region is usually regulated by controlling either the amount of current or the voltage applied to the stimulating electrodes. A problem arises in controlling both current and voltage because resistance values across the electrodes do not remain constant. (Recall Ohm's law: voltage is equal to the product of the current and the resistance.) Electronically, it is easier to regulate the applied voltage. However, without knowing the resistance, the amount of charge delivered (the time integral of the current) is not controlled. On the other hand, if a constant current is delivered, large voltages can arise if resistance values become small.

Whether the stimulus is quantitated in terms of a constant voltage or a constant current, there is a relationship between the strength of the stimulus and the application time required to elicit a response. The actual values of the strength-duration curve depend on the recording situation, whether threshold or maximal stimulation is desired, and on a variety of other factors. Examples are shown in Figures 6–4 and 6–5. The "rheobase" is the minimum stimulus strength required to elicit a threshold response. Below this strength, charge dissipates into the surrounding tissues without sufficiently depolarizing the neural membrane.

Not all fibers are affected equally by the application of a particular stimulus.[15] Following strong stimuli, conduction block may occur (Fig. 6–6). Many of the same factors that affect the shape of the AP at the recording site (to be described) play a role in determining which fibers are depolarized sufficiently to produce an AP during stimulation. The distance between the axonal membrane and the stimulating electrodes and the electrical properties of the intervening nonneural tissue control the spread of charge from the extracellular electrodes to the region of the axonal membranes.

In addition to contributing variability to the magnitude of the stimulation required to elicit a response, these effects alter attempts

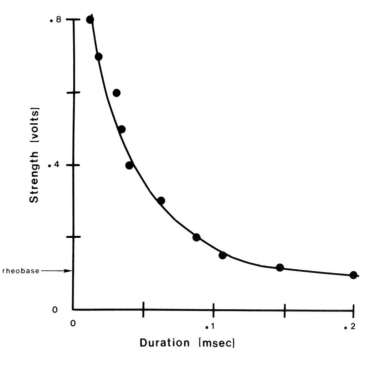

Figure 6–4. Strength-duration curve. This figure shows the approximate reciprocal relationship between the stimulus intensity and duration, to elicit a threshold response. Data were recorded from the sciatic nerve of a frog using 26-gauge wire electrodes. The "rheobase" is the minimum strength required to elicit a CAP during a prolonged stimulus.

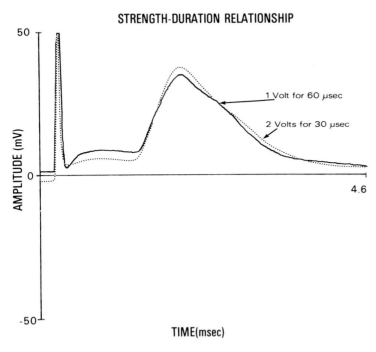

Figure 6–5. Relationship between stimulus strength and duration. The solid line represents the response following a stimulus strength of 1 volt for 60 μsec. A similar response (dashed line) is obtained following a stimulation of 2 volts for 30 μsec. Both responses are submaximal.

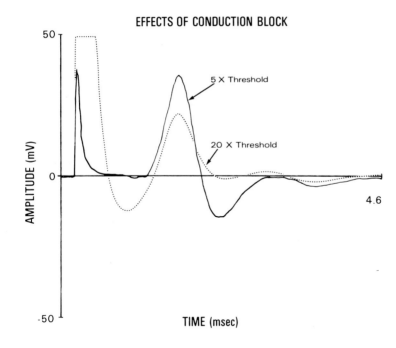

Figure 6–6. Effects of conduction block. If too great a stimulus is applied, it is possible to actually block conduction by causing hyperpolarization in the region surrounding the area of excitation. Partial conduction block has occurred in the response shown by a dashed line (20 × threshold stimulation).

to measure conduction velocity. The CAP may be initiated at some distance from the cathode (negative electrode). This effect is illustrated in Figure 6–7. Volume conducted stimulation can be a significant source of error in estimating the propagated distance, especially when recording from short segments of nerve.

An extremely intense stimulus may actually reduce the amplitude of the response by blocking conduction in the surrounding region. An example of the effects of conduction block is shown in Figure 6–6. It is even possible to elicit a CAP at the anode (positive electrode) by means of "rebound stimulation," which evokes a voltage-dependent permeability change in the membrane.

Generally, large axons are more readily stimulated than smaller fibers. This effect can sometimes be seen as one or more "bumps," which appear on the trailing side of the CAP as the stimulus intensity is increased (Fig. 6–8). As populations of smaller fibers are recruited, their slower conduction results in distinct contributions to the CAP.

The final stimulus parameter, accompanying *intensity* and *duration*, is the *frequency* of application. This affects the response produced by the CAP if one stimulus is presented during the refractory period of another. Following an AP, time is required to re-establish the conductance of the membrane (to Na^+ and K^+) back toward normal

levels. During this time, it is impossible (absolute refractory period) or more difficult (relative refractory period) to elicit an AP.

Different fiber types have different refractory periods, lasting upward from 1 msec. This not only limits the physiologic "bandwidth" of the nervous system but also limits the maximum frequency of stimulus application. If stimuli are presented during the refractory period, the amplitude of the CAP will be reduced, or more intense stimuli will be required to elicit a CAP with the same magnitude as the first response. Effects due to the refractory period are illustrated in Figure 6–9. By stimulating at more than one site, a number of other effects are possible. These are generally referred to as "collision" responses.

Propagation of the Compound Action Potential

The AP can be viewed as a localized region of excitation in which the interior of a cell has a net positive charge compared with the negative interior in the rest of the cell.[11, 12] In addition to the electrochemical gradient across the cell membrane, there is a longitudinal charge separation at either end of the region of excitation. With only the small internal resistance to the cell to impede flow, longitudinal currents flow to neutralize the

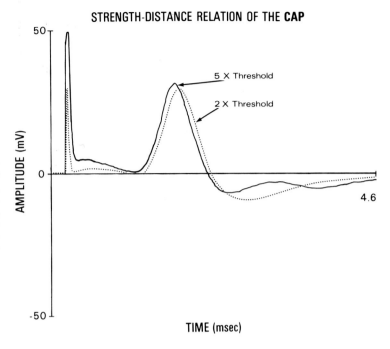

STRENGTH-DISTANCE RELATION OF THE CAP

Figure 6–7. APs evoked at a distance from the stimulating electrode. This figure shows the effects of increased stimulus on the arrival time of the CAP. As stimulus intensity is increased, APs are evoked at locations farther from the stimulating electrode and closer to the recording electrode. The reduced distance of the conduction pathway results in an earlier arrival of the CAP. This apparent decrease in conduction time and apparent increase in conduction velocity could lead to misinterpretation of the CAP, especially over shorter distances.

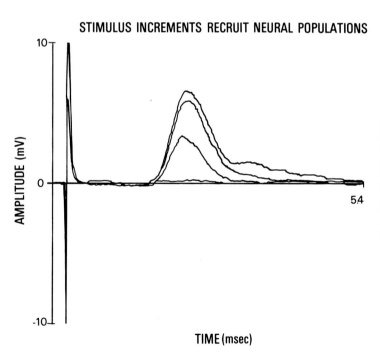

STIMULUS INCREMENTS RECRUIT NEURAL POPULATIONS

Figure 6–8. Effects of stimulus intensity on the CAP. This figure shows a series of CAPs in response to different stimulus intensities. The smallest response is near threshold and the largest CAP shows a maximal response. The appearance of a second "bump" on the maximal response shows the recruitment of a population of more slowly conducting nerve fibers.

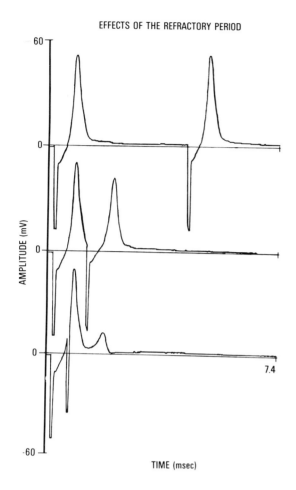

EFFECTS OF THE REFRACTORY PERIOD

AMPLITUDE (mV)

TIME (msec)

Figure 6–9. CAPs recorded following various interstimulus intervals. If stimuli are presented too rapidly, the refractory period affects the shape of the CAP. This figure shows a series of paired CAPs recorded from the sciatic nerve of a frog. In the upper panel the interstimulus interval is sufficient to allow full recovery, resulting in identical CAP waveforms. In the middle panel some fibers remained refractory during the application of the second stimulus, resulting in a reduced amplitude of the CAP waveform. In the lower panel most of the fibers were refractory during the application of the second stimulus, resulting in a greatly reduced amplitude of the CAP.

charge separation (capacitive discharge). This slightly depolarizes the membrane ahead of the region of excitation, which in turn results in the permeability changes to sodium and potassium that have been described. The membrane potential then strongly depolarizes (ionic flow), and the entire process is repeated in the next forward segment. Without active propagation, the potential would simply dissipate.

Many factors that have not been considered in this simplified view of nerve conduction can affect the rate of propagation of the AP. However, from the previous paragraph, it can been seen that the conduction velocity (CV) will increase if the internal resistance (r_i) of the cell is reduced. Similarly, if less current leaks across the membrane, the interior of the cell will charge more rapidly for a given current. In other words, the CV will increase as the membrane resistance (r_m) increases. The proportionality is:

$$CV = K\sqrt{r_m/(r_i + r_e)}$$

where K is a constant and r_e is the resistance of the extracellular medium. Under most conditions, the resistance in the extracellular medium (r_e) is small compared with the interior of the cell (r_i) and can be ignored.

Many of the principles governing the development of the peripheral nervous system can be discussed based on this equation. Optimal criteria for the function of the peripheral nervous system are minimal volume to promote metabolic efficiency, maximum velocity to reduce conduction delays, and reliable transmission. The internal resistance (r_i) can be reduced by increasing the cross-sectional area of the axon. Therefore, smaller fibers conduct more slowly.

Increasing the CV by increasing the diameter of the nerve fibers compromises the total volume occupied by the peripheral nervous system. Thus, the myelin sheath was developed in many vertebrate axons to increase the effective membrane resistance (r_m). The myelin sheath is a multilayer specialized structure of the membrane of the Schwann cell (the satellite cell of the axon), which segmentally surrounds the nerve fiber. The sheath is interrupted every few millimeters by zones about 1 μm long where the axonal membrane is exposed. These zones, termed nodes of Ranvier, allow for the normal regenerative processes of the AP to take place. However, between the nodes the membrane resistance (r_m) can be up to 10,000 times higher than normal. This greatly increases the conduction velocity between the nodes. The AP conducts rapidly or "jumps" between nodes of Ranvier. Thus, propagation along a myelinated fiber is often termed saltatory conduction.

Nodes from different fibers are not aligned uniformly within a nerve bundle. Therefore, the summed waveform of the extracellularly recorded signal from a bundle of such fibers does not show any direct effect due to saltatory conduction. However, the conduction velocity is increased up to 100 m/sec as a result of myelination. Whereas the conduction velocity in an unmyelinated fiber is proportional to the square root of the fiber's diameter, the velocity of a myelinated fiber is roughly proportional to the diameter, as a result of the increase in r_m.

Factors That Affect the Shape of the Compound Action Potential

Some factors that affect the shape of the CAP are due to the physiologic condition of the conducting fibers. However, many parameters are affected by the recording situation and have no bearing on the overall function of the peripheral nervous system. Thus, although the presence or absence of a CAP is perhaps the most useful piece of information in a clinical situation, estimates of the magnitude of the response must be accompanied by careful attention to the recording setup.

One factor that affects the shape of the CAP is the diversity of conduction velocities in different nerve fibers.[5] This progressively broadens the CAP as conduction proceeds (Fig. 6–10). An analogy would be groups of automobiles that travel at different speeds from the same starting point. Close to the starting point (site of stimulation) the density of automobiles (either per length of highway or per unit of time) is great, whereas at some later time the automobiles become progressively separated and the density is reduced.

However, if one were to remain at any position long enough, the total number of automobiles that pass would remain the same. For this reason, the magnitude of the response of the CAP is often quantitated in terms of the total area (the sum of the magnitudes at all times) in order to counteract the effects of waveform broadening.

A second effect that is caused by the diversity of CVs is the appearance of groupings within the CAP. This is due to populations of similar fiber types (e.g., large myelinated versus small unmyelinated) serving an area of the body. Although there appears to be a continuum of fiber sizes and degrees of myelination, populations of similar types result in "bumps" appearing on the CAP corresponding to groups of fibers with similar CVs. This effect is shown in Figures 6–2 and 6–3.

Fiber types contribute unequally to the CAP response.[2, 6] Under similar conditions, a large axon will generate a larger response than a small axon recorded at the same distance. Large, rapidly conducting fibers dominate the CAP. The distribution of fiber diameters, CAP, and cross-sectional view from a sciatic nerve of a frog are shown in Figure 6–11. The contribution by small (0.2 to 1.0 μm diameter) unmyelinated type C fibers is usually so slight that averaging must be used to visualize these responses.

Similarly, the size of the recording electrode determines the volume of cells whose potential will be summed. Larger electrodes (i.e., with more surface area in electrical contact with the nerve) can "sense" responses from a larger volume of cells. Smaller electrodes sense from smaller regions. One extreme, which has already been mentioned, is the intracellular micropipette (with a tip diameter less than 1 μm) that can sense the potential generated by an individual cell (see Fig. 6–1).

Both the distance between the active fiber and the recording electrode and the conductance properties of the intervening tissue play a role in determining the magnitude of a contribution by an individual axon. A fiber deep within a nerve bundle will contribute less than one on the surface near the recording electrode. Scar formation, vascular supply, and the ratio of neural to non-neural tissue all affect both the magnitude and the shape of the CAP.

The intervening tissues do not equally affect different frequencies contained in any

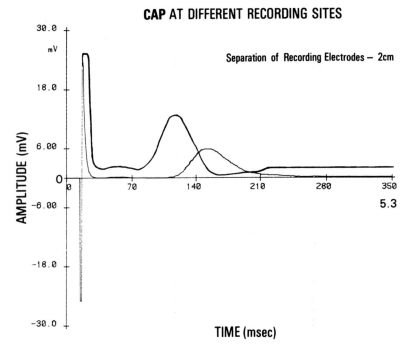

CAP AT DIFFERENT RECORDING SITES

Separation of Recording Electrodes — 2cm

Figure 6–10. CAP recorded at different sites. This figure illustrates a CAP recorded at two sites separated by 2 cm along the sciatic nerve of a frog. The second waveform is broadened and reduced in amplitude as a result of the dispersion of conduction velocities (and possibly also as a result of some branching). If the second waveform is subtracted from the first, the result would be similar to a bipolar recording. (From Publicover, N., and Terzis, J. K.: Clin. Plast. Surg., *11*:42, 1984.)

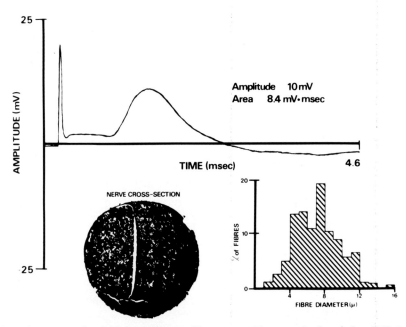

Figure 6–11. Contribution to the CAP by different fiber types. The magnitude of the CAP is dominated by contributions due to large myelinated axons. However, there is a wide range of different axons which make up a nerve bundle. This figure shows a CAP, cross-section, and distribution of fiber diameters, all taken from the same sciatic nerve of a frog. (From Publicover, N., and Terzis, J. K.: Clin. Plast. Surg., *11*:43, 1984.)

response. An extremely rapid event is not conducted through non-neural tissue as well as a prolonged event. This is because cellular membranes behave like a capacitor (i.e., they have the ability to store charge temporarily). Instead of producing a measurable response, high frequency signals are dissipated by rapidly charging and discharging tissue membranes. The net result is an attenuation or "filtering" of high frequency components in the CAP.

In addition to filtering by non-neural tissues and fluids, selective attenuation can also occur because of filtering in the recording apparatus itself. Some amount of attenuation occurs as a result of the electrodes. In addition, the "bandwidth" or frequency response of the recording apparatus is limited (or filters are often included specifically to reduce electronic noise). The attenuation of high frequencies without affecting low frequencies is called a "low-pass" filter (i.e., low frequencies are allowed to pass).

The effect of a low-pass filter is to rid the signal of rapid fluctuations. This is desirable as long as the CAP itself is not affected. As the cutoff frequency of the low-pass filter is reduced, the distinct "bumps" in the CAP merge into one, and the total amplitude of the CAP may be reduced.

On the other hand, a high-pass tends to keep the baseline of the response near zero. This is also desirable, except that there may be a tendency toward the baseline during the CAP itself. This may also reduce the total amplitude of the CAP and distort the response.

Thus, a compromise must be chosen between the desirable effects of filters and the amount of distortion of the CAP. There are a number of more subtle effects of filters, such as phase-shifting and interactions during bipolar responses. Some of these are illustrated in Figure 6–12. A frequency response that includes at least the range between 20 Hertz (cycles per second) and 20,000 Hertz should be suitable for most recordings of the CAP.

There are a variety of other factors that can affect the shape of the CAP without altering the physiologic condition of individual fibers. Recording near the location of a nerve branch may significantly affect the shape of the waveform. The presence of blood vessels,

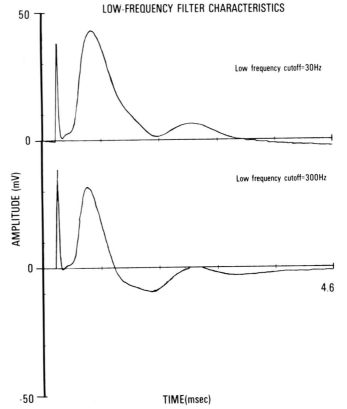

Figure 6–12. Effects of a high-pass filter. The two responses shown are identical, except that in the upper trace frequencies below 30 Hertz have been filtered, whereas in the lower trace frequencies below 300 Hertz have been filtered. (The low-pass cutoff has been set at 30,000 Hertz.) The reduced bandwidth illustrated in the lower trace causes a reduction in the amplitude of the CAP and the appearance of a polyphasic response. These effects could lead to misinterpretation of the CAP.

CAP ASSESSMENT OF REPAIR

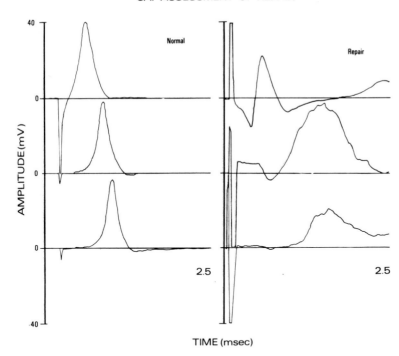

Figure 6–13. Assessment of repair using the CAP. The left panel shows three recordings taken at various distances along an uninjured ulnar nerve of a baboon. The right panel shows the CAP recorded at approximately the same locations from a nerve that has been severed and repaired using microsurgical techniques. The upper trace shows the recording from the nerve segment proximal to the repair. In the middle trace, the recording electrode has been placed just distal to the repair. The lower trace shows a recording 4 cm distal to the repair. The slowing of the CAP across the repair is evident. (From Publicover, N., and Terzis, J. K.: Clin. Plast. Surg., *11*:44, 1984.)

the effect of tapering, and the dryness of the neural surface all play a role in determining the magnitude of the response.

Factors That Affect the Velocity of the Action Potential

As reviewed in a previous section, the major determinant of the conduction velocity along an axon is the ratio of the membrane resistance (r_m) to the internal resistance (r_i) (assuming a low resistance extracellular medium).[5, 11] This is determined primarily by the size and type of fiber and by the physiologic condition of the axon. Sites of injury often show a marked slowing of the CAP because of constriction or demyelination. An example of this is illustrated in Figure 6–13. Velocity is a key factor in determining the location of an injury in which conduction continues to occur (e.g., clinical compression neuropathies).

There is a range of "normal" conduction velocities for each type of fiber. However, various factors other than the geometry of the cell can also influence propagation without affecting long-term viability of the peripheral nerve. Temperature has a dramatic effect on both CV and the refractory period. The effect of temperature on CV is roughly

2 m/sec per degree Centigrade, although higher values are reported. In one example of a 19-year-old male, Buchthal and Rosenfalck[3] reported that the absolute refractory period varied from 0.7 msec at 36°C to 2.0 msec at 24°C. Within a certain range, the effects of temperature are completely reversible.

Buchthal and Rosenfalck[3] also report that conduction velocities slow down with aging. They suggest that at least one third of this slowing can be explained by a decrease in the temperature of the extremities of older subjects. Other possibilities include the selective loss of larger fibers,[19] peripheral segmental demyelination,[14] or the effects of tapering in the distal segments of nerve fibers.[7]

A number of other factors associated with surgical procedures can affect conduction. Mechanical trauma and interruption of the vascular supply (also affecting temperature) are often unavoidable. Conduction can be temporarily slowed or even blocked totally (neurapraxia) during prolonged surgical procedures. This is usually not serious, as patients report a return of sensory and motor function within hours or days following surgery. The condition is serious, however, if it is interpreted intraoperatively as a permanent conduction block and an attempt is made to resect and repair otherwise healthy tissue. Attention must also be paid to the type of anesthetic used. For these reasons it is imperative that surgeons understand the complexities and consequences of the CAP signal so that rational interpretation and diagnosis are achieved.

References

1. Aminoff, M. J.: Electrodiagnosis in Clinical Neurology. New York, Churchill Livingstone, 1980.
2. Brazier, M. A. B.: The Electrical Activity of the Nervous System. London, Pitman Medical Publishing Company, Ltd., 1968.
3. Buchthal, F., and Rosenfalck, A.: Evoked action potentials and conduction velocity in human sensory nerves. Brain Res., 3:1–122, 1966.
4. Butikofer, R., and Lawrence, P. D.: Electrocutaneous nerve stimulation. 1. Model and experiment. IEEE Trans. Biomed. Engineering, *BME-25*:526–531, No. 6, 1978.
5. Dorfman, L. J., Cummins, K. L., and Leifer, L. J.: Conduction Velocity Distributions. New York, Alan R. Liss, Inc., 1981.
6. Erlanger, J., and Gasser, H. S.: The compound nature of the action current of nerve as disclosed by the cathode ray oscillograph. Am. J. Physiol., *70*:624–666, 1924.
7. Gassel, M. M., and Trojaborg, W.: Clinical and electrophysiological study of the pattern of conduction times in the distribution of the sciatic nerve. J. Neurol. Neurosurg. Psychiatry, 27:351–357, 1964.
8. von Haller, A.: Elements physiologiae corporis humani. Grasset, Lausanne, 4:596, 1762.
9. von Helmholtz, H.: Messungen uber den zeitlichen Verlauf der Zuckung animalischer Muskeln und die Fortpflanzungsgeschwindigkeit der Reizung in den Nerven. Joh. Muller's Arch. Anat. Physiol., 1850, pp. 276–364.
10. Hodgkin, A. L., Huxley, A. F., and Katz, B.: Ionic currents underlying activity in the giant axon of the squid. Arch. Sci. Physiol., 3:129–150, 1949.
11. Jack, J. J. B., Nobel, D., and Tsien, R. W.: Electric Current Flow in Excitable Cells. London, Oxford University Press, 1975, pp. 5–260.
12. Katz, B., and Miledi, R.: Propagation of electric activity in motor nerve terminals. Proc. Roy. Soc. Lond. (Biol.), *161*:453–482, 1965.
13. Kline, D. C., and Nulsen, F. E.: The neuroma in continuity. Its preoperative and operative management. Surg. Clin. North Am., *52*:1189–1209, 1972.
14. Lascelles, R. G., and Thomas, P. K.: Changes due to age in internodal length in the sural nerve in man. J. Neurol. Neurosurg. Psychiatry, 29:40–44, 1966.
15. Rauck, J. B. Jr.: Which elements are excited in electrical stimulation of mammalian central nervous system: a review. Brain Res., *98*:417–440, 1975.
16. Smorto, M. P., and Basmajian, J. V.: Clinical Electroneurography, An Introduction to Nerve Conduction Tests. Baltimore, The Williams & Wilkins Company, 1972.
17. Smorto, M. P., and Basmajian, J. V.: Electrodiagnosis, A Handbook for Neurologists. Hagerstown, Maryland, Harper & Row, Publishers, 1977.
18. Stein, R. B., Charles, D., Davis, J., Jhamandas, J., Mannard, A., and Nichols, T. R.: Principles underlying new methods for chronic neural recording. Can. J. Res. Sci. Neurol., August, 1975, pp. 235–244.
19. Swallow, M.: Fibre size and content of the anterior tibia nerve of the foot. J. Neurol. Neurosurg. Psychiatry, *29*:205–213, 1966.
20. Terzis, J. K., Dykes, R. W., and Hakstian, R. W.: Electrophysiological recordings in peripheral nerve surgery: a review. J. Hand Surg., *1*:52–66, 1976.
21. Terzis, J. K.: Sensory mappings. Clin. Plast. Surg., *3*:59–64, 1976.
22. Terzis, J. K., and Felker, B.: A computerized study of the intraneural organization of the median nerve. J. Hand Surg. (submitted).
23. Williams, H. B., and Terzis, J. K.: Single fascicular recordings: an intraoperative diagnostic tool for the management of peripheral nerve lesions. Plast. Reconst. Surg., *57*:562–569, 1976.

7

Epineurial Versus Perineurial Repair of Peripheral Nerves

■

Michael G. Orgel, M.D., M.Sc.

The surgical repair of a transected nerve would ideally allow as many axons as possible to enter the distal stump and proceed to their correct end-organ reinnervation. However, studies[1, 35, 36] have demonstrated a failure of regeneration of the intrinsic perineurium after nerve transection. A new perineurial structure is simulated by endoneurial fibroblasts and Schwann cells. Additionally, the internal fascicular structure at the suture line undergoes a dynamic disorganization. These phenomena occur after suture of the epineurium or the perineurium and may make it impossible for individual axons to reach their previous endoneurial tubes. Therefore, can the technique of nerve repair affect the attainment of optimal functional restoration?

Suture of the external epineurium has been the traditional method of repair of transected peripheral nerves since the late 1800s.[20] However, this technique has been disputed because a significant percentage of patients treated by this method do not regain useful postoperative function.[34, 43] Anatomic data have been presented that have led many surgeons to conclude that epineurial suture also has certain theoretical disadvantages. Edsage[12] showed that this method could cause malalignment and buckling or displacement of fascicles. In addition, Sunderland[43] has demonstrated that nerve trunk funiculi repeatedly divide and fuse to form plexuses. This process occurs over short distances and may cause disparate fascicular patterns of cross sections more than a few centimeters apart. However, Jabaley et al.[23a] have re-

peated this work in the nerves of the forearm and have found considerably less branching than shown in the previous work. Therefore, with some loss of nerve substance, an epineurial repair could guide many axons into the epineurial tissues or incorrect distal endoneurial tubes—both leading to useless regeneration.

Langley and Hashimoto[27] and Sunderland[42] were early advocates of suture of the perineurium, but this method was largely disregarded, since the technical refinements allowing its skillful performance were not yet available. However, since the advent of the operating microscope for peripheral nerve surgery,[25, 40] a strong interest in perineurial repair of lacerated nerves has been renewed.

CLINICAL STUDIES

Numerous reports have appeared in the clinical literature[4, 10, 12, 16, 19, 21-23, 26, 29, 31-33, 39-41, 44-46] advocating various methods for treating peripheral nerve injuries. Many of these studies have been difficult to assess accurately because there has been no consistent agreement regarding what constitutes an adequate epineurial or perineurial repair; certain authors have formed a personal bias not based on scientific data; patients have often been grouped together without regard for the many factors that can influence the success of a nerve repair; or one type of repair has been compared with another performed by a different group (usually at an earlier time). To date, a detailed electrophysiologic

97

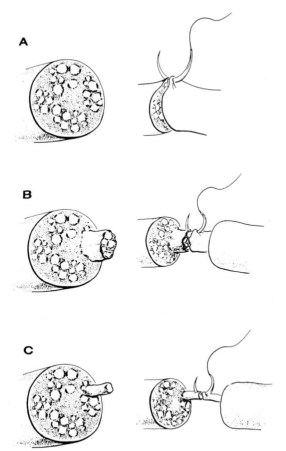

Figure 7–1. Three types of peripheral nerve coaptation techniques. *A,* Epineurial suture. Note that the suture is inserted in the outer epineurial sheath. *B,* Group fascicular suture. Coaptation in this case is accomplished by suturing the interfascicular epineurium of a group of fascicles. *C,* Perineurial suture. This fascicular suture technique invades the perineurial sheath in an effort to coapt individual fascicles. (From Orgel, M. G.: Clin. Plast. Surg., *11*:102, 1984.)

study combined with a careful prospective clinical assessment of a randomized sample of patients has yet to be performed.[38]

There is no consensus that one method of nerve suture is superior to another. Since sutures placed directly into the perineurium have the potential for causing greater damage to nerve fibers,[23, 30] the issue may be whether to suture the outer or inner epineurium.[23, 44] Several authors have noted that epineurial and perineurial suture techniques are not in competition, but rather that there are indications for each[23, 26, 33, 44] (Fig. 7–1). Jabaley[23] has succinctly defined these indications. First, monofascicular nerves are repaired by outer epineurial suture. Second, "group funicular suture"[42] is best utilized where branches representing unique functions are

"well formed and identifiable within the main trunk." In addition, it is generally held that outer epineurial suture should be done in the case of an acute, clean, sharply transected nerve at any level.[26, 33, 44]

Another facet of this problem concerns the identification of motor and sensory fascicles in the proximal and distal stump of a severed polyfascicular nerve. No method has been universally accepted, although most authors prefer the anatomic technique[23, 33, 44] utilizing the extensive work of Sunderland.[43] Other methods have included the use of electrophysiologic[15, 18, 45a] and histochemical[13, 17] parameters, but these have inherent deficiencies that have limited their acceptance. Until a method is developed that can accurately predict correct fascicular orientation, this problem will remain a significant clinical variable. In fact, this question may be insolvable, as Dykes and Terzis[11] have found a large percentage of sensory axons in the deep motor branch of the ulnar nerve and caution against looking at any fascicle as being purely motor or sensory.

ANIMAL RESEARCH STUDIES

Research studies addressing the subject of epineurial versus perineurial suture techniques have been dismissed as having little value.[33] There are inherent disadvantages in attempting to relate the results of experimental studies to the treatment of humans. These include different rates of nerve regeneration, dissimilar scarring potential, and the simpler fascicular patterns found in lower animals. On the other hand, research studies have certain intrinsic advantages. Their major resource is the limitation of variables not possible in most clinical studies. A single surgeon cannot compare the two techniques performed in precisely the same way for treatment of exactly the same injury. In addition, laboratory studies can present quantitative data utilizing techniques not possible or acceptable in humans.

Until recently there has been no consensus in the research literature concerning the relative merits of either technique of nerve repair.[2, 3, 8, 14, 15, 28, 47, 48] In addition, these studies have used disparate means for determining results including subjective assessment of functional return, histologic observation, biochemical assay, nerve conduction, muscle tension, and electromyography.

Currently available investigative tools have made it possible to study both structural and functional nerve regeneration by quantitative means. The combination of quantitative electrophysiology and neurohistology in a "blinded" model allows objective assessment not previously available. Utilizing these techniques, no statistical differences have been found in transected nerves repaired by either epineurial or perineurial suture, although a superiority of perineurial suture was evident in both the morphologic and the neurophysiologic data.[37]

In a further attempt to resolve the controversies found in both human and experimental reports, Kline et al.[24] have repeated a comparison of epineurial and perineurial repairs in polyfascicular nerves in primates. In addition, they have combined quantitative morphology and electrophysiology in assessing the results. Their findings confirm another primate study[9] and demonstrate conclusively that in nonhuman primates perineurial suture of a lacerated polyfascicular nerve confers no advantage over the standard epineurial repair.

It has more recently become possible to assess the central ramifications of nerve transection and repair. In an elegant series of experiments utilizing the retrograde transfer of horseradish peroxidase, Brushart and Mesulam and colleagues[5-7] have demonstrated abnormalities in connections between muscle and anterior horn motoneurons and reorganization of dorsal horn projections from muscle after peripheral nerve repair. An epineurial repair of the sciatic nerve in the rat led to disturbances in position, quantity, and size distribution of the anterior horn cells serving a specific muscle group.[5] Perineurial repair of the same nerve resulted in fewer misconnections.[6] Aberrant muscle projections into the dorsal horn of the spinal cord have also been found.[7] These projections were wider and more variable after epineurial repair but were not eliminated by individual fascicular suture. The latter technique is therefore unable to prevent axonal disorganization within the fascicle itself.

SUMMARY AND CONCLUSIONS

A survey of clinical and experimental work concerning the efficacy of epineurial versus perineurial suture techniques for the treatment of peripheral nerve disruption has been presented. It seems that little difference results from the utilization of either of these methods. Therefore, suture of the outer epineurium is the technique of choice for most acute nerve lacerations, since it is easier, faster, and requires less manipulation of the delicate internal neural structure. Clinical indications for outer epineurial or inner epineurial (group funicular) repair have also been discussed.

The reasons why these techniques lead to similar results remain unclear. However, it would seem to be impossible to align individual axons if their vast numbers and the dynamic disruptive phenomena that occur after nerve transection are taken into account.

It is now recognized that peripheral nerve regeneration studies must address events occurring at the level of the injury and additionally in the periphery and the cell body itself. The answer to the clinical problem of nerve transection will lie in our ability to manipulate axonal regeneration from the central nervous system to correct peripheral end-organs. This question will not be solved by the position in which suture material is placed.

References

1. Behrman, J. E., and Ackland, R. D.: Experimental study of the regenerative potential of perineurium at a site of nerve transection. J. Neurosurg., 54:79–83, 1981.
2. Bora, F. W.: Peripheral nerve repair in cats: the fascicular stitch. J. Bone Joint Surg., 49A:659–666, 1967.
3. Bora, F. W., Pleasure, D. E., and Didizian, N. A.: A study of nerve regeneration and neuroma formation after nerve suture by various techniques. J. Hand Surg., 1:138–143, 1976.
4. Brunelli, G.: Nerve suture. Int. Surg., 65:499–501, 1980.
5. Brushart, T. M., and Mesulam, M.-M.: Alteration in connections between muscle and anterior horn motoneurons after peripheral nerve repair. Science, 208:603–605, 1980.
6. Brushart, T., Tarlov, E., and Mesulam, M.-M.: A comparison of motoneuron pool organization after epineurial and perineurial repair of the rat sciatic nerve. Ortho. Trans., 4:19–20, 1980.
7. Brushart, T. M., Henry, E. W., and Mesulam, M.-M.: Reorganization of muscle afferent projections accompanies peripheral nerve regeneration. Neuroscience, 6:2053–2061, 1981.
8. Cabaud, H. E., Rodkey, W. G., McCarroll, H. R., et al.: Epineurial and perineurial fascicular nerve repairs: A critical comparison. J. Hand Surg., 1:131–137, 1976.
9. Cabaud, H. E., Rodkey, W. G., and McCarroll, H. R.: Peripheral nerve injuries: Studies in higher nonhuman primates. J. Hand Surg., 5:201–206, 1980.

10. Donoso, R. S., Ballantyne, J. P., and Hansen, S.: Regeneration of sutured human peripheral nerves: an electrophysiological study. J. Neurol. Neurosurg. Psychiatry, 42:97–106, 1979.

11. Dykes, R. W., and Terzis, J. K.: Functional anatomy of the deep motor branch of the ulnar nerve. Clin. Orthop., 128:167, 1978.

12. Edsage, S.: Peripheral nerve suture. A technique for improved intraneural topography. Acta Chir. Scand. (Suppl.), 331:1–104, 1964.

13. Engel, J., Ganel, A., Melamed, R., et al.: Choline acetyltransferase for differentiation between human motor and sensory nerve fibers. Ann. Plast. Surg., 4:376–380, 1979.

14. Goto, Y.: Experimental study of nerve autografting by funicular suture. Arch. Jpn. Chir., 36:478–494, 1967.

15. Grabb, W. C., Bement, S. L., Kaepke, G. H., et al.: Comparison of methods of peripheral nerve suturing in monkeys. Plast. Reconstr. Surg., 46:31–38, 1970.

16. Graham, J. K.: Microsurgery IV: Microneural repair of nerve injuries. J. Louis. St. Soc., 131:71–73, 1979.

17. Gruber, H., Freilinger, G., Holle, J., et al.: Identification of motor and sensory funiculi in cut nerves and their selective reunion. Br. J. Plast. Surg., 29:70–73, 1976.

18. Hakstian, R. W.: Funicular orientation by direct stimulation: an aid to peripheral nerve repair. J. Bone Joint Surg., 50A:1178–1186, 1968.

19. Hakstian, R. W.: Perineurial neurorrhaphy. Orthop. Clin. North Am., 4:945–956, 1973.

20. Hueter, K.: Die allgemeine Chirurgie. Leipzig, Vogel Verlag, 1873.

21. Ikeda, K.: Timing and technique of peripheral nerve repair. Neurol. Med. Chir. (Tokyo), 20:759–767, 1980.

22. Ito, T., Hirotani, H., and Yamamoto, K.: Peripheral nerve repairs by the funicular suture technique. Acta Orthop. Scand., 47:283–289, 1976.

23. Jabaley, M. E.: Current concepts of nerve repair. Clin. Plast. Surg., 8:33–44, 1981.

23a. Jabaley, M. E., Wallace, W. H., and Heckler, F. R.: Internal topography of major nerves of the forearm and hand: a current view. J. Hand Surg., 5:1, 1980.

24. Kline, D. G., Hudson, A. R., and Bratton, B. R.: Experimental study of fascicular nerve repair with and without epineurial closure. J. Neurosurg., 54:513–520, 1981.

25. Kurze, T.: Microtechniques in neurological surgery. Clin. Neurosurg., 11:128–137, 1964.

26. Kutz, J. E., Shealy, G., and Lubbers, L.: Interfascicular nerve repair. Orthop. Clin. North Am., 12:277–286, 1981.

27. Langley, N. N., and Hashimoto, M.: On the suture of separate nerve bundles in a nerve trunk and on internal plexuses. J. Physiol., 51:318, 1917.

28. Levinthal, R., Brown, W. J., and Rand, R. W.: Comparison of fascicular, interfascicular and epineural suture techniques in the repair of simple nerve lacerations. J. Neurosurg., 47:744–750, 1977.

29. Lilla, J. A., Phelps, D. B., and Boswick, J. A.: Microsurgical repair of peripheral nerve injuries in

the upper extremity. Ann. Plast. Surg., 2:24–31, 1979.

30. Lundborg, G.: The intrinsic vascularization of human peripheral nerves. J. Hand Surg., 4:35–41, 1979.

31. Millesi, H.: The interfascicular nerve-grafting of the median and ulnar nerves. J. Bone Joint Surg., 54A:727–750, 1972.

32. Millesi, H.: Microsurgery of peripheral nerves. Hand, 5:157–160, 1973.

33. Millesi, H.: Reappraisal of nerve repair. Surg. Clin. North Am., 61:321–340, 1981.

34. Moberg, E.: Evaluation and management of nerve injuries in the hand. Surg. Clin. North Am., 44:1019–1029, 1964.

35. Morris, J. H., Hudson, A. R., and Weddell, G.: A study of degeneration and regeneration in the divided rat sciatic nerve based on electron microscopy. II. The development of the "regenerating unit." Z. Zellforsch., 125:103–130, 1972.

36. Morris, J. H., Hudson, A. R., and Weddell, G.: A study of degeneration and regeneration in the divided rat sciatic nerve based on electron microscopy. IV. Changes in fascicular microtopography, perineurium and endoneurial fibroblasts. Z. Zellforsch., 124:165–203, 1972.

37. Orgel, M. G., and Terzis, J. K.: Epineurial vs. perineurial repair: An ultrastructural and electrophysiological study of nerve regeneration. Plast. Reconstr. Surg., 60:80–91, 1977.

38. Peripheral-nerve repair (Editorial). Lancet, 1:812, 1979.

39. Salvi, V.: Problems connected with the repair of nerve sections. Hand, 5:25–32, 1973.

40. Smith, J. W.: Microsurgery of peripheral nerves. Plast. Reconstr. Surg., 33:317–329, 1964.

41. Snyder, C. C.: Epineurial Repair. Orthop. Clin. North Am., 12:267–276, 1981.

42. Sunderland, S.: Funicular suture and funicular exclusion in the repair of severed nerves. Br. J. Surg., 40:580–587, 1953.

43. Sunderland, S.: Nerves and Nerve Injuries. 2nd ed. Edinburgh, Churchill Livingstone, 1978.

44. Sunderland, S.: The anatomic foundation of peripheral nerve repair techniques. Orthop. Clin. North Am., 12:245–266, 1981.

45. Terzis, J. K., and Strauch, B.: Microsurgery of the peripheral nerve: A physiological approach. Clin. Orthop. Rel. Res., 133:39–48, 1978.

45a. Terzis, J. K., Dykes, R. W., and Hakstian, R. W.: Electrophysiological recordings in peripheral nerve surgery: a review. J. Hand Surg., 1:52–66, 1976.

46. Vahvanen, V., Gripenberg, L., and Nuutinen, P.: Peripheral nerve injuries of the hand in children. Scand. J. Plast. Reconstr. Surg., 15:49–51, 1981.

47. Wise, A. J., et al.: A comparative analysis of macro and microsurgical neurorrhaphy techniques. Am. J. Surg., 117:566–572, 1969.

48. Yamamoto, K.: A comparative analysis of the process of nerve regeneration following funicular and epineurial suture for peripheral nerve repair. Arch. Jpn. Chir., 43:276–301, 1974.

8

The Anatomy of Free Vascularized Nerve Grafts

■

Julia K. Terzis, M.D., Ph.D.
Warren Breidenbach, M.D.

In many ways the improvement in nerve grafting may be related to an increased understanding of blood supply. This, of course, is an oversimplification since it belittles the obviously important role played by improvements in techniques (fascicular repair), technology (microsuture, microscope, microinstruments), and anatomy (internal topography). Early investigators understood the importance of blood supply to nerve grafting. However, other problems were so much more evident (method of repair, type of suture, amount of tension, etc.) that little direct attention was given to vascular supply.

The purpose of the section on Historical Perspective in this chapter is to demonstrate the central role that adequate blood supply has played in nerve grafting. Afterwards we shall discuss the theoretical advantages of vascularized nerve grafts, our general understanding of blood supply to nerves, and finally the specific anatomy of vascularized free nerve grafts.

HISTORICAL PERSPECTIVE

The first nerve grafts were done by Phillipeaux and Vulpian[19] in 1870 and Albert in 1885.[1] From this period through World War I, nerve grafting remained controversial. It normally was limited to use in only the most desperate situations. In 1919, Platt[20] reviewed 430 peripheral nerve injuries. Fifteen of these were treated with nerve grafting and all resulted in failure.

Platt's results, along with similar reports in the British literature, greatly influenced post–World War I views on nerve grafting.[22] Most argued that nerve grafting did not work. However, the problem was understanding why. Some felt that nerve grafting was an exercise in biologic futility and would never work. Others believed that grafting was theoretically sound and failures were secondary to imperfection in technique.

Retrospectively, we can see that the latter theory was correct. Better techniques (magnification, microsuture, microinstruments) have improved results. However, this is not the only explanation. The importance of blood supply to nerve grafts was incompletely understood. Therefore, Platt wrapped his 15 nerve grafts with a fascial envelope. We now know that these protective covers increase fibroblastic activity, probably by blocking revascularization. Thus, these 15 grafts were doomed to failure regardless of technique.

During the interim between the World Wars, considerable experimental evidence accumulated supporting the theoretical feasibility of nerve grafting. There were also some positive clinical reports. Successful results with grafting of the facial nerve in the middle ear were reported by Ballance and Duel[3] in 1932. Bunnell[6] in 1927 reported good results with grafting of digital nerves.

In 1939, Bunnell and Boyes[7] introduced the concept of "cable grafting" for reconstruction of large peripheral nerves. They used multiple strands of a sensory cutaneous nerve bound into a cable of equal diameter to the nerve to be constructed and presented both experimental and clinical evidence that these cable grafts would work. Bunnell and Boyes correctly surmised that the survival of these grafts would be better than that of a single large graft of equal diameter (trunk graft) because of increased rapidity of revascularization of the former. Subsequent experimental and clinical evidence demonstrated that trunk grafts undergo central necrosis once surpassing a critical size.[5, 22, 29] Cable grafting was the first attempt to improve the results of nerve grafting by increasing the blood supply.

In spite of these reports, nerve grafting was approached with considerable caution. Primary closure was attempted at all costs. Mobilization, rerouting, transposition, joint positioning, nerve stretching, and even bone shortening were used in order to achieve end-to-end anastomosis. Only after failure of these methods was nerve grafting contemplated (i.e., in the most desperate cases).[28]

During World War II, primary closure was the approach to nerve injury. Spurling et al.[25] in 1945 did a retrospective study on 1500 battlefield injuries. Nerve grafting was used in only 1% of these cases and results were predictably poor. Grafting was used only in the most difficult cases, often involving large defects and poorly vascularized beds.

Following World War II, nerve grafting remained circumspect. In 1945, St. Clair Strange[26] reported on the first vascularized nerve pedicle for reconstruction of large nerve gaps. The ulnar nerve was transferred in two stages to reconstruct the median nerve. The nerve pedicle maintained its blood supply through its proximal end until the blood supply was re-established from the recipient nerve. The advantages of this method were twofold. First, it allowed the donor nerve to be vascularized. Second, it allowed a larger diameter graft to be transferred without fear of central necrosis. The disadvantage was that it required sacrifice of a major (sensory and motor) nerve, thereby limiting its use to extensive compound injuries. Although controversial, many advocated and even expanded the principle of pedicle nerve grafting.[8] Seddon[22] and Alpar and Brooks[2] reported cases of median nerve reconstruction with full recovery of thenar eminence muscles. They definitely felt that pedicle grafts were superior to trunk or cable grafts because of the former's increased blood supply.

The next important step in peripheral nerve reconstruction was the recognition that tension might play a detrimental role at the repair site. This was accomplished by two independent investigators. Millesi[15, 16] first offered morphologic evidence that increased tension led to increased fibrosis at the repair site. A separate study by Terzis et al.[32] resulted in the same conclusion; this study assessed nerve regeneration across a gap by electrophysiologic means. Both studies suggested that it was more advantageous for the regenerating axon to cross two repair sites without tension. What often went unstated in these studies was the relationship between tension and blood supply. Presumably, tension at the repair site compromised the delicate blood supply, causing ischemia and fibroplasia.

These studies radically changed the approach to nerve gap reconstruction. Up until these reports, primary closures were acceptable even under considerable tension. Challenging the acceptability of tension at the repair site automatically elevated the importance of nerve grafting. Realizing this, Millesi et al.[17] advocated the use of grafts in nerve gaps greater than 2 cm. Furthermore, they advocated the use of interfascicular grafts as opposed to cable grafts. The former method arranged small cutaneous nerves in parallel strands as in cable grafting. However, unlike cable grafting, these interfascicular grafts were anatomically aligned with appropriate fascicles.

Millesi suggested that interfascicular grafting would have certain advantages over cable grafting. First, appropriate fascicles were aligned.[17] Second (and this is often left unstated in the published reports), revascularization is presumably more complete and rapid.[18] Since interfascicular grafting uses more and smaller nerve strands than cable grafting, this may result in easier revascularization.

One problem with trunk, cable, or interfascicular grafts was their limited effectiveness in a scarred recipient bed. A technique that addressed the problem of a compromised bed was offered by Taylor and Ham in 1976.[30] For the first time, they transferred a nerve with its blood supply using microvascular techniques. The superficial branch of the radial nerve with the radial artery was used to reconstruct a median nerve damaged by Volkmann's ischemic contracture. A 22-cm defect in the median nerve was repaired in an area of poorly vascularized tissue. Axonal regeneration occurred at a rate much faster than expected, and after 9 months, protective sensation returned; however, the most striking feature was the return of sympathetic reinnervation.

Use of the superficial radial nerve as a free vascularized nerve graft offered a new solution to the problem of a scarred donor bed. The disadvantage of this procedure was the mandatory sacrifice of the radial artery.

In 1981, Franchinelli et al.[9] reported on the use of free vascularized sural nerve grafts. These were used in several cases to reconstruct median nerves damaged by Volkmann's ischemic contracture. The sural nerve has its own direct blood supply and does not require sacrifice of a major artery.

In summary, nerve grafting has made tremendous strides since its initial rejection following World War I. Many of these advances are secondary to technical improvements (magnification, microsuture) and a better understanding of nerve physiology (the role of tension) and anatomy (fascicular patterns).

Improvements have also been made in our understanding of the importance of blood supply. Initial attempts at nerve grafting produced poor results. This was in part due to the use of trunk grafts, which underwent central necrosis, and fascial envelopes, which blocked revascularization.

One of the first major steps toward solving the problems of nerve grafting was the introduction of cable grafting by Bunnell and Boyes.[7] Long before the introduction of any new techniques (microsuture, microinstruments, and magnification), this simple concept offered an improvement in grafting results simply by improving the blood supply. Unfortunately, this idea, although recognized, was not universally embraced.

Strange's pedicle nerve graft technique improved grafting results by guaranteeing adequate blood supply to a trunk graft.[26] However, this technique has found limited use, since it requires sacrifice of a major upper extremity nerve.

The next major step was understanding the detrimental role of tension at the repair site. This led to grafting smaller defects than were previously accepted. At the same time, interfascicular grafting was introduced and

enhanced by the development of the operating microscope and microsurgical instruments. Without a doubt, technical improvements have aided the advances made in nerve grafting. However, it should not be overlooked that each advancement in grafting (trunk grafts to cable grafts to pedicle nerve grafts to interfascicular grafts to free vascularized nerve grafts) was associated with increasing the nerve's blood supply.

The next advancement in nerve reconstruction may be the use of vascularized nerve grafts. These grafts are mandatory when the recipient bed has inadequate blood supply. There may be a further role for vascularized nerve grafts when the lesion is proximal, the nerve gap is large, and the blood supply of the recipient bed is compromised but not inadequate. This presumption is based on the theoretical advantages that increased blood supply may bring to the nerve graft.

THEORETICAL ADVANTAGES OF VASCULARIZED NERVE GRAFTS

Wallerian degeneration produces axonal and myelin sheath degeneration distal to the site of injury. The remaining Schwann cells proliferate, and fibroblasts (probably of Schwann cell origin) infiltrate the endoneurial tubes. Therefore, the regenerating axon does not meet a "favorable" endoneurial tube to reinnervate. Instead, it encounters a fibrotic "unfavorable" distal stump containing Schwann cells and fibroblasts.[21] If proximal axonal regeneration is unduly delayed, the fibroblasts almost completely replace the Schwann cells, leaving a scarred endoneurial tube and a fibrotic distal nerve. Thus, rapidity of axonal growth is a prime consideration in proximal lesions when the distances to the end-organs are great.

Early vascularization of the nerve graft may decrease the extent of fibroblast infiltration and therefore decrease endoneurial scarring. It may also provide an optimal environment for an increased rate and amount of axonal regeneration. However, no one has scientifically compared the rate of axonal regeneration by means of vascularized grafts with that of nonvascularized nerve grafts to determine if these theories are correct. Studies of vascularized nerve grafts have been hampered by two factors. First, there is no experimental evidence that a proximal lesion, compromised recipient bed, or large defects are better treated with free vascularized grafts. At present, the only accepted clinical setting for vascularized grafts is a completely compromised recipient bed in which conventional grafts will definitely fail. Second, even if one wishes to use vascularized grafts in a wider clinical setting, the options are limited. The vascular anatomy of only two peripheral nerves has been reported in terms of free vascularized nerve transfer.

The following sections discuss the general concepts of nerve blood supply and specifically report four new potential vascularized nerve grafts.

BLOOD SUPPLY TO NERVES

General Principles

Nerves have both an extrinsic and an intrinsic blood supply.[12] The extrinsic system consists of arteries and veins that accompany the nerve close to but not incorporated within the epineurium. This longitudinal extrinsic system may accompany the nerve for a portion or all of its length. There are several different patterns of relationships between the extrinsic system and the nerve. The nerve may be accompanied for a majority of its length by one artery and one vein. The nerve may be accompanied at different points by different extrinsic systems (e.g., the ulnar nerve, which is supplied superiorly by the superior ulnar collateral; in the region of the medial epicondyle by the supratrochlear and posterior ulnar recurrent arteries, and in the forearm by the ulnar artery). Finally the nerve may be supplied by one or more longitudinal systems that accompany the nerve for part of its course, but then veer away, leaving segments at the nerve without any extrinsic system.[4, 27]

The interface between the extrinsic and the intrinsic system is that of the vasa nervorum. These are the short vessels connecting the extrinsic longitudinal vessels with the intrinsic system. There, nutrient vessels (arteriae nervorum) pass to the nerve through a sheet of thin areolar tissue referred to as the mesoneurium. All vessels to large nerves enter through this mesoneurium and nothing enters from the remainder of the nerve's circumference.[23, 24]

The nutrient vessels are distributed in an arcade fashion through the mesoneurium, much like the arteries in the mesentery of the bowel. It is presumed that the mesoneurium allows complex movement of the extremities (flexion, extension, pronation, supination) without loss of blood supply to the nerve.

All of the large peripheral nerves have areas of mesoneurium, but the mesoneurium is not necessarily incorporated along the entire length of the nerve. On the contrary, there may be long lengths of nerves without any extrinsic blood supply, and some of the small peripheral nerves are completely lacking extrinsic vessels.[4, 23, 24]

The intrinsic system consists of epineural, perineural, and endoneural vascular plexuses running longitudinally. There are extensive anastomoses between all of these systems. Under normal conditions, only parts of the vessels are patent at any one time. However, trauma may result in vasodilatation of the closed channels and even reversal in direction of flow. Therefore, it is clear that the intrinsic system maintains a plasticity of both amount and direction of flow to accommodate trauma. Teleologically, this may have developed as a method of preventing ischemia caused by transection, compression, or ischemia.[10, 11]

The extrinsic and intrinsic systems are, in part, functionally independent. Using the sciatic tibial nerve of rabbits, Lundborg et al.[13, 14] showed that the nerve could be mobilized (i.e., separated from the extrinsic blood supply) along its entire length without any disturbance in intraneural circulation. The width:length ratio was 1:100. When the distal segment was transected, the microcirculation remained normal to the midpoint of the nerve. This represented a length:width ratio of 1:45. This has obvious implications for application of pedicle grafting, free vascularized nerve grafts, and extent of mobilization in order to relieve tension. It shows that a nerve may be separated from its extrinsic blood supply and still survive by means of its intrinsic system. However, there are limits as to how much nerve the intrinsic system can support.

Classification

Two hundred twenty-nine dissections were carried out on 25 fresh cadavers, examining the 13 nerves listed in Table 8–1. The relationship between the nerves and

Table 8–1. POTENTIAL VASCULARIZED
NERVE GRAFTS EXAMINED BY CADAVER
DISSECTION

Upper Extremity:
  1. Superficial radial
  2. Ulnar
  3. Medial brachial cutaneous
  4. Lateral antebrachial cutaneous
  5. Medial antebrachial cutaneous

Lower Extremity:
  1. Sural
  2. Anterior tibial
  3. Superficial peroneal
  4. Saphenous
  5. Posterior cutaneous nerve of the thigh
  6. Lateral cutaneous nerve of the thigh
  7. Femoral cutaneous nerves

Trunk:
  1. Intercostal

their intrinsic and extrinsic blood supply was recorded. It was noted that there are two types of extrinsic vessels: (1) those that arise from musculocutaneous perforators and fascia, are small in caliber, and enter the nerve directly; and (2) large-caliber axial vessels that run with the nerve for a portion of its length. Although both of these are referred to as extrinsic vessels, we prefer to identify the latter as a dominant system. The presence or absence of a dominant system is the basis of the following classification.

Peripheral nerves may have (1) no dominant system, (2) one dominant system, or (3) multiple dominant systems (Fig. 8–1).

Those nerves that have no dominant system receive their blood supply from numerous small musculocutaneous perforators and/or branches from the surrounding fascia. These enter the nerve directly, joining immediately with the intrinsic system. Obviously, these nerves are not suitable for use as vascularized nerve grafts since there is no extrinsic system large enough upon which they may be based. The dominant system may run the entire length, or for most of the length, of the nerve. In this situation (one dominant system) the nerve is supplied by the vasa nervorum connecting the extrinsic and intrinsic systems. This type of arrangement is ideal for a vascularized nerve graft. The nerve may be based on the one dominant system and easily divided into separate segments, each segment guaranteed a blood supply by the dominant system through the vasa nervorum.

The dominant system may not run along a major portion of the length of the nerve. The portion of the nerve without dominant vessels receives its blood supply from musculocutaneous perforators, fascial vessels, and the intrinsic system. If such a nerve is used as a vascularized nerve graft, the portion of the nerve without a dominant system must survive by its intrinsic system. This is even further compromised if the nerve is used in interfascicular grafting. In this case, the nerve must be divided, leaving part of the epineurium intact. Therefore, the portion of the nerve without a blood supply from a dominant system must survive by means of the intrinsic vessels coming only through the epineurium. It therefore becomes obvious that not all nerves with one dominant system have the same potential for use as vascular-

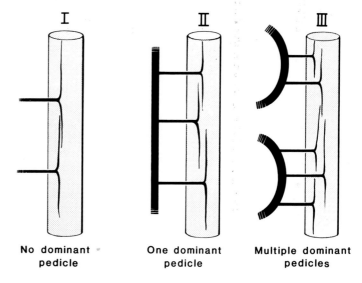

Figure 8–1. Terzis and Breidenbach's classification of blood supply to nerves.

I   II   III

No dominant   One dominant   Multiple dominant
pedicle   pedicle   pedicles

ized grafts. Those that have a dominant system running along a major portion of the nerve length will be superior to those with a system running only a small portion of the nerve length. Interfascicular grafts in the former case will receive their blood supply via the vasa nervorum directly from the dominant system. In the latter case, some of the grafts must depend on only the intrinsic epineurial blood supply.

The final situation is a nerve that has multiple dominant systems. Theoretically, these nerves may be transferred on their multiple dominant systems. However, this would be impractical since it would involve multiple anastomoses, increased operating time, and often sacrifice of major vessels. Therefore, these nerves are more practically used when based on the entire dominant system, which can most easily be spared. However, this converts the nerve from one with multiple dominant systems to one with a single dominant system running for most of the nerve length.

In summary, there are three patterns of extrinsic blood supply to nerves (no dominant, one dominant, and multiple dominant). Two of these (one dominant and multiple dominant) may be used as vascularized nerve grafts. Only the nerve in which there is a complete absence of a dominant blood supply is unsuitable for free vascularized nerve graft transfer.

DONOR VASCULARIZED NERVE GRAFTS

Several different factors have limited the use of free vascularized nerve grafts. First, they are long, complicated, and difficult procedures. Second, there is no definite evidence that a vascularized graft is superior to conventional grafting except when the recipient bed is severely scarred. Finally, there is a paucity of available donor nerves for free vascularized nerve grafts.

Increasing the availability of donor nerves might encourage more liberal use of free vascularized nerve grafts. This in turn would eventually lead to comparative studies of both grafting methods.

With this in mind, 229 dissections were carried out on the 13 nerves listed in Table 8–1. Each was classified according to its extrinsic blood supply and then considered regarding its potential as a free vascularized nerve graft. Those nerves that may be used as free vascularized nerve grafts will be presented in considerably more detail, including discussion of: (1) measurements from fresh cadaver dissections, (2) injection studies, and (3) clinical cases.

Anatomic Studies

Nerves with No Dominant System

The following nerves were found to have no dominant blood supply and therefore to be unsuitable for free vascularized nerve graft transfer: medial brachial cutaneous nerve, medial antebrachial cutaneous nerve, lateral cutaneous nerve of the thigh, and femoral cutaneous nerves. On isolated occasions, extrinsic vessels were noted that ran with the nerve for a very short distance. There were no cases that were suitable for free vascularized nerve transfer.

Nerves with One Dominant System

The medial sural, superficial radial, posterior cutaneous nerve of the thigh, intercostal, anterior tibial, lateral antebrachial cutaneous

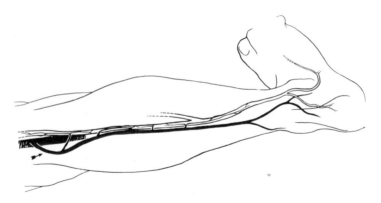

Figure 8–2. Diagram of medial sural nerve and blood supply. Arrow points to superficial sural artery.

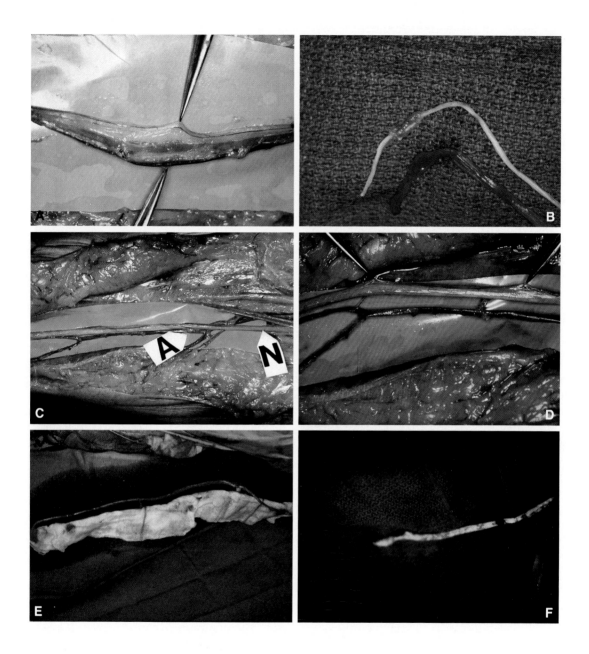

A, Cadaver dissection of the medial sural nerve and accompanying superficial sural vessels. The superficial sural artery is injected with green acrylic. The vein is in the middle. B, Intraoperative photograph of a vascularized sural nerve graft (*lower*) and a nonvascularized sural nerve graft (*upper*). Note the obvious difference in vascularity. C, Cadaver dissection of right arm showing view of acrylic-injected superior ulnar collateral artery (A) and ulnar nerve (N). D, Close-up view of same cadaver dissection as in Plate C. The ulnar nerve is held superiorly; the acrylic-injected superior ulnar collateral artery is below. Two arteriae nervorum are present. E, Intraoperative photograph of ulnar nerve isolated on the superior ulnar collateral artery and vein. Bleeding is noted from both ends. F, Intraoperative photograph of the distal portion of the ulnar nerve shown in Plate E. The photograph was taken 5 minutes after 1 gm of fluorescein was administered intravenously. Fluorescein was noted the entire length of the nerve.

nerve of the forearm, and superficial peroneal nerves all have one dominant blood supply. They are discussed in detail below.

Medial Sural Nerve. Use of this nerve as a vascularized nerve graft was first reported by Franchinelli et al.[9] The superficial sural artery runs with the nerve for most of its length (Fig. 8–2 and Plates *A* and *B*). This vessel arises from the posterior tibial artery or the right or left sural artery. Both the vein (1.3 mm) and the artery (1.2 mm) are suitable for microsurgical anastomosis.

There are several disadvantages in the use of this nerve. First, surgical exposure requires that the patient be in a prone position. Most upper extremity reconstructions require that the patient be supine. Therefore, operating time and nerve ischemia time are increased by an intraoperative position change. Second, histology studies indicated that sufficient neural tissue is available for transfer. However, there is considerable loss of neural tissue (when considered from a distal to proximal direction) compared with other nerves. Finally, and most important, the arteriovenous complex may be absent in a high percentage of cases. Franchinelli et al.[9] reported that in 33% of their dissections, there was no pedicle. In 70% of our dissections, no pedicle was present.

Superficial Radial Nerve. The first vascularized nerve graft was reported by Taylor and Ham[30] using the superficial radial nerve. This nerve arises from the radial nerve at the proximal portion of the brachioradialis muscle. It runs down the forearm under cover of this muscle and is joined on its medial side by the radial artery (Figs. 8–3 and 8–4). Distally the nerve turns away from the artery and passes under the tendon of the brachioradialis. The full length of the superficial radial nerve from the posterior interosseous nerve to the bifurcation just above the wrist may be used as a graft. The vascularized nerve graft is based on the radial artery and venae comitantes. The vascular supply is

constant (present in 100% of dissections), is of large size (artery 3.6 mm, vein 3.8 mm), and has a long pedicle (artery 6.4 cm, vein 6.4 cm). The extrinsic system runs with this nerve only for about half of the total graft length. This nerve has both proximal and distal segments without a dominant system (average graft length of 23.3 cm versus the length that vessels run with the nerve of 11.8 cm).

Posterior Cutaneous Nerve of the Thigh. The posterior cutaneous nerve of the thigh arises from the sciatic nerve under the gluteus maximus muscle and receives its blood supply from a continuation of the inferior gluteal vessels. This complex runs with the nerve under the muscle and out into the subcutaneous tissue of the posterior thigh. As a graft, the nerve is used at the point where it exits under the gluteus maximus. Dissections revealed that the vessels were dependable, but the nerve length was short (less than 20 cm); the neural tissue area was small (see section on Histologic Studies); and the nerve was highly branched. Therefore, because of characteristics of the nerve, this complex was rejected as a possible vascularized graft.

Intercostal Nerve. The intercostal nerve runs in the intercostal space under the edge of the rib. At the posterior axillary line it gives rise to a cutaneous portion, which exits from the intercostal space. The remaining predominantly motor portion continues on to supply the intercostal muscles. Dissections revealed a dependable blood supply that ran only with the nerve in the intercostal space. The cutaneous portion has no dominant blood supply. The size of the nerve and amount of neural tissue were small.

Anterior Tibial Nerve. The anterior tibial nerve arises below the head of the fibula from the common peroneal nerve. It passes under the peroneus longus, through the intramuscular septum, and under the extensor digitorum and passes down the leg, lying

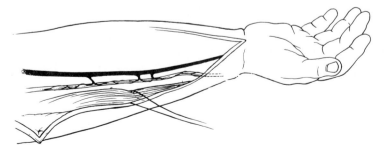

Figure 8–3. Diagram of superficial radial nerve and radial artery.

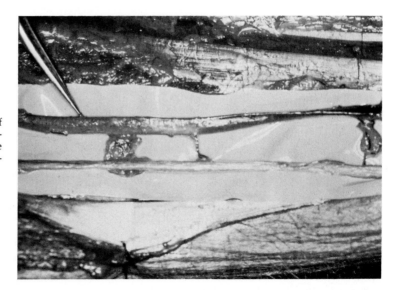

Figure 8–4. Cadaver dissections of superficial radial nerve with accompanying radial artery. Three arteriae nervorum are evident. Mesoneurium has been resected.

between the extensor hallucis longus and tibialis anterior muscles. Four to eight centimeters from its origin the nerve is joined by the anterior tibial artery and venae comitantes. This nerve may be used as a vascularized nerve graft based on the anterior tibial artery and veins (Fig. 8–5).

Surgical exposure is obtained by finding the plane distally between the tibialis anterior and extensor hallucis longus. This is traced proximally until the nerve and vascular complex separate. Each of the motor branches must be identified and preserved.

The nerve is used as a graft after it gives

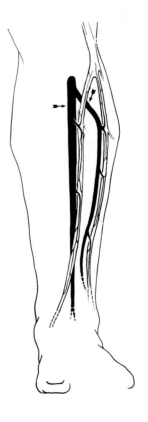

Figure 8–5. Diagram of the superficial peroneal and anterior tibial nerves with their respective blood supplies. Arrow on the right points to the superficial peroneal artery; arrow on the left points to the anterior tibial artery.

off its last motor branch to the anterior lateral compartment muscles. Therefore, the short extensors in the foot are sacrificed. This leaves a graft of moderate length (24.5 cm). The artery and veins are of large size (4.4 mm and 3.4 mm, respectively). The vascular complex is dependable (present in 100% of the dissections), but the level of the last motor branch may vary. In one dissection, the last motor branch came off the nerve low in the leg, thus leaving a very short graft. This could be avoided only by extensive intraneural neurolysis or sacrificing the motor branch. This particular dissection was rejected as a possible vascularized graft. However, 95% of the dissections were suitable for free vascularized transfer.

Lateral Antebrachial Cutaneous Nerve of the Forearm. The musculocutaneous nerve arises from the lateral cord and passes through the coracobrachialis into the lateral aspect of the arm, lying between the biceps and brachialis. Here it gives off motor branches to these muscles. The continuation of this nerve, after the motor branches are given off, is the lateral antebrachial cutaneous nerve of the forearm.

An artery and vein arise from the brachial vessels, pass under the biceps, and join the nerve in the region of the last motor branch. This arteriovenous complex runs with the nerve for a variable distance of 1 to 9 cm before turning away to supply the biceps. The remaining distal portion of the nerve has no extrinsic blood supply. Theoretically, the lateral antebrachial cutaneous nerve of the forearm could be used as a vascularized graft, based on the vessel complex arising from the brachial artery. The artery and vein are also of adequate caliber for microsurgical anastomosis. However, only 25% of the dissections were suitable for free vascularized nerve grafting. In four cases, no vessels were present; in nine cases, the vessels accompanied the nerve for only a short distance; and in one case, the last motor branch was distal to the extrinsic blood supply.

Superficial Peroneal Nerve. The superficial peroneal nerve arises from the common peroneal nerve below the head of the fibula. The nerve runs under the peroneus longus, giving off a motor branch to this muscle, and comes to lie in a plane between the peroneus longus and brevis and the extensor digitorum. Six to twelve centimeters from its origin, the nerve receives a vascular pedicle. This complex arises from the anterior tibial artery and vein and runs deep to the extensor digitorum to join the superficial peroneal nerve. It accompanies the nerve for 3 to 18 cm. The graft may be taken proximally from the last motor branch (1 to 12 cm from the origin) to the bifurcation distally at the level of the ankle. The length of the graft ranges from 14 to 30 cm (Fig. 8–5).

Surgical exposure is gained by finding the superficial peroneal nerve at the level of the ankle in the subcutaneous tissue. The nerve is traced, distal to proximal, into the muscle plane between the peroneus muscles and the anterior lateral compartment muscles. The extrinsic vessels always lie on the medial side of the nerve. They join the nerve 10 cm below the head of the fibula. The vessels are then traced through the fascia separating the lateral and anterior lateral compartments and under the extensor digitorum muscle to their junction with the anterior tibial vessels. This must be done to gain adequate length of the vascular pedicle. Care should be taken in this area, since the anterior tibial nerve passes under this vascular pedicle.

The vessels are of adequate size for microsurgical transfer, and the graft is of moderate length (23.6 cm). The extrinsic vessels run with the nerve for 9.1 cm. The far proximal and distal portions of the graft have no extrinsic blood supply and must survive on the intrinsic system.

Nerves with Multiple Dominant Systems

Ulnar Nerve. Proximally the ulnar nerve is supplied by the superior ulnar collateral artery (Fig. 8–6 and Plates C and D). In the region of the medial epicondyle, it is supplied by the posterior ulnar recurrent and supratrochlear arteries. Below the elbow, it is nourished by the ulnar artery.

Under normal circumstances the ulnar nerve is not available for nerve grafting. However, in certain traumatic amputations or in brachial plexus injuries where roots C8 and T1 have been avulsed, the ulnar nerve may be used as a vascularized graft. In these cases, the nerve is based upon the superior ulnar collateral artery and vein. The distal and proximal portions of the nerve must survive on the intrinsic blood supply.

Injection and fluorescein studies were carried out to investigate the relationship between the extrinsic and intrinsic systems. In cadavers, the nerve was elevated and based

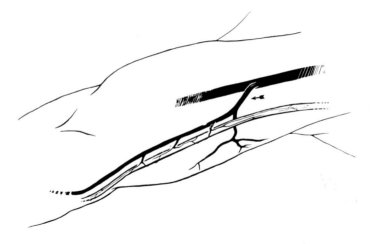

Figure 8–6. Diagram of ulnar nerve and superior ulnar collateral artery. Arrow points to origin of the superior ulnar collateral artery from the brachial artery.

only on the superior ulnar collateral artery. This was injected and the dye was followed from the extrinsic into the intrinsic system. The dye filled the intrinsic system for only a short distance. However, this was probably an artefact of the cadavers' age (all were dissected 12 hours or later after death) and not a true indication of intrinsic blood supply. When the same procedure was done intraoperatively using fluorescein, the entire length of the nerve fluoresced. This indicates that blood enters through the extrinsic system and is then carried to both ends of the nerve through the intrinsic system (Plates *E* and *F*).

The surgical exposure of the nerve is initiated at the cubital tunnel and is then followed proximally. The superior ulnar collateral artery and vein, which were present in 100% of dissections, always run with the nerve on its deep side. The superior ulnar collateral artery arises from the brachial artery 14 to 22 cm above the medial epicondyle. Therefore, it may arise as high as the axilla. The vein starts in the same region or slightly lower, coming from a plexus formed by the basilic and brachial veins. These vessels then proceed in a medial direction to join the nerve. They run with the nerve on its deep side for 4 to 15 cm before turning away, always above the cubital tunnel.

The entire length of the ulnar nerve may be used, giving a very long graft averaging 55.6 cm. The proximal and distal portions, without extrinsic blood supply, should be carefully dissected, leaving a cuff of surrounding tissues to protect the epineurial vessels. If these vessels are damaged, the portion of graft without extrinsic blood supply will not survive.

Saphenous Nerve. The saphenous nerve has a multiple dominant system of blood supply. Proximally it is supplied by the femoral artery. In the region of the knee, it is supplied by the saphenous artery. Below the knee, there is no dominant system. The saphenous nerve may be used as a vascularized graft based on the saphenous artery and vein (Figs. 8–7 and 8–8). The sartorius muscle is identified in the proximal thigh and reflected laterally, exposing the femoral artery and nerve. The saphenous nerve is a medial component of the femoral nerve and comes to lie directly to the lateral side of the femoral artery. The nerve and artery proceed down the leg into Hunter's canal, maintaining this relationship. In Hunter's canal the saphenous nerve crosses lateral to medial over the femoral artery, and in this region the saphenous artery and vein leave the femoral vessels and run 2 to 6 cm to join the saphenous nerve. These vessels join the nerve 27.4 cm from its origin in the groin. The vessels and nerve pass between the sartorius and gracilis tendons out into the subcutaneous tissue of the distal thigh. At this point the sartorius is pulled medially so that the nerve may be followed in its subcutaneous course. At the level of the knee the nerve and vessels start to split into branches.

The saphenous nerve may be used as a graft from the groin to below the knee. Graft length averages 40.9 cm. The vascular complex accompanies the nerve for about 13.2 cm of the total length. When elevated on the saphenous artery, the nerve is converted from a multiple extrinsic system to one extrinsic system.

The vascular supply to this nerve may present problems. In 20% of the dissections,

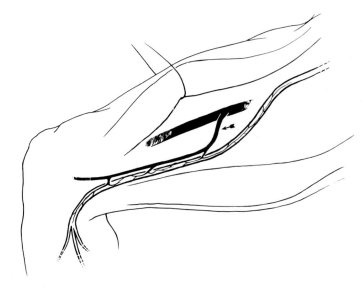

Figure 8–7. Diagram of the saphenous artery and nerve. Arrow points to the origin of the saphenous artery from the femoral artery.

it was absent, thus precluding free vascularized nerve graft transfer. The junction of the nerve and blood supply is quite variable, i.e., 17 to 42 cm from origin of the nerve. This is because in 15% of the dissections the blood supply arose not from the femoral artery but more distally from the popliteal artery (Fig. 8–9).

Summary of Anatomic Studies

Nine of the 13 nerves examined had dominant systems adequate enough to be considered as possible vascularized nerve grafts (superficial radial, ulnar, lateral antebrachial cutaneous, sural, anterior tibial, superficial peroneal, saphenous, posterior cutaneous nerve of the thigh, and intercostal). Of these, both the intercostal and the posterior cutaneous nerve of the thigh supply a small amount of neural tissue for transfer (see Histology Studies) and therefore are not suitable as vascularized grafts. The lateral antebrachial cutaneous nerve was a suitable donor nerve in only 25% of cases.

Therefore, six nerves were acceptable as vascularized donor nerves. These are listed in Table 8–2.

Histologic Studies

The purpose of a nerve graft is to provide an environment (Schwann cells and endo-

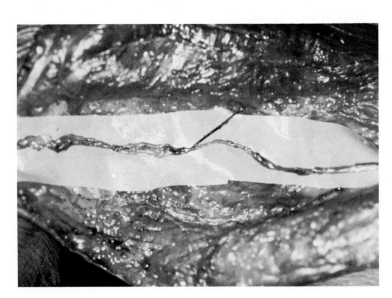

Figure 8–8. Cadaver dissection of the saphenous nerve proximal to the knee. Acrylic-injected saphenous artery is seen joining the nerve.

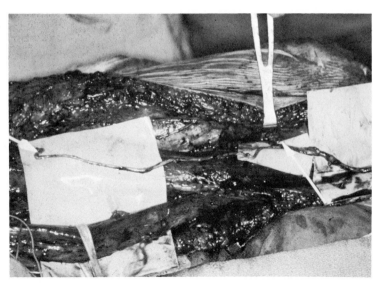

Figure 8–9. Intraoperative photograph of the left saphenous nerve. The gracilis muscle is pulled inferiorly by a Penrose drain. Weck spear on the right points to the vascular pedicle of the saphenous nerve. In this dissection the pedicle is more distal, arising from the popliteal vessels. In the cadaver dissection shown in Figure 8–8, the pedicle arises more proximally from the femoral artery.

neurial tubes) through which the regenerating axons may grow. Presumably, more of such an environment is present when the amount of neural tissue in a graft is plentiful. Therefore, neural tissue area is one criterion to be considered when selecting a donor nerve.

Values for the area of neural tissue were obtained for each of the 13 nerves studied. Nine of these nerves had potential for use as free vascularized grafts. The intercostal nerve and posterior cutaneous nerve of the thigh had small neural areas, thus limiting their usefulness. The lateral antebrachial cutaneous nerve is not a suitable donor nerve because the pedicle is absent 75% of the time. Therefore, its neural tissue area is not considered. The remaining six nerves were carefully analyzed by comparing neural area.

These six nerves were matched for neural tissue area according to position. That is, all of the nerves' neural areas were compared in the proximal position, next in the middle, and finally distally. Only the ulnar nerve was significantly different from the remaining nerves.

Next the average neural areas (proximal, middle, and distal averaged together) were compared. This indicated that none of the nerves were statistically different.

Examination of the average neural area in square millimeters has the following regression: ulnar $(3.00 + 1.18)$, superficial radial (0.88 ± 0.33), superficial peroneal (0.81 ± 0.25), sural (0.72 ± 0.30), anterior tibial (0.57 ± 0.21), saphenous (0.54 ± 0.22). Caution must be exercised when interpreting these results. They appear to imply that the superficial radial is a better graft than the anterior tibial. However, strict analysis reveals that the difference is not statistically significant. The problem is that there was wide variation of the neural area values. This is because nerves were compared from many different cadavers of different gender, size, and weight.

Therefore, this study *cannot* be used as clear evidence (except for the ulnar nerve) that in a given individual any one nerve will uniformly supply more neural tissue than another. In order to do this, one must repeat the studies on cadavers matched for sex, height, weight, and age.

With a conventional nerve graft, consider-

Table 8–2. NERVES AND VESSELS THAT MAY BE USED FOR VASCULARIZED NERVE GRAFTS

Nerve		Blood Supply
Superficial radial	←——→	Radial
Ulnar	←——→	Superior ulnar collateral
Sural	←——→	Superficial sural
Anterior tibial	←——→	Anterior tibial
Superficial peroneal	←——→	Superficial peroneal
Saphenous	←——→	Saphenous

able attention is given to the percentage of neural tissue and the number of fascicles. Revascularization from the surrounding tissue is greatly aided when the graft is composed of many small fascicles with a paucity of connective tissue. With a vascularized nerve graft, these factors may not be meaningful, since the vascular supply is assured regardless of neural tissue:connective tissue ratios. However, technically an interfascicular neurography may be easier when there is little connective tissue present. The external epineurium may be quickly removed, exposing the internal epineurium through which the sutures are placed.

Examination of the results for the six vascularized donor nerves reveals that the average percentage of neural tissue is very similar in all the nerves: ulnar (36.2 ± 10.3), superficial radial (34.9 ± 8.4), superficial peroneal (39.3 ± 12.9), sural (37.2 ± 15.0), anterior tibial (38.0 ± 12.5), and saphenous (34.4 ± 9.6).

Frequent branching should be avoided when selecting a donor nerve. An evaluation of the extent of branching may be obtained from these results by subtracting the neural area distally from the proximal value. This produces the following values: superficial radial (0), anterior tibial (0.09), superficial peroneal (0.18), sural (0.18), saphenous (0.17), and ulnar (1.06). As expected, there is essentially no branching in the superficial radial and anterior tibial nerves. The sural, superficial peroneal, and saphenous nerves show a moderate amount of branching. Note that for the sural nerve, proximal values were subtracted from the distal. This is because the addition of the lateral sural makes the distal nerve larger than the proximal nerve. It may at first seem surprising that there is branching in the superficial peroneal nerve. The graft was taken from below the motor branches to above the bifurcation at the ankle. However, frequently there was a small cutaneous branch observed above the bifurcation, which would account for some neural loss. The value obtained for the saphenous nerve represents the qualitative difference between grafts taken from the groin and the level of the knee.

The Ideal Vascularized Nerve Graft

Sunderland[28] listed a series of criteria for conventional donor nerve grafts. With vas-

cularized nerve grafting, a new set of criteria must be considered. The following are the characteristics evaluated when selecting a vascularized donor nerve.

1. *Type of vascular supply:* Obviously, a nerve with no dominant system will not work as a vascularized graft. The ideal vascularized nerve graft is one with one dominant system running along a major portion of its length.

2. *Neural tissue area:* There is no sense in using the posterior cutaneous nerve of the thigh to reconstruct a trunk of the brachial plexus. The amount of neural tissue transferred by the donor graft should ideally approximate the neural tissue to be reconstructed.

3. *Length of nerve graft:* The donor nerve must be sufficiently long so that, when cut into the appropriate number of strands, it will still bridge the gap.

4. *Consistency of vascularized potential:* In some cases because of absent vessels, short vascular length running with the nerve, or early branching, the nerve could not be transferred as a vascularized nerve graft. Some nerves showed a high degree of undependability (sural), whereas others were very dependable (superficial radial).

5. *Accessibility of donor nerve:* Dissection of a vascularized donor nerve is technically demanding and may be time consuming. Ideally the nerve to be reconstructed and the donor nerve should be on the same surface (anterior or posterior). In this way two teams can work at the same time and the patient need not be turned intraoperatively.

Certain factors are given less attention with a vascularized free graft than with conventional grafts. With conventional grafting, the connective tissue:neural tissue ratio was important in determining the extent of vascularization. However, with a vascularized free graft, this ratio is no longer crucial to survival.

The number and size of fascicles are also not considered. In a vascularized nerve graft, the vascular supply is guaranteed, regardless of fascicular size and number.

The ideal graft would have adequate length, be accessible, have sufficient neural tissue area, and have one dominant system running along the whole length of the nerve. In some cases, it may be necessary to sacrifice one factor for another.

We have found the saphenous nerve good for upper extremity peripheral nerve reconstruction. It is anteriorly situated and has a good graft length with a moderately dependable vascular supply. Since 1981, we have done six saphenous vascularized nerve grafts, all for upper extremity reconstruction. Five nerves were successfully transferred. In one case, a microsurgical error led to graft failure. In all cases, a pedicle was present. In one case, the pedicle came off in the popliteal fossa, as was noted in 15% of our dissections. The only postoperative complication was a seroma and subsequent infection, which resolved with conservative treatment in the case presented in Figure 8–9. The dissection for the saphenous nerve is extensive and must be adequately drained to avoid this problem.

We avoid use of the superficial radial nerve. It has many advantages, including a large amount of neural tissue area, minimal branching, anterior surface position, and one dominant dependable vascular supply (radial artery). However, there now are alternative nerves, as elucidated by this study, which do not require sacrifice of a major vessel. Also, the superficial radial nerve supplies only a graft of moderate length. The senior author (JKT) successfully used the superficial radial nerve twice as a vascularized free nerve graft for upper extremity reconstruction and simultaneously reconstructed the radial artery with an interposition vein graft.

The medial sural nerve has a very unreliable vascular supply. It is located in a posterior position and has considerable neural area loss (distal to proximal). We have used this nerve only once. At the present time we feel the saphenous nerve is a better alternative.

The lateral antebrachial cutaneous nerve of the forearm was rejected as a possible donor nerve because of its unreliable blood supply. However, the percentage suitable for microvascular transfer was similar for the sural nerve and lateral antebrachial cutaneous nerve of the forearm (30% for the former and 25% for the latter). The sural nerve was listed as a possible donor nerve, and the lateral antebrachial cutaneous nerve was rejected only in deference to a previous report.[9] This showed that a higher percentage (60%) of sural nerves were available for microsurgical transfer. The discrepancy between results is as yet unexplained.[9]

In August 1983 the senior author (JKT) used the superficial peroneal nerve as a free vascularized graft. This was the first time this nerve was used clinically. We feel that this nerve has many advantages, including anterior position, dependable blood supply, and sufficient neural tissue area.

The anterior tibial nerve may have a place in isolated cases. However, we are reluctant to sacrifice a major lower extremity vessel.

We have found the ulnar nerve ideal for brachial plexus reconstruction when roots C8 and T1 have been avulsed. It has sufficient neural tissue, dependable blood supply, and surgically is just an extension of the regular brachial plexus exploration. Since 1981, we have successfully attempted twelve vascularized or pedicle transfers of the ulnar nerve based on the superior ulnar collateral artery.

SUMMARY

With the advent of vascularized nerve graft transfer, a new method of managing nerve gaps was introduced. Theoretical considerations plus limited clinical and experimental evidence indicate advantages to these grafts in certain situations. However, investigation has been limited by the need for further clarification of nerve intrinsic and extrinsic blood supply, a paucity of available donor nerves, and technical problems in creating cable grafts. This chapter reviews our work in addressing these problems. First, a new classification of nerve blood supply is presented that helps predict those nerves best suited for microsurgical transfer. Second, six potential donor nerves are reviewed, including their surgical exposure, and when applicable, our clinical experience. Finally, methods of technically creating cable grafts while maintaining blood supply are discussed. Much work still remains to be done clarifying the indications for vascularized nerve grafts and determining the extent or absence of their benefits.

References

1. Albert, E.: Einige Operationen an Nerven. Wien. Med. Presse, 26:1285, 1885.
2. Alpar, E. K., and Brooks, D. M.: Long-term results of ulnar to median nerve pedicle grafts. Hand, 10:61, 1978.
3. Ballance, C., and Duel, A. B.: The operative treatment of facial palsy by the introduction of nerve grafts. Arch. Otolaryngol., 15:1, 1932.
4. Breidenbach, W. B., and Terzis, J. K.: Vascularized Nerve Grafts. A.S.P.R.S. Essay Contest, 1983.
5. Brooks, D.: The place of nerve grafting in orthopedic surgery. J. Bone Joint Surg., 37-A:299, 1955.

6. Bunnell, S.: Surgery of the nerves of the hand. Surg. Gynecol. Obstet., *44*:145, 1927.

7. Bunnell, S., and Boyes, J. H.: Nerve grafts. Am. J. Surg., *44*:64, 1939.

8. Edgerton, M. T.: Cross arm nerve pedicle flap for reconstruction of major defects of the median nerve. Surgery, *64*:248, 1968.

9. Franchinelli, A., Masquelet, A., Restrepo, J., and Gilbert, A.: The vascularized sural nerve. Int. J. Microsurg., *3*:57, 1981.

10. Lundborg, G.: Ischemic nerve injury. Experimental studies on intraneural microvascular pathophysiology and nerve function in a limb subjected to temporary circulatory arrest. Scand. J. Plast. Reconstr. Surg., Supplement 6:1, 1970.

11. Lundborg, G.: Structure and function of the intraneural microvessels as related to trauma, edema formation and nerve function. J. Bone Joint Surg., *57-A*:938, 1975.

12. Lundborg, G.: Intraneural microvascular pathophysiology as related to ischemia and nerve injury. *In* Daniel, R. K., and Terzis, J. K. (eds.): Reconstructive Microsurgery. Boston, Little, Brown and Co., 1977, p.334.

13. Lundborg, G., and Branemark, P. I.: Microvascular structure and function of peripheral nerves. Vital microscopic studies of the tibial nerve in the rabbit. Adv. Microcirc., *1*:66, 1968.

14. Lundborg, G., and Rydevik, B.: Effects of stretching the tibial nerve of the rabbit. A preliminary study of the intraneural circulation and the barrier function of the perineurium. J. Bone Joint Surg., *55-B*:390, 1973.

15. Millesi, H.: Microsurgery of peripheral nerves. Hand *5*:157, 1973.

16. Millesi, H.: Healing of nerves. Clin. Plast. Surg., *4*:459, 1977.

17. Millesi, H., Meissl, G., and Berger, A.: The interfascicular nerve grafting of the ulnar and median nerve. J. Bone Joint Surg., *54-A*:727, 1972.

18. Millesi, H.: Personal communication.

19. Phillipeaux, J. M., and Vulpian, A.: Note sur les essais de greffe d'un proncox de nerf lingual entre les deux bouts de 17 hypoglosse. Arch. Physiol. Norm. Path., *3*:618, 1870.

20. Platt, H.: On the results of bridging gaps in injured nerve trunks by autogenous fascial tubulization and autogenous nerve grafts. Br. J. Surg., *7*:384, 1919.

21. Remensnyder, J.: Physiology of nerve healing and nerve grafts. *In* Krizek, T. (ed.): Symposium on Basic Science in Plastic Surgery. St. Louis, C. V. Mosby, 1976, p. 1960.

22. Seddon, H. J.: Nerve grafting. J. Bone Joint Surg., *45-B*:447, 1963.

23. Smith, J. W.: Factors influencing nerve repair. Blood supply of peripheral nerves. Arch. Surg., *93*:335, 1966.

24. Smith, J. W.: Factors influencing nerve repair. Collateral circulation of peripheral nerves. Arch. Surg., *93*:433, 1966.

25. Spurling, R. G., Lyons, W. R., Whitcomb, B. B., and Woodall, B.: The failure of whole fresh homogenous nerve grafts in man. J. Neurosurg., *2*:79, 1945.

26. Strange, F. G. St. C.: An operation for nerve pedicle grafting. Preliminary communications. Br. J. Surg., *34*:423, 1947.

27. Sunderland, S.: Blood supply of nerves of the upper limb in man. Arch. Neurol. Psychiatry, *54*:280, 1945.

28. Sunderland, S.: Nerves and Nerve Injuries, 2nd ed. Edinburgh, Churchill-Livingstone, 1978.

29. Tarlov, I. M., and Epstein, J. A.: Nerve grafts: The importance of an adequate blood supply. J. Neurosurg., *2*:49, 1945.

30. Taylor, I. G., and Ham, F. J.: The free vascularized nerve graft. Plast. Reconstr. Surg., *57*:413, 1976.

31. Taylor, I. G.: Nerve grafting with simultaneous microvascular reconstruction. Clin. Orth. Rel. Res., *133*:56, 1978.

32. Terzis, J. K., Faibisoff, B., and Williamson, H. B.: The nerve gap: Suture under tension vs. graft. Plast. Reconstr. Surg., *56*:166, 1975.

9

Vascularized Sural Nerve Graft

■

Alain Gilbert, M.D.

Nerve grafts are the surgeon's solution to a fair number of difficult situations, allowing him or her to fill in lengthy tissue losses and obtain satisfactory results. However, some patients are difficult to treat, especially those in whom a loss of nerve tissue is associated with multiple lesions causing intense fibrosis and in whom there is a poor vascularization of the bed along which the graft is to be laid. In these patients, the risk of failure because of graft necrosis is high. Various factors determine graft survival:[10]

1. The quality of the underlying bed.

2. The diameter of the graft. This was the fundamental cause of failures in the past, when attempts were made to transplant entire nerve trunks.

3. The internal organization of the graft. Sunderland maintains that grafts made up of many small nerve bundles survive better than those made up of large bundles.

4. The size of the graft. A short graft will be revascularized from its ends more quickly than a long graft that needs a blood supply throughout its entire length.

Guidelines governing the use of nerve grafts have gradually evolved in response to these different requirements:

1. Trunk grafts are no longer used. They have been replaced by cable grafts from small-diameter sensory nerves; these grafts provide good revascularization under satisfactory conditions.[13]

2. Most surgeons prefer to lengthen the graft through healthy tissue rather than take the shortest route through an area of fibrosis.

Despite this progress and the excellent results obtained, some conditions in which fibrosis is extensive (Volkmann's contracture, radiation injury) have not been satisfactorily treated. In some anatomic sites (e.g., the brachial plexus) the number and length of required nerve grafts are greater than the available pool of sensory nerves. In such cases, the surgeon is forced to sacrifice nerve trunks (e.g., the ulnar nerve trunk), which is associated with a considerable risk of ischemic necrosis.

These two situations constitute one of the most formidable challenges in nerve surgery. In the past, use of pedicled nerve grafts, which retained their blood supply, was occasionally successful. These grafts were used to reconstruct the median nerve[2, 9] or the sciatic nerve.[5] However, surgery had to be staged over several different operative procedures and involved the sacrifice of a major nerve.

With the advances in microsurgery, Taylor and Ham[14] proposed the concept of nerve grafts that are revascularized by nerve-artery anastomoses.[14] This eventually led to the solution of managing the two difficult situations mentioned above.

VASCULAR ARCHITECTURE OF NERVES

The vascular architecture of nerves was studied as early as the seventeenth century by van der Spiegel (1627) and in the eighteenth century by various anatomists (von Haller, 1752; Isenglamm, 1768; Ruysch, 1791). Reference should also be made to the remarkable work of Ranvier (1878), who described the anastomoses between the intra- and epineural systems. However, the pathologic aspects of blood supply to the nerves had not been studied until the mid-twentieth century. Sunderland[11] (1945) made a special study of the relationships between the blood supply of different human nerves, and more recently Lundborg[6] (1970) determined the physiology of this blood supply based on in vivo studies.

Embryologically, the nerve-artery pedicle lies along the axis of the developing limb. In the upper limb, the interosseous artery gives off a large branch that follows the median nerve and supplies blood to the hand during part of embryonic life. This artery regresses when its role is taken over by the radial and ulnar arteries, but it remains a relatively important structure in the adult.

The vascular system of nerves is made up of a longitudinal intraneuronal network running in the perineurium and an epineuronal network, also longitudinal, that receives a supplementary blood supply at regular intervals from the nutrient arteries. There are multiple anastomoses between these two systems. Indeed it is because of these multiple connections that a nerve can be freed over a considerable length and its blood supply maintained intact despite the section of several nutrient arteries.[6] Conversely, the existence of one nutrient artery is enough to maintain normal flow in an isolated segment of nerve.[6] This allows a vascularized nerve to be divided into strands.[4]

DONOR SITES

Since the time that Taylor[14] first used the superficial branch of the radial nerve, a variety of other sites for vascularized nerve grafts have been proposed. They must possess the qualities required of a nerve graft, defined by Sunderland,[10] and have a well-established, easily transplantable blood supply that does not require sacrifice of a major limb artery. Very few nerves meet these criteria.

The Sural Nerve

Without any doubt the sural nerve most closely fulfills the criteria outlined above and is the nerve most commonly used for grafts. It is long (35 to 40 cm) and has a well-recognized bundle structure. Its blood supply was described by Faschinelli and his co-workers[4] (Fig. 9–1). The superficial sural artery (Figs. 9–2 and 9–3) arises either directly from the popliteal artery or from the sural arteries. It gives off several cutaneous branches and follows the sural nerve along almost its entire length, usually ending in the lower third of the leg by anastomosing with an ascending branch of the posterior tibial artery. The superficial sural artery sup-

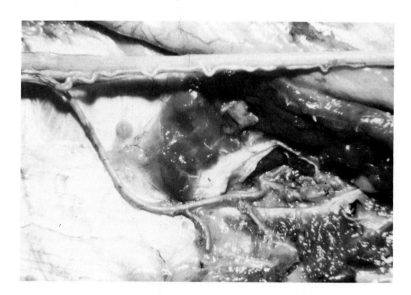

Figure 9–1. The superficial sural artery and the sural nerve. (From Gilbert, A.: Clin. Plast. Surg., 11:75, 1984.)

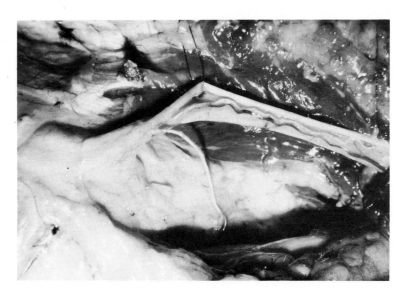

Figure 9–2. The artery and vein of the sural nerve. (From Gilbert, A.: Clin. Plast. Surg., *11*:75, 1984.)

plies the nerve with an average of seven nutrient arteries, with a gap of 4 or 6 cm between each. At its origin the diameter of the artery varies between 0.6 and 2.0 mm. In 80 per cent of cases, the artery is wider than 1 mm or else arises from a twin artery and can therefore be used for transfer of the nerve.

The surgical approach is made through a longitudinal posterior incision with the patient in the prone position. In the popliteal fossa the vascular pedicle is easily identified and followed to its origin. Its size and anatomic shape can then be determined and a decision made as to whether transfer is possible. If it is, the dissection is very easy and requires removing the nerve and its perineural structures (artery and satellite veins). The nerve is divided at both ends and is left pedicled to its blood vessels. On release of the tourniquet, its blood supply can be checked.

If the loss of tissue is fairly small and several strands are needed, the blood supply can be preserved by dividing the nerve while maintaining the vascular pedicle intact.

Of nine attempts to transfer the sural nerve with its blood supply, eight proved possible. In one case, the artery was very narrow (0.2 mm) and arose directly from the popliteal artery (Fig. 9–4).

Other Donor Sites

As mentioned previously, the sural nerve is the best cutaneous nerve available for grafting from the point of view of its blood supply and easy transfer; I have not had much personal experience working with any other nerve. However, other donor sites have been described and could possibly be used.

The Superficial Radial Nerve. The anatomy of this nerve was described by Taylor,[14] who was the first to use it for grafting. The superficial radial nerve is supplied by direct branches of the radial artery. It makes an excellent nerve graft, but its use is limited by

Figure 9–3. The origins of the superficial sural artery: JI = medial sural artery, JE = lateral sural artery, P = popliteal artery, and SE = superficial sural artery. (From Gilbert A.: Clin. Plast. Surg., *11*:74, 1984.)

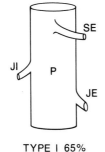

TYPE I 65%

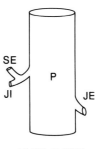

TYPE II 20%

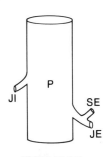

TYPE III 8%

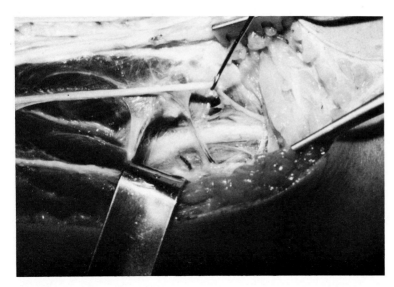

Figure 9–4. In some cases, the artery is very small and is not suitable for transfer. (From Gilbert, A.: Clin. Plast. Surg., *11:*76, 1984.)

insufficient length (17 to 28 cm) and above all by the fact that its transfer involves sacrifice of the radial artery.

The Medial Cutaneous Nerve of the Arm. This nerve was used for grafting by Comtet et al.,[3] who also studied its vascular anatomy. The nerve runs with the vena basilica, and its arterial blood supply comes from the brachial artery via either the superior ulnar collateral artery or the inferior ulnar collateral artery or from a muscle branch of the brachial artery (Fig. 9–5).

The Saphenous Nerve. The anatomy of the blood supply of the saphenous nerve is described in Chapter 8. The saphenous artery comes from the femoral artery at the level of the adductor ring. It gives off a descending cutaneous branch and a small artery that divides into a short ascending branch and a long descending branch.

The saphenous nerve is a long nerve, but its vascular dissection is somewhat difficult and only the distal half of the nerve is always supplied by the saphenous artery.

The Anterior Tibial Nerve. This nerve is larger than the purely cutaneous nerves. Only the distal two thirds can be removed, since the proximal third of the anterior tibial nerve gives off some important muscle branches. This proximal part of the nerve is supplied by a tributary of a large muscle branch of the anterior tibial artery. Over its distal two thirds, the nerve is supplied by multiple nutrient arteries arising directly

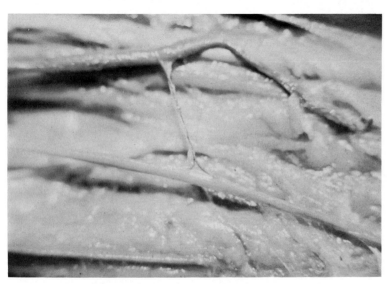

Figure 9–5. The medial cutaneous nerve of the forearm is vascularized by a branch of the superior ulnar collateral artery.

from the anterior tibial artery (Figs. 9–6 and 9–7).

The advantages of this nerve for grafting are its length, its size, and the absence of any branches in the distal two thirds. However the drawbacks are not inconsiderable and include the need to sacrifice a muscle in the foot (the extensor digitorum brevis) and, above all, the necessity of sacrificing a major limb artery.

The Ulnar Nerve. The use of the ulnar nerve for grafting purposes has always been tempting when one is faced with lesions involving the entire brachial plexus. However, in the majority of lesions, the C8 and T1 roots have been avulsed and there is no hope for functional recovery of the ulnar nerve. Furthermore, the use of the hand is still possible in the absence of the ulnar nerve as long as there is return of median nerve function. Thus, Strange[9] sacrificed the ulnar nerve in order to preserve the median nerve.

The ulnar nerve has a complex blood supply. As described by Sunderland,[10] it contains several components. In the axilla and the

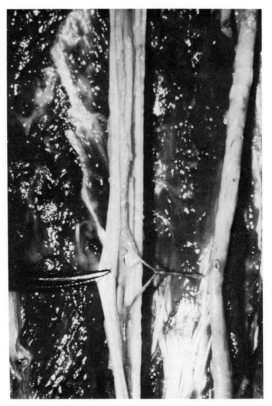

Figure 9–7. The distal part of the anterior tibial nerve is vascularized by direct branches of the anterior tibial artery.

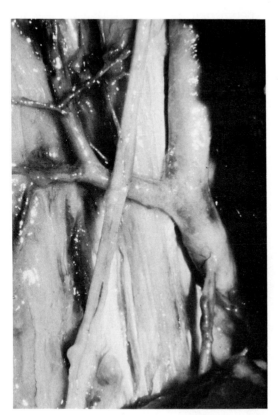

Figure 9–6. The superior part of the anterior tibial nerve is vascularized by a branch arising from the large muscular branch of the anterior tibial artery.

upper third of the arm, the ulnar nerve is supplied by direct branches of the axillary artery and by the superior ulnar collateral artery. In the elbow and in the lower third of the arm, blood supply comes from an anastomotic network made up of the posterior ulnar recurrent artery and the inferior ulnar collateral artery (Fig. 9–8). Finally, in the forearm, blood supply is shared by the posterior ulnar recurrent artery and direct branches of the ulnar artery.

The ulnar nerve in the forearm based on the ulnar artery has been used for repairs of the brachial plexus by Jamieson (personal communication, 1981). Since 1981 Terzis has used the whole length of the ulnar nerve as a free vascularized graft based on the superior ulnar collateral artery, thus avoiding sacrifice of a major artery to the upper extremity (see Chapter 8). Although this is undoubtedly a most interesting concept, it does mean that the surgeon must be absolutely certain of the avulsion of roots C8 and T1. The nerve can be taken only after direct exploration and visual confirmation of the avulsion.

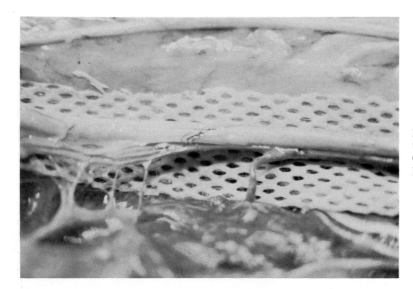

Figure 9–8. At the distal part of the arm, the ulnar nerve is vascularized by branches from the posterior ulnar recurrent artery.

The Sciatic Nerve. As studied by Sunderland,[10] this nerve has an extensive blood supply, mainly from the inferior gluteal artery and perforators from the deep femoral artery (Fig. 9–9).

My own anatomic studies[7] have shown that in the buttock the nerve is supplied by the greater sciatic artery, which is a branch of the inferior gluteal artery and which follows the nerve down to the popliteal fossa. In the thigh, the nutrient arteries arise from the second and third perforating arteries. The largest pedicle is provided by the third perforator; it has an average diameter of 2 mm and is about 7 cm long.

EXPERIMENTAL STUDIES

Very few experimental studies involving vascularized nerve grafts have been done; in fact, no complete study has yet been published. One difficulty is in finding a reliable experimental model for vascularized grafts. The ideal animal for statistical analysis of nerve regeneration is the rat; I have perfected a model for the vascularized graft of the sciatic nerve in the rat. Unfortunately, in this model, under the proper conditions of a well-vascularized bed, a nonvascularized graft becomes revascularized in 3 to 5 days. This is the time it takes for the axons to grow

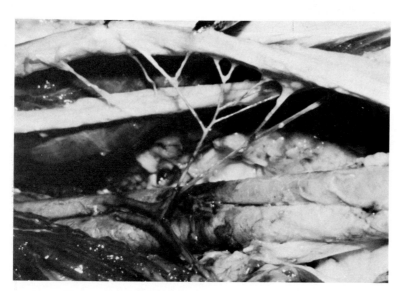

Figure 9–9. At the level of the division, the sciatic nerve is vascularized by branches from the third perforating artery.

through the proximal suture line and thus the graft is always revascularized when the axons reach this point. This means either that larger animals have to be used (animals whose nerves do not become revascularized as quickly, e.g., monkey, pig, dog) or that the process of revascularization of the sciatic nerve in the rat has to be prevented. In the former case, statistical analysis loses precision, whereas in the latter, there are still technical problems to be solved. However, it is logical to suppose that survival of the graft is ensured by its blood supply, and therefore, it is also logical to attempt these vascularized grafts in clinical situations in which the classic type of graft is certain to fail.

CLINICAL APPLICATIONS

Indications for vascularized nerve grafts are rare at present, but essentially they concern two clinical areas: nerve grafts in a highly unfavorable bed and use of trunk nerve grafts.

Nerve Graft in an Unfavorable Bed

This technique has proved useful in the treatment of Volkmann's contracture. Experience has shown that long grafts to replace the median nerve after its destruction have almost always failed. I have been able to use vascularized grafts of the sural nerve eight times—seven times in the reconstruction of the median nerve and once in reconstruction of the posterior tibial nerve.

The following is a typical case:

Case 1

A 5-year-old boy developed Volkmann's contracture of the right forearm after a fracture of the radius and ulna at age 4. A large graft was carried out by means of a Scaglietti procedure. Subsequently, there was total paralysis of the median and ulnar nerves in the hand, with hypoesthesia and trophic changes. On August 10, 1979, a second Scaglietti procedure was carried out through a forearm approach. The median nerve was divided at the distal third of the forearm, as was the ulnar artery. The gap due to loss of tissue measured 6 cm.

With the patient in the prone position, the right sural nerve was excised. The arterial pedicle came from the inferior sural artery and was 1 mm in width. On release of the tourniquet, there was

excellent revascularization. The nerve was positioned in the forearm, arteries and veins were sutured, and revascularization occurred. The nerve had been divided into four strands, each one 7 cm long, while preserving the continuity of the nutrient artery. Eighteen months later protective sensory perception reappeared in the distribution of the median nerve and the trophic changes had disappeared. There was no return of motor function.

What is remarkable about this case is not only the apparent ease of axon progression with the recovery of useful sensation, but also the speed of this regeneration, quite as though it had occurred under the most favorable local conditions.

Nerve Trunk Grafts

Basically this means using a sacrificed nerve trunk to replace considerable tissue loss. The following case illustrates what can be achieved using this approach:

Case 2

A 20-year-old woman lost both legs and suffered total left brachial plexus paralysis as a result of a traffic accident on February 9, 1981. Since she showed no signs of recovery in the left arm, she was operated upon on June 17, 1981. Roots C5, C6, and C7 were found to be divided and roots C8 and T1 were torn away. Given the extent of tissue loss (18 cm) and the unavailability of nerve grafts, it was decided to use the left sciatic nerve. With the patient in the prone position, the distal 18 cm of the sciatic nerve was removed, together with the bifurcation. Blood supply to the nerve was provided by a large vascular pedicle from the third perforator. The artery was 1.2 mm wide, the vein 2 mm. On release of the tourniquet, revascularization of the nerve was observed.

The sciatic nerve was positioned behind the clavicle. The trunk was sutured to roots C5, C6, and C7 and the bifurcation: common peroneal nerve to the axillary nerve and posterior tibial nerve to the median and the musculocutaneous nerves. Vascular anastomoses were used for the greater pectoral pedicle.

One year later the results were as follows: deltoid = 2, biceps = 0, and flexor digitorum sup. = 3. DTP (distal tingling percussion/Tinel's sign) for the median nerve was below the elbow. This is, of course, an unusual case, and it is not often that the surgeon is able to use the sciatic nerve for a vascularized graft. However, in this case, there was practically no other solution to this dramatic problem.

It is difficult to assess the results of these grafts. They are certainly not better than those of classic strand grafts carried out on

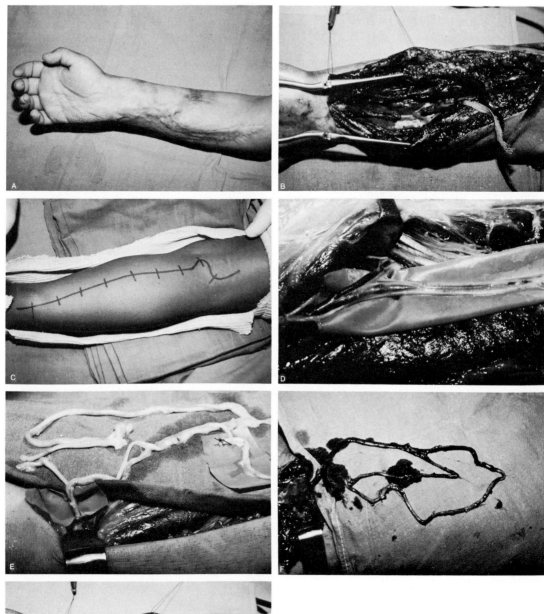

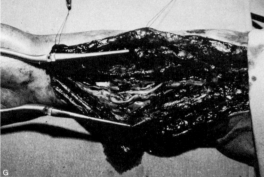

Figure 9–10. Case 1 (see text). *A*, Volkmann's contracture in a 5-year-old boy. *B*, There is a 6 cm loss of substance of the median nerve. *C*, Approach to the sural nerve. *D*, The large vascular pedicle. *E*, The nerve is cut and left on its pedicle. *F*, After tourniquet release, the nerve is revascularized. *G*, The nerve has been divided into four grafts.

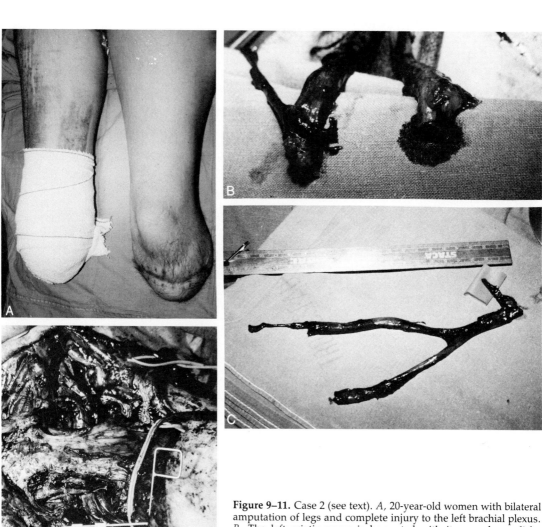

Figure 9–11. Case 2 (see text). *A,* 20-year-old women with bilateral amputation of legs and complete injury to the left brachial plexus. *B,* The left sciatic nerve is harvested with its vascular pedicle. Good bleeding was obtained from the extremities. *C,* The graft with the vascular pedicle. *D,* The anastomosis with the pectoralis major artery and vein. The sciatic nerve is seen passing under the clavicle.

an excellent bed. The patients who come to this kind of operation often have long-standing disorders with considerable destruction of tissue, and such conditions must influence the results. What counts is that there is even a slight degree of recovery, given that satisfactory repair is impossible using established methods.

Vascularized nerve grafts have their place in the practice of microsurgery. This place is not yet well defined because of the lack of experimental studies. The main indications at the present time for such grafts are tissue loss in an unfavorable bed and the use of large nerve trunks in very extensive lesions.

References

1. Adams, W. E.: The blood supply of nerves. Historical review. J. Anat., 76:323, 1942.
2. Barnes, R., Bacsich, P., and Wyburn, G.: A histological study of a pre-degenerated nerve graft. Br. J. Surg., 33:130, 1945.
3. Comtet, J. J., Bertrand, H., Moyen, B., and Condamine, J.: Greffe nerveuse vascularisée utilisant le brachial cutané interne transplanté avec un pédicule vasculaire.
4. Faschinelli, A., Masquelet, A., Restrepo, J., and Gilbert, A.: Int. J. Microsurg., 3:57, 1981.
5. MacCarthy, C. S.: Two stage autograft for repair of extensive damage to the sciatic nerve. J. Neurosurg., 8:318, 1951.
6. Lundborg, G.: Ischemic nerve injury. Scand. J. Plast. Reconstr. Surg., Suppl. 1970.
7. Restrepo, J., and Gilbert A.: Vascularization of the trunk of the sciatic nerve. Clinical application. Int. J. Microsurg., Vol. 4, 1982.
8. Seddon, H. J.: Surgical Disorders of the Peripheral Nerves. Edinburgh, Churchill-Livingstone, 1972.
9. Strange, F. G.: An operation for nerve pedicle grafting. Br. J. Surg., 34:423, 1947.
10. Sunderland, S.: Nerves and Nerve Injuries. Edinburgh, Churchill-Livingstone, 1972.
11. Sunderland, S.: Blood supply of the peripheral nerves. Arch. Neurol. Psychiatry, 54:283, 1945.
12. Sunderland, S.: The blood supply of the sciatic nerve. Arch. Neurol. Psychiatry, 54:280, 1945.
13. Sunderland, S., and Ray L.: The selection and use of autografts for bridging gaps in injured nerves. Brain, 70:75, 1947.
14. Taylor, G. I., and Ham, F.: The free vascularized nerve graft. Plast. Reconstr. Surg., 57:413, 1976.

CLINICAL ASPECTS OF TRAUMATIC NEUROPATHIES

PART 2

10

Modulation of Nociception and Analgesia—Localization of Spinal Mechanisms

■

George E. Goode, Ph.D.

Presently, there is no unified theory that explains man's conscious appreciation of pain. Although we maintain an ability to modulate this sensation, the mechanisms that are responsible for normal or abnormal modulation of nociception have not been elucidated. Although the pattern theory of visceral and somatic sensibility incorporates some of our notions of nociceptive mechanisms, we are certain that the stimulus-specificity of peripheral nerves must be an integral part of a unified theory. A unified theory must account for several other factors. It must explain why nociceptive information may be interpreted differently from visceral and body wall structures, e.g., why there are differences in our conscious awareness of painful stimuli from different tissues within visceral or body wall compartments, such as epidermis, dermis, or periosteum, or within the layers of one tissue type. In addition, we suspect that the relative proportion of fiber types in the peripheral nerves affects pain threshold and that degeneration in the central nervous system may produce intractable pain and alter endogenous inhibitory mechanisms located in the spinal cord dorsal horn, the brain stem reticular core, and the forebrain. Nociceptive mechanisms localized in the substantia gelatinosa (SG) of the spinal cord have received special attention in recent years.

The SG of the spinal cord receives primary afferent projections from the dorsal roots, dorsal columns, and dorsolateral fasciculus.

In addition, segmental and suprasegmental axons terminate here. The SG and its associated lamina form a complex structure. It has been involved in the localization and manipulation of a variety of active components, including neurotransmitters and modulators, acetylcholine, gamma-aminobutyric acid, biogenic amines, and several neuropeptides. In addition, opiate receptors have been localized here, as have active enzymes, including acetylcholinesterase and fluoride-resistant acid phosphatase. Small cells in the marginal zone (lamina I) and SG (lamina II) receive few axosomatic contacts. In contrast, their processes are reportedly involved in axodendritic, axoaxonic, dendrodendritic, and dendroaxonic interactions. One center for these synaptic interactions is localized in a complex synaptic array or glomerulus, in which the individual components may arise from different sources. This complex neuropil poses technical problems for current physiologic investigations as well as anatomic analyses.

There is also considerable controversy concerning the distribution of small dorsal root fibers (mainly the A-delta and C-fibers) within the dorsal horn of the spinal cord. This controversy in part arises from technical limitations inherent in previous attempts to study the anatomy and physiology of the small fiber systems of the central nervous system. It has been shown that by using Fink-Heimer impregnation the degenerating central processes of ganglionic cells can be identified by transecting their peripheral processes.[32, 41, 80] This reaction of ganglionic cells to peripheral trauma has also been demonstrated at the ultrastructural level in the spinal cord.[28, 29] The issues remain as to whether this central change is a transganglionic effect or a product of ganglionic cell death and to what extent these changes affect sensory function. For example, limb removal has been shown not only to affect the dorsal root ganglia, but also to cause cell loss in the second-order neurons of the dorsal column nuclei in the adult.[37]

In spite of the anatomic and physiologic limitations thus far encountered, it is believed that some of the major neuroanatomic and physiologic substrates that modulate spinal nociception reside in the dorsal horn, specifically in laminae I, II, and III, and the base of the dorsal horn, i.e., in lamina V (for more recent reviews see references 6a, 26, 39, 54, and 56).

PRIMARY AFFERENT LOCALIZATION

Much of the classic anatomy of Cajal[64] and of Ranson[65, 66] concerning the primary afferent systems that project to the dorsal horn, as well as the anatomy of the substantia gelatinosa and its intrinsic circuitry, has been reviewed and updated by Szentagothai,[73] the Scheibels,[69] and more recently by Kerr[39] and Beals and Fox.[8] There is general agreement that at least two different axonal systems, based on fiber size, are distributed within the gelatinous substance. These data are derived primarily from Golgi-impregnated material.[8, 64, 69, 73] First, the flame-shaped arbors of Cajal are well known in neonatal material. In the adult these myelinated fibers enter the gelatinous substance from its ventral aspect. The second component is made up of small A-delta and C-fibers, which course mainly in the dorsolateral fasciculus (Lissauer's tract) and form a capping plexus over the dorsal horn neuropil. The latter fiber system enters the SG at its dorsal extreme and overlaps the terminal distribution of the looping flame-shaped arbors in laminae II and III of the dorsal horn. A third afferent component also appears to exist and is referred to as Cajal's marginal collaterals. This third system is said to enter the capping plexus of lamina I and is thought to terminate there.

The distribution of primary afferents to laminae I, II, and III has been difficult to

evaluate experimentally because of the capricious silver staining of degenerating axoplasm.[12, 18, 33, 71, 72] Although all of these studies report some degeneration in laminae I and II after dorsal root transection, the existence of a strong, organized dorsal root projection to these areas has been demonstrated only recently. Brown et al.[10, 11] and Takahachi and Otsuka[74] showed that the highest concentration of substance P, a small peptide, is localized in the dorsal laminae of the dorsal horn. This concentration decreases on the central side of a ligature of the dorsal roots, whereas it accumulates on the ganglion side. Hokfelt et al.[35] have shown that two different populations of small cells in the dorsal root ganglion contain different peptides, somatostatin and substance P. These small peptides are also present in the dorsal horn, but their distribution differs. Substance P is localized in laminae I, II, and III, over the dorsomedial bend of the dorsal horn, around the central canal, and to a lesser extent in the base of the dorsal horn. Somatostatin is almost exclusively localized to laminae II and III. These data correlated with the organization of small fiber afferents to the marginal and SG layers, as originally described by Cajal[64] in 1911. There may be a correlation between the localization of substance P and somatostatin with the different zones of termination for the small fiber systems in the dorsal horn. In addition, based on experimental degeneration and autoradiography studies, LaMotte[44] suggested that the C-fiber afferents project mainly to laminae II and III, whereas the A-delta afferents terminate in lamina I and the dorsal half of lamina II. It has also been demonstrated[3] that an opiate antagonist, H diprenorphine, binds to the neuropil of laminae I and II,[3] and LaMotte et al.[45] suggest that the opiate receptors are on the primary afferent terminals in the same laminae. All of these results support the notion that some of the major neuroanatomic and physiologic substrates of nociception reside in the dorsal laminae of the dorsal horn and that the specific synaptic relationships of the small primary afferents in this region must be determined.

The electron microscope has been of significant advantage to the study of primary afferents to the dorsal horn. Ralston[61] was one of the first to report the synaptic relationships of degenerating profiles in the dorsal horn following dorsal root section. Heimer and Wall[33] reported that the central axon terminals of complex synaptic clusters in the SG degenerate following rhizotomies of 1 to 3 days' survival time. The identification of primary afferent terminals in some glomeruli of the SG has been confirmed by Ralston[61] in the cat, Coimbra et al.[74] and Knyihar et al.[40] in the rat, and Goode[28, 29] in the opossum spinal cord. These data correlate well with the ultrastructural analysis of the neuropil of the subnucleus caudalis of the spinal trigeminal system and the identification of the terminals of primary afferents that serve nociception, which terminate in the SG glomeruli of that nucleus.[22-25]

NORMAL STRUCTURE OF DORSAL HORN (Figs. 10-1 to 10-4)

The normal structure of laminae I to III does not differ in any major way from previous descriptions of these laminae outlined by Gobel[22-25] for the mammalian dorsal horn of the caudal medulla. Therefore, a detailed description of the ultrastructure of the dorsal horn will not be presented here. Although the components of the neuropil of these three laminae is similar, each layer has distinctive characteristics. Lamina I (marginal layer) caps the dorsal horn of the spinal cord. This layer may exceed 100 μ in thickness laterally, but is attenuated medially as it forms the dorsomedial bend of the dorsal horn to join lamina I from the contralateral side over the central canal. This continuity is broken in the enlargements by the neural elements of laminae IV–VII.

The large projection cells (Waldeyer cells) are limited to the marginal layer and the outer half of lamina II. Their proximal dendrites course longitudinally in lamina I and in the dorsal extensions of lamina II. These

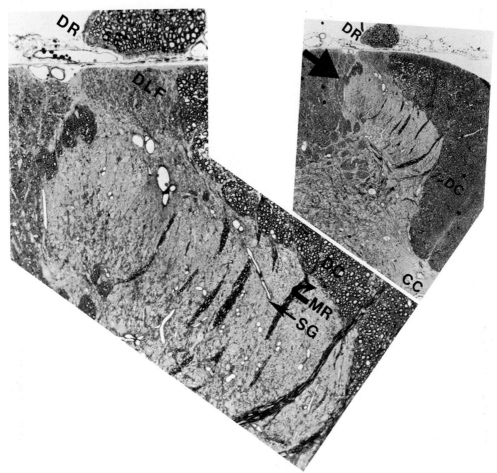

Figure 10–1. Low-power magnifications of the dorsal horn, photographed from 1.0 μ plastic sections. Solid block arrows indicate the location of the substantia gelatinosa. CC = central canal, DR = dorsal rootlet, DLF = dorsolateral fasciculus, DC = dorsal columns, MR = marginal zone, SG = substantia gelatinosa.

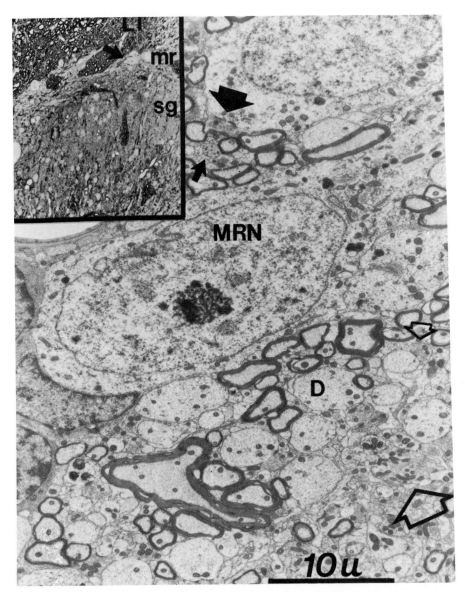

Figure 10–2. Low-power electron micrograph of the marginal layer (lamina I). MRN = marginal neuron cell body, D = dendrite. The larger solid arrow indicates the location of an axosomatic synapse (rare); the smaller solid arrow points to a presynaptic terminal filled with dense core vesicles. The large open block arrow indicates a synaptic glomerulus; small open arrow localizes an axodendritic synapse (frequently seen). *Insert,* the black arrow indicates the location from which the electron micrograph was taken.

dendritic profiles are frequently seen in electron micrographs, in addition to dense bundles of unmyelinated axons, scattered myelinated axons, and synaptic terminals containing dense core and clear vesicles. Many of these axon terminals originate from primary afferents as well as from multiple suprasegmental sources, i.e., brain stem reticular formation, raphe nuclei, locus coeruleus, and midbrain tegmentum[29–31] and terminate on dendritic shafts and spines in the marginal layer. The small myelinated axons

that give a "peppered" appearance to the marginal layer extend ventrally and form parallel arrays in laminae II and III and delimit columns of lightly stained neuropil.

Laminae II and III share a distinctive characteristic, namely, a specialized synaptic structure called a complex synaptic array by Ralston,[61] or a synaptic glomerulus by Kerr,[39] Coimbra et al.,[15] and Gobel.[23] This structure is made up of large central *boutons en passage,* surrounded by five to eight smaller synaptic elements enclosed by glial processes. Postsynaptic elements include dendritic shafts, racemose appendages, and spines from dendrite 1 from SG interneurons and from projection neurons in laminae I and V. Some of these dendritic shafts and racemose dendritic appendages associated with the central terminal have packets of clear vesicles.

The origins of many of the various components of the SG glomeruli and its surrounding neuropil have not been identified, although several investigators have worked on the problem.[15, 23–25, 28, 29, 33, 38–41, 61–63, 67] It appears, however, that the central endings in some SG glomeruli originate from small primary afferents and that the major postsynaptic elements of primary afferent terminals are glomerular and extraglomerular dendrites as well as dendritic appendages. Our own

data suggest that the latter processes arise from (1) small marginal interneurons and large Waldeyer's cells, (2) cells of the SG proper, and (3) cells in more ventral laminae, principally dendrites of laminae IV and V cells. At least two of the proposed postsynaptic cells (lamina I neurons and cells in the base of the dorsal horns IV and V) have been shown to transmit nociceptive information through the spinothalamic tract.[1, 2, 14, 19, 42, 75, 81, 82] The third group of postsynaptic cells (i.e., the SG cells) are thought to be interneurons of laminae I–III. The suggested inhibitory role of some of these SG interneurons[79] has gained support from studies that localize glutamate decarboxylase, the enzyme related to the inhibitory neurotransmitter GABA, in the neuropil of laminae I–III.[4–6, 52]

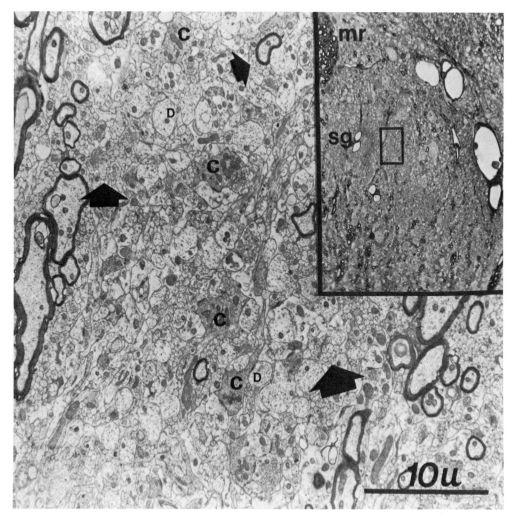

Figure 10–3. This electron micrograph was taken fron the SG open block in the insert. Note the vertical display of central axons (C), which synapse in glomeruli. D = dendrite, mr = marginal zone. Solid black arrows indicate the location of bundles of nonmyelinated axons.

Preliminary work has concentrated on the synaptology of the glomerular fields of the SG. The identification of some of the brain stem afferents to the neuropil of laminae I and II has begun also. The first three laminae of Rexed from the lumbar enlargement have been studied by light and electron microscopy. In most species thus far studied, the marginal layer (lamina I) forms an incomplete cap over the dorsal horn and extends a variable distance into the dorsal horn (usually 75 ± 10 μ). Its neuropil is rich in longitudinal bundles of small (0.10–0.25 μ) unmyelinated axons, scattered profiles of myelinated axons, and large dendrites (measuring up to 7 μ). Marginal neurons have small (8–12 μ) spindle-shaped perikaryons, and many of their dendrites course over the neuropil of laminae I and II. Axodendritic contacts are frequently encountered in lamina I and the terminals contain both clear and dense-cored synaptic vesicles. In addition to the small neuronal population, the marginal layer also contains a limited number of giant Waldeyer cells.

Although most cells of laminae I, II, and III and some cells of laminae IV contribute neuronal processes to the neuropil of the SG, some of these dendritic processes have appendages that arise as thin pedicles and terminate in spheroidal bodies 1 to 3 μ in diameter. These appendages have the configuration of impregnated axons, although, unlike axons, they issue from the dendrite singly, in clusters, or as a "string of beads." Processes such as these have been reported in other nuclear groups that receive primary afferents from cranial nerves.[20, 60] Profiles of the ultrastructural corollaries to these Golgi impregnations are shown in Figure 10–4, and they form the basis for the identification of these processes in the glomerulus of the SG.

In mammals, the SG of the lumbar spinal cord is characterized by fields of glomeruli (Figs. 10–3 and 10–4). These complex syn-

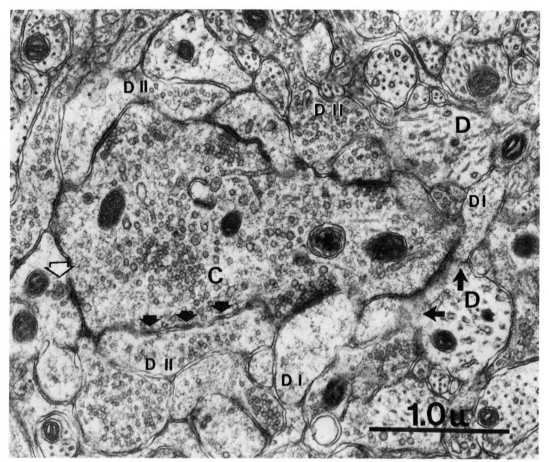

Figure 10–4. High-power electron micrograph of the synaptic glomerulus in the SG. The central axon terminal (C) is presynaptic to both type 1 (DI) and type 2 (DII) dendritic spines.

aptic arrays contain a central (C) primary afferent terminal surrounded by multiple pre- and postsynaptic elements. The C-terminal is presynaptic to dendritic shafts and two types of dendritic spines. Type I dendritic spines are the major postsynaptic elements in the glomerulus. They participate in dendrodentritic synapses with type 2 dendritic spines, which contain ovoid synaptic vesicles. Some C-terminals degenerate within 24 hours following dorsal rhizotomy and "darken" 2 weeks after *peripheral nerve lesions.*

In addition to glomeruli, the marginal and SG layers of the dorsal horn contain many extraglomerular terminals with granular synaptic vesicles. Some of these terminals degenerate 48 hours after (1) cervical hemisection, (2) raphe magnus lesions, and (3) rostral

pontine or midbrain lesions. These dense-cored, vesicle-containing terminals contact small-diameter dendritic shafts in the marginal and dorsal half of the SG layer.

It is important to continue the analysis of the suprasegmental components of the SG neuropil and their synaptic interaction with primary afferents in order to understand a massive, although controversial, physiologic and pharmacologic literature concerned with central nociceptive facilitation and inhibition.

CENTRAL CHANGES FOLLOWING PERIPHERAL NERVE LESIONS
(Figs. 10–5 to 10–8)

The origin of the central terminals of the SG glomeruli was determined by using two

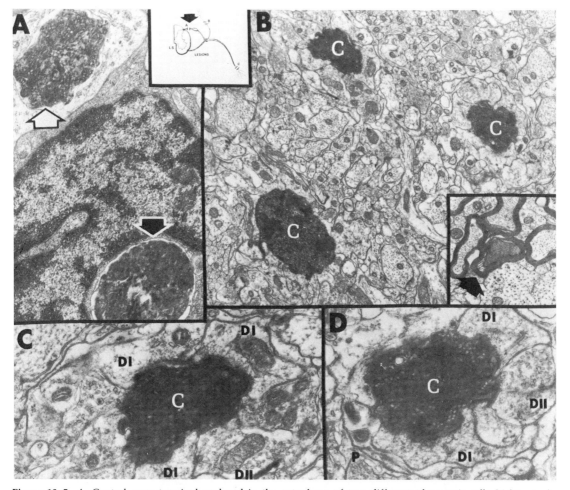

Figure 10–5. *A,* Central axon terminal enclosed in the cytoplasm of two different phagocytic cells 24 hours after dorsal rhizotomy (*insert*). *B,* Some degenerating central terminals (C) are still in contact with the glomerulus 48 hours after rhizotomy. *Insert,* degenerating small myelinated axon in the SG. *C* and *D,* High-power electron micrographs of degenerating central axon terminals following dorsal rhizotomy. DI = dendritic spine, type 1; DII = dendritic spine, type 2; P = peripheral terminal.

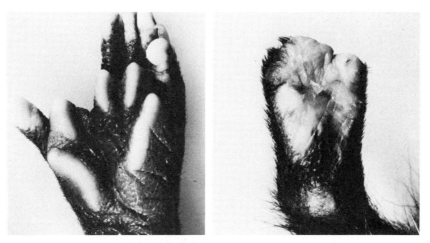

Figure 10–6. *A*, Normal hindpaw of opossum *Didelphis marsupialis virginiana*. *B*, Thirty day experimental lesion of opossum hindpaw.

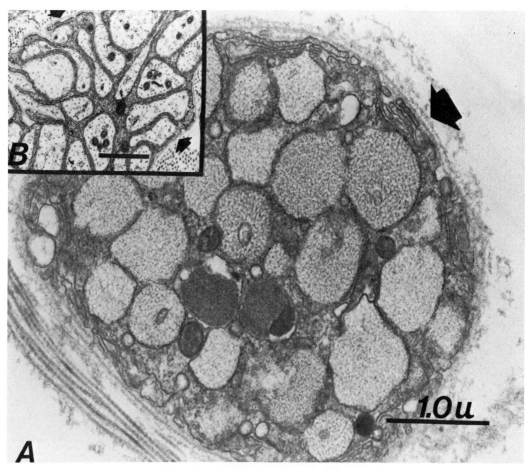

Figure 10–7. *A*, Electron micrograph of degenerating unmyelinated bundle at the dorsal root entry zone in the opossum seen after peripheral lesion (see Fig. 10–6). *B*, Normal Remak bundle. Arrows indicate location of basal lamina.

experimental techniques—dorsal rhizotomy and peripheral axotomy. Within 24 to 48 hours after dorsal rhizotomy, some of the central terminals of the SG glomerulus degenerated, although darkened synaptic profiles were most often associated with glial cytoplasm in all three dorsal layers of the spinal cord. In contrast, darkened unmyelinated and myelinated axonal fragments remained isolated in the neuropil. At these survival times, the degenerating central terminal is either of normal dimensions or slightly crenated. The mitochondria and synaptic vesicles (both clear and dense cored) are closely packed in a dense axoplasm. The synaptic cleft is widened and elongated.

Following experimental foot cautery or distal amputation, no electron microscopic changes were observed in the SG until 2 weeks after surgery. Observable changes in the *central processes* of ganglion cells were limited to unmyelinated axon bundles in the dorsal rootlets and a few small fragmented myelinated axons in the dorsal root entry zone. Reactive unmyelinated bundles (Remak bundles) identified in the dorsal rootlets were still surrounded by Schwann cell cytoplasm and associated basal lamina. The axons appeared disorganized and swollen, and their dense core vesicles, tubules, and mitochondria were absent. Most myelinated axons were filled with a flocculent material, although a few were dark and granular. Darkened myelinated axon profiles were limited to the dorsal root entry zone and the capping plexus of the marginal layer. In two rats in which the entire hindlimb was amputated (autocannibalism), darkened and fragmented axons were observed in the dorsal columns as well as in the dorsal roots, capping plexus, and dorsal horn matter.

The dark reaction of central terminals in glomeruli after peripheral insult is distinctly different compared with that seen after dor-

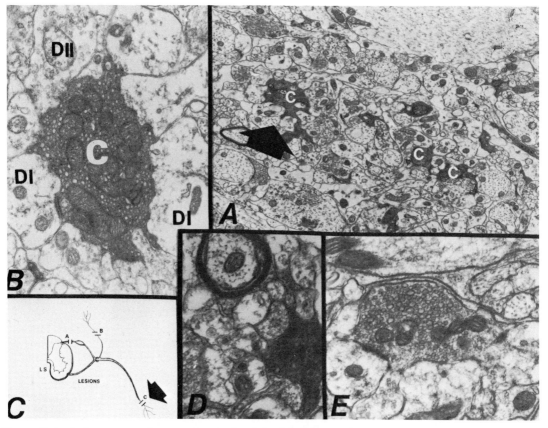

Figure 10–8. *A,* Low-power electron micrograph of the SG following long survival time after peripheral lesion indicated in *C* and in Figure 10–6*B*. *B,* Higher power electron micrograph of darkened central terminal (C) in a synaptic glomerulus. *C,* Solid arrow indicates location of the lesion. *D* and *E,* Darkened extraglomerular terminal includes both dense core vesicle terminals (D) and terminals with clear synaptic vesicles (E). DI = dendritic spine, type 1, DII = dendritic spine, type 2.

sal rhizotomy. The reaction is most intense following foot cautery. Although the axoplasm is dense and the synaptic vesicles are swollen, the mitochondria do not fragment. There is a high incidence of adherent junctions and a lack of glial engulfment of these terminals. Small degenerating myelinated axons, darkened unmyelinated axons, and preterminal and terminal segments filled with dense core and clear vesicles were observed in lamina I and II of the dorsal horn bilaterally, although contralateral degeneration was rare.

In summary, although many spinal ganglion cells terminate centrally as axodendritic contacts in the dorsal horn gray matter, a number of primary afferents are involved in complex synapses of the glomeruli in the SG and associated lamina. Within the SG we have experimentally demonstrated transganglionic changes at the ultrastructural level in the spinal cord. This "darkening" of the central processes of ganglionic cells after peripheral lesions is observed in the small myelinated and unmyelinated axon profiles in the marginal and SG layers and in some of the central terminals of the SG glomerulus. Degeneration has not been seen in the dorsal column system following our peripheral lesions. However, if ligature and transection of the peripheral nerve is accomplished closer to the ganglion, dorsal column degeneration can be elicited.[55]

Our hypothesis is that this "darkening" is the response of a select population of ganglionic cells, specifically the small cells that project their central processes to laminae I, II, and III of the dorsal horn. Peripheral lesions may be useful to (1) selectively study the response of the small ganglionic cells and (2) demonstrate the distribution and termination of their central processes.

This central change after peripheral manipulation may be related to degenerative atrophy of these neurons and, conceivably, of the same neurons in which Hokfelt et al.[35] demonstrated the presence of somatostatin and substance P. Although the physiologic role of these peptides is unclear, Henry[34] suggested that substance P may play a role in the excitation of spinal neurons that transmit nociception, whereas Hokfelt[35] stated that somatostatin exerts inhibitory actions in the several tissue types in which it has been isolated (e.g., in hypothalamus, in the extrahypothalamic brain regions, including primary afferent neurons, and in several peripheral tissues). Whether somatostatin and substance P, as well as other neuropeptides, play inhibitory and excitatory transmitter roles in nociceptive mechanisms remains to be elucidated. However, the presence of these peptides in peripheral tissues, as well as in the cell bodies and processes of primary afferent neurons, may be related to the response of some spinal ganglion cells to peripheral manipulations.

Peripheral nerve manipulation has distinct advantages over dorsal rhizotomies to study primary afferent pathways. Such manipulation does not interfere with the blood supply to the spinal cord, as has been reported to occur when laminectomy is needed, and does not produce a rapid glial response with phagocytosis of degenerating axon terminals. The use of peripheral nerve manipulations better reflects the physiologic and pathologic states of nociception encountered in practice. For example, the termination of dorsal versus ventral primary rami may be determined by anatomic dissection. Likewise, visceral and somatic afferents may be differentiated with peripheral manipulation not only in a dermatome, but also over a peripheral nerve field with distributions to several neighboring spinal segments. The overlap of primary afferent distribution in the dorsal horn may play an important role in normal sensibility, especially for pain sensation.[56] It is this overlap of primary afferents to the SG that may be important to our understanding of the pain states following spinal cord injury.

SUPRASEGMENTAL PROJECTIONS TO THE DORSAL HORN (Fig. 10–9)

Many brain stem nuclei send axons to terminate in the dorsal horn. By retrograde tracing techniques using horseradish peroxidase, axons that terminate in the SG and associated lamina are found to originate from the nucleus of Edinger-Westphal, ventral lateral periaqueductal gray, locus coeruleus and subcoeruleus, ventral gigantic and magnocellular reticular formation, and raphe nuclei. Most of these sources of suprasegmental projections to the dorsal horn have been confirmed by radioautographic methods.[7, 30] Degeneration produced by small electrolytic lesions in these nuclei can be seen in the SG with the electron microscope. Axons from the brain stem terminate on small dendritic shafts and spines, as well as on other axons.

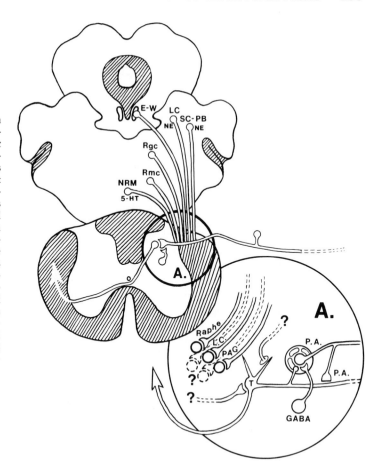

Figure 10–9. Schema of dorsal horn synaptic organization at *A*. Primary afferents (P.A.) terminate as axodendritic extraglomerular and complex glomerular components. Gabanergic neurons also terminate on the primary afferent terminals (GABA). Suprasegmental axons terminate as axodendritic contacts on undefined neurons. Suprasegmental axons that terminate in the dorsal horn originate from the ventromedial periaqueductal gray (E-W and PAG), the locus ceruleus (LC) and subcorrelus (SC) and parabrachial (PB) nuclei. Reticulospinals originate from the magnocellular and gigantocellular reticular nuclei raphe and from the raphe–nucleus raphe magnus (NRM). All suprasegmental inputs to the SG thus far studied terminate outside the glomerulus. NE = noradrenergic, T = transmitter neuron.

The terminals form asymmetrical contacts and contain both clear and dense-cored vesicles. No terminals are found associated with the complex glomeruli. Although degenerating myelinated axons from these lesions descend in all spinal funiculi, many reach the SG by way of the dorsal half of the lateral funiculus.[30]

PHYSIOLOGIC AND PHARMACOLOGIC SUBSTRATES OF NOCICEPTION AND ANALGESIA

The identification of suprasegmental afferents to the dorsal horn is important in light of recent physiologic and pharmacologic findings. Several brain stem nuclei in the dorsal midbrain have been identified that modulate the transmission of nociception, although other sites include the more rostral periaqueductal regions and sites adjacent to the third ventricle.[49–51] Similar investigations have been carried out on the cat, the rhesus monkey, and humans. Serotonergic projections from the nucleus raphe dorsalis and

nucleus raphe magnus, as well as adrenergic projections from locus coeruleus and subcoeruleus, terminate in lamina I, II and III of the spinal gray.

The analgesic effects of these neuronal systems have been demonstrated by the tail flick test, by direct stimulation,[36, 57, 58, 68] and by microinjection of narcotic analgesics. Analgesia can be interrupted by a putative serotonin blocker, by administration of the narcotic antagonist naloxone,[58] and by interference with the descending pathways in the dorsolateral funiculus of the spinal cord. Analgesia has also been measured directly by stimulating the nucleus of the dorsal raphe and recording the inhibitory response of dorsal horn nociceptive cells to noxious skin stimuli.

In addition to the brain stem stimulus–dependent system, other brain stem sites are thought to be involved in the modulation of nociception. For example, stimulation of the midbrain and medullary reticular formation is known to inhibit spinal cord flexion reflexes. These spinal withdrawal reflexes and pain perception are thought to be integrated mechanisms.[59] Stimulation of the medullary reticular formation also inhibits nociceptive responses of spinothalamic neurons, and stress analgesia (grid shock or rotation) is reported to be independent of the integrity of the dorsolateral funiculus and not reversible by naloxone. These studies suggest that there may be reticular afferents to the spinal cord that also modulate nociception.[13, 21, 83]

With the recent advances in peptide neurochemistry, specifically with the location of endogenous enkephalins, substance P, and somatostatin in addition to cholecystokinin, vasoactive intestinal polypeptide, octapeptide, pancreatic polypeptide, gastrin, and neurotensin within the brain stem, spinal ganglia, and dorsal horn neuropil, it has become important to understand the cell-to-cell organization of these neurons and their processes at the ultrastructural level.[47, 70, 76, 77] Ultrastructural studies are required to elucidate the synaptic organization of small fiber pathways, because primary spinal afferents (e.g., those of cranial nerve origin) may terminate in synaptic glomeruli that are too small for current electrophysiologic probes. Although it is still not possible to assess the precise effect of axodendritic and dendrodendritic activity in the glomerulus upon the transmission of nociception to consciousness, there is good evidence for the suprasegmental control of nociception in the dorsal horn. We must now identify the synaptic organization of the dorsal horn not only in three dimensions, but by neurotransmitter and neuropeptide localization, receptor binding interactions, and pathophysiologic states following interruption of normal inhibitory mechanisms.

INTRACELLULAR MARKING OF DORSAL HORN NEURONS

In an attempt to understand the synaptic organization of the SG, we have labeled neurons of the cat dorsal horn intracellularly. This study is directed toward one subpopulation of neurons in lamina I, namely, the large marginal neurons or Waldeyer cells. These cells receive direct nociceptive information from primary afferent terminations on their dendrites in the marginal zone.[38, 39] Do they participate in the glomerular complex?

Thirty-five unconditioned adult cats weighing 2.5 to 3.5 kg were anesthetized with sodium pentobarbital (Nembutal) and secured in a stereotactic apparatus (manufactured by David Kopf). Surgical procedures included cannulation of the femoral vein and trachea, dissection of the right hindlimb cutaneous nerves, denervation of the major muscle groups of the hindlimb, and L4–S1 laminectomy. Temperature was maintained between 36 and 38°C, and some animals were paralyzed with gallamine triethiodide (Flaxedil) and were given artificial respiration. Neurons in laminae I–IV were impaled on glass micropipettes containing a 4% solution of sigma type VI horseradish peroxidase (HRP) in 0.5 M potassium chloride tris buffer (pH 7.6) with resistances of 20 to 150 megohms. The HRP was iontophoresed with 100 to 200 msec depolarizing current pulses of 3 to 5 nA delivered at 3 to 5/second for 3 to 5 minutes. Following post-injection survival times of 1 to 5 hours, the cats were perfused through the ascending aorta with 1 liter of saline injected in line with 1.0 ml of 2% lidocaine hydrochloride (Xylocaine) followed by 1.5 liters of 1% paraformaldehyde and 1% glutaraldehyde in phosphate buffer (pH 7.4). Vibratome serial sections, measuring 8 μ, from four animals were processed for electron microscopy.

The sections were cut parasagittally or coronally, collected in buffer, intensified with 5% $CaCl_2$, processed for reaction product with diaminobenzidine tetrahydrochloride and hydrogen peroxide, and rinsed in buffer. These sections were mounted and coverslipped from a 0.5% gelatin solution and kept moist during localization and photography. Sections with single marginal neurons and normal morphology were placed in 2% osmium tetroxide for 1 hour, rinsed in buffer, and dehydrated through graded acetones and embedded in Maraglas. Thick and thin sections were obtained from an LKB Ultratome II. Thin sections were stained with uranyl acetate–lead citrate and photographed with a Phillips 300 electron microscope.

The pyramidal-shaped neuron appears to have apical and basal dendrites that cap the dorsal neuropil, whereas some of its thick basal dendrites project toward the SG. Note the characteristics of the processes filled with reaction product, the clarity of their edges, and the lack of any large, unusual excretions on their surfaces (Fig. 10–10). The presynaptic elements, which are unlabeled, form serrated or scalloped borders with the labeled cell processes. The characteristics and distri-

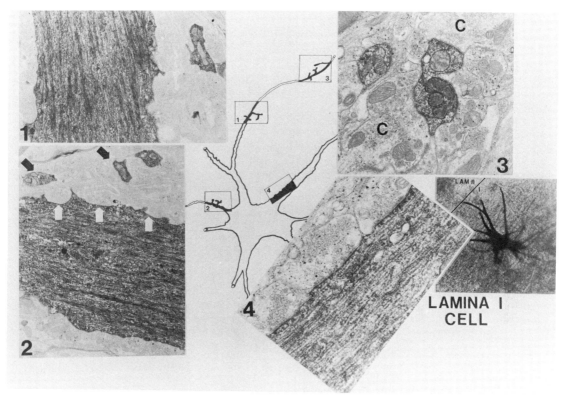

Figure 10–10. A collection of electron micrographs from serial ultrathin sections of a marginal neuron labeled by an intracellular injection of horseradish peroxidase. The location of each micrograph from the labeled neuron is indicated in the inserted boxes 1 to 4 on the central line drawing. This labeled marginal cell has extensive axodendritic contacts on its proximal dendritic shaft at 2 (block arrows). Its distal dendritic spines participate in a complex synaptic array (glomerulus) at 3. C = central axon terminal from primary afferent neuron.

bution of the HRP reaction product inside the cell are similar to those described by others[9] and will not be repeated here.

There are at least three different types of terminals that contact the soma, based on synaptic vesicle size and shape. Terminals with either large (350 to 380 μ) or small (320 to 340 μ) spherical vesicles predominate; some have a subpopulation of dense-cored vesicles. Other terminals contain large pleomorphic vesicles. Some synaptic terminals that contact the soma are more complex and, in addition to axosomatic and axodendritic contacts, form axoaxonic active zones at the branching points of soma and dendrite.

A remarkable change in synaptic density and type takes place on some of the distal tips and dendritic appendages of these large marginal neurons. The distal dendrites and their appendages are involved in complex synaptic arrays with primary afferent neurons. This glomerular site is also the location of gabanergic presynaptic inhibitory contacts on primary afferent axon terminals.

It may now be possible to combine intracellular marking of physiologically identified single units with other contemporary techniques (e.g., immunocytochemistry) to further understand the organization of this part of the nervous system. These data have important health-related implications directed toward an understanding of nociceptive mechanisms related to such surgical and nonsurgical phenomena as phantom limb pain and central and peripheral trauma. It can be reasoned that peripheral nerve lesions induce degenerative atrophy in the central processes of spinal and cranial nerve ganglia, which may be related to or responsible for many paresthetic and causalgic phenomena.

More important, as Knyihar[41] and Crutcher[16, 17] point out, are the recent studies that reveal degenerative atrophy followed by a regenerative or sprouting proliferation in the central nervous system. Plastic phenomena (e.g., collateral sprouting) are at present a major focus under investigation in the neurosciences. These studies of normal synaptic organization will serve as a basis for further investigations concerning regeneration in the central nervous system, as well as establishing a basis for study of ganglionic cell response to chronic diseases of other tissues, including the cardiovascular, endocrine, and autonomic nervous systems.

References

1. Albe-Fessard, D., Levant, A., and Lamour, Y.: Origin of spinothalamic tract in monkeys. Brain Res., 65:503–509, 1974.
2. Applebaum, A. E., Beall, J. E., Foreman, R. D., and Willis, W. D.: Organization and receptive fields of primate spinothalamic tract neurons. J. Neurophysiol., 38:572–586, 1975.
3. Atweh, S. F., and Kuhar, M. J.: Autoradiographic localization of opiate receptors in spinal cord and lower medulla of the rat. Neurosci. Abstr., 2:809, 1976.
4. Barber, R. P., McLaughlin, B. J., Saito, K., and Roberts, E.: Light microscopic localization of glutamate decarboxylase in boutons of rat spinal cord before and after dorsal rhizotomy. Neurosci. Abstr., 127, 1974.
5. Barber, R. P., Saito, K., and Roberts, E.: Effects of deafferentation upon GAD positive terminals in rat spinal cord. Anat. Rec., 184:352, 1976.
6. Barber, R. P., Vaughan, J. E., Saito, K., McLaughlin, B. J., and Roberts, E.: FABAergic terminals are presynaptic to primary afferent terminals in the substantia gelatinosa of the rat spinal cord. Brain Res., 141:35–55, 1978.
6a. Basbaum, A. I., and Fields, H. L.: Endogenous pain control systems: Brainstem spinal pathways and endorphin circuitry. Ann. Rev. Neurosci., 7:309–338, 1984.
7. Basbaum, A. I., Clanton, C. H., and Fields, H. L.: Three bulbospinal pathways from the rostral medulla of the cat; an autoradiographic study of pain modulating systems. J. Comp. Neurol., 178:209–224, 1978.
8. Beals, J. A., and Fox, C. A.: Afferent fibers in the substantia gelatinosa of the adult monkey (*Macaca mulatta*): A Golgi study. J. Comp. Neurol., 168:113–144, 1976.
9. Bishop, G. A., and King, J. S.: Tracing neural connections with horseradish peroxidase histochemistry intracellular injection. In Mesulam, M. M. (ed.): IBRO Handbook Series: Methods in Neuroscience. New York, John Wiley and Sons, 1981.
10. Brown, A. G., Rose, P. K., and Snow, P. J.: The morphology of hair follicle afferent fibre collaterals in the spinal cord of the cat. J. Physiol. (Lond.), 272:779–797, 1977.
11. Brown, A. G., Rose, P. K., and Snow, P. J.: Morphology and organization of axon collaterals from afferent fibres of slowly adapting type I units in cat spinal cord. J. Physiol. (Lond.), 277:15–27, 1978.
12. Carpenter, M. B., Stein, B. M., and Shriver, J. E.: Central projections of spinal dorsal roots in the monkey. II. Lower thoracic, lumbosacral and coccygeal dorsal roots. J. Comp. Neurol., 123:75–118, 1968.
13. Carstens, E., Tulloch, I., and Zieglgansberger, W.: Presynaptic excitability changes induced by morphine in single cutaneous C and A fibers. Pflügers Arch., 379:143–147, 1979.
14. Christensen, B. N., and Perl, E. R.: Spinal neurons specifically excited by noxious or thermal stimuli: the marginal zone of the dorsal horn. J. Neurophysiol., 33:293–307, 1970.
15. Coimbra, A., Sodre-Borges, B. P., and Magalhaes, M. M.: The substantia gelatinosa Rolandi of the rat. Fine structure, cytochemistry (acid phosphatase) and changes after dorsal root section. J. Neurocytol., 3:199–217, 1974.
16. Crutcher, K. A., and Collins, F.: In vitro evidence for two distinct hippocampal growth factors: Basis of neuronal plasticity. Science, 217:67–68, 1982.
17. Crutcher, K. A.: Cholinergic denervation of rat neocortex results in sympathetic innervations. Exp. Neurol., 74:324–329, 1981.
18. Culbertson, J. L., and Kimmel, D. L.: Primary afferent fiber distribution at brachial and lumbosacral spinal cord levels in the opossum (*Didelphis marsupialis virginiana*). Brain Behav. Evol., 12:229–246, 1975.
19. Dilly, P. N., Wall, P. D., and Webster, K.: Cells of origin of the spinothalamic tract in the cat and rat. Exp. Neurol., 21:550–562, 1968.
20. Famiglietti, E. V., and Peters, A.: The synaptic glomerulus and the intrinsic neuron in the dorsal lateral geniculate nucleus of the cat. J. Comp. Neurol. 144:285–334, 1972.
21. Giesler, G. J., Gerhart, K. D., Yezierski, R. P., Wilcox, T. K., and Willis, W. D.: Postsynaptic inhibition of primate spino-thalamic neurons by stimulation in the nucleus raphe magnus. Brain Res., 204:184–188, 1981.
22. Gobel, S., and Purvis, M. B.: Anatomical studies of the organization of the spinal V nucleus: The deep bundles and the spinal V tract. Brain Res., 48:27–44, 1972.
23. Gobel, S.: Synaptic organization of the substantia gelatinosa glomeruli in the spinal trigeminal nucleus of the adult cat. J. Neurocytol., 3:219–243, 1974.
24. Gobel, S.: Golgi studies of the substantia gelatinosa neurons in the spinal trigeminal nucleus. J. Comp. Neurol., 162:397–415, 1975.
25. Gobel, S.: Dendroaxonic synapses in the substantia gelatinosa glomeruli of the spinal trigeminal nucleus of the cat. J. Comp. Neurol., 167:165–176, 1976.
26. Gobel, S.: Neural circuitry in the substantia gelatinosa of Rolando: anatomical insights. In Bonica, J. J. et al. (eds.): Advances in Pain Research and Therapy. Vol. 3. New York, Raven Press, 1979, pp. 175–195.
27. Goode, G. E.: An electron microscopic study of rubrospinal projections to the lumbar spinal cord of the opossum. Neurosci. Abstr., 1:172, 1975.
28. Goode, G. E.: The substantia gelatinosa of the American opossum: Fine structure and changes after dorsal rhizotomy and peripheral lesions. Anat. Rec., 184:412–413, 1976.
29. Goode, G. E.: The ultrastructural identification of primary and suprasegmental afferents in the marginal and gelatinous layers of lumbar spinal cord following central and peripheral lesions. Neurosci. Abstr., 2:975, 1976.
30. Goode, G. E., Humbertson, A. O., and Martin, G.

F.: Projections from the brain stem reticular formation to laminae I and II of the spinal cord. Studies using light electron microscopic techniques in the North American opossum. Brain Res., *189*:327–342, 1980.

31. Goode, G. E., and Sreesai, M.: An electron microscopic study of rubrospinal projection to the lumbar spinal cord of the opossum. Brain Res., *143*:61–70, 1978.

32. Grant, G., and Arvidsson, J.: Transganglionic degeneration in trigeminal primary sensory neurons. Brain Res., *95*:265–279, 1975.

33. Heimer, L., and Wall, P. D.: The dorsal root distribution to the substantia gelatinosa of the rat with a note on distribution in the cat. Exp. Brain Res., *6*:89–99, 1968.

34. Henry, J. L.: Substance P excitation of spinal nociception neurons. Neurosci. Abstr., *1*:390, 1975.

35. Hokfelt, T. R., Elder, R., Johansson, O., Luft, R., Nilsson, G., and Arimura, A.: Immunohistochemical evidence for separate populations of somatostatin-containing and substance P-containing primary afferent neurons in the rat. Neurosci. Abstr., *1*:131–136, 1976.

36. Hosobuchi, Y., Adams, J. E., and Linchintz, R.: Pain relief by electrical stimulation of the central gray matter in humans and its reversal by maloxone. Science, *197*:183–186, 1977.

37. Johnson, J. I., Hamilton, T. C., and Hsung, J.: Gracile nucleus absence in adult opossums after leg removal in infancy. Brain Res., *38*:421–424, 1972.

38. Kerr, F. W. L.: The ultrastructure of the spinal tract of the trigeminal nerve and the substantia gelatinosa. Exp. Neurol., *16*:359–376, 1966.

39. Kerr, F. W. L.: Neuroanatomical substrates of nociception in the spinal cord. Pain, *1*:325–356, 1975.

40. Knyihar, E., Laszlo, I., and Lornyos, S.: Fine structure and fluoride resistant acid phosphatase activity of electron dense sinusoid terminals in the substantia gelatinosa Rolandi of the rat after dorsal root transection. Exp. Brain Res., *19*:529–544, 1974.

41. Knyihar, E.: Effect of peripheral axotomy on the fine structure and histochemistry of the Rolando substance: Degenerative atrophy of central processes of pseudo-unipolar cells. Exp. Brain Res., *26*:73–87, 1976.

42. Kumazawa, T., Perl, E. R., Burgess, P. R., and Whitehorn, D.: Ascending projections from marginal zone (lamina I) neurons of the spinal dorsal horn. J. Comp. Neurol., *162*:1–12, 1975.

43. Laemle, L. K.: Neuronal populations of the human. Periaqueductal gray nucleus lateralis. J. Comp. Neurol., *186*:93–108, 1979.

44. LaMotte, C.: Distribution of Lissauer's tract and dorsal root fibers in the primate spinal cord. Neurosci. Abstr., *2*:966, 1976.

45. LaMotte, C., Pert, C. B., and Snyder, S. H.: Opiate receptor-binding in primate spinal cord: distribution and changes after dorsal root section. Brain Res., *112*:407, 1976.

46. Lewis, V. A., and Gebhart, G. F.: Morphine induced and stimulation produced analgesias at coincident periaqueductal central gray loci: evaluation of analgesic congruence, tolerance and crosstolerance. Exp. Neurol., *57*:934–955, 1977.

47. Loren, I., Alumets, J., Hakanson, R., and Sundler, F.: Cell Tissue Res., *200*:179–186, 1979.

48. Mantyh, P.: The midbrain periaqueductal gray in

the rat and monkey: a Nisse, Weiland and Golgi analysis. J. Comp. Neurol., *204*:349–363, 1982.

49. Mayer, D. J.: Endogenous analgesia systems: neural and behavioral mechanisms. *In* Bonica, J. et al. (eds.): Advances in Pain Research and Therapy, Vol. 3. New York, Raven Press, 1979.

50. Mayer, D. J., and Liebeskind, J. C.: Pain reduction by focal electrical stimulation of the brain: an anatomical and behavioral analysis. Brain Res., *68*:73–93, 1974.

51. Mayer, D. J., Wolgle, T. L., Akil, H., Carder, B., and Liebeskind, J. C.: Analgesia from electrical stimulation in the brainstem of the rat. Science, *174*:1351–1354, 1971.

52. McLaughlin, B. J., Barber, R., Saito, K., and Roberts, E.: Immunocytochemical localization of glutamate decarboxylase in rat spinal cord. J. Comp. Neurol., *164*:305–322, 1975.

53. Melzack, R.: The Puzzle of Pain. New York, Basic Books, 1973.

54. Melzack, R., and Wall, P. D.: Pain mechanisms: A new theory. Science, *150*:971–979, 1965.

55. Moradian, G. P., and Rustioni, A.: Transganglionic degeneration in the dorsal horn and dorsal column nuclei of adult rat. Anat. Rec., *187*:660, 1977.

56. Nathan, P. W.: The gate-control theory of pain. Brain, *99*:123–158, 1976.

57. Oliveras, J. L., Besson, J. M., Guilband, G., and Liebeskind, J. C.: Behavorial and electrophysiological evidence of pain inhibition from midbrain stimulation in the cat. Exp. Brain Res., *20*:32–44, 1974.

58. Oliveras, J. L., Redjemi, F., Guilband, G., and Besson, J. M.: Analgesia induced by electrical stimulation of the inferior centralis of the raphe in the cat. Pain, *1*:139–145, 1975.

59. Price, D. D.: Characteristics of second pain and flexion reflexes indicative of prolonged central summation. Exp. Neurol., *37*:371–387, 1972.

60. Rafols, J. A., and Valverde, F.: The structure of the dorsal lateral geniculate nucleus in the mouse. A Golgi and electron microscopic study. J. Comp. Neurol., *150*:303–332, 1973.

61. Ralston, H. J.: Dorsal root projections to dorsal horn neurons. J. Comp. Neurol., *132*:303–329, 1968.

62. Ralston, H. J.: The synaptic organization in the dorsal horn of the spinal cord and in the ventrobasal thalamus in the cat. *In* Cubner, R., and Kawamura, Y. (eds.): Oral-Facial Sensory and Motor Mechanisms. New York, Appleton-Century-Crofts, 1971, pp. 229–250.

63. Ralston, H. J., III, and Ralston, D. D.: The distribution of dorsal root axons in laminae I, II and III of the *Macaque* spinal cord: a quantitative electron microscope study. J. Comp. Neurol., *184*:643–684, 1979.

64. Ramon y Cajal, S.: Histologie du systeme nerveux de l'homme et des vertebres. Trans. by L. Azoulay, Maloine, Paris.

65. Ranson, S. W.: The course with the spinal cord of the non-medullated fibers of the spinal dorsal roots: A study of Lissauer's tract in the cat. J. Comp. Neurol., *23*:259–274, 1913.

66. Ranson, S. W.: The tract of Lissauer and the substantia gelatinosa Rolandi. Am. J. Anat., *16*:97–126, 1914.

67. Rethelyi, M., and Szentagothai, J.: The large synaptic complexes of the substantia gelatinosa. Exp. Brain Res., *7*:258–274, 1969.

68. Richardson, D. E., and Akil, H.: Pain reduction by electrical brain stimulation in man. J. Neurosurg., 47:178–183, 1977.

69. Scheibel, M. E., and Scheibel, A. B.: Terminal axonal patterns in the cat spinal cord. II. The dorsal horn. Brain Res., 9:32–58, 1968.

70. Sims, K. B., Hoffman, D. L., Said, S. J., and Zimmerman, E.: Vasoactive intestinal polypeptide (VIP) in mouse and rat brain: an immunocytochemical study. Brain Res., 186:165–183, 1980.

71. Sprague, J. M., and Ha, H.: The terminal fields of dorsal root fibers in the lumbosacral spinal cord of the cat, and the dendritic organization of the motor nuclei. Progr. Brain Res., 11:120–154, 1964.

72. Sterling, P., and Kuypers, H. G. J. M.: Anatomical organization of the brachial spinal cord of the cat. I. The distribution of dorsal root fibers. Brain Res., 4:1–15, 1967.

73. Szentagothai, J.: Neuronal and synaptic arrangements in the substantia gelatinosa Rolandi. J. Comp. Neurol., 122:219–240, 1964.

74. Takahachi, T., and Otsuka, M.: Regional distribution of substance P in the spinal cord and nerve roots of the cat and the effect of dorsal root section. Brain Res., 87:1–11, 1975.

75. Trevino, D. L., Maunz, R. A., Bryan R. N., and Willis, W. D.: Location of cells of origin of the spinothalamic tract in the lumbar enlargement of the cat. Exp. Neurol., 34:64–77, 1972.

76. Uhl, G. R., Goodman, R. R., and Snyder, S. H.: Neurotensin-containing cell bodies, fibers and terminals in the brain stem of the rat: immunohistochemical mapping. Brain Res., 167:77, 1979.

77. Vanderhaeghen, J. J., Lotstra, F., DeMey, J., and Gilles, C.: Immunohistochemical localization of cholecystokinin and gastrin-like peptides in the brain and hypophysis of the rat. Proc. Natl. Acad. Sci., 77:1190–1194, 1980.

78. Wall, P. D., Merrill, E. G., and Yaksh, T. L.: Responses of single units in laminae 2 and 3 of cat spinal cord. Brain Res., 160:245–260, 1979.

79. Westlund, K., and Coulter, J. D.: Descending projections from the locus coeruleus in monkey. Anat. Rec., 193:718, 1979.

80. Westrum, L. E., Canfield, R. C., and Black, R. G.: Transganglionic degeneration in the spinal trigeminal nucleus following removal of tooth pupils in adult cats. Brain Res., 101:137–140, 1976.

81. Willis, W. D., Kenshalo, D. R., Jr., and Leonard, R. B.: The cells of origin of the primate spinothalamic tract. J. Comp. Neurol., 188:543–574, 1979.

82. Willis, W. D., Maunz, R. A., Foreman, R. D., and Coulter, J. D.: Static and dynamic responses of spinothalamic tract neurons to mechanical stimuli. J. Neurophysiol., 38:587–600, 1975.

83. Zorman, G., Hental, I. D., Adams, J. E., and Fields, H. L.: Naloxone-reversible analgesia produced by microstimulation in the rat medulla. Brain Res., 219:137–148, 1981.

11

Management Techniques for the Painful Upper Extremity

■

George E. Omer, Jr., M.D., M.Sc. (Orthop. Surg.)

Pain is an unpleasant sensory and emotional experience associated with actual or potential tissue damage or described in terms of such damage.[76] The most common reason for patients seeing a physician is pain,[25] and approximately 75 million Americans are afflicted with pain every year.[14]

Chronic pain is defined as pain that persists or recurs at intervals for months or years.[14] It is caused not only by pathologic processes in the nervous system, but also by psychopathologic and environmental influences. Chronic pain is a pernicious energy that imposes excessive psychologic, social, and economic stresses on the patient. Over 40 million Americans are either partially or totally disabled by chronic pain, and as a result nearly 700 million work days are lost annually, which together with health care costs and compensation total approximately 50 billion dollars each year.[14]

There is no objective method to measure pain. The recognition of pain is subjective and depends upon the intensity of the peripheral stimulus, the central summation, and the personality of the patient. The treatment of chronic pain problems is very difficult and complex, since pain is such an intensely personal reaction that Aristotle and Plato considered pain to be a "passion of the soul."[32]

NEUROPHYSIOLOGY

Current investigation suggests that pain is a specific sensory event and not merely excessive stimulation of other sensory modalities. There are specific pain receptors in the skin, viscera, and deep somatic structures. All of these receptors respond to innocuous stimulation, whether mechanical, thermal, electrical, or chemical. A significant portion of the bare nerve endings are termed nociceptors and respond only to strong stimulation that is potentially damaging to tissue.[13] In the peripheral nervous system, the small myelinated axons are called A-delta (class III) and conduct at 12 to 80 m per second (m/sec). Approximately 25% of these axons are nociceptors and are stimulated by temperatures above 45°C or below 10°C and by intense mechanical stimulation. The even smaller unmyelinated axons are termed C-delta (class IV) and conduct at 0.4 to 1.0 m/sec. Approximately 50% of these axons are nociceptors. Iggo[51] has defined the characteristics of the nociceptors as very high thresholds to mechanical or thermal stimuli, relatively small receptive fields, and persistent after-discharges for any suprathreshold stimulus. There are three groups of nociceptors: high-threshold mechanoreceptors, heat nociceptors, and "polymodal" nociceptors responsive to both noxious mechanical and noxious thermal stimuli.[9] Polymodal and heat nociceptors can be sensitized after repeated or prolonged stimulation or during regeneration following section of a nerve, so that their thresholds for activation can be lowered to levels of stimulus intensity that are ordinarily innocuous. This could account for the pain states following burns or nerve injury.[120]

The sympathetic nervous system of the

upper extremity is concentrated in the thoracic portion of the spinal cord. Myelinated sympathetic axons exit via the anterior nerve root, then separate to form the white rami that enter the thoracic ganglia. A synapse occurs, and the postganglionic unmyelinated axons exit from the thoracic ganglia and enter the peripheral nerve. Since preganglionic axons form plexuses and synapses with many different postganglionic axons, a sympathetic discharge may affect several different target organs represented in more than one dermatome. Activation of a sympathetic discharge may elicit either an excitatory or an inhibitory response in different target organs, based on the relative potencies of the various catecholamines released at the neuroeffector junction. During an abnormal process, such as reflex sympathetic dystrophy, there may be great variations in the extremity, such as vasodilatation or vasoconstriction, increased redness or pallor, sweating or dryness, and coolness or heat, depending upon the severity or the state of involvement of target organs.

Injured nerve axons are excited by norepinephrine, which is the substance released at the neuroeffector junction by efferent impulses in the sympathetic nervous system. In the normal intact sensory nerve, sympathetic transmitters do not evoke obvious injury signals, although they may modulate sensitivity. Partially damaged nerve membrane and the unmyelinated axons (sprouts) within a neuroma are highly sensitive to norepinephrine. Stimulation of myelinated axons releases local endorphins, which dampen or stop the oversensitive spontaneous activity of these unmyelinated axons at the spinal cord level. When tissue is injured, the nociceptors are influenced by the sympathetic efferents, chemical environment, vasculature, temperature, and high-frequency antidromic impulses.

The study of peripheral receptors led to an understanding of the relationship between humoral mediators and pain. Acute inflammation induces an exudative response that results in hydrolysis of extracellular macromolecules and breakdown of intracellular compounds.[112] The immediate mediators include histamine, released from basophils and mast cells, and serotonin, released from platelets. At the same time, plasma precursors are activated to form materials with low molecular weight that provoke acute vascular inflammation and pain. All injured cells release prostaglandins and thromboxanes. These mediators are also liberated by mechanical, electrical, radiation, or thermal injury. They induce pain in two ways: (1) by direct irritation or stimulation of the nociceptors, and (2) by sensitizing the nociceptors to the pain-provoking effect of kinins and similar substances. The humoral mediators lower the threshold to pain transmission and increase the intensity of the stimulus.

We would suffer unrelenting pain if there were no endogenous defense against these humoral mediators. The mechanisms that limit their activity are being identified. For example, histaminase is produced to break down histamine and peptidases to degrade the kinins. Specific drugs can interrupt metabolic reactions such as injury to cells that results in formation of prostaglandins and thromboxane. The clinical value of nonsteroidal anti-inflammatory agents, such as aspirin or indomethacin, is that they block the metabolic pathway for the formation of prostaglandins and thromboxanes.[139]

The action potential produced by stimulation of the nociceptors passes to the dorsal horn of the spinal cord, which has six laminae of cell networks that process as well as transmit the impulses.[105] There appear to be two types of pain-related sensory neurons in the dorsal horn. Class 1 nociceptive neurons are located in the most superficial layer of the dorsal horn (lamina I). Class 1 neurons are responsive to injurious levels of stimulation.[20] Class 2 nociceptive neurons are located primarily in lamina V and respond to low intensity stimulation, but as the intensity of the stimulation is increased, these neurons follow with more vigorous and sustained discharge.[144] Class 2 neurons are impinged upon by both somatic and visceral sources and may be involved in visceral referred pain.[44] Melzack and Wall[73] postulated a dynamic interaction (control gate) among large and small afferent neurons, mediated through the small cells of the substantia gelatinosa (laminae II and III). Large afferent neurons excite the cells of the substantia gelatinosa and increase presynaptic inhibition (closing the gate) to noxious impulses incoming on small afferent neurons. Small afferent neurons inhibit the cells of the substantia gelatinosa, thus decreasing the presynaptic inhibition (opening the gate). Pain is perceived when a threshold level of nociceptive action potential is attained by the central transmission neurons.

Nociceptive impulses are transmitted from the dorsal horn of the spinal cord to all levels of the central nervous system. The neurons in laminae I, IV, V, and VI of the dorsal horn connect to the spinothalamic system, the neospinothalamic tract, and the paleospinothalamic tract.[17, 138] The neospinothalamic tract runs to the thalamus, where it synapses with central neurons that pass to the somatosensory cortex. This tract conveys information for perception of sharp, well-localized pain. The older paleospinothalamic tract projects to the spinal cord and the thalamus, where it synapses with neurons that connect with the limbic forebrain structures. This tract conveys information for the perception of poorly localized, dull, aching, burning pain. Impulses transmitted by this tract provoke suprasegmental reflex responses concerned with circulation, respiration, and endocrine function. In addition, there are multisynaptic afferent systems, including the spinoreticular system, spinocervicothalamic system, dorsal intracornu system, and other complex tracts. These pain tracts may be altered or destroyed by injury or loss of other peripheral sensory systems, and the central pain summation may result from abnormal control mechanisms rather than from increased intensity of the peripheral stimulus. In this infinitely duplicated system for the reception, transmission, and perception of pain, there is specificity at the periphery, but in the central nervous system the specificity is lost completely.

Supraspinal descending neural systems modify the nociceptive impulses. The pyramidal tracts, rubrospinal tracts, and reticulospinal tracts influence transmission in the dorsal horn.[42, 121] The descending fibers from the cortex of the brain affect transmission in the thalamus, reticular formation, dorsal column of the cord, and other relay stations.

In 1969, Reynolds[106] stimulated cells in the periaqueductal periventricular gray matter and produced profound analgesia at the spinal cord level. This stimulation-produced analgesia can completely inhibit the pain-evoked discharges of class 2 dorsal horn neurons, without affecting their responsiveness to nonpainful stimuli.[83] This appears to be the same descending circuit that is affected by morphine to produce analgesia.[70] One particular spinal pathway conveying these descending pain modulatory impulses is the dorsolateral funiculus, which terminates in the dorsal horn of the spinal cord. The neu-

rotransmitter carried by these cells and released in the spinal cord is serotonin.[3, 120] Either chemical or dietary depletion of brain serotonin levels increases sensitivity to pain. Tolerance develops to stimulation-produced analgesia, and cross-tolerance is found between morphine and stimulation-induced analgesia.[71] The morphine antagonist naloxone reverses stimulation-produced analgesia when the stimulator is ventral within the periaqueductal gray matter,[2] but does not block analgesia when the stimulator is more dorsal.[4]

There are stereospecific receptors for the alkaloids from the opium poppy in the brain.[39] These receptors are confined to nerve tissue and perhaps influence the transmission of pain.[97] Hughes and colleagues[50] extracted a peptide of low molecular weight from the brain that acted as an agonist at opiate receptor sites, and its action was prevented by narcotic antagonists. The peptide was named enkephalin. Others noted that the amino acid sequence of enkephalin was identical to that of beta-lipotropin C-fragment, a pituitary peptide. A higher opiate activity was exhibited by the beta-lipotropin in C-fragment peptide than by enkephalin.[15] The C-fragment is now named beta-endorphin. When injected intravenously, beta-endorphin produces analgesic effects three to four times as potent as morphine.[127] Pretreatment with naloxone eliminates the analgesia. A possible neurotransmitter or neuromodulator role for these neuropeptides is suggested by studies showing they affect the action or release of dopamine and acetylcholine.[52, 63, 79] At spinal levels, enkephalin release appears to be able to suppress pain transmission by interfering with the release of substance P, another peptide found in terminals of sensory afferents and the dorsal horn of the spinal cord. Acupuncture analgesia may be mediated by morphine-like hormones or neuropeptides released by the pituitary.[100] Thus, it may be possible that the physiologic role of opiates and endogenous opiate-like neuropeptides involves the transmission of pain. The endogenous opiate-like neuropeptides may act on both presynaptic and postsynaptic opiate receptors in the spinal cord and brain. The same substance may be used as a neurotransmitter in one instance, a neuromodulator in another, and a hormone in still another situation.[41, 84]

In addition to the endogenous opioid mechanism for analgesia, there may also be a nonopioid mechanism. Mayer and colleagues[70] reported that naloxone blocked acupunctural analgesia, but not hypnotic analgesia, in humans. Stimulation-produced analgesia is effective when the stimulator is in one portion of the periaqueductal gray matter, but is not effective when the stimulator is moved to nearby sites.[4] Mayer and Price[72] have proposed that the descending pain inhibitory mechanism may involve both a serotonergic and an enkephalin-like neurotransmitter system. Endorphins (enkephalins) may act as hormone-releasing or hormone-inhibiting factors in peripheral target organs such as the adrenal medulla and the pancreas.[5] Electrical or chemical stimulation of either system produces analgesia, whereas chemical or surgical blockade of either prevents analgesia.

In summary, the factors involved in the intensity of the peripheral nociceptive stimulus are the chemical environment at the site of injury and abnormal sympathetic overactivity. The factors in central summation are neuron-inhibiting "gating" systems, neurojunction inhibitors, and multisynaptic ascending and descending pain tracts.

PERCEPTUAL PARAMETERS AND PERSONALITY

The pain threshold is the least stimulus at which a subject perceives pain.[76] The pain tolerance level is the greatest stimulus intensity causing pain that a subject is prepared to tolerate.[76] In the experimental setting, pain threshold and tolerance can be determined by several techniques and show high reliability.[22, 120, 130, 131, 146] Age, sex, race, ethnic group, religion, and other factors influence pain tolerance.[109]

Personality is the unique blend of intellectual and emotional qualities reflected in our individual behavior.[11, 133] A number of traits are characteristic facets of personality, such as anxiety, expressiveness, depression, and hypochondriasis.[58] Clinicians may believe that the patient who complains about pain more than "average" has a low pain threshold, but this is an error. The readiness to communicate the pain is a function of expressiveness, and this in turn is associated with a degree of extroversion.[120] In experimental studies, Lynn and Eysenck[67] found that pain tolerance of college students was negatively correlated with neuroticism and positively correlated with extroversion. Social learning influences expressiveness as well, including that related to pain communication. In clinical situations, anxiety is associated with acute pain and the anticipation of body harm, whereas depression is associated with chronic pain and intrapunitive anger. Sternbach and associates[119] found that patients with low back pain of less than 6 months' duration obtained Minnesota Multiphasic Personality Inventory (MMPI) profiles within normal limits, whereas those patients with low back pain of longer duration had markedly elevated scores for depression, hypochondriasis, and hysteria.

Basic personality attributes may be measured by two tests, the Eysenck Personality Inventory (EPI) and the MMPI. The EPI measures two dimensions of personality regarded as fundamental because they are related directly to physiologic activity of the central nervous system. These dimensions are stability/neuroticism (N) and introversion/extroversion (E). The higher the patient's N score, the greater the emotional vulnerability shown. The higher the E scale, the more the individual will be found to be gregarious and cheerful and have high levels of energy. In general, thresholds for pain are lower for introverts than for extroverts. The EPI can be completed in 10 to 15 minutes.[11] The MMPI is a checklist of physical and emotional symptoms, including those from the past and those present at the time of examination. High scores indicate the presence of an emotional disturbance. For patients with chronic pain, significantly higher scores are found on those items measuring hypochondriasis, depression, and hysteria. Patients with acute pain show high scores for hypochondriasis and hysteria, but not for depression. One of the attractions of the MMPI is that the personality profiles permit the identification of groups of characteristics, and patients with pain problems may be categorized on this basis.[11] There is a reported clinical correlation of 86.3% between the topographic pain drawing[27] and the MMPI score.

Experienced surgeons who spend time with their patients and make thoughtful decisions based on objective findings plus clinical impressions usually obtain good results with elective surgery, even in patients who have abnormal MMPI scales.[129] However, the MMPI aids in confirming clinical impressions of a patient's psychologic status and serves as a useful diagnostic device when the clinician is insecure concerning his or her decision for surgery. In a practical sense, the attending surgeon or therapist must learn to identify the unstable emotional personality. In these patients the "pain state" becomes a permanent "memory bank," and the total personality may become focused on the pain. These patients will require much more time and explanation in order to cope with their pain.

The pattern for development of a chronic pain syndrome follows a sequence: nociceptive stimulus → to sensation of pain → to suffering → to pain behavior—which may continue in the absence of tissue damage. It is also important to delineate psychosocial factors. Some characteristics of an established pain syndrome include: (1) symptoms longer than 6 months; (2) minimal objective physical findings; (3) evidence of medication abuse; (4) somatic preoccupation, with poor appetite, loss of energy, insomnia, and diminished ability to concentrate; and (5) attempts to manipulate the surgeon, family, and environment.

For elective surgical procedures, an important concept is the prevention of pain.[89] It is obvious that nerve injury, such as accidental laceration of a cutaneous nerve, should be avoided. If a cutaneous nerve, such as the superficial radial nerve, is partially cut, the appropriate procedure is prompt suture of the laceration. In extensive injuries, venous repair is important for the prevention of edema. Surgical release of fascial sheaths is performed when indicated. During the early postoperative period, one should attempt to prevent edema. The extremity should be immobilized in longitudinally oriented nonconstrictive bulky dressings and elevated. Early motion must be initiated, such as shoulder exercises when the fingers are not allowed to be moved. Early motion is essential to prevent joint contractures and muscle atrophy, and active motion is begun before pain is appreciated by the patient.

Medications during the early postoperative period should include aspirin and perhaps a tranquilizer. Aspirin blocks the metabolic pathway from injured cells to the formation of prostaglandins and thromboxanes.[43, 139] A mild tranquilizer, such as hydroxyzine pamoate, reduces the incidence of analgesic side effects, including nausea and vomiting, and promotes the inhibition of anxiety.[71]

These medications are most effective during the first 24 to 72 hours after surgery.

Postoperative pain should be evaluated promptly; one should never wait for the full development of an established pain syndrome before initiating aggressive treatment. For example, the osteoporosis of Sudek's atrophy is not evident by radiography for 5 to 8 weeks' postinjury,[98] but the patient has pain from the time of injury.

DIFFERENTIAL DIAGNOSIS

In the upper extremity it is necessary to evaluate the potential cause of pain from the hand to the spinal cord. A detailed history and a thorough physical examination should be obtained. The history is obviously important in problems such as brachial plexus neuropathy,[126] diabetes, or paresthesia of the hand following radiation therapy for lung cancer.[56] Routine laboratory studies, such as the sedimentation rate, are useful. Roentgenographic evaluation may require plain radiographs in multiple planes, computed tomography, cinefluoroscopy, arthrography, discography, and computed tomographic metrizamide myelography. Technetium and gallium radionuclide scans are used to confirm clinical observations. It is impossible to differentiate the functional activity of the nervous system from that of the vascular system; e.g., the Doppler examination[10] is a flow detector, whereas plethysmography is a volumetric analysis of flow.[143] Thermography can be employed to identify sensory root involvement.[55, 99] Electrodiagnostic studies include nerve conduction velocities and electromyography. Nerve conduction testing is useful in localizing the level of dysfunction, distinguishing partial and complete lesions, and differentiating muscle from nerve pathology.[26]

Diagnostic confusion lies in the numerous sources from which painful symptoms may arise, with massive overlap and similarities in the clinical picture. For example, hypertrophic osteoarthritis of the cervical spine may produce pain in several ways: (1) direct nerve compression of either the nerve roots or the spinal cord, which results in muscle weakness and sensory abnormalities over specific dermatomes; (2) vertebral artery insufficiency and compression of the posterior cervical sympathetic plexus by osteophytes from the apophyseal joints or joints of Luschka, resulting in potential cervical migraine or neck or arm pain; (3) thoracic outlet compression from spasm of the scalene muscles; and (4) irritation of the joint capsules with their intrinsic innervation, which may result in paresthesia in the neck, tip of the shoulder, lateral aspect of the arm, or hand.[23]

It is useful to divide the pattern of subjective symptoms into categories: (1) nociceptive peripheral increased stimulus; (2) summation of the reflex sympathetic overflow; (3) inflammatory or systemic pain, which may be generalized; (4) central pain; (5) cancer pain; and (6) personality dysfunction.[94]

There are only two principles in the treatment of an established pain syndrome involving the upper extremity: (1) relieve the subjective pain experience, and (2) institute active function of the involved extremity.[87-89]

Subjective Pain Relief Techniques

Peripheral Nociceptive Stimulus

Pain may develop after local trauma for many reasons. The damaged portion of the nerve may develop intraneural fibrosis, or external adhesions may transfix the nerve to its bed. Friction upon a nerve will result in inflammatory changes and further fibrosis. The compressed nerve will have venous stasis, capillary leakage, and perineurial edema.[108] Decreased blood flow can be associated with pain, as in any compression syndrome.[33] Any procedure producing vasodilatation may relieve this pain.

The peripheral nociceptive stimulus is often associated with trigger points. A trigger point or area is a small hypersensitive region from which impulses bombard the central nervous system and give rise to referred pain.[125] Trigger points are most often associated with myofascial pain syndromes,[74] and charts have been developed showing trigger points of the head, neck, and upper extremities.[74, 107, 117, 125] The termination of pain by either local injection of an anesthetic or hyperstimulation will normalize function and help prevent recurrent abnormal neural activity.[75] Methods of hyperstimulation analgesia have included intense cold, intense heat, chemical irritation, dry needling, and acupuncture.[74] Moxa, or moxibustion, has a purpose similar to acupuncture and involves applying combustible cones of powdered leaves of *Artemisia vulgaris* to the skin.[93] The

cones are placed in charted spots and set on fire; they are extinguished after a blister is formed. There are special charts for moxa points, but the cones can also be applied to the acupuncture points. Many Korean patients in Eighth U.S. Army hospitals during the 1950s had the complication of a series of small, round burns from initial Korean hanyak (Chinese, yin-yang) therapy.[93] Western authors have recommended massage and stretching the underlying muscles after trigger point injection.[107, 110, 117]

A peripheral nerve responds to injury, whether partial or complete, with proliferation of connective tissue and regeneration of damaged axons to form a neuroma. The neuroma becomes symptomatic depending upon the quality of regeneration and is influenced by the extent of fibrosis, vascularity, infection, foreign material, and other local factors. Neuromas with inadequate numbers of large myelinated axons or outer fibrous layers develop hyperpathia, which is a painful syndrome characterized by over-reaction and after-sensation to stimuli.[76] The patient characteristically has extreme sensitivity directly over the neuroma, altered sensibility in at least part of the area supplied by the nerve, and sustained, widely distributed, poorly localized pain.[145]

Percutaneous injection about the painful neuroma should provide local anesthesia. Bupivacaine hydrochloride has a longer duration of anesthesia than lidocaine hydrochloride.[78] Percutaneous injection of triamcinolone acetonide about the neuroma after a cutaneous block with 2% lidocaine hydrochloride has been reported to relieve the pain symptoms in 50% of patients after one injection and in 80% of patients after multiple injections.[115]

Percussion or massage of painful neuromas has been a clinical procedure in amputes since World War I. Controlled clinical studies have indicated that the technique is useful in selected cases.[40] Rubber mallets, mechanical vibrators, or ultrasonic treatments will provide the repetitious percussion. Anesthesia may be necessary over a trigger area at the onset of treatment, but later the percussion or massage should be done without local anesthesia.

A chemical peripheral sympathetic block may be performed in the patient's room.[85, 86] A 16-gauge needle is inserted just proximal to the "trigger point," and a flexible 18-gauge polyethylene intravenous catheter is inserted through the needle. The needle is removed, leaving the catheter in place. A solution of 0.5 ml of 0.5% lidocaine hydrochloride is injected. If the pain is relieved, the catheter is capped and taped in place, allowing exercise activity. Additional periodic injections of lidocaine solution are based on the length of time of pain-free activity. The periodic infusion has been continued for a few days up to 2 weeks. If there is more than one "trigger point," separate catheters should be used. This method has not been as effective in those patients in whom the pain has been untreated for 3 or more months.

A neuroma can be classified as a terminal bulb or a neuroma in continuity. Kline[54] states that partial nerve transection occurs in the majority of civilian injuries. A painful partial nerve disruption may benefit from internal neurolysis and graft repair of some fascicular groups.[87, 118] If there is no useful distal sensory or motor function, an end-to-end anastomosis should be performed after removal of the neuroma in continuity.[91] Terminal bulb neuromas typically occur in amputation stumps.[90, 92] Although many procedures have been reported, present methods include simple resection of the neuroma, capping the terminal portion of the neuroma with silicone, or transposing the entire neuroma to a new site.[47, 123, 128] The most reliable procedure is transfer of the neuroma, attached to the proximal nerve stump, to a new site where compression is unlikely and traction is minimal. The neuroma should be placed in an area of good circulation with a thick subcutaneous layer that is free of scar.[29, 57] Success has been reported in 82% of patients treated with this technique.

Traction injuries to the brachial plexus are often painful initially, but the pain should progressively subside.[145] An increase in pain may represent fibrous tissue involvement. The pain from nerve root avulsion is severe, having the characteristics of causalgia or maximum reflex sympathetic summation.[147] Mesencephalic tractotomy gave lasting pain relief in three of six patients in one reported series.[148]

Summation of Reflex Sympathetic Overflow

Many clinical syndromes have been described that include burning pain, abnormal vasomotor response, and dystrophy. Classic causalgia may have variants that are termed Leriche's post-traumatic pain syndrome (minor causalgia), Sudek's atrophy, or shoulder-arm-hand syndrome.[58] Phantom pain is identical to reflex sympathetic dystrophy but also includes postural cramping or squeezing. Reflex sympathetic dystrophy may not develop immediately but gradually increases to dominate the clinical picture.

The loss of vascular, sudomotor, pilomotor, and muscle tone controls will result in profound nutritional (trophic) changes. There is atrophy of subcutaneous tissue, skin, muscle, and bone. In the early stages, the residual limb is markedly swollen and warm. There is hyperesthesia to light touch and sensitivity to cold. After 2 to 3 months, fibrotic brawny edema develops. Contractures become fixed owing to lack of active motion. Roentgenograms of the distal bones show patchy osteopenia. A bone scan (99m technetium etidronate sodium) will be positive before the bone resorption is visible on plain films. Six to nine months after the onset of pain, the extremity becomes pale and cool with either hyperhidrosis or dryness. Pain may dominate, or the extremity may be totally ignored by the patient.

This syndrome is thought to be a prolongation of the normal sympathetic response to injury.[12] The pain impulses to the cortex are greatly amplified, causing intense discomfort. The hypothesis that a partial injury to a major nerve can result in abnormal cross-stimulation between sympathetic and sensory fibers has clinical support.[28] Others have postulated the liberation of a vasodilator substance (neurokinin) at the periphery as the basis for the pain.[7, 19]

In patients with vasospastic disorders or Raynaud's symptoms associated with pain, it is important to measure digital blood flow.[6] We follow Porter and colleagues'[101] method: the patient sits quietly for 30 minutes in a warm room with temperature ± 24°C. The digital pulp temperature is determined with an electronic telethermometer. The patient's hands are then immersed in an ice water mixture for 20 seconds, and the digital pulp temperature is measured until the temperature returns to the baseline value for 45 minutes. Normal temperature recovery time is 10 minutes, with a range from 5 to 20 minutes. The digital temperature test can be supplemented with arteriography to differentiate arterial spasm from organic obstructive disease.

The arteriovenous communications and

the precapillary arterioles of the extremities are sympathetically innervated, and a variety of drugs that decrease sympathetic activity should be beneficial for the patient with painful Raynaud's symptoms. Various drugs have been proposed for intra-arterial injection, including the alpha-receptor blocking drugs tolazoline hydrochloride (Priscoline) and phenoxybenzamine hydrochloride, the beta-adrenergic receptor blocking drug propranolol hydrochloride, and the neuronal norepinephrine depletors reserpine, methyldopa, and guanethidine. Griseofulvin has also been used because it has a direct vasodilator action exclusive of sympathetic innervation. Acevedo et al.[1] injected 1.25 mg of reserpine in 10 ml of normal saline into the brachial artery over 1 minute and reported beneficial results both in patients without surgical treatment and in those who previously underwent preganglionic sympathectomy. Porter and associates[101] obtained excellent responses in patients with Raynaud's symptoms by repeated brachial artery injections of reserpine (0.25 mg) at approximately 2- to 3-week intervals. Porter et al. also treated 23 patients with oral guanethidine, 10 mg daily, and then increased the level by 10 mg each week until either hypotension or symptomatic improvement occurred. Two patients could not tolerate guanethidine, even at the minimal dose of 10 mg daily, because of hypotension, and their medication was changed to phenoxybenzamine, 10 mg daily. After an average follow-up of 12 months, 19 of the 23 patients had significant reduction in the frequency and severity of Raynaud's attacks.[101] Similar results have been reported for propranolol hydrochloride in oral dosages of 40 mg every 4 hours[111] and prazosin hydrochloride in oral dosages of 1 mg twice daily.[135]

Chronic small vessel digital ischemia, associated with pain, severe cold intolerance, and occasional finger tip ulceration, is often found in patients with frostbite, post-traumatic crush injuries, and chronic vascular diseases. A residual group of these patients do not improve with direct intra-arterial vasodilators, tobacco abstinence, and central ganglionic blocking agents and may benefit from digital sympathectomy. This procedure consists of isolating the terminal branches of the sympathetic nerves that travel with the peripheral nerves, dividing these branches, and stripping the adventitia of the digital arteries.[31] These patients should be evaluated

first with radioisotope imaging of the distal circulation, peripheral pulse volume recordings, cold stress testing, and distal chemical sympathetic blockade of the digital nerves.[142] Surgical digital sympathectomy has been reported to reduce pain and increase pulp temperature.[31, 142]

Chuinard and associates[21] have reported the use of reserpine administered intravenously to relieve pain in large vessel spasm and sympathetic overflow. The technique is the same as that used for intravenous regional anesthesia. Reserpine, 1 mg, diluted in 50 ml of normal saline solution is injected, and the tourniquet is released after 15 minutes. The authors reported that 21 of 25 patients obtained pain relief.

Hannington-Kiff[45, 46] introduced the regional intravenous sympathetic block technique with guanethidine. Wynn Parry[147] records that guanethidine blocks are very effective and provide instantaneous pain relief. Under tourniquet control, 20 mg of guanethidine in 20 ml of normal saline is injected slowly into a dorsal wrist vein. The tourniquet is deflated in 20 minutes.

Early treatment includes chemical central interruption of the abnormal sympathetic reflex, and a cervical sympathetic block should be performed as a diagnostic test as well as a therapeutic procedure.[30] We use solutions of either lidocaine hydrochloride, 1%, or mepivacaine hydrochloride, 1%, to produce peripheral warming and loss of sweating, as well as relief of pain. The anterior approach is preferred for the isolated stellate block, using the technique described by Kleinert et al.[53] A series of four or five blocks should be given on consecutive days; one placebo of normal saline solution given during the series will confirm the value of the sympathetic block. Leffert and colleagues[60] at the Massachusetts General Hospital have developed a technique for continuous sympathetic blockade that utilizes an indwelling catheter for injection about the stellate ganglion. The initial technique for periodic chemical sympathetic blocks involved the lumbar area.[124]

Prognosis can be related to the effect of the sympathetic block: (1) one block may give total relief; (2) one block may give tolerable relief; (3) the duration of the first block may exceed that expected, and subsequent blocks may give progressively longer relief; (4) the duration of the first block may exceed that expected, but subsequent blocks may give progressively shorter relief; and (5) the block may give relief only for the duration expected from the anesthetic agent used.[86] For the first three responses, a series of chemical central sympathetic blocks should lead to resolution of the pain syndrome, and further treatment, other than physical therapy, may not be necessary.

Surgery should be performed when the burning pain completely responds to chemical central sympathectomy but requires repeated blocks for the long-term relief of pain. The effectiveness of sympathectomy is not related to interrupting a sensory pathway from the extremity, but to eliminating the sympathetic efferent discharge to the peripheral arteries and sweat glands. Surgical sympathectomy will relieve only burning pain; associated painful neuromas or arthritic pain will not be altered. We favor the transaxillary approach over the posterior transcostal approach, with removal of the sympathetic chain from the fourth thoracic level superior to include the lower half of the stellate ganglion. Horner's syndrome often does not develop after the transaxillary approach, which permits removal of only the lower half of the stellate ganglion, but it is more often present following the supraclavicular approach and can be very annoying to the patient. For a satisfactory result, precise postoperative sudomotor function tests should demonstrate complete sympathetic denervation of the involved extremity.

Permanent improvement by sympathetic block should not be expected in patients with response number four or five to the chemical cervical block.[86] Transcutaneous electrical nerve stimulation should be considered for those patients whose pain persists after chemical central sympathetic block. Three sites of electrode placement are utilized: (1) over a large nerve trunk proximal to the pain site; (2) at the periphery of a painful area if the lesion appears primarily cutaneous; or (3) directly over a pain site if proximal nerve trunks are not readily stimulated.[38] The intensity should be varied by the patient, because stimuli that are too intense overcome the inhibition mechanism and produce additional pain. Pain relief is complete in less than one third of patients,[37, 38, 62, 64] and the best results are obtained when the transcutaneous electrical stimulation is initiated within 3 months of the onset of pain.

In 1967, White and Sweet[140] implanted electrodes directly on the median and ulnar nerves of a patient with traumatic hyper-

pathia. Nashold and associates[82] reported 38 peripheral nerves in 35 patients stimulated with electrodes over periods from 4 to 9 years. There was successful relief of pain in 53% of patients with upper extremity pain. Direct peripheral nerve stimulation is more effective in the upper extremity than in the lower extremity. Researchers are currently implanting electrodes to stimulate cells in the periaqueductal, periventricular gray matter to release beta-endorphin and obtain analgesia.[48, 66]

Acupuncture is an ancient technique involving point pressure to relieve pain.[74, 107, 117, 125] Traditional teaching identifies 365 to 400 acupuncture points along the 12 meridian channels that contain the yin-yang forces that control the energy of life.[93, 134] Modern laboratory studies imply that acupuncture analgesia is transmitted by the nervous system and requires an intact functional nervous system to be successful.[69, 113, 132] If an intact dynamic interaction (control gate) among large and small afferent neurons is required, acupuncture should be ineffective in a disrupted nerve, such as a terminal bulb neuroma, and should be more effective in reflex sympathetic summation than in peripheral nociceptive stimulus.

An additional neurophysiologic explanation of acupuncture is that some humoral agent may be responsible, and this may explain the generalized alterations in pain threshold that have been reported in humans.[122] Sjolund and Eriksson[114] have shown that naloxone, an opiate antagonist, reverses the analgesia of acupuncture-like transcutaneous electrical nerve stimulation (TENS), but not that of traditional TENS.[18] Acupuncture-like TENS has a frequency of 2 Hz, whereas traditional TENS has a frequency of 50 to 100 Hz. Acupuncture or low frequency TENS is associated with a gradual onset of both analgesia and elevation of pain threshold, which may last for hours after the stimulation has stopped.[18, 116]

Inflammatory or Systemic Pain

Rheumatoid arthritis, diabetes, and other systemic conditions may result in stiffness and pain. Corticosteroids are useful for the patient undergoing a massive episode of painful inflammatory stiffness.[35, 36] Treatment includes a tourniquet and intravenous regional block with 30 ml of lidocaine hydrochloride, 1%, and 40 mg of methylprednisolone sodium succinate.[141] During the 20 to 30 minutes of analgesia, stiff joints can be manipulated and contracted web spaces stretched. An alternative technique is a 10-day program in which approximately 25 mg of prednisone is given orally each day for 5 days, and then the dosage is decreased 5 mg each day for 5 days. A similar 10-day program could utilize 250 mg of hydrocortisone sodium succinate intravenously each day for 5 days, then decreasing the dosage to 100 mg each day for 5 days. These drugs must be monitored and the patients evaluated for adverse reactions. As the pain subsides, the patient is encouraged to employ a gentle lanolin massage and warm water baths. Salicylates should be given to abort ongoing inflammatory metabolic pathways.

Osteoarthritis is managed with aspirin, splinting, physical therapy, and intra-articular steroids as clinically indicated. Compression and massage therapy may be helpful adjuncts, and tissue vibrators at frequencies of 100 to 140 Hz can activate joint mechanoreceptors that have inhibitory influences in the dorsal horn of the spinal cord. Transcutaneous electrical nerve stimulation can activate afferent circuits and induce inhibitory influences. Septic complications require appropriate antibiotics.

Central Pain

Severe pain is frequently cited by patients as the most incapacitating characteristic of their central nervous system postinjury (stroke or trauma) syndrome.[24] Pain of central origin is generally hyperpathic, paroxysmal, and spontaneous—descriptions used by patients include burning, searing, crawling, crushing, and gripping.[16] This monstrous agony may command all of the patient's attention and thus seriously interfere with all attempts at rehabilitation. Central pain is not often resolved by any singular treatment program, and a multifaceted approach provides the best result.[68, 102]

Beneficial medical treatment includes anticonvulsants, principally phenytoin sodium (Dilantin) and carbamazepine (Tegretol), or tricyclic antidepressant drugs such as amitriptyline hydrochloride (Elavil) or doxepin hydrochloride (Sinequan).[141] Phenytoin may be given up to 300 to 500 mg daily in divided or single doses taken with food. Amitriptyline may be given as 25 mg at bedtime and at intervals during the day for up to 150 mg

maximum daily dosage. Phenytoin and amitriptyline may be used together.[137] Amitriptyline and doxepin facilitate serotonin utilization in the central nervous system, a process involved in the transmission of pain-suppressing signals.[102] Benson[8] also advises a phenothiazine such as fluphenazine hydrochloride (Prolixin), which potentiates any narcotic, possesses an analgesic property of its own, and depresses the response to peripheral stimuli. Recommended dosage is 1 mg three times daily; this may be increased to a total of 10 mg per day.[8, 145]

Carbamazepine is the more effective drug but is prone to cause toxic symptoms such as nausea, vomiting, or unsteady gait. Because it is more often a toxic drug, carbamazepine should be increased slowly from a starting dose of 200 mg a day, gradually increasing up to a maximum of 1500 mg in divided doses. In the event that toxic symptoms occur, increasing the dose should be temporarily postponed and the dosage "plateaued" for a few days at previously tolerated levels and then gradually increased again until pain is relieved or toxic symptoms appear once more.[43, 81] Because of hematopoietic suppression, it is appropriate to follow patients on carbamazepine with monthly hemoglobin and white blood cell counts.

An occasional sedative hypnotic for a particular situation may be effective. Hydroxyzine pamoate (Vistaril), in doses of 25 to 50 mg four times a day, does not produce dependence or withdrawal effects. Narcotics are not indicated for chronic pain syndromes.

In addition to medication, electrical stimulation and psychotherapy have been effective in carefully selected cases. A neurostimulator may be inserted into the medial or lateral thalamus for pain that is diffuse, extremely agonizing, and of the highest central origin. Stimulation may reduce the pain by 50% or more in about half the patients with stroke, trauma, or quadriplegia.[103, 104]

Cancer Pain

Patients should be considered for an invasive operation when their pain is proved to be intractable to more conservative pain relief techniques.

Spinal dorsal sensory root rhizotomy through a laminectomy is indicated for patients who have unilateral pain involving the brachial plexus if the involved extremity is functionally useless. Leavens[59] has reported long-standing anesthesia in 50 of 71 patients undergoing this procedure. Other reports of rhizotomy have indicated limited success and disappointing long-term results.[49, 61, 95] Cordotomy is indicated when the pain is diffuse and involves areas innervated by many roots in a functioning upper extremity. In one study unilateral cervical cordotomy was done in 37 patients, 15 of whom experienced some pain relief until death from their disease occurred an average of 3 months after surgery.[59] Twelve of the 37 patients developed pain in the previously nonpainful side an average of 1½ months after surgery.[59] Destructive lesions in the thalamus, brain stem, and frontal lobes have been employed for many years to control pain. Cingulumotomy is the one technique that is still used for patients in whom anxiety and depression are major factors.[65]

None of these procedures provides long-lasting pain relief,[34] and all are most useful in patients who are expected to live no more than 1 year. The return of pain after surgery is related to the increased activity of polysynaptic systems (paleospinothalamic or spinoreticulothalamic) that are widespread in the brain stem and thalamus. These polysynaptic systems are infinitely complex and diffuse and eventually frustrate any ablation procedure.

Personality Dysfunction

Personality dysfunction is a component of all the symptom categories, yet may become the primary stimulus for chronic pain. There are a number of clinical conditions that demonstrate personality dysfunction, such as (1) the clenched fist syndrome, (2) factitious lymphedema, and (3) the SHAFT syndrome.[136] When a patient with a very unstable personality acquires a chronic pain syndrome, the result often is medication abuse and psychosis before treatment can be undertaken. Optimal management requires a multifaceted and highly individualized program. These patients' general physical condition may have deteriorated because of inadequate sleep, improper diet and exercise, medication abuse, or other complications. Depression may progress to the point that these patients develop an attitude of hopelessness.

Often such patients become narcotic addicts, with the following symptoms: (1) increased dose tolerance, (2) psychic craving, (3) withdrawal syndrome, and (4) inability to

sustain abstinence. These patients should be admitted as in-patients for 48 hours to establish a "drug profile," whereby they are permitted to take medications as required as long as the medications are accurately recorded by the nursing staff. The amounts of medications taken are then converted into narcotic and sedative-hypnotic equivalents, and by using arithmetic computations, an equivalent dose of one narcotic drug (methadone) and one sedative-hypnotic (phenobarbital) can be calculated and all addicting medications can be replaced.[43] These drugs are then given in a masking vehicle such as a "pain cocktail" or "pain capsules." This is an effective way of reversing drug dependency, and medication may be administered through appropriate routes, such as heparinlock, and titrated to prevent apprehension. This technique may be based on respiration rate. Once established on a medication regimen of time-contingent methadone and/or phenobarbital in their masking vehicle, these patients are often more manageable. Gradual reduction of the narcotic and/or sedative-hypnotic by 10% per day permits elimination of the dependency-producing drugs.[43, 81]

Electromyographic biofeedback may be utilized to relieve tension. Pain declined significantly in 12 of 18 patients with tension headaches studied at the University of Washington in Seattle,[96] but significant pain relief was obtained in only one of eight patients with back pain. To be effective, this modality must be utilized in conjunction with maximal therapist support.

In the latter part of the eighteenth century, the German physician Franz Anton Mesmer developed modern techniques for hypnosis. Experiments using hypnosis have shown that subjects can distort perception as well as motor movements, and by means of hypnosis one can produce partial to total anesthesia. Successful acupuncture and hypnosis both require the cerebral cortex to activate complex conditioned reflexes that raise pain thresholds, remove anxiety and tension, and relieve depression.[80]

Extremity Function Techniques

The second principle in the treatment of an established pain syndrome is functional activity. This portion of the management program is supervised by the health care team, but must be accomplished by the patient!

Passive modalities will improve circulation, decrease edema, and prepare the patient for voluntary participation in active modalities such as athletics. Passive modalities include massage, vibrators, stump wrapping, faradic muscle stimulation, ice packs, hot packs, paraffin packs, microwaves, ultrasound, and inflatable splints with positive-negative pressure. In the apprehensive patient, use of these modalities may have to be preceded by very delicate techniques, such as stroking the skin with a feather. Some passive modalities may be contraindicated, such as the whirlpool bath, which is heat dependent and may increase edema. The passive program should maintain joint motion, prevent contracture, and desensitize hyperesthetic areas.[145]

The more important phase is voluntary functional activity. Active modalities will build strength and develop dexterity. Special care should be directed to warming-up key areas of circulation, such as the rotator cuff muscles in a shoulder-arm-hand syndrome. Total body conditioning is important, and the patient should be ambulatory if possible. Function can be developed with repetitive exercises, diversional games, athletics, activities of daily living, and assigned work. It is important that the health care team be compassionate, yet obtain maximal effort from the patient. The best functional activity occurs when the patient returns to daily work. Patients who continue functional activity will ultimately "cure" themselves.

References

1. Acevedo, A., Reginato, A. J., and Schnell, A. M.: Effect of intra-arterial reserpine in patients suffering from Raynaud's phenomenon. J. Cardiovasc. Surg., 19:77–84, 1978.
2. Adams, J. E.: Naloxone reversal of analgesia produced by brain stimulation in the human. Pain, 2:161–166, 1976.
3. Akil, H., and Liebeskind, J. C.: Monoaminergic mechanisms of stimulation-produced analgesia. Brain Res., 94:279–296, 1975.
4. Akil, H., Mayer, D. J., and Liebeskind, J. C.: Antagonism of stimulation-produced analgesia by naloxone, a narcotic antagonist. Science, 191:961–962, 1976.
5. Amir, S., Brown, Z. W., and Amit, Z.: The role of endorphins in stress: Evidence and speculations. Neurosci. Behav. Rev., 4:77–86, 1980.
6. Balas, P., Tripolitis, A. J., Kaklamanis, P., Mandalaki, T., and Paracharalampous, N.: Raynaud's phenomenon. Primary and secondary causes. Arch. Surg., 114:1174–1177, 1979.
7. Barnes, R.: The role of sympathectomy in the treatment of causalgia. J. Bone Joint Surg., 35B:172–180, 1953.
8. Benson, W. F.: Treatment of the painful extremity. American Society for Surgery of the Hand, Newsletter 50, 1977.
9. Bessou, P., and Perl, E. R.: Response of cutaneous sensory units with unmyelinated fibers to noxious stimuli. J. Neurophysiol., 32:1025–1043, 1969.
10. Blair, W. F., Greene, E. R., and Omer, G. E., Jr.: A method for the calculation of blood flow in human digital arteries. J. Hand Surg., 6:90–96, 1981.
11. Bond, M. R.: Pain. Its Nature, Analysis, and Treatment. Edinburgh, Churchill Livingstone, 1979, pp. 35–40.
12. Bonica, J. J.: Causalgia and other reflex sympathetic dystrophies. Postgrad. Med. J., 53:143–148, 1976.
13. Bonica, J. J.: Neurophysiologic and pathologic aspects of acute and chronic pain. Arch. Surg., 112:750–761, 1977.
14. Bonica, J. J.: Current status of pain therapy. In Perry, S. (Chairman): The Interagency Committee on New Therapies for Pain and Discomfort. Report to the White House. U.S. Dept. of Health, Education, and Welfare, Public Health Service, Bethesda, Md., National Institutes of Health, May, 1979, pp. 111–114.
15. Bradbury, A., Smyth, D., Snell, C., Deakin, J., and Wendlant, S.: Comparison of the analgesic properties of lipotrophin C-fragment and stabilized enkephalins in the rat. Biochem. Biophys. Res. Commun., 74:478–754, 1977.
16. Burke, D. C.: Traumatic spinal paralysis in children. Paraplegia, 11:268–276, 1974.
17. Casey, K. L.: Pain: A current view of neural mechanisms. Am. Sci., 61:194–200, 1973.
18. Chapman, C. R., and Benedetti, C.: Analgesia following transcutaneous electrical stimulation and its partial reversal by a narcotic antagonist. Life Sci., 21:1645–1648, 1977.
19. Chapman, L. F., Ramos, A. O., Goodell, H., and Wolff, H. G.: Neurohumoral features of afferent fibers in man. Arch. Neurol., 4:49–82, 1961.
20. Christensen, B. N., and Perl, E. R.: Spinal neurons specifically excited by noxious or thermal stimuli: marginal zone of the dorsal horn. J. Neurophysiol., 33:293–307, 1970.
21. Chuinard, R. G., Dabezies, E. J., Gould, J. S., Murphy, G. A., and Mathews, R. E.: Intravenous reserpine for treatment of reflex sympathetic dystrophy. ASSH proceedings. J. Hand Surg., 5:289, 1980.
22. Craig, K. D., Best, H., and Ward, L. M.: Social modelling influences on psychophysical judgments of electrical stimulation. J. Abnorm. Psychol., 84:366–373, 1975.
23. Craun, G. G., and Riley, L. H., Jr.: The evaluation of neck and associated arm pain. Surg. Pract. News, 11:(November)13–27, 1982.
24. Davis, R.: Pain and suffering following spinal cord injury. Clin. Orthop., 112:76–80, 1975.
25. de Jong, R. H.: Commentary: Defining pain terms. J.A.M.A., 244:143, 1980.
26. Delagi, E. F.: Electrodiagnosis in peripheral nerve lesions. In Omer, G. E., Jr., and Spinner, M. (eds.): Management of Peripheral Nerve Problems. Philadelphia, W. B. Saunders Company, 1980, pp. 30–43.
27. Dennis, M. D., Rocchio, P. O., and Wiltse, L. L.:

The topographical pain representation and its correlation with MMPI scores. Orthopaedics, 5:432–434, 1981.

28. Doupe, J., Cullen, C. H., and Chance, G. Q.: Post-traumatic pain and causalgic syndrome. J. Neurol. Neurosurg. Psychiatry, 7:33–48, 1944.
29. Eaton, R. G.: Painful neuromas. In Omer, G. E., Jr., and Spinner, M. (eds.): Management of Peripheral Nerve Problems. Philadelphia, W. B. Saunders Company, 1980, pp. 195–202.
30. Eriksen, S.: Duration of sympathetic blockage: Stellate ganglion versus intravenous regional guanethidine block. Anaesthesia, 36:768–771, 1981.
31. Flatt, A. E.: Digital artery sympathectomy. J. Hand Surg., 5:550–556, 1980.
32. Geldard, F. A.: The Human Senses, 2nd Ed. New York, John Wiley and Sons, Inc., 1972.
33. Gelberman, R. H., Hergenroeder, P. T., Hargens, A. R., Lundborg, G. H., and Akeson, W. H.: The carpal tunnel syndrome. A study of carpal tunnel pressure. J. Bone Joint Surg., 63A:380–383, 1981.
34. Gildenberg, P. L.: Central surgical procedures for pain of peripheral nerve origin. In Omer, G. E., Jr., and Spinner, M. (eds.): Management of Peripheral Nerve Problems. Philadelphia, W. B. Saunders Company, 1980, pp. 303–314.
35. Glick, E. N.: Reflex dystrophy (algoneurodystrophy): Results of treatment by corticosteroids. Rheumatol. Rehabil., 12:84–88, 1973.
36. Glick, E. N., and Helal, B.: Post-traumatic neurodystrophy. Treatment by corticosteroids. Hand, 8:45–47, 1976.
37. Goldner, J. L.: Pain: Extremities and spine—Evaluation and differential diagnosis. In Omer, G. E., Jr., and Spinner, M. (eds.): Management of Peripheral Nerve Problems. Philadelphia, W. B. Saunders Company, 1980, pp. 119–175.
38. Goldner, J. L., Nashold, B. S., and Hendrix, P. C.: Peripheral nerve electrical stimulation. Clin. Orthop., 163:33–41, 1982.
39. Goldstein, A., Lowney, L. I., and Pal, B. K.: Stereospecific and nonspecific interactions of the morphine congener levorphanol in subcellular fractions of mouse brain. Proc. Nat. Acad. Sci. U.S.A., 68:1742–1747, 1971.
40. Grant, G. H.: Methods of treatment of neuromata of the hand. J. Bone Joint Surg., 33A:841–848, 1951.
41. Guillemin, R.: Discussion. In Reichlin, S., Baldessarini, R. J., and Martin, J. B. (eds.): The Hypothalamus. New York, Raven Press, 1978, p. 215.
42. Hagbarth, K. E., and Kerr, D. I. B.: Central influences on spinal afferent conduction. J. Neurophysiol., 17:295–307, 1954.
43. Halpern, L. M.: Analgesic drugs in the management of pain. Arch. Surg., 112:861–869, 1977.
44. Handwerker, H. O., Iggo, A., and Zimmerman, M.: Segmental and supraspinal actions on dorsal horn neurons responding to noxious and non-noxious skin stimuli. Pain, 1:147–165, 1975.
45. Hannington-Kiff, J. G.: Intravenous regional sympathetic block with guanethidine. Lancet, 1:1019–1020, 1974.
46. Hannington-Kiff, J. G.: Relief of Sudek's atrophy by regional intravenous guanethidine. Lancet, 1:1132–1133, 1977.
47. Herndon, J. H., Eaton, R. G., and Littler, J. W.: Management of painful neuromas in the hand. J. Bone Joint Surg., 58A:369–373, 1976.
48. Hosobuchi, Y., Possier, J., Bloom, F. E., and Guil-

lemin, R.: Stimulation of human periaqueductal grey matter for pain relief increases immuno-reactive beta-endorphin in ventricular fluid. Science, 203:279–281, 1979.
49. Hosobuchi, Y.: The majority of unmyelinated afferent axons in human ventral roots probably conduct pain. Pain, 8:167–180, 1980.
50. Hughes, J., Smith, T. W., Morgan, B. A., and Fothergill, L. A.: Purification and properties of enkephalin—the possible endogenous ligand for the morphine receptor. Life Sci., 16:1753–1758, 1975.
51. Iggo, A.: Pain receptors. In Bonica, J. J., Procacci, P., and Pugni, C. A. (eds.): Recent Advances on Pain: Pathophysiology and Clinical Aspects. Springfield, Ill., Charles C Thomas, 1974, pp. 3–35.
52. Jhamandos, K., Swaynok, J., and Sutak, M.: Enkephalin effects on release of brain acetylcholine. Nature, 269:433–439, 1977.
53. Kleinert, H. E., Cole, N. M., and Wayne, L.: Post-traumatic sympathetic dystrophy. Orthop. Clin. North Am., 4:917–927, 1973.
54. Kline, D. G.: Timing for exploration of nerve lesions and evaluation of the neuroma-in-continuity. Clin. Orthop., 163:42–49, 1982.
55. Koob, S.: Thermography in hand surgery. Hand, 4:64–67, 1972.
56. Kori, S. H., Foley, K. M., and Posner, J. B.: Brachial plexus lesions in patients with cancer: 100 cases. Neurology, 31:45–50, 1981.
57. Laborde, K. J., Kalisman, M., and Tsi, T.-M.: Results of surgical treatment of painful neuromas of the hand. J. Hand Surg., 7:190–193, 1982.
58. Lankford, L. L.: Reflex sympathetic dystrophy. In Omer, G. E., Jr., and Spinner, M. (eds.): Management of Peripheral Nerve Problems. Philadelphia, W. B. Saunders Company, 1980, pp. 216–244.
59. Leavens, M. E.: Neurosurgical relief of pain in cancer patients. Cancer Bull. 33:98–100, 1981.
60. Leffert, R. D., Lenson, M. A., and Todd, D. P.: The use of continuous sympathetic blockade in the treatment of reflex dystrophy. Personal communication, June 19, 1978.
61. Loeser, J. D.: Dorsal rhizotomy for the relief of chronic pain. J. Neurosurg., 36:745–750, 1972.
62. Loeser, J. D., Black, R. G., and Christman, A.: Relief of pain by transcutaneous stimulation. J. Neurosurg., 43:308–314, 1975.
63. Loh, H., Brase, D., Sampath-Khanna, S., Mar, J., Way, E., and Li, C.: Beta-endorphin in vitro inhibition of striatal dopamine release. Nature, 264:567–568, 1976.
64. Long, D. M.: Electrical stimulation for the control of pain. Arch. Surg., 112:884–888, 1977.
65. Long, D. M.: Relief of cancer pain by surgical and nerve blocking procedures. J.A.M.A., 244:2759–2761, 1980.
66. Long, D. M.: Neuromodulation for the control of chronic pain. Surg. Rounds, 5:25–34, 1982.
67. Lynn, R., and Eysenck, H. J.: Tolerance for pain, extraversion and neuroticism. Percept. Motor Skills, 12:161–162, 1961.
68. Marshall, J.: Sensory disturbances in cortical wounds with special reference to pain. J. Neurol. Neurosurg. Psychiatry, 14:187–204, 1951.
69. Matsumoto, T., and Levy, B. A.: Acupuncture for Patients. Springfield, Ill., Charles C Thomas, 1975.
70. Mayer, D. J., Wolfle, T. E., Akil, H., Carder, B.,

and Liebeskind, J. C.: Analgesia from electrical stimulation in the brainstem of the rat. Science, *174*:1351–1354, 1971.

71. Mayer, D. J., and Hayes, R.: Stimulation-produced analgesia: development of tolerance and cross-tolerance to morphine. Science, *188*:941–943, 1975.

72. Mayer, D. J., and Price, D. D.: Central nervous system mechanisms of analgesia. Pain, *2*:379–404, 1976.

73. Melzack, R., and Wall, P. D.: Pain mechanisms: A new theory. Science, *150*:971–979, 1965.

74. Melzack, R., Stillwell, D. M., and Fox, E. J.: Trigger points and acupuncture points for pain: correlations and implications. Pain, *3*:3–23, 1977.

75. Melzack, R.: Myofascial trigger points: Relation to acupuncture and mechanisms of pain. Arch. Phys. Med. Rehab., *62*:114–117, 1981.

76. Mersky, H.: Pain terms: A list with definitions and notes on usage. International Association for the Study of Pain (IASP) Subcommittee on Taxonomy. Pain, *6*:249–252, 1979.

77. Momose, T.: Potentiation of post-operative analgesic agents by hydroxyzine. *In* Bonica, J. J. (ed.): Considerations in Management of Acute Pain. New York, Hospital Practice Publishing Company, 1976, pp. 22–27.

78. Moore, D. C., Bridenbaugh, L. D., Bridenbaugh, P. O., and Tucker, G. T.: Bupivacaine: A review of 2,077 cases. J.A.M.A., *214*:713–718, 1970.

79. Moroni, F., Cheney, D., and Costa, E.: Beta-endorphin inhibits ACH turnover in nuclei of rat brain. Nature, *267*:267–268, 1977.

80. Murphy, T. M., and Bonica, J. J.: Acupuncture analgesia and anesthesia. Arch. Surg., *112*:896–902, 1977.

81. Murphy, T. M.: The pharmacology of pain relieving drugs. Symposium, American Society for Surgery of the Hand, Boston, October 17–19, 1982.

82. Nashold, B. S., Goldner, J. L., Mullen, J. B., and Bright, D. S.: Long-term pain control by direct peripheral-nerve stimulation. J. Bone Joint Surg., *64A*:1–10, 1982.

83. Oliveras, J. L., Besson, J. M., Guilbraud, G., and Liebeskind, J. C.: Behavioral and electrophysiological evidence of pain inhibition from midbrain stimulation in the cat. Exp. Brain Res., *20*:32–44, 1974.

84. Olson, G. A., Olson, R. D., Kastin, A. J., and Coy, D. H.: The opioid neuropeptides enkephalin and endorphin and their hypothesized relation to pain. *In* Smith, W. L., Mersky, H., and Gross, S. C. (eds.): Pain, Meaning and Management. New York, SP Medical and Scientific Books, 1980, pp. 21–53.

85. Omer, G. E., Jr., and Thomas, S. R.: Treatment of causalgia. Review of cases at Brooke General Hospital. Tex. Med., *67*:93–96, 1971.

86. Omer, G. E., Jr., and Thomas, S. R.: The management of chronic pain syndromes in the upper extremity. Clin. Orthop., *104*:37–43, 1974.

87. Omer, G. E., Jr., and Spinner, M.: Peripheral nerve testing and suture techniques. Instruct. Course Lecture, Am. Acad. Orthop. Surg., Vol. 24, 1975, pp. 122–143.

88. Omer, G. E., Jr.: Management of pain syndromes in the upper extremity. *In* Hunter, J. M., Schneider, L. H., Mackin, E. J., and Bell, J. A. (eds.): Rehabilitation of the Hand. St. Louis, The C. V. Mosby Company, 1978, pp. 341–349.

89. Omer, G. E., Jr.: Management of the painful extremity. *In* Ahstrom, J. P., Jr. (ed.): Current Practice in Orthopaedic Surgery, Vol. 8. St. Louis, The C. V. Mosby Company, 1979, pp. 86–98.

90. Omer, G. E., Jr.: Nerve, neuroma, and pain problems related to upper limb amputations. Orthop. Clin. North Am., *12*:751–762, 1981.

91. Omer, G. E., Jr.: The neuroma-in-continuity. *In* Strickland, J. W., and Steichen, J. B. (eds.): Difficult Problems in Hand Surgery. St. Louis, The C. V. Mosby Company, 1982, pp. 369–373.

92. Omer, G. E., Jr.: The painful neuroma. *In* Strickland, J. W., and Steichen, J. B. (eds.): Difficult Problems in Hand Surgery, St. Louis, The C. V. Mosby Company, 1982, pp. 319–323.

93. Omer, G. E., Jr.: An American surgeon in Korea: Han Yak medicine, Unpublished observations.

94. Omer, G. E., Jr.: Present thoughts on the management of pain in the upper extremity. Clin. Plast. Surg., *11*:85–93, 1984.

95. Onofrio, B. M., and Campa, H. K.: Evaluation of rhizotomy. Review of 12 years' experience. J. Neurosurg., *36*:751–755, 1972.

96. Peck, C. L., and Kraft, G. H.: Electromyographic biofeedback for pain related to muscle tension. Arch. Surg., *112*:889–895, 1977.

97. Pert, C., and Snyder, S.: Opiate receptor: Demonstration in nervous tissue. Science, *179*:1011–1014, 1973.

98. Plewes, L. W.: Sudek's atrophy in the hand. J. Bone Joint Surg., *38B*:195–203, 1956.

99. Pochaczevsky, R.: Assessment of back pain by contact thermography of extremity dermatomes. Orthop. Rev., *12*:45–58, 1983.

100. Pomeranz, B., Cheng, R., and Law, P.: Acupuncture reduces electrophysiological and behavioral responses to noxious stimuli: Pituitary is implicated. Exp. Neurol., *54*:172–178, 1977.

101. Porter, J. M., Snider, R. L., Bardana, E. J., Rosch, J., and Eidemiller, L. R.: The diagnosis and treatment of Raynaud's phenomenon. Surgery, *77*:11–23, 1975.

102. Ray, C. D.: Pain of central nervous system injury origin. Surg. Pract. News, Vol. *11*:(September) 7–19, 1982.

103. Ray, C. D.: Control of pain by electrical stimulation: a clinical follow-up review. *In* Penholz, H. (ed.): Brain Hypoxia: Pain: Papers presented at the 26th Annual Meeting of the Deutsche Gesellschaft fur Neurochirurgie, Heidelberg, May 1–3, 1975, Berlin, New York: Springer-Verlag, pp. 216–224.

104. Ray, C. D.: Spinal epidural electrical stimulation for pain control: Practical details and results. Appl. Neurophysiol., *44*:194–206, 1981.

105. Rexed, B.: The cytoarchitecture organization of the spinal cord of the cat. J. Comp. Neurol., *96*:415–496, 1952.

106. Reynolds, D. V.: Surgery in the rat during electrical analgesia induced by focal brain stimulation. Science, *164*:444–445, 1969.

107. Rubin, D.: Myofascial trigger point syndromes: an approach to management. Arch. Phys. Med. Rehab., *62*:107–110, 1981.

108. Rydevik, B., Lundborg, G., and Bagge, U.: Effects of graded compression on intraneural blood flow. J. Hand Surg., *6*:3–12, 1981.

109. Schachtel, H. J.: Pain and religion. Cancer Bull. *33*:84–85, 1981.

110. Simons, D.: Myofascial trigger points: A need for

understanding. Arch. Phys. Med. Rehab., 62:107–110, 1981.

111. Simson, G.: Propranol for causalgia and Sudek atrophy (Letter). J.A.M.A., 227:327, 1974.

112. Singer, S. J.: Architecture and topography of biologic membranes. *In* Weissman, G., and Claiborne, R. (eds.): Cell Membranes: Biochemistry, Cell Biology, and Pathology. New York, Hospital Practice Publishing Company, 1975, pp. 35–44.

113. Sjolund, B., Terenius, L., and Eriksson, M.: Increased cerebrospinal fluid levels of endorphins after electro-acupuncture. Acta Physio. Scand., 100:382–384, 1977.

114. Sjolund, B. H., and Eriksson, M. B. E.: The influence of naloxone on analgesia produced by peripheral conditioning stimulation. Brain Res. 173:295–301, 1979.

115. Smith, J. R., and Gomez, N. H.: Local injection therapy of neuromata of the hand with triamcinolone acetonide, a preliminary study of twenty-two patients. J. Bone Joint Surg., 52A:71–83, 1970.

116. Snyder, S. H.: Opiate receptors and internal opiates. Sci. Am., 236(March):44–56, 1977.

117. Sola, A. E., and Williams, R. L.: Myofascial pain syndromes. Neurology (Minneapolis), 6:91–95, 1956.

118. Spinner, M.: Injuries to the Major Branches of Peripheral Nerves of the Forearm, 2nd Ed. Philadelphia, W. B. Saunders Company, 1978, pp. 54–63.

119. Sternbach, R. A., Wolf, S. R., Murphy, R. W., and Akeson, W. H.: Traits of pain patients: the low-back "loser." Psychosomatics, 14:226–229, 1973.

120. Sternbach, R. A.: Modern concepts of pain. *In* Dalessio, D. J. (ed.): Wolff's Headache and Other Head Pain, 4th Ed. New York, Oxford University Press, 1980, pp. 9–23.

121. Stilz, R. J., Carron, H., and Sanders, D. B.: Reflex sympathetic dystrophy in a 6-year-old: Successful treatment by transcutaneous nerve stimulation. Anesth. Analg., 56:438–443, 1977.

122. Sufian, S., Pavlides, C., Fischer, C. R., III, Matulewski, T., and Matsumoto, T.: Acupuncture for chronic pain and anesthesia. Surg. Rounds, 5:38–49, 1982.

123. Swanson, A. B., Boeve, N. R., and Lumsden, R. M.: The prevention and treatment of amputation neuromata by silicone capping. J. Hand Surg., 2:70–78, 1977.

124. Thomason, J. R., and Moritz, W. H.: Continuous lumbar paravertebral sympathetic block maintained by fractional installation of procaine. Surg. Gynecol. Obstet., 89:447–453, 1949.

125. Travell, J., and Rinzler, S. H.: The myofascial genesis of pain. Postgrad. Med., 11:425–434, 1952.

126. Tsairis, P., Dyck, P. J., and Mulder, D. W.: Natural history of brachial plexus neuropathy. Arch. Neurol., 27:109–117, 1972.

127. Tseng, L. F., Loh, H., and Li, C.: Beta-endorphin as a potent analgesic by intravenous injection. Nature, 263:239–240, 1976.

128. Tupper, J. W., and Booth, D. M.: Treatment of painful neuromas of sensory nerves in the hand:

A comparison of traditional and newer methods. J. Hand Surg., 1:144–151, 1976.

129. Turner, R. S., and Leiding, W. C.: Correlation of MMPIs with lumbosacral spine fusion results: Prospective and retrospective groupings. A five-year study of 155 patients. (Personal correspondence, October 10, 1981.)

130. Tursky, B., and O'Connell, D.: Reliability and interjudgment predictability of subjective judgments of electrocutaneous stimulation. Psychophysiology, 9:290–295, 1972.

131. Tursky, B.: Physical, physiological, and psychological factors that affect pain reaction to electric shock. Psychophysiology, 11:95–112, 1974.

132. Ulett, G. H.: Acupuncture treatments for pain relief. J.A.M.A., 245:768–769, 1981.

133. Vaux, K. L.: Pain: The moral dimensions. Cancer Bull. 33:86–87, 1981.

134. Veith, I.: Acupuncture in traditional Chinese medicine. Calif. Med., 118:70–79, 1973.

135. Waldo, R.: Prazosin relieves Raynaud's vasospasm. J.A.M.A., 241:1037, 1979.

136. Wallace, P. F., and Fitzmorris, C. S., Jr.: The S-H-A-F-T syndrome in the upper extremity. J. Hand Surg., 3:492–494, 1978.

137. Ward, N. G., Bloom, V. L., and Friedel, R. D.: The effectiveness of tricyclic antidepressants in the treatment of co-existing pain and depression. Pain, 7:331–341, 1979.

138. Webster, K. E.: Somaesthetic pathways. Br. Med. Bull., 33:113–120, 1977.

139. Weissman, G.: Pain mediators and pain receptors. *In* Bonica, J. J. (ed.): Considerations in Management of Acute Pain. New York, Hospital Practice Publishing Company, 1977.

140. White, J. C., and Sweet, W. H.: Pain and the Neurosurgeon. A Forty Year Experience. Springfield, Ill., Charles C Thomas, 1969, pp. 895–896.

141. Wiley, A. M., Poplawski, Z. B., and Murray, J.: Post-traumatic dystrophy of the hand. Orthop. Review, 6:59–61, 1977.

142. Wilgis, E. F. S.: Evaluation and treatment of chronic digital ischemia. Ann. Surg., 193:693–698, 1981.

143. Wilgis, E. F. S.: Techniques for diagnosis of peripheral nerve loss. Clin. Orthop., 163:8–14, 1982.

144. Willis, W. D., Trevino, D. L., Coulter, J. D., and Maunz, R. A.: Responses of primate spinothalamic tract neurons to natural stimulation of the hindlimb. J. Neurophysiol., 37:358–372, 1974.

145. Wilson, R. L.: Management of pain following peripheral nerve injuries. Orthop. Clin. North Am., 12:343–359, 1981.

146. Wolff, B. B., and Jarvik, M. E.: Variations in cutaneous and deep somatic pain sensitivity. Can. J. Psychol., 17:37–44, 1963.

147. Wynn Parry, C. B.: Brachial plexus lesions, causalgia, and Sudek's atrophy. American Society for Surgery of the Hand, Newsletter 2, 1981.

148. Zorub, D. S., Nashold, B. S., Jr., and Cook, W. A., Jr.: Avulsion of the brachial plexus: I. A review with implications on the therapy of intractable pain. Surg. Neurol., 2:347–353, 1974.

12

The Painful Stump Neuroma and Its Treatment

■

H. Bruce Williams, M.D.

Symptomatic neuromas continue to be an enigma to the treating surgeon—their symptomatology is poorly understood and their successful treatment is often difficult.

PATHOLOGY AND CLINICAL SYMPTOMS

A post-traumatic neuroma may be defined as a tumor mass that is composed of nerve and connective tissue and is usually situated terminally at the end of a completely severed nerve or in continuity if the nerve injury itself is incomplete. Grossly, it is composed of rubbery to firm, usually well-circumscribed white tissue that may be adherent to adjacent structures. This surrounding scar, which resulted from the primary injury, may involve the adjacent skin, muscle, tendon, or periosteum. Pain is usually the presenting symptom and the neuroma may be exquisitely sensitive to touch or to percussion. Proximal or distal radiation of the pain is often an associated finding. With careful examination, a trigger area can often be detected, thus accurately identifying the location of the neuroma. Histologically, there is an admixture of nerve elements and fibrous tissue arranged in a haphazard fashion. The axonal elements may be arranged in a whorl-type pattern and are surrounded by proliferating Schwann cells and fibroblasts with varying amounts of collagen and fibrous tissue (Fig. 12–1).

NERVE INJURY AND NEUROMA CLASSIFICATION

Nerve injuries may be complete or incomplete. Seddon's classification[14] divided the nerve injuries into three types: (1) neurapraxia, (2) axonotmesis, and (3) neurotmesis. Neurapraxia is a temporary loss of conduction without loss of continuity of the nerve. This injury usually results after contusion of a nerve, or it can be associated with tourniquet ischemia. Axonotmesis is a more severe form of nerve injury with severance of the axon but with preservation of the endoneurial sheaths. Neurotmesis is complete severance of the nerve with loss of continuity of the entire structure.

Sunderland[15] contributed a further subdivision of nerve injuries and listed five grades according to their severity: grade I, loss of conduction in the axons; grade II, loss of continuity of the axons without affecting the endoneurium; grade III, loss of continuity of the nerve fibers (endoneurium affected); grade IV, loss of continuity of the fascicles (perineurium affected); and grade V, loss of continuity of the entire nerve.

These two classifications can be compared for purposes of description. For example, grade I injuries of Sunderland correspond to neurapraxia in Seddon's classification; similarly, grade II injuries (Sunderland) correspond to axonotmesis (Seddon), and grades III, IV, and V injuries of Sunderland represent gradations in severity of Seddon's neurotmesis. Proximal pseudoneuromas, as seen

161

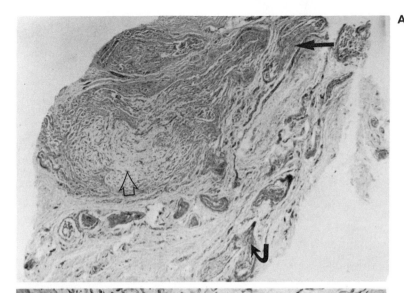

A

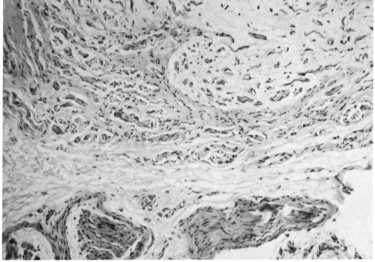

B

Figure 12–1. *A,* Digital nerve neuroma (hematoxylin and eosin, × 20). Note the marked perineural fibrosis and the haphazard arrangement of nerve tissue admixed with intraneural scar tissue. One area of myxoid degeneration is seen (*open arrow*), and the digital nerve stump is seen entering the neuromatous tissue (*arrow*). A misdirected nerve remnant is seen within the scar tissue below (*curved arrow*). (From Williams, H. B.: Clin. Plast. Surg., *11:*80, 1984.) *B,* Same specimen at high power (× 100). Multiple small whorl-like axonal fascicles are seen surrounded by internal nerve fibrosis.

in nerve compression problems such as the carpal tunnel syndrome or the cubital tunnel syndrome, can range in severity from grade I to grade III in Sunderland's classification and may represent either neurapraxia or axonotmesis in Seddon's classification. True neuromas form following complete nerve disruption and are therefore classified under neurotmesis (Seddon) or as grade V lesions (Sunderland).

CHANGES IN THE NERVE FOLLOWING SEVERANCE

Both the proximal and the distal segments of a severed nerve should be considered in a discussion of nerve injuries. The changes seen at the proximal end of the cut nerve are obviously of greatest importance when neuroma formation is under consideration.

Proximal Nerve Segment. The parent cell, either in the anterior horn of the spinal cord (motor nerves) or in the posterior root ganglia (sensory nerves), shows changes in its cell body, nucleus, and nucleolus. The cells swell, the Golgi apparatus fragments, and the Nissl granules may dissolve. This histologic change is known as chromatolysis and should likely be regarded as a preparation for regeneration rather than as a degenerative phenomenon. The nerve fiber itself (axon) degenerates in a retrograde fashion to the next intact node of Ranvier. Within a few hours to days, each individual axon forms several branches that grow distally. The

Schwann cells of each involved endoneurial tube proliferate, as do the fibroblasts of the endoneurium, perineurium, and epineurium. This process continues unchecked in an unrepaired nerve until a bulbous neuroma is formed at the end of the injured nerve and is often associated with considerable adhesions to all surrounding structures.

Distal Nerve Segment. Following nerve severance, changes are clearly evident in the distal segment within 24 hours. In the early stages, there is swelling followed by fragmentation of the neurofibrils and separation of the myelin sheaths. All traces of the axons disappear by the second or third week. The myelin sheath itself fragments into droplets, and the Schwann cells show proliferation within 48 hours. The myelin fragments, axonal remnants, and debris are removed in the process of phagocytosis by either the active Schwann cells or the tissue macrophages. This entire process, called Wallerian degeneration, was initially described by A. V. Waller, an English physiologist, in 1850. All that survives in the distal segment of the severed nerve is a syncytial strand of cells, reinforced by the endoneurial connective tissue sheath. Electrical stimulation of the distal segment gives a positive response for 3 to 5 days, depending on the speed of axonal degeneration.

NEUROMA FORMATION

A terminal neuroma or a stump neuroma will form when the nerve is completely cut,

and a neuroma in continuity will result from an incomplete nerve lesion. Painful neuromas are also seen following surgical repair of severed nerves, particularly nerves that show little evidence of recovery, which may in part be related to faulty surgical technique. The management of neuromas in continuity has been covered in other publications.[21, 22] This discussion will be directed toward the management of painful terminal or stump neuromas.

Symptoms. There seems little doubt that all severed nerves will form neuromas at their cut ends. However, only a small percentage of neuromas become painful, and there appears to be a relationship between the development of pain and the location of the nerve that is injured. For example, cut digital nerves commonly produce painful neuromas, as does damage to the superficial radial nerve at the level of the wrist or distal forearm (Fig. 12–2). This seems to be a particularly associated finding when the nerve is inadvertently cut during surgical procedures such as ganglionectomy or following tendon release in de Quervain's syndrome. It is also thought that median nerve neuromas are more common than those following injuries of the ulnar nerve, and, in addition, a significant number of patients with stump neuromas following amputations will have pain and other signs of localized symptomatology.

The pain from neuromas will be described as burning, sharp, or aching in nature, and a trigger area can usually be identified that is the central focus for the pain stimulus. Some patients with neuromas may even de-

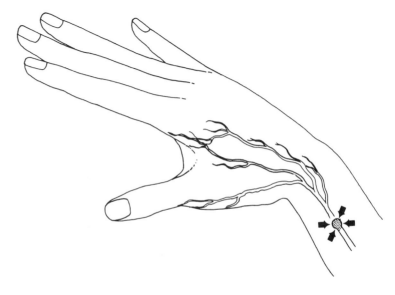

Figure 12–2. Symptomatic neuroma over the superficial radial nerve at the wrist. Arrows indicate the exquisitely tender "trigger" area that can be located with careful examination. (From Williams, H. B.: Clin. Plast. Surg., *11*:80, 1984.)

velop reflex sympathetic dystrophic changes, and other patients with partial nerve injuries may exhibit a fullblown causalgia-like syndrome. The pain mechanism is difficult to explain and there appears to be great patient specificity. For example, some patients will have severe debilitating pain symptoms, whereas others with the same injury remain completely asymptomatic. At times, it is difficult to determine if there is a relationship between the patient's personality and neuroma symptoms. Patients who tend to be labile with passive-aggressive personalities seem to develop symptomatology, or perhaps their personality changes are secondary to the injury and its sequelae. The symptoms related to neuromas should likely be differentiated from true causalgia, although both may show evidence of sympathetic overactivity. The diagnosis of causalgia, as defined by Granit et al.,[7] should likely be restricted to partial nerve injuries that permit efferent sympathetic discharge to activate afferent pain fibers through a breakdown in insulation at the point of injury. This would correspond to the original description of causalgia by Weir Mitchell.

MANAGEMENT OF NEUROMAS

Prevention. Prophylaxis against neuroma formation is of vital importance in the surgical management of wounds. Following amputation, each nerve end should be identified, dissected free, and then allowed to retract into healthy tissue. In this manner, a large number of painful neuromas can be prevented, and, similarly, great care should be taken with all surgical procedures that might damage local nerves in the process of exploration. This particularly applies to operative procedures such as ganglion excisions at the wrist, in decompression in de Quervain's syndrome, or tendon explorations and repairs. Older methods of nerve end management, such as crushing, coagulation, and injection of chemicals, likely add very little to the prevention of neuroma formation.

Local Treatment and Desensitization. Massage, percussion, tapping, and active physiotherapy with use of the injured part often help in alleviation of neuroma symptoms. In many ways, this is similar to the counterirritant type of treatment.

Transcutaneous Electrical Nerve Stimulation. Transcutaneous electrical nerve stimulation (TENS) has progressed in technical sophistication and effective application over the past several years. It is used most commonly for chronic pain problems or as a "last resort" modality, but may also be useful for certain acute pain problems. Many TENS devices are available, and an understanding of the reliability and safety of each instrument is of great importance. Different ranges of current amplitude, pulse width duration, and pulse rate are offered, and desensitization is performed by providing sensory rather than motor stimulation.

With careful patient selection, properly applied TENS may be extremely useful as an adjunctive modality in controlling pain associated with post-traumatic neuromas (Fig. 12–3).

Scar Release. Dissection and excision of the neuroma with neurolysis and freeing of the adherent scar from the surrounding tissue will allow for proximal retraction of the nerve into normal tissue. This localized treatment will provide relief in approximately 60% of symptomatic neuromas.

Nerve Capping. Nerve capping was introduced in an attempt to prevent recurrence of neuromas by walling off the nerve end from surrounding tissues. A number of materials have been used for nerve capping, including Millipore by Campbell et al.[1] and Micropore by Freeman and associates.[5, 6] Gold foil and tantalum have also been used in the past, and more recently silicone capping has been introduced and reported upon by Tauras and Frackelton,[17] Swanson and associates,[16] and others. The silicone capping method allows for epineurial healing over the severed fascicles within the chamber and will, hopefully, lessen the chances of painful neuroma formation (Fig. 12–4). Using this technique, the nerve is dissected free from all adjacent scar and the epineurium is brought distally over the ends of the fascicles; using the two suture ends, the nerve is passed into the silicone cap and anchored well away from the area of injury (Fig. 12–5). This method of neuroma management has been successful in about 70% of reported cases.

Funiculectomy and Epineurial Sleeves. With this technique, the epineurium is first retracted under microscopic control, and each fascicle (funiculus) is cut short and allowed to retract within the epineurial sleeve. The epineurium is then brought out to full length and a double or triple ligature is placed around the epineurial sleeve, allowing

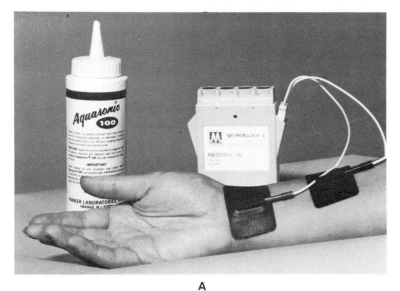

A

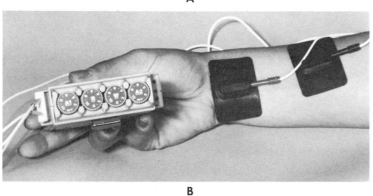

B

Figure 12–3. *A,* Transcutaneous electrical nerve stimulation (TENS). The pad electrodes are applied to the skin over the painful neuroma. (Stimulator by Medelco Ltd., 4478 Chesswood Drive, Downsview, Ontario, Canada; Conductive gel by Aquasonic, Parker Laboratories, Orange, New Jersey). (From Williams, H. B.: Clin. Plast. Surg., *11*:82, 1984.) *B,* Control dials for stimulation, amperage, and duration can be regulated by teaching personnel or by the patient after suitable training.

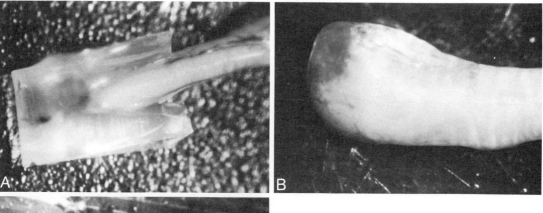

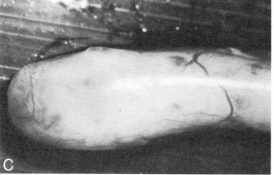

Figure 12–4. *A,* Silicone nerve capping (experimental rat model) demonstrating the smooth resurfaced distal cut end of the nerve with minimal neuroma formation. *B,* Bulbous neuroma 3 weeks following nerve section without silicone capping. *C,* The 3-week specimen following silicone capping demonstrates limited neuroma formation and rich vasculature of the resurfaced epineurium.

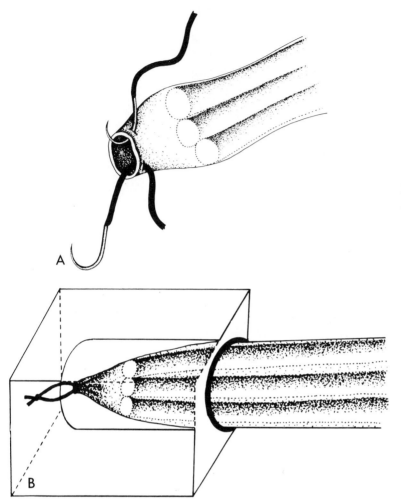

Figure 12–5. Silicone capping technique. *A,* The epineurium is brought distal to the shortened fascicles, and two sutures are placed for positioning of the nerve end into the silicone cap. *B,* Silicone cap in position with sutures tied after passage through silicone cap. (From Williams, H. B.: Clin. Plast. Surg., *11*:82, 1984.)

nerve healing to take place within its epineurial space. In this way, it is postulated that less fibroblastic proliferation will occur, and the resultant reduction in scar tissue will lessen the chances of neuroma formation (Fig. 12–6).

Chapple[2] reported on the use of epineurial sleeves in 1917. More recently, Tupper[19] reported on the combination of epineurial sleeves and funiculectomy and offered a comparison between these results and treatment using silicone caps. He reviewed 172 patients with 348 painful neuromas and showed that excisional neurectomy alone was successful in 65% of patients and silicone capping did not significantly improve the results. Funicular resection with epineurial ligation in 45 patients gave as good results as excisional neurectomies.

Combined Funiculectomy, Epineurial Sleeves, and Silicone Capping. It should also be stressed that silicone capping can be com-

bined with funiculectomy and epineurial sleeves, and this combination has been used in a number of our patients with improved results. Our personal experience indicates that this combined method of treatment should likely be reserved for recurrent or resistant neuromas, particularly in those patients with considerable scar tissue at the site of injury (Fig. 12–7).

Sympathetic Blockade with Guanethidine. Guanethidine displaces norepinephrine from the sympathetic nerve endings and produces a continuous sympathetic blockade lasting from several days to 3 weeks. It apparently binds to the norepinephrine storage vesicles and releases this substance from the nerve endings. Guanethidine has been used for the management of hypertension for several years and has recently been reported as a method of regional sympathetic block using the intravenous route and a tourniquet. With this technique, the limb to be blocked is

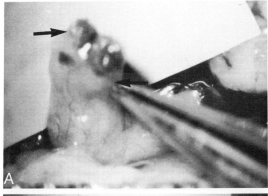
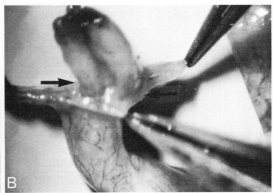
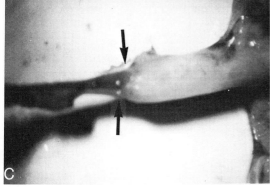

Figure 12–6. Funiculectomy and epineurial sleeve technique. *A,* The epineurium is grasped distally (*arrows*) for proximal retraction and shortening of fascicles. *B,* The epineurium is retracted (*arrows*). The distally placed fascicles will be excised, thus allowing the epineurial sleeve to be brought distally. *C,* Following resection of the distal fascicles, the epineurium is brought out to length and fine sutures may then be used for ligation of this epineurial sleeve (*arrows*).

elevated for 3 to 5 minutes for drainage of blood and is then further exsanguinated by means of an Esmarch bandage. A double cuff tourniquet is then applied and the pressure is elevated to 250 mg Hg. Through an intravenous needle that had previously been inserted into a peripheral vein of the limb to be blocked, a dose of 15 to 20 mg of guanethidine (in the arm) or 20 to 30 mg (in the leg) is injected. The guanethidine is diluted with 20 to 40 ml of normal saline solution or 0.5% mepivacaine, depending on the limb to be blocked and the size of the patient. The total dose and volume of drugs injected can be reduced if, for example, only the hand is isolated. The tourniquet is then kept inflated for 10 to 15 minutes after the injection in order to allow the guanethidine to become fixed within the tissues of the extremity and to reduce any tendency toward hypotension upon the release of the guanethidine into the circulation when the tourniquet is deflated. Patients are monitored in the recovery room for 2 hours following the block. The efficacy of sympathetic blockade is judged by measuring skin temperature and comparing this with temperature of the unblocked extremity.

Most of our microsurgical replantation pa-

Figure 12–7. Drawing to demonstrate the combined method of treatment with funiculectomy, epineurial sleeve technique, and silicone capping. (From Williams, H. B.: Clin. Plast. Surg., *11*:83, 1984.)

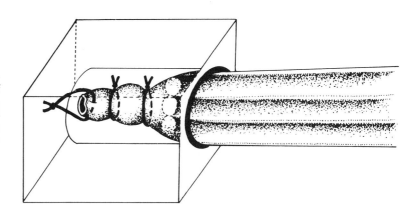

tients for the past 8 years have been treated with guanethidine in an attempt to provide a sympathetic block for 7 to 10 days following replantation, thus improving localized blood flow to the replanted parts. Recently this technique has been expanded to include the treatment of patients with symptomatic neuromas.

Neuroma Excision and Nerve Grafting. Precise microsurgical techniques for nerve repair will usually prevent the formation of neuromas. However, the occasional patient is seen who exhibits marked discomfort or even intractable pain at the site of surgical repair that is not amenable to the usual forms of therapy. These patients may travel from one surgeon to another searching for a cure and may well have undergone a wide variety of treatment modalities such as brachial blocks, visits to pain clinics, acupuncture, injections, prolonged physiotherapy and occupational therapy, and perhaps even neurolysis, all without success. Such patients present a formidable task for those interested in the problem, and surgical excision under controlled conditions followed by nerve grafting may be the only sensible form of treatment. This may well be feasible for intractable pain such as that found with superficial radial neuromas and with neuromas of the median nerve. I have found that an added sympathetic blockade with guanethidine is extremely helpful in managing these difficult problems.

CASE REPORTS

Case 1

A 34-year-old woman had an amputation through the middle phalanx of the right index finger. She had not returned to work in a textile factory for 18 months following injury because of intractable pain over the amputation stump. One scar revision and neuroma resection was performed at 9 months after injury without any improvement in her symptoms. At surgery, the adherent scar over the stump was excised, and the bilateral stump neuromas were dissected free of the surrounding tissues (Fig. 12–8A and B). A funiculectomy was performed along with ligation of the epineurial sleeve, and a small silicone cap was placed on each nerve. The patient has remained asymptomatic since operation and has returned to her occupation. This represents the combined treatment of funiculectomy, epineurial sleeve, and silicone capping (Fig. 12–8C and D).

Case 2

A 28-year-old man had severe pain on touch and pressure over a superficial radial nerve neuroma at the right wrist. The symptoms followed surgical tendon release in de Quervain's syndrome when the superficial radial nerve was completely severed. Two attempts at neuroma excision and transposition of the nerve end were unsuccessful, and the patient was unable to return to his work as a laborer for 2½ years. He was returned to the operating room, and a small sural graft was used to bridge the gap following resection of the neuroma and freeing of the distal segment (Fig. 12–9). The patient progressed well following this third operative procedure, and although he continued to have mild local symptoms at the site of surgery, he was able to return to his former occupation 6 weeks following surgery. This patient represents an example of neuroma treatment using microsurgical techniques and nerve grafting.

Case 3

This 38-year-old woman presented with a 5-year history of intractable pain over the distal right forearm, hand, and radial 3½ digits following a repair of a severed median nerve. Distal recovery was minimal, with a two-point discrimination of 15 mm over the median nerve distribution, and the patient showed evidence of a sympathetic dystrophy with a red, swollen hand and diffuse atrophy and osteoporosis on radiographic study. She had previously been treated with neurolysis without improvement, and a period of desensitization was started using electrical stimulation. Local massage and percussion of the neuroma area did not help her symptoms, and prolonged physiotherapy and occupational therapy were of little benefit. The patient was rapidly becoming a recluse with an almost fullblown causalgia syndrome (Fig. 12–10A).

She was treated with a series of guanethidine blocks and continued with transcutaneous electrical desensitization. The nerve was then surgically explored, and the large median nerve neuroma in continuity was completely resected (operation performed by Dr. H. C. Brown). The large resultant nerve defect was treated using microsurgical techniques with four sural nerve grafts, and her initial good postoperative result continued during a long-term follow-up. Her sensory recovery was not impressive. She showed only a 12-mm moving two-point discrimination, and there was no evidence of thenar muscle recovery. The patient, however, was free of pain in the hand 2 years following the surgical procedure, and it was possible to discontinue all other forms of treatment. She continued to have localized discomfort on palpation in the nerve graft area, but this did not interfere with her return to work.

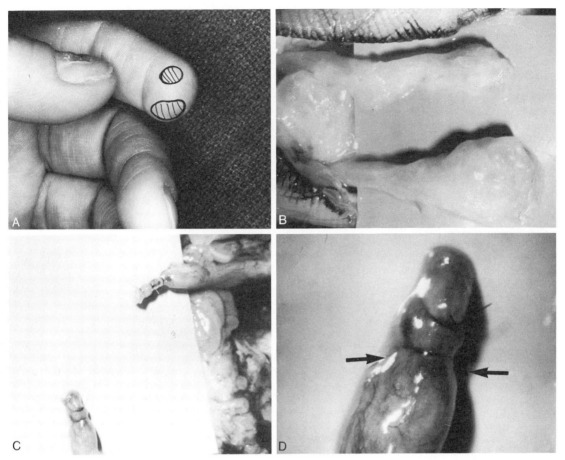

Figure 12–8. Case 1 (see text). *A,* Painful neuromas, distal left index finger amputation stump. Ulnar "trigger" area was larger, as outlined in black ink. *B,* Following exploration, these two neuromas are demonstrated with extensive scar adherence. Note the larger neuroma on the ulnar side. *C,* Following neuroma excision, both digital nerves were managed with funiculectomy, epineurial sleeve suture ligation, and silicone capping. *D,* Close-up to show two sutures closing the epineurial sleeve following funiculectomy *(arrows)*. A silicone cap will now be applied.

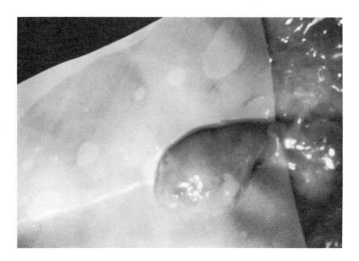

Figure 12–9. Case 2 (see text). Neuroma, superficial radial nerve, right wrist.

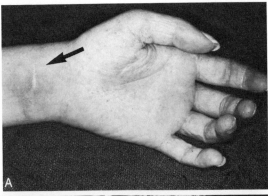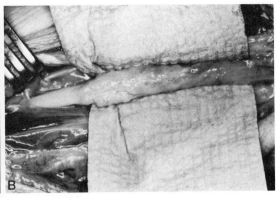

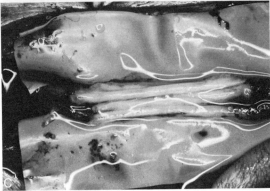

Figure 12–10. Case 3 (see text). *A,* Patient with severe sympathetic dystrophic changes following right median nerve severance. Positive Tinel's sign (*arrow*) corresponded to large neuroma at site of injury. Note thenar wasting and color changes over finger tips. *B,* After dissection a large neuroma of the median nerve is exposed, showing lack of fascicular continuity and marked surrounding scar. *C,* Multiple sural nerve grafts in place following resection of the median nerve neuroma.

This method of patient management is an example of neuroma excision in a major nerve with nerve grafting and sympathetic blockade. It could be considered for patients with long-term disorders of over 2 to 3 years' duration, particularly when all other forms of treatment have been unsuccessful.

SUMMARY

Successful clinical management of symptomatic neuromas continues to present a challenge to the responsible surgeon. Why some patients with neuromas are completely asymptomatic whereas others exhibit debilitating symptoms remains unexplained.

Prevention of neuromas is paramount, with precise attention to severed nerves following amputations or other surgical procedures. Once neuromas are established, treatment consists of careful patient counseling, local massage, and desensitization procedures. Sympathetic blockade with guanethidine may be beneficial in some patients. When necessary, surgical excision of the neuroma along with a combination of funiculectomy, epineurial sleeve suture ligation, and silicone capping offers the best chance for eradication. In intractable or recurrent cases and following careful patient selection, neuroma excision followed by nerve grafting combined with sympathetic blockade using guanethidine can be successful in a significant number of patients.

References

1. Campbell, J. G., Bassett, C. A. L., and Bohler, J.: Frozen irradiated homografts shielded with microfilter sheaths in peripheral nerve surgery. J. Trauma, 3:303, 1963.
2. Chapple, W. A.: Re-amputation. Br. Med. J., 2:242, 1917.
3. Davies, K. H.: Guanethidine sympathetic blockade: Its value in reimplantation surgery. Br. Med. J., 2:876, 1976.
4. Frackelton, W. H., Yeasley, J. L., and Tauras, A.: Neuromas in the hand treated by nerve transposition and silicone capping. J. Bone Joint Surg., 53:813, 1971.
5. Freeman, B. S.: Adhesive neural anastomoses. Plast. Reconstr. Surg., 35:167, 1965.

6. Freeman, B. S., Perry, J., and Brown, D.: Experimental study of adhesive surgical tape for nerve anastomosis. Plast. Reconstr. Surg., 43:174, 1969.
7. Granit, R., Leksell, L., and Skoglund, C. R.: Fiber interaction of injured or compressed region of nerve. Brain, 67:125, 1944.
8. Hannington-Kiff, J. G.: Intravenous regional sympathetic block with guanethidine. Lancet, 1:1019, 1974.
9. Holland, A. J. C., Davies, K. H., and Wallace, D. H.: Sympathetic blockade of isolated limbs by intravenous guanethidine. Can. Anaes. Soc. J., 24:597, 1977.
10. Lampe, G. N.: Introduction to the use of transcutaneous electrical stimulation device. Am. Physiotherapy Assoc. (Special Issue), 58:14, 1978.
11. McMinn, R. M. H., and Pritchard, J. J.: Tissue Repair. New York, Academic Press, 1969.
12. Mannheimer, J. J.: Electrical placements for transcutaneous electrical nerve stimulation. Am. Physiotherapy Assoc. (Special Issue), 58:19, 1978.
13. Orgel, M., Aguayo, A., and Williams, H. B.: Nerve regeneration in skin grafts. J. Anat., 111:121, 1972.
14. Seddon, H.: Surgical Disorders of the Peripheral Nerves. Edinburgh, Churchill Livingstone, 1972.
15. Sunderland, S.: Nerves and Nerve Injuries. Baltimore, Williams and Wilkins Company, 1968.
16. Swanson, A. B., Boeve, N. R., and Lumsden, R. M.: The prevention and treatment of amputation neuromata by silicone capping. J. Hand Surg., 2:70, 1977.
17. Tauras, A. P., and Frackelton, W. H.: Silicone capping of nerve stumps in the problem of painful neuromas. Surg. Forum, 18:504, 1967.
18. Terzis, J., and Williams, H. B.: Functional aspects of reinnervation of skin grafts. Surg. Forum, 25:518, 1974.
19. Tupper, J. W.: Treatment of painful neuromas of sensory nerves in the hand: A comparison of traditional and newer methods. J. Hand Surg, 1:144, 1976.
20. White, J. C., and Hamlin, H.: New uses of tantalum in nerve suture; control of neuroma formation. J. Neurosurg., 2:402, 1945.
21. Williams, H. B.: Neuromas, diagnosis and management. In Fredricks, S., and Brody, G. (eds.): Neurological Aspects of Plastic Surgery. St. Louis, C. V. Mosby Company, 1978.
22. Williams, H. B., and Terzis, J.: Single fascicular recordings: An intraoperative diagnostic tool for the management of peripheral nerve lesions. Plast. Reconstr. Surg., 57:562, 1976.
23. Woolsley, R. L., and Niew, A. S.: Drug therapy (guanethidine). N. Engl. J. Med., 295:1053, 1976.
24. Youmans, J. R.: Neurological Surgery, 2nd Ed. Philadelphia, W. B. Saunders Company, 1982.

13

Nerve Injection Injuries*

■

Alan R. Hudson, M.B., Ch.B., F.R.C.S.(C)

Permanent motor and sensory deficit may result from the inadvertent injection of a large number of drugs into various peripheral nerves.[14] The management of patients suffering from nerve injection injuries requires a basic understanding of the neuropathology of these lesions and the management of lesions in continuity, as described by Kline et al.[6, 9, 10] The medico-legal implications of such accidents are obvious, so that there is a tendency not to publicize the case material.

PATHOLOGY OF NERVE INJECTION INJURY

Gentili et al.[1] have reported on their and other investigators' animal experiments that indicate that, in the vast majority of cases, a direct intrafascicular injection of the offending agent is required to cause nerve damage. The same drug that causes severe nerve fiber damage following intrafascicular injection may cause no significant neural injury as a result of injection in the immediate proximity of a peripheral nerve. This is an important point, as frequently the person who performed the injection will claim that the needle insertion was well away from the course of a peripheral nerve and that the substance must have "tracked down a fascial plane." A major variable affecting the severity of nerve injury appears to be the drug itself, and animal models have shown clear differences in the impact on nerve fiber integrity according to the particular drug injected (Table 13–1).

Not unexpectedly, there is a drug-dose relationship to the severity of injury. The offending agent directly injures both myelinated and unmyelinated nerve fibers and also causes a breakdown in blood-nerve barrier function. Thus, the environment within which the damaged fibers lie is altered.

Pathologic alteration in nerve fibers is evident within 30 minutes of injection, and the mechanism of injury appears to be a direct neurotoxic effect on both the axon and the Schwann cell.[4] It should be emphasized that some local anesthetics that are injected directly into the nerve will cause nerve fiber injury.[3] Mackinnon et al.[11] have studied the effect of commonly injected steroid preparations that may cause severe damage if inadvertently injected into a nerve fascicle. Controlled studies in animals demonstrated that the nerve injury is related to the drug injected and not to the trauma of needle insertion or complicating hemorrhage (Fig. 13–1).

The extent of nerve regeneration is unpredictable in humans, as there is no way of knowing the quantity of drug that was injected within the substance of the nerve as opposed to that injected adjacent to the nerve. Regeneration seen in rat experiments should be correlated with the human experience with care, as rats have an incredible ability to regenerate nerves following total degeneration of all nerve fibers.

MANAGEMENT OF PATIENTS WITH NERVE INJECTION INJURY

The history of the incident is quite characteristic. The patient will complain of im-

*Supported in part by MRC Grant MA 7279.

Table 13–1. DRUGS INJECTED IN ANIMAL EXPERIMENTS CAUSING NERVE FIBER DAMAGE*

Drug	Intrafascicular Injection	Extrafascicular Injection
Saline	–	–
Blood	+	–
Dexamethasone (Decadron, Merck Sharp & Dohme)	+	–
Bupivacaine hydrochloride, 0.5% (Marcaine, Winthrop)	+	–
Gentamicin (Garamycin, Schering)	+ +	–
Cephalothin (Keflin, Eli Lilly)	+ +	–
Chloramphenicol (Chloromycetin, Parke-Davis)	+ +	–
Iron-dextran (Imferon, Fisons)	+ +	–
Triamcinolone acetonide (Kenalog, Squibb)	+ +	–
Methylprednisolone (Depo-Medrol, Upjohn)	+ +	–
Lidocaine hydrochloride, 1% ± epinephrine (Xylocaine, Astra)	+ +	–
Lidocaine hydrochloride, 2% ± epinephrine (Xylocaine, Astra)	+ +	–
Bupivacaine hydrochloride, 0.5% + epinephrine (Marcaine, Winthrop)	+ +	–
Benzylpenicillin (Penicillin G, Ayerst)	+ + +	+
Diazepam (Valium, Roche)	+ + +	+
Chlordiazepoxide (Librium, Roche)	+ + +	+
Chlorpromazine (Largactil, Poulenc)	+ + +	+
Meperidine (Demerol, Winthrop)	+ + +	–
Dimenhydrinate (Gravol, Horner)	+ + +	+
Hydrocortisone (Solu-Cortef, Upjohn)	+ + +	–
Triamcinolone hexacetonide (Aristospan, Lederle)	+ + +	–
Lidocaine hydrocarbonate, 2l% (Xylocaine, Astra)	+ + +	–
Procaine hydrochloride, 2% (Novocain, Winthrop)	+ + +	–
Tetracaine hydrochloride, 1% (Pontocaine, Winthrop)	+ + +	–

*See original publications for details of osmolarity and dosage schedules.[1, 3, 4, 11]
Key: + = mild, + + = moderate, + + + = severe.

mediate local pain at the site of injection and subsequent radiation of the pain in the appropriate distribution of that nerve. In our reported clinical experience and in subsequent unreported cases, this history is repeatedly elicited and is of importance in the medico-legal review of the case, as the incident stands out clearly in a conscious patient's memory in contradistinction to the various spurious alternative suggestions, usually proposed by the person who performed the injection.[2, 7] The motor-sensory dysfunction is immediately apparent and follows the distribution of the injected nerve. Usually the diagnosis is perfectly straightforward, and the smoke screen created by anxious medical, nursing, and administrative staff is quickly dispersed by the very simple

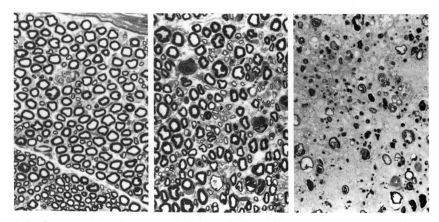

Figure 13–1. *Left,* Cross section of normal sciatic nerve. *Center,* Twelve days after intrafascicular injection of dexamethasone. *Right,* Twelve days after intrafascicular injection of triamcinolone hexacetonide. The center section shows minor damage and the section on the right shows severe, widespread axonal and myelin degeneration (toluidine blue, × 336). (From Mackinnon, S. F., Hudson, A. R., Gentili, F., et al.: Plast. Reconstr. Surg., *69*:482, 1982.)

explanation of nerve injection injury. Animal experiments suggest that there is nothing to be gained by any immediate surgical maneuver currently available. Thus, the experimental model suggests that washing of the nerve or decompression of surrounding tissues would have no effect on the outcome, and we do not advise such emergency measures.[4]

The long-term outcome may be one of complete recovery or total failure of recovery. Partial or no recovery may be associated wtih extremely severe pain syndromes. I have had the experience of seeing patients with total radial nerve palsy associated with meperidine injection who had total clinical recovery within a year without any treatment whatsoever. This experience would tend to encourage a conservative approach, but the main practical clinical problem is that of practitioners waiting far too long in the face of lack of improvement of nerve function. There is no point in waiting several years for recovery that never occurs and then attempting to formulate a plan of surgery for the peripheral nerve. By that stage, end-organ atrophy is so severe that recovery, even with reinnervation, is impossible.[13]

Suggested Plan of Management

1. Details of the incident should be sought. The patient can frequently point to the exact site at which the needle entered the arm or leg. The exact dosage and nature of the drug injected should be recorded. Standard motor-sensory examination reveals whether or not function of the particular nerve is completely or partially lost and appropriate records are made. Arrangements are made for appropriate splinting and passive movements for the affected joints. Anesthetic areas must be guarded to prevent burns and other injuries.

2. It is essential that the patient be referred immediately to an expert in peripheral nerve injuries. Failure to do this is subsequently regarded as an attempt to "cover up the incident." At subsequent medico-legal review it is far better to note that the appropriate consultations were immediately obtained and that the nature of the problem was explained to the patient by an experienced nerve surgeon who neither attempted to mislead the patient as to what happened nor prejudiced the position of his colleagues by careless or unproven allegations. "They were trying to hide something from me,"

"he told me it was all in my head," "he tried to pretend I had had a stroke," "I was told my nerve must have been in the wrong place," "I injected in the correct place, therefore, you cannot have a nerve injury," "you must have been incorrectly positioned on the operating table, because I gave the pre-med. in the correct place," are statements frequently heard in this situation. These terminological inexactitudes merely aggravate the sense of injustice, disappointment, and outrage felt by patients when they subsequently understand the reality of the situation and bolster their determination to both extract compensation and obtain revenge.

3. A 3-month period of examination is appropriate, during which the peripheral nerve surgeon looks for evidence of recovery. For example, in a radial nerve injection injury one would repeatedly test the brachioradialis muscle in the hope of finding some evidence of clinical return of function. During this time, it is appropriate to see the patient approximately every 3 weeks to look for evidence of recovery and also to reassure the patient that he has not been abandoned following the accident. It is far preferable that the management of the case be conducted by an expert and not by those responsible for the original accident. Thus, the fear of a malpractice suit, the anxiety surrounding the problem, and all other extraneous factors are removed and a straightforward doctor/patient relationship is established.

4. If at 3 months there is no evidence of motor, sensory, or autonomic recovery, a full appraisal of the situation should be made. It is appropriate to have electrical studies performed at approximately 6 weeks and again at 12 weeks after the event. The main judgment as to whether or not recovery is occurring is based on clinical appraisal. In practical terms, the most common failure in management is that of waiting too long in an irreparable situation. If a physician does not refer a patient for consultation early because he hopes that spontaneous recovery will occur and hence the accident not be publicized, he will compound the initial error. It is difficult to respond to the patient's or lawyer's question "why did he not do something for all that time, when there was still a chance of repairing the nerve?" Electrophysiologic information should be interpreted with care, and the surgeon should review reports only of expert electromyographers in his overall appraisal of the situation.[8] Minor electrical

evidence of recovery is not necessarily associated with useful limb function in the future.

5. The exact duration of the waiting period varies with the particular site of nerve injection and the distance from that site to the first target muscle, but, as a general rule, if there is no evidence of recovery by 4 months, the patient should undergo peripheral nerve exploration.

6. The nerve is exposed according to standard peripheral nerve surgery techniques, using general anesthesia with spontaneous respiration. No tourniquet is used. It is important to have adequate exposure, as the drug may have tracked longitudinally within the substance of the nerve (Fig. 13–2). The site of injury is usually easily established by inspection, and a circumferential epineurectomy is performed (Fig. 13–3). It is essential that the operator have available some form of assessing axonal transmission through the lesion (either nerve potential or evoked potential equipment). Thus, information of trans-lesion axonal regeneration is available before end-organ reinnervation has occurred. The appearance of a significant nerve action potential transmission signals that the operation should be terminated and that return of function can be expected with a fair degree of confidence (Fig. 13–4). Failure to elicit electrical evidence of axonal transmission through the lesion indicates that resection is required. It is imperative to resect the entire length of the injured nerve, and this may be quite substantial, owing to intraneural tracking of the offending agent (Fig. 13–5). Therefore, the surgeon must be aided by a pathologist skilled in interpreting frozen sections of peripheral nerve specimens. It must also be appreciated that microsurgical internal neurolysis may reveal intact fascicles and yet the nerve may be permanently damaged. Sophisticated techniques for assessing function of fascicles intraoperatively have been described by Terzis et al.[15] The two stumps bearing normal fascicular patterns on their cut faces are then restored, using whatever peripheral nerve technique is appropriate.[12] Sural nerve grafting has been found to be necessary in the majority of our cases. Good to excellent results are possible in even extensive (12 cm) radial nerve grafts, but we have had only poor to bad results from any suture technique involving the peroneal component of the sciatic nerve.

7. Appropriate soft tissue and bone reconstructive procedures are indicated in the event of incomplete or absent recovery after nerve surgery. We advise the just described sequence of nerve surgery first, as it may reduce the extent of subsequent reconstructive procedures usually performed 2 years after the nerve surgery.

Pain

Pain may be a debilitating symptom in the later phases. Its true assessment may be difficult in the medico-legal setting. Patients should receive physiotherapy and be encouraged to use, and not overprotect, the partially denervated limb. All limbs in which reinnervation is occurring are uncomfortable, and this discomfort can achieve cataclysmic proportions by psychogenic focus on the prob-

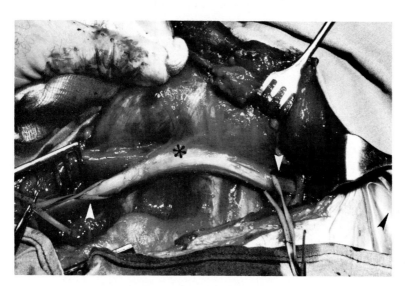

Figure 13–2. Sciatic nerve penicillin nerve injury. Site of injury (∗) is clearly demarcated by the adherence of the sciatic nerve to the elevated gluteal lid. ▲ Distal sciatic nerve. ▼ Proximal sciatic nerve. (From Hudson, A. R.: Clin. Plast. Surg., *11*:28, 1984.)

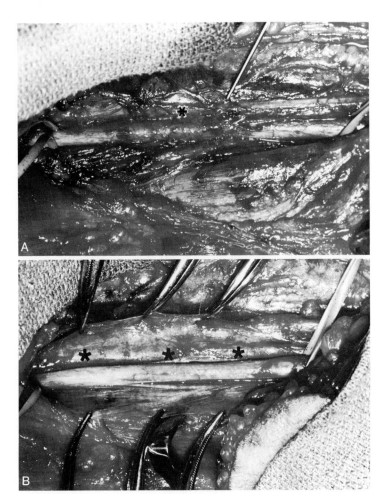

Figure 13–3. Median nerve local anesthetic injury suffered by an orthopedic surgeon. Axillary plexus block was presumably delivered into the median nerve in an attempt to obtain anesthesia for repair of a severed extensor tendon. *A*, Exposure. Injection point (*). *B*, 360° external neurolysis. Hemostats are on the cut edge of the scar tissue (* * *). At this state, stimulation and recording of nerve action potentials are obtained.

lem area. It is axiomatic that local nerve pain requires local nerve surgery and not sympathectomy, so that if all appropriate conservative maneuvers have been exhausted, we advise external and, if appropriate, internal neurolysis. We have been reasonably encouraged by this technique (which is safely performed by an experienced operator under high magnification) even in later stages, at which time significant motor or sensory recovery would not be expected.[5]

PREVENTION

All appropriate personnel should be aware of the surface markings of the specific nerves. The radial and sciatic nerves are those most commonly at risk, but injection injuries have been reported in many other nerves.[14] We advise caution, particularly in patients who have either small or flabby muscles (Fig. 13–6). It is probably wisest to avoid buttock injections altogether in children and to give these injections into the vastus lateralis. When performing regional anesthetic blocks, it is important to place the local anesthetic around the appropriate nerve or plexus and not intraneurally. This is particularly important in both supra- and infraclavicular plexus blocks, and I have seen examples of permanent nerve damage in both sites following regional blocks with local anesthetics. If there is any reason to inject steroids close to the known course of a peripheral nerve, it is probably reasonable not to employ local anesthesia so that the injector can be warned if the needle tip approaches the major peripheral nerve prior to the steroid injection. If the patient complains of excessive pain on needle placement, in any circumstance, it is wise not to inject at that site. Nurses giving these injections have frequently been both experienced and very busy. Possibly, the less experienced injector is more aware of recently learned surface anatomy and injection technique.

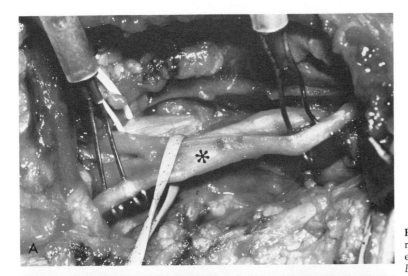

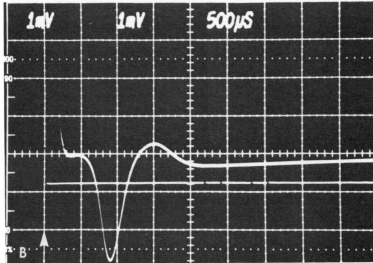

Figure 13–4. *A*, Stimulating and recording electrodes placed on either side of lesion-in-continuity. *B*, Oscilloscope tracing of nerve action potential. Arrow points to stimulus position. (From Hudson, A. R.: Clin. Plast. Surg., *11*:29, 1984.)

Figure 13–5. Ulnar nerve injection injury caused by attempted self-administration of amphetamines into axillary veins. ▲ Distal ulnar nerve. ▼ Proximal ulnar nerve.

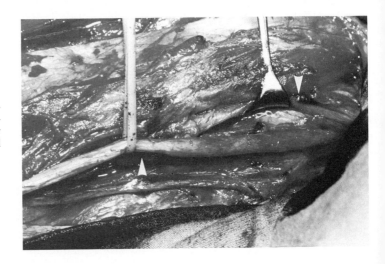

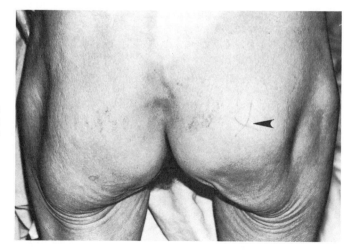

Figure 13–6. Elderly, wasted severe diabetic patient. Arrows points to site of penicillin injection, which resulted in total sciatic nerve palsy.

CONCLUSIONS

Nerve injection injury is preventable. There is now a reasonable basis for management of the unfortunate victims if an accident does occur. Practitioners who follow the basic steps of management will aid their patients and also can give a better account of themselves in the medico-legal setting.

References

1. Gentili, F., Hudson, A. R., Kline, D. G., et al.: Peripheral nerve injection injury. Neurosurgery, 4:3, 1979.
2. Gentili, F., Hudson, A. R., and Hunter, D.: Clinical and experimental aspects of injection injuries of peripheral nerves. Can. J. Neurol. Sci., 7:143–151, 1980.
3. Gentili, R., Hudson, A. R., Hunter, D., and Kline, D. G.: Nerve injection injury with local anesthetic agents: A light and electron microscopic, fluorescent microscopic, and horseradish peroxidase study. Neurosurgery, 6:263–272, 1980.
4. Gentili, F., Hudson, A. R., Kline, D. G., and Hunter, D.: Early changes following injection injury of peripheral nerves. Can. J. Surg., 23:177–182, 1980.
5. Gentili, F., Hudson, A. R., Kline, D. G., and Hunter, D.: Morphological and physiological alterations following internal neurolysis of normal rat sciatic nerve. In Gorio, A., Millesi, H., and Mingrino, S. (eds.): Posttraumatic Peripheral Nerve Regeneration. New York, Raven Press, 1981, pp. 183–196.
6. Hudson, A. R., and Kline, D. G.: Progression of partial experimental injury to peripheral nerve. Part II. Light and electron microscopic studies. J. Neurosurg., 42:1–15, 1975.
7. Hudson, A. R., Kline, D. G., and Gentili, F.: Injection injury of nerve. In Omer, G. E., Jr., and Spinner, M. (eds.): Management of Peripheral Nerve Problems. Philadelphia, W. B. Saunders Company, 1980, pp. 639–653.
8. Hudson, A. R., Berry, H., and Mayfield, F.: Chronic injuries of peripheral nerves by entrapment. In Youmans, J. R. (ed.): Neurological Surgery, 2nd Ed. Philadelphia, W. B. Saunders Company, 1982, pp. 2430–2474.
9. Kline, D. G., Hudson, A. R., Hackett, E., and Bratton, B.: Progression of partial experimental injury to peripheral nerve. Part I. Periodic measurements of muscle contraction strength. J. Neurosurg., 42:1, 1975.
10. Kline, D. G., and Hudson, A. R.: Neuropathology and neurophysiology of the lesion in continuity. In Gorio, A., Millesi, H., and Mingrino, S. (eds.): Posttraumatic Peripheral Nerve Regeneration. New York, Raven Press, 1981, pp. 175–181.
11. Mackinnon, S., Hudson, A. R., Gentili, F., Kline, D. G., and Hunter, D.: Peripheral nerve injection injury with steroid agents. Plast. Reconst. Surg., 69:482–490, 1982.
12. Omer, G. E., and Spinner, M. (eds.): Management of Peripheral Nerve Problems. Philadelphia, W. B. Saunders Company, 1980.
13. Richter, H.: Impairment of motor recovery after late nerve suture: Experimental study in the rabbit. Parts I and II. Neurosurgery, 10:70–85, 1982.
14. Stöhr, M.: Iatrogene Nervenläsionen. Stuttgart, Georg Thieme Verlag, 1980.
15. Terzis, J. K., Dykes, R. W., and Hakstian, R. W.: Electrophysiological recordings in peripheral nerve surgery—A review. J. Hand Surg., 1:52, 1976.

14

Functional Sensation and Its Re-Education

■

A. Lee Dellon, M.D.

Rehabilitation of the hand presupposes an understanding of its function. For the sensory component of hand function, this remains an elusive goal. To re-educate sensation, we must have in mind not only how sensation is used in hand function, but also which sensory modality—pain, temperature, or touch—is essential to that function. Furthermore, we need to be able to evaluate that sensibility and measure it. Over the past two decades, by means of basic science and clinical investigations in the neurosciences, the subpopulations of nerve fibers that mediate pain, temperature, and touch have been defined, and the sensory receptors that transduce mechanical stimuli have been identified. With this knowledge, we can devise a rational plan for evaluation of the sensibility required for hand function and develop a rehabilitation plan for re-education of sensation in the hand.

The primary sensory modality required for hand function is touch. The sensory aspect of hand function can be subdivided into a static and an active component. For example, the ability to hold a sewing needle between the fingers requires the recognition that something is being held in constant contact with the fingers and the perception of how heavy it is, so that we know how much pressure to apply. This is termed "static grip." The ability to identify an object held between the fingers, requiring movement of the fingers over the object, is a more active sensory function. It is this ability to recognize an object (object identification) that we term "tactile gnosis." Depending upon what type of function (static, active, or both) will be required of the hand, plans can be made for sensory re-education. Evaluating the sensibility before and during rehabilitation is essential as a guide to instituting specific sensory exercises at the appropriate time during recovery.

The purpose of this chapter is to briefly describe our present concept of the neurophysiology of the touch modality, outline a rational approach to evaluation of sensibility, and describe the technique and results of sensory re-education. Each of these areas has been expanded greatly in a recent monograph.[13]

NEUROPHYSIOLOGIC CORRELATES OF TOUCH

The nerve fibers that mediate the perception of touch are the group A (myelinated) beta fibers (10 to 15 μ diameter). These may be subdivided based upon their adaptation to a constant-touch stimulus into slowly adapting and quickly adapting fiber/receptor systems. The slowly adapting fiber/receptor system continues to transmit neural impulses throughout the duration of the stimulus, with a slow decline in impulse frequency. This system will increase the frequency of neural impulses in proportion to the intensity (pressure) of the constant-touch stimulus.

The quickly adapting fiber/receptor system essentially has no significant response to constant-touch or pressure stimuli (except the "on response" during the ramp phase of the stimulus) but does respond significantly to oscillating mechanical stimuli, such as vibration, or to moving-touch. During these stimuli, the nerve will respond in a manner related to the stimulus frequency. Although each quickly adapting fiber will respond to a wide range of frequencies, a frequency exists at which it is most sensitive, i.e., its threshold is the lowest. This system may be subdivided into a group with fibers that are most sensitive to low frequency stimuli and a group most sensitive to high frequency stimuli. For clinical purposes (and considering the availability of tuning forks), the low frequency group may be tested with a 30-cps tuning fork and the high frequency group with a 256-cps tuning fork.[5, 6, 14, 21, 25] A slowly adapting fiber will respond to a vibrating stimulus, but its response requires high stimulus intensity and cannot be entrained.

The correlation of these touch fibers with their appropriate sensory receptors is now more certain. Pacinian corpuscles are sufficiently large to be recorded from directly and are the receptors for the high frequency, quickly adapting group. The touch pad of the cat and the Merkel cell rete papilla of the racoon are analogous morphologic structures and sufficiently large for single-unit recordings. They are slowly adapting. The Merkel cell–neurite complex is the analogous recep-

tor in the human. The remaining sensory "corpuscles" in glabrous skin are the Meissner corpuscles, located in the dermal papillae. Application of topical anesthetic to the skin raises the threshold for the low frequency group of quickly adapting fibers. The Meissner corpuscle is the receptor for this group.[5, 6, 14, 16, 21]

These relationships and sensory correlates are given in Table 14–1. This entire subject recently has been reviewed extensively.[13]

EVALUATION OF FUNCTIONAL SENSIBILITY

For more than two decades, the concepts of sensory testing proposed by Erik Moberg have guided our efforts away from the purely academic tests of sensibility and toward functional tests.[19, 20] Moberg demonstrated that perception (i.e., pain, temperature, cotton wool stroking, cogwheel) did not correlate with a patient's ability to use his hand. However, he defined hand function in terms of static grips. The functional test with which he correlated the academic tests was the pickup test in which objects were picked up (not identified) and placed into a receptacle. The classic Weber two-point discrimination test correlated best with the ability of the hand to perform this precision sensory grip.[19] Since this is a static grip and (as described in the preceding section) the static two-point discrimination test measures the innervation

Table 14–1. NEUROPHYSIOLOGIC AND SENSORY CORRELATES*

Nerve Fiber Property	Peripheral Receptor	Neurophysiologic Correlate	Clinical Test	Sensation
Slowly adapting	Merkel cell– neurite complex	Stimulus Threshold Innervation density	Fingertip touch von Frey hair Classic two-point discrimination	Constant-touch Pressure "Tactile gnosis" (static)
Quickly adapting	Meissner corpuscle	Stimulus	Fingertip stroking or 30 cps tuning fork	Moving-touch
		Threshold Innervation density	Vibrometer Moving two-point discrimination	Flutter Tactile gnosis (active)
Quickly adapting	Pacinian corpuscle	Stimulus	Fingertip stroking or 256 cps tuning fork	Moving-touch
		Threshold Innervation density	Vibrometer Moving two-point discrimination	Vibration Tactile gnosis (active)

*From Dellon, A. L.: Evaluation of Sensibility and Reeducation of Sensation in the Hand. Baltimore, Williams and Wilkins, 1981, with permission.

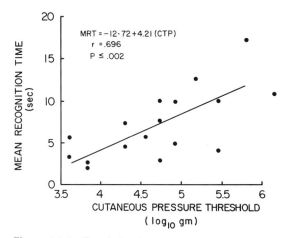

Figure 14–1. Correlation between cutaneous pressure threshold and mean recognition time.

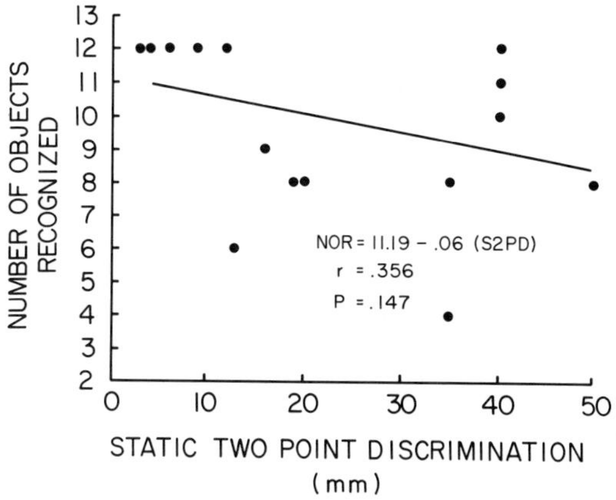

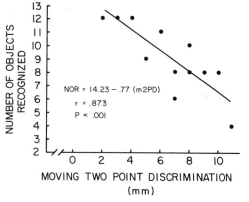

Figure 14–3. Correlation between classic static (Weber) two-point discrimination and tactile gnosis.

density of this slowly adapting fiber/receptor system, Moberg's findings now have a firm neurophysiologic basis.

Many careful clinical observers, however, have found that patients with "no useful" static two-point discrimination greater than 12 to 15 mm are nevertheless using their hand well.[11] Moberg's studies predict that for a value between 15 and 30 mm only "gross grip" is possible and that true tactile gnosis (the ability to "see" with our fingertips) is not possible.[19] The paradox is answered when we understand that tactile gnosis requires fingertip movement; this activates the quickly adapting fiber/receptor system, which is not evaluated by the classic Weber test. This fiber/receptor system is evaluated by the moving two-point discrimination test (Table 14–1).[11]

When the moving two-point discrimina-

tion test was first described, it was not correlated with a test of tactile gnosis. If we define hand function as active and tactile gnosis as object recognition, then a study similar to Moberg's design is required in which all contemporary tests of sensibility are evaluated and judged by their ability to predict the patient's success in identifying a series of objects. This study was presented to members of the American Association of Plastic Surgery at their May, 1981, meeting.[15] The results, presented in part in Figures 14–1 to 14–4, demonstrate that neither cutaneous pressure threshold determinations (von Frey hairs or Semmes-Weinstein monofilaments), cutaneous vibratory threshold measurements (using the vibrometer[6]), nor static two-point discrimination correlated with the ability of a patient with median nerve sensory impairment to identify objects correctly. The mov-

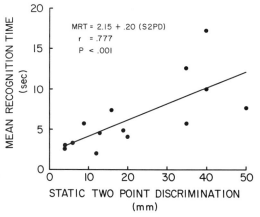

Figure 14–2. Correlation between classic static (Weber) two-point discrimination and mean object recognition time.

Figure 14–4. Correlation of moving two-point discrimination and tactile gnosis. (From Dellon, A. L., and Kallman, C. H.: J. Hand Surg., 8:865, 1983.)

ing two-point discrimination test correlated best (p<0.001) with object identification.[15]

Case 1

An example of the functional difference just discussed is patient J.C. He was evaluated 3 years after a median nerve repair at the wrist. He had normal thenar motor function and normal perception of pain and temperature, 30- and 256-cps tuning fork, constant- and moving-touch. Over the index finger and thumb, his cutaneous pressure threshold markings were 5.1 and 4.9, compared with a control value of 3.84; vibratory threshold was 1.0 and 1.0, compared with a control value 0.25 μ; and static two-point discrimination was 40 and 40, compared with a control value of 3 mm. All of these were grossly abnormal. His moving two-point discrimination was 4 and 4 mm, compared with a control value of 2 mm; this value was almost normal. He could identify all 12 of the test objects correctly, requiring an average of 9.8 seconds per object to do so (control value is 2 seconds per object). As he tried to identify the smallest objects in the test (metal hex versus square nuts, 6 mm per side), the object would often fall from between his thumb, index, and middle fingers' three-point pinch. This is because there was insufficient sensibility (slowly adapting fiber/receptor system) to permit perception of how hard to press to maintain the grip. But there was sufficient sensibility (innervation density of the quickly adapting fiber/receptor system) to permit object recognition if the object was kept moving between the fingers.

From this example, it is clear that although moving two-point discrimination is the best predictor of active hand function (object recognition), if poor static two-point discrimination is present, the time of object recognition is prolonged. Since one must know how hard to press an object to keep it from falling from the fingers, cutaneous pressure threshold correlates with the object recognition *time*. Thus, static two-point discrimination, the innervation-density correlate of this slowly adapting system, gives additional predictive value beyond moving two-point discrimination in terms of both precision-grip functions and speed of object recognition functions.[15]

Since the most important neurophysiologic sensory predictor of hand function is how many functional fiber/receptor units are present in a given area of skin (innervation density), is it ever necessary to test sensory thresholds? If a nerve is subjected to any injury other than complete transection, it may still function but will require a higher stimulus intensity to achieve that function. Thus, threshold measurements will reveal abnormal nerve function prior to innervation density measurements. For example, with peripheral nerve compression, this has been demonstrated for vibratory stimuli (tuning fork) in the carpal tunnel syndrome[12, 14] and cubital tunnel syndrome.[14] Recording a patient's response to tuning fork perception, however, is not quantitative. Similar results were obtained with a vibrometer.[6] The Semmes-Weinstein nylon monofilaments can give similar quantitative threshold measurements for the slowly adapting fiber/receptor system. The actual recording of the cutaneous pressure threshold is laborious, and its relative disadvantages were discussed recently.[13] Threshold measurements permit sequential monitoring of clinical conditions and lend themselves to research studies requiring quantitation. There may be a specific indication for cutaneous pressure threshold measurements in patchy-type peripheral neuropathy, such as leprosy, in which the lesion may not affect the nerve evenly.[5]

One remaining concern in sensibility evaluation is that it is possible that increasingly advanced neurophysiologic testing techniques may permit such a "high-power" microscopic view of neural events that we begin to doubt our clinical ability to assess sensibility at all.[4] For example, critical analysis reveals that when an examiner tests static two-point discrimination, the test stimulus is, in fact, not constant in either the location on the skin or the degree of stimulus intensity because of movement in both the examiner's and the patient's hand. Note that in this situation the critical analyzer is the oscilloscope screen—not the patient. The patient's conscious response, his perception, is that something is being pressed upon his finger steadily. The answer must be in choosing the testing instrument according to the question being asked. The paper clip can tell us if the repaired nerve has recovered, the tuning fork can determine whether or not the nerve is compressed, and the microelectrode and oscilloscope can answer more precise single-unit neurophysiology questions.

CONCEPT OF SENSORY RE-EDUCATION

Sensory re-education is a group of techniques or methods that allow a patient to achieve the maximum potential for functional recovery following nerve suture.[10, 15] Sensory re-education permits a narrowing of the gap between the technical expertise in the operating room and the limited functional recovery still observed all too often in the examining room (Fig. 14–5). Sensory re-education is practiced by the surgeon at each office visit, the hand therapist at each therapy session, and the patient in the quiet of his own home. Sensory re-education is instituted at the appropriate time in the recovery process, and the exercises instituted are specific for the stage in the recovery of sensation.[9, 13]

After even the most precise microsurgical nerve suture, the following problems will lead inevitably to an altered profile of neural impulses. A certain number of regenerating axons will enter the epineurial or perineurial tissue and fail to regenerate distally but will become misdirected into a different topographic area so that an axon that formerly innervated the distal thumb may, upon regeneration, reinnervate the palm or index finger. A certain number of axons will regenerate into the correct topographic location but will fail to reinnervate their appropriate sensory end-organ so that a quickly adapting fiber that previously innervated a Meissner corpuscle may regenerate and either will fail to reinnervate an end-organ or will reinnervate a Merkel cell–neurite complex. These types of problems lead to a finger in which a previously well-defined stimulus, such as stroking the finger, will now initiate a set of neural impulses that are altered from the set that would have been initiated prior to the nerve injury. This occurs even if a sufficiently

long period has been allowed to elapse from the time of nerve suture until evaluation of sensibility. This altered profile of neural impulses reaches the somatosensory cortex, and the patient may become aware that his finger has been stimulated but may fail to be able to match this altered profile with a previous pattern of neural impulses in his "association cortex." Thus, although the patient may be aware that something is touching his hand, he may be unable to identify or recognize that object. Sensory re-education attempts to retrain the patient so that he may utilize his reinnervated peripheral sensory mechanisms to their maximum advantage, even though they may, in fact, be deficient in many ways.

Sensory re-education is not new. As the literature is reviewed, there are many examples of what we would now term "sensory re-education" that have simply not been recognized as such. For example, the ultimate capacity for tactile discrimination in the normal hand remains to be defined. In attempting to establish normal values for the classic Weber two-point discrimination test, Onne[23] and Dellon[9] both observed that in the patient's nonoperated or control hand (or in nonoperated patient control groups), repeat sensory evaluation would often demonstrate improvement in the first tested normal two-point discrimination. For example, when a patient's control hand is tested at the first evaluation session, a value of 6 mm might be found. Upon subsequent testing during later evaluation sessions, this value may have decreased to 3 mm. Furthermore, the ability of the normal hand to undergo sensory re-education is emphasized by the capacity of

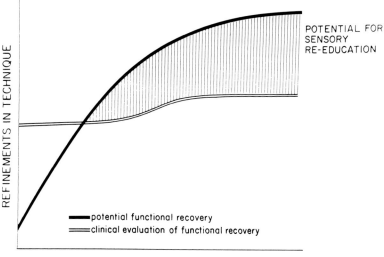

Figure 14–5. Sensory re-education gives the patient the opportunity to fulfill the sensory potential provided by the surgery. (From Dellon, A. L.: Evaluation of Sensibility and Re-education in the Hand. Baltimore, Williams and Wilkins, 1981.)

POTENTIAL FOR SENSORY RE-EDUCATION

REFINEMENTS IN TECHNIQUE

potential functional recovery
clinical evaluation of functional recovery

TIME

formerly sighted (blind) individuals to read braille. Heinrichs and Moorehouse[18] evaluated two-point discrimination in nondiabetic blind people. Whereas the normal value in their control group was 3 to 5 mm, the blind braille readers had a two-point discrimination of 1.5 mm. These findings have been supported by an independent study by Almquist.[1]

The first formal program for sensory re-education of patients following nerve repair was that published by Wynn Parry in his monograph in 1966.[17] Dellon et al.[8] presented their work on re-education of sensation to members of the American Society for Surgery of the Hand at their 1971 meeting. This material was ultimately published in manuscript form in 1974.[10] Sensory retraining had begun, however, at least 10 years before in hemiplegics[17] and 30 years before in animals, in which it was demonstrated that removal of the parietal lobe resulted in a stereognosis and that these animals could subsequently be retrained.[24] An example of sensory re-education applied to the visual system is the work of Bach-y-Rita et al.[2, 7] in developing the tactile visual substitution system. This group's previous experience in working with patients with brain lesions has demonstrated to them a remarkable capacity for cerebral reorganization. Critical, however, to this reorganization has been the need for sensory re-education.[3]

The program of sensory re-education we use is based upon initiating a series of specific sensory exercises at the appropriate time in the recovery process following nerve suture. Dellon et al.[9] evaluated the pattern of sensory recovery utilizing moving-touch, constant-touch, and vibratory stimuli at 30 and 256 cps. These sensory evaluation techniques were based upon the neurophysiologic studies described previously. Dellon et al.[9] observed the following sequence of recovery of sensation based upon these testing techniques. The first to recover was the perception of the 30-cps vibratory stimulus. This was followed quickly by the ability to perceive a moving-touch stimulus, as tested simply by finger stroking with the examiner's finger. Then, after a considerable delay, the ability to perceive constant-touch returned, and finally the ability to perceive the 256-cps vibratory stimulus was recovered. Far ahead of all of these was recovery of the ability to perceive pain and temperature.

This pattern of sensory recovery should be thought of as the timetable on which to base the introduction of sensory exercises. Initiating an exercise before the appropriate fiber/receptor system has been reunited can only lead to frustration and failure. Instituting the exercise at the appropriate time speeds patient recovery, builds patient confidence, and facilitates recovery of maximum function in a minimal time period.[13]

EARLY PHASE SENSORY RE-EDUCATION

When 30-cps vibratory stimulus and moving-touch have returned to an area, e.g., the palm, early phase re-education may begin for moving touch. It is most critical to begin by the time recovery has reached the proximal phalanx. The goal at this stage is (1) to re-educate submodality specific perception, movement vs. constant-touch and pressure, and (2) to re-educate misdirected or incorrect localization. The exercise simply involves the patient's use of a soft instrument, such as a pencil eraser, to stroke up and down the length of the area being re-educated. The patient observes what is happening, shuts his eyes and concentrates on what he is perceiving, and then opens his eyes to confirm again what is really happening. He should verbalize to himself what he is perceiving as specifically as he can, i.e., "I feel something moving up (or down) my index finger into the palm."

When the patient can perceive constant-touch, the same type of early phase re-education is done for this touch submodality.

Remembering that the newly reunited fiber/receptor system is "immature" and its threshold is high early during the recovery of sensation, a greater stimulus intensity must be used for perception to occur. Therefore, press the moving or immobile eraser as hard as necessary for the patient to perceive moving-touch or constant-touch. However, the stimulus intensity should never be great enough to evoke the perception of pain.

In evaluating a patient, the situation may arise in which both tuning forks may be perceived at the end of a fingertip but neither moving- nor constant-touch can be appreciated there. In this situation, the patient has re-established the necessary fiber/receptor system for the perception of moving-touch at the fingertip, but a "potential" gap exists. Within 2 to 3 weeks of intensive early phase re-education, this gap can be overcome. In these situations, the tuning fork is your guide to instituting specific sensory exercises. Early phase re-education should be introduced to the fingertip 4 to 6 months following a median nerve or ulnar nerve suture at the level of the wrist.[13]

LATE PHASE SENSORY RE-EDUCATION

Late phase sensory re-education should begin early, as soon as moving-touch and constant-touch can be perceived definitely and unambiguously at the fingertip with good localization. In our experience, this often can be as early as 6 to 8 months after median or ulnar nerve repair at the wrist.[13]

It is never too late, however, to begin late phase sensory re-education. In addition, beginning it too early can lead to patient failure at the recognition tasks and can heighten patient and therapist frustration. It is important to inform the patient of this at the beginning of this phase of re-education. The goal of late phase sensory re-education is to guide the patient to recovery of tactile gnosis—nothing less. If we expect less, we'll get less.[13]

Sensory re-education cannot induce axonal regeneration; it can only help the patient achieve the fullest potential provided by the nerve repair. The specific exercises in this stage must involve object identification. Tactile discrimination recovers progressively over time as measured by both classic and moving two-point discrimination.[13]

Late phase sensory re-education is begun with a set of familiar household objects, differing widely in shape, size, and texture. Again, the following sequence is utilized: object grasp with eyes open, then eyes shut with concentration on perception, then eyes open for reinforcement. After the patient has practiced with the objects, the therapist may test him, using the number of objects identified correctly or the time required in seconds (measured with a stopwatch) for object identification. Records such as this provide evidence to the patient, therapist, and referring physician that progress is occurring. It gives the patient a goal "to beat" next time and assists in patient motivation.[13]

Late phase sensory re-education is continued by progressing to objects differing largely in texture and then to objects that are smaller, differing in size and shape but not in texture and requiring subtle discrimination. At this stage, the patient will be clinically recovering classic two-point discrimination, and moving two-point discrimination will be less than 7 mm. As moving two-point discrimination drops below 5 mm, the patient will be able to identify the smallest objects correctly, although the objects may fall from the patient's grasp because the slowly adapting fiber/receptor system has not recognized and matured sufficiently.[15] It should be obvious that late phase sensory re-education also provides motor re-education.

Object identification tasks during late phase sensory re-education can be geared to the patient's job or household activities so that specific job retraining can be incorporated into the generalized sensory re-education program.

RESULTS OF SENSORY RE-EDUCATION

Does sensory re-education work? If the proof of success is the general acceptance of a technique, then we maintain that sensory re-education does indeed work. Sensory re-education has been described in detail in seven books, described briefly in nine books, and discussed as part of the methodology employed in twelve scientific reports. Sensory re-education has appeared on the program of at least one, and usually more than one, nationally publicized hand symposium for the past 10 years. There are active sensory re-education programs throughout the United States and in Australia, Austria, Canada, England, France, India, Japan, Sweden, and Switzerland.

Nevertheless, there are very few published reports with actual data demonstrating the results of sensory re-education. Wynn Parry has published his results, not only in his book, but also in a more recent publication.[28] Wynn Parry, however, does not indicate the number of patients studied nor over what period of time his patients obtained the results published. If the grading system of Highet is used, Wynn Parry indicates that 33% of his patients with median and ulnar nerve repairs recovered to grade S3+. Wynn Parry reports that 50% of his median and 25% of his ulnar nerve patients recovered

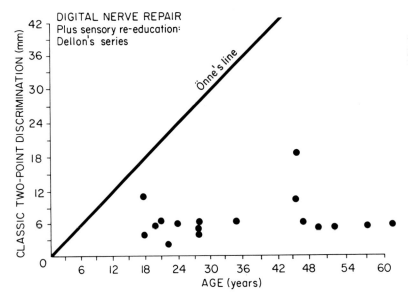

Figure 14–6. Onne's line represents the ideal, i.e., result obtained at 5 years after primary nerve repair. The result is age related. A patient's results are plotted on graph so that the dot falling below the line represents an improvement due to sensory re-education compared with previous ideal results. This graph depicts results of patient with digital nerve repair at just 2 years following surgery. (From Dellon, A. L.: Evaluation of Sensibility and Re-education in the Hand. Baltimore, Williams and Wilkins, 1981.)

Figure 14–7. See Figure 14–6 for a description of "Onne's line." This graph depicts results of patients with median nerve repair at just 2 years following surgery. (From Dellon, A. L.: Evaluation of Sensibility and Re-education in the Hand. Baltimore, Williams and Wilkins, 1981.)

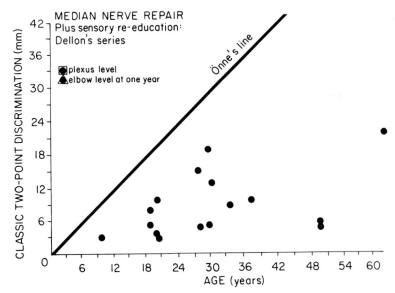

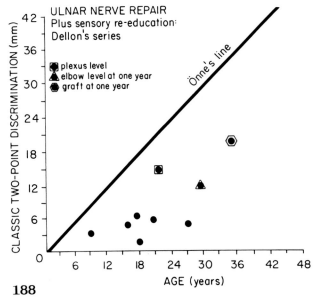

Figure 14–8. See Figure 14–6 for a description of "Onne's line." This graph depicts results of patients with ulnar nerve repair at just 2 years following surgery. (From Dellon, A. L.: Evaluation of Sensibility and Re-education in the Hand. Baltimore, Williams and Wilkins, 1981.)

near normal sensation (level S4). When these results are compared with the results of nerve repair based on historic controls, they are quite an improvement, as essentially no adult civilian patients have been reported to have recovered to level S4 following nerve suture. The only other reported late phase sensory re-education results are those of Wilgis and Maxwell[26] for patients with digital nerve grafts. Wilgis and Maxwell reported 33% of their patients recovering to level S3+ and 67% of their patients to S4. These results were for adult patients, and this represents a very dramatic improvement over the historic controls for digital nerve grafts in patients who have not received sensory re-education. Dellon[13] has recently published his personal series of adult nerve suture patients who have undergone sensory re-education. In this group, at less than 2 years following nerve suture, 39% of median and 20% of ulnar nerve suture patients recovered to level S3+, and 54% of median and 80% of ulnar nerve suture patients recovered to S4. In Dellon's series of patients with digital nerve repairs who received sensory re-education, 12% of the patients recovered to level S3+ and 82% to level S4 by 2 years after nerve suture. In comparison to an historic control group, Dellon's results of sensory re-education demonstrated an improvement that was highly statistically significant at the p<0.001 level (Figs. 14–6 to 14–8).

In summary, the success of sensory re-education in patients recovering from nerve repair has been demonstrated in general by the worldwide acceptance of the technique and in particular by the results published in the few studies available. The success achieved with sensory re-education is in both the percentage of patients achieving the highest level of recovery (S4) and the savings in time (1 to 2 years instead of 5 years) in which this level is achieved.

References

1. Almquist, E.E.: The effect of training on sensory function. *In* Michon, J., and Moberg, E. (eds.): Traumatic Nerve Lesions of the Upper Limb. Edinburgh, Churchill Livingstone, 1975, pp. 53–54.
2. Bach-y-Rita, P.: Visual information through the skin—a tactile vision substitution system. Trans. Am. Acad. Ophthmol. Otol., *78*:OP729–740, 1974.
3. Bach-y-Rita, P.: Plastic brain mechanisms in sensory substitution. *In* Zulch, K.J., Creutzfeldt, O., and Galbraith, G.C. (eds.): Cerebral Localization. Berlin, Springer-Verlag, 1975, pp. 203–216.
4. Bell, J.: Time-force relationships of sensory testing. Proceedings of the American Society for Surgery of the Hand Meeting, July, 1982 (Abstracts).
5. Bell, J.: Personal communication, 1983.
6. Brown, A.G., and Iggo, A.: A quantitative study of cutaneous receptor and afferent fibers in the cat and rabbit. J. Physiol., *193*:707, 1967.
7. Collins, C.C., and Bach-y-Rita, P.: Transmission of pictorial information through the skin. Adv. Biol. Med. Phys., *14*:285–315, 1973.
8. Dellon, A.L., Curtis, R.M., and Edgerton, M.T.: Re-education of sensation in the hand following nerve injury. J. Bone Joint Surg., *53A*:812, 1971 (Abstract).
9. Dellon, A.L., Curtis, R.M., and Edgerton, M.T.: Evaluating recovery of sensation in the hand following nerve injury. Johns Hopkins Med. J., *130*:235, 1972.
10. Dellon, A.L., Curtis, R.M., and Edgerton, M.D.: Re-education of sensation in the hand following nerve injury. Plast. Reconstr. Surg., *53*:297, 1974.
11. Dellon, A.L.: The moving two-point discrimination test: clinical evaluation of the quickly-adapting fiber receptor system. J. Hand Surg., *3*:474, 1978.
12. Dellon, A.L.: Clinical use of vibratory stimuli to evaluate peripheral nerve injury and compression neuropathy. Plast. Reconstr. Surg., *65*:466–476, 1980.
13. Dellon, A.L.: Evaluation of Sensibility and Re-Education of Sensation in the Hand. Baltimore, Williams and Wilkins Company, 1981.
14. Dellon, A.L.: The vibrometer. Plast. Reconstr. Surg., *71*:427–431, 1983.
15. Dellon, A.L., and Kallman, C.H.: Evaluation of functional sensation in the hand. J. Hand Surg., *8*:865–870, 1983.
16. Dellon, A.L., and Munger, B.L.: Correlation of histology and sensibility after nerve repair. J. Hand Surg., *8*:871–878, 1983.
17. Foster, R.M., and Shields, C.D.: Cortical sensory defects causing disability. Arch. Physic. Med., *40*:56–61, 1959.
18. Heinrichs, R.W., and Moorehouse, J.A.: Touch perception in blind diabetic subjects in relation to the reading of Braille type. N. Engl. J. Med., *280*:72–75, 1979.
19. Moberg, E.: Objective methods for determining the functional value of sensibility in the skin. J. Bone Joint Surg., *40B*:454, 1958.
20. Moberg, E.: Reconstructive hand surgery in tetraplegia, stroke and cerebral palsy: some basic concepts of physiology and neurology. J. Hand Surg., *1*:29, 1976.
21. Mountcastle, V.B., Talbot, W.H., Darian-Smith, I., et al.: A neural base for sense of flutter vibration. Science, *155*:597, 1967.
22. Munger, B.L., Pubols, L.M., and Pubols, B.H.: The Merkel rete papilla—a slowly-adapting sensory receptor in mammalian glabrous skin. Brain Res., *29*:47, 1971.
23. Onne, L.: Recovery of sensibility and sudomotor function in the hand after nerve suture. Acta Chir. Scand. Suppl., *300*, 1962.
24. Ruch, T.C., Fulton, J.F., and German, W.J.: Sensory discrimination in monkey, chimpanzee and man after lesions of the parietal lobe. Arch. Neurol. Psychiatry, *39*:919–938, 1938.
25. Werner, G., and Mountcastle, V. B.: Neural activity

in mechanoreceptive afferents: stimulus response relationships, Weber functions and information transmission. J. Neurophysiol., *28*:359, 1965.

26. Wilgis, E.F.S., and Maxwell, G.P.: Distal digital nerve grafts; clinical and anatomic studies. J. Hand Surg., *4*:439–443, 1979.

27. Wynn Parry, C.B.: Rehabilitation of the Hand. London, Butterworths, 1966, pp. 92, 107–109, 112–113.

28. Wynn Parry, C.B., and Salter, M.: Sensory re-education after median nerve lesions. Hand, *8*:250–257, 1976.

15

Rehabilitation of the Hand

■

Christine A. Moran, M.S., R.P.T.
Gretchen L. Maurer, B.S., O.T.R.

Recent advances in microsurgery have greatly increased the number of patients with good prognosis for functional recovery following upper extremity peripheral nerve injuries. The advances also accentuate the importance of carefully planned rehabilitation of these patients by trained physical and occupational therapists. This chapter presents the basic principles of management.

IMMEDIATE POSTOPERATIVE MANAGEMENT

Postoperative management of patients with peripheral nerve injuries begins immediately after the removal of surgical dressings and the surgeon's inspection of the wound. The process begins with fitting the patient with a static splint and an upper extremity sling. A special immobilizer sling (Fig. 15–1) is used for patients with brachial plexus repairs. All patients receive instructions about elevation of the limb for control of postoperative edema.

IMMOBILIZATION

All joints of the operated upper extremity are immobilized during the first postoperative week. The timing of immobilization of some of these joints depends upon the repair technique used. According to Millesi and colleagues,[69, 70] patients who have undergone nerve grafting can begin motion after 10 days of immobilization. Tupper[93] recommends 3 weeks of immobilization followed by graded active motion for patients with end-to-end repair.[93] Graded active motion is usually increased weekly in stages of 10 to 15 degrees; joint positions are maintained by static splints that are not removed until the patient can achieve full active motion. The rehabilitation process following end-to-end repair requires close coordination between therapist and surgeon to ensure that the nerve ends remain approximated.

Our clinic uses a specific protocol for all patients with brachial plexus repairs. First, the repaired shoulder is immobilized for 4 weeks. Gentle movement, active or passive, of the distal joints of the limb is encouraged 2 weeks after surgery. At 4 weeks, passive shoulder flexion and abduction are begun by the therapist, leading to 45 degrees of shoulder motion by the sixth postoperative week; the next 2 weeks are spent increasing passive motion to 90 degrees. The third postoperative month is used to restore full passive shoulder flexion and abduction.

SCAR REMODELING

Scar remodeling techniques begin within a day after removal of the sutures. Arem and Madden[1] have shown that rat skin scars respond to controlled stress during the remodeling phase. Warren et al.[98] showed that heat increased the responsiveness of rat tail to stretching. Laboratory studies of the effects of ultrasound on skin, muscle, and scar suggest that heat and mechanical vibration produce elongation of these tissues.[21, 30, 31, 36, 40, 56, 57, 61, 67, 75, 76, 81, 87] Comparable data on

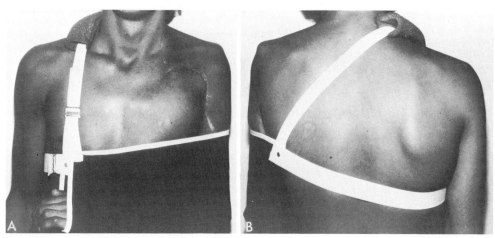

Figure 15–1. The brachial plexus postoperative sling, anterior (*A*) and posterior (*B*) views. An additional strap keeps the operated extremity against the chest wall and assists in minimizing the subluxation of the glenohumeral joint.

humans are not available, but indirect measurements of human tissue extensibility suggest that heat is beneficial for tissue elongation and scar remodeling in clinical practice.

A scar remodeling protocol should be designed to place graduated specific stress on the incisional scar and to increase the range of motion secondarily. Heat, friction massage, mechanical vibration, and ultrasound all form part of the regimen. Treatment begins with warm packs, paraffin, or ultrasound to increase circulation and accelerate scar remodeling (Fig. 15–2). The efficacy of massage and vibration in scar remodeling is unproved, but clinical results support the use of both techniques. In addition, elastomer, molded over the scar and worn either under the splint or with Ace wraps, can be used to apply constant pressure and to stress the scar

by reducing its blood supply and reducing PO_2 levels.[53]

Treatment continues until dermotenodesis is no longer evident and the scar is smooth and pliable. Gentle stretching is begun during and after heat treatment if the scar area remains dense for more than 3 to 4 weeks after surgery.[56, 97] An electromyographic biofeedback unit is used to encourage motion against the scar and control the amount of motion during treatment sessions.

RANGE OF MOTION

Active and passive range of motion is necessary in the rehabilitation of patients with peripheral nerve injuries in order to avoid joint and muscle contractures,[26, 78, 88] but motion must be controlled to protect the nerve repair. Patients must be made to understand the importance of preserving joint function during the period of nerve regeneration and muscle reinnervation.

Patients should maintain joint motion both in the office or clinic and at home. In certain situations patients can be taught techniques of joint mobilization[66] to help maintain soft tissue extensibility and joint mobility. This complements the static and/or dynamic splinting that is being used to maintain joint mobility and tissue extensibility during nerve reinnervation. In addition, joint mobilization is used to restore passive range of motion to all involved joints. Specific textbooks and courses relating to joint mobilization are available, and therefore this technique will

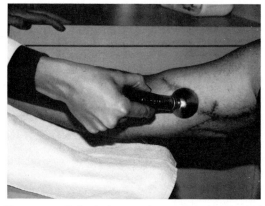

Figure 15–2. Pulsed ultrasound is used as a scar remodeling technique postoperatively.

not be discussed in any greater detail in this chapter.

Some loss of function is virtually inevitable in these patients. Hills and Byrd[44] demonstrated that after 30 days of plaster immobilization even individuals with healthy extremities experience a 25% decrease in range of motion and a 44% decrease in grip strength, as well as muscle atrophy and localized edema. To avoid this, all patients with peripheral nerve injuries are taught conditioning exercises that can be performed both in the office or clinic and at home.

MANAGEMENT OF EDEMA

Untreated edema from venous stasis will become chronic, and the patient may develop muscle and connective tissue fibrosis.[94] We begin corrective measures at once if a patient develops hand or arm edema in the immediate postoperative period. The usual techniques to assist venous return are retrograde massage and active or passive motion (when appropriate) performed in an elevated position.[90, 94] Elastic gloves or Ace wraps may prove useful in patients with persistent edema.[105]

A tape measure can demonstrate changes in the circumference of an edematous arm. Changes in hand volume can be determined with a volumeter.[12, 36]

MUSCLE STIMULATION

Some investigators and practitioners have questioned the need for muscle stimulation. The literature is replete with laboratory evidence of its effect on reducing muscle atrophy; however little clinical evidence of the effectiveness of muscle stimulation has been reported.[20, 41, 43, 45, 47, 48, 68, 82, 89, 96] Jackson and Seddon[47] published a report of stimulation performed on patients with median and ulnar nerve injuries in whom they measured a delay in atrophy via volumeter readings. Whereas Wakim and Krusen[97] reported both delay in atrophy and in increase in measurable output of work. The significance of multiple short sessions every day was established by Stillwell and Wakim in 1962.[89] In 1974 and 1977, Rosselle and colleagues[85] reported a large series of studies showing that stimulation of denervated muscle results in electro-

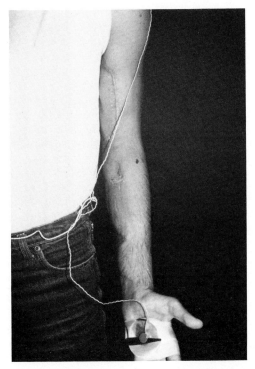

Figure 15–3. Galvanic (slow pulse) stimulation is used postoperatively for this patient with a brachial plexus repair. The positive electrode pad is placed on the shoulder (not shown), while the negative electrode pad is placed in the palm.

myographic change and earlier resumption of voluntary contractions.

Galvanic (slow pulse) electrical stimulation to all denervated muscles should be applied prior to nerve repair if possible and postoperatively during the period of nerve regeneration up to the time of reinnervation. For effective stimulation, the duration or pulse width is determined by chronaxy and is usually 50 to 100 msec at a rate of one pulse per 10 seconds.[59] The muscle contracts four times better in the longitudinal direction of stimulation of its fibers than transversely. Therefore, bipolar electrode placement is preferred for denervated muscle. In patients with complete lesions that have involved several large muscles, the positive electrode pad is placed on the shoulder in our clinic. The negative pad is placed on the wrist or palm for stimulation (Fig. 15–3). Stimulation of denervated muscles should be performed for 30 minutes at a time. As suggested by Liberson,[59] we at the Norfolk Hand Clinic are currently stimulating large muscles up to 5 hours a day, with ten separate 30-minute sessions. For children, stimulation should be performed for only 15 minutes at a time. The most important factor in determining time is the patient's skin tolerance to the current.

For nerve injuries occurring at the wrist level, a hand-held, battery-operated unit can be used for stimulation of the small intrinsic muscles (Fig. 15–4). Longitudinal stimulation can be accomplished by placing the positive pad proximally to the muscle with the stimulating probe applied distally. The probe is enlarged with the use of a saline-soaked 4 × 4 pad to better disperse the current.

Stimulation of the denervated muscles should begin approximately 2 to 3 weeks after surgery and continue until suspected reinnervation is imminent. Muscle stimulation will maintain muscle fiber and delay the onset of fibrosis.[85] However, it may reduce extrajunctional hypersensitivity to acetylcholine, thus inhibiting reinnervation.[68] Therefore, discontinuation of stimulation prior to suspected reinnervation is advisable.

MOTOR RE-EDUCATION

Formal motor re-education begins after reinnervation has been demonstrated by electromyographic studies, manual muscle testing, or clinical observation. This re-education program is divided into three areas: (1) faradic stimulation, (2) electromyographic biofeedback, and (3) functional activities.

Faradic (brief) stimuli, which depolarizes the nerve at a higher frequency per unit of time,[41] is both comfortable for the patient and effective in early retraining (Fig. 15–5). For effective stimulation of innervated muscles, the pulse width is about 100 μsec at a rate of

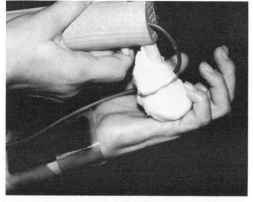

Figure 15–4. A patient with low ulnar nerve injury using a hand-held galvanic stimulator. Again, the positive electrode is placed proximally and the negative electrode distally. A saline-soaked 4 × 4 pad disperses the current over a larger area.

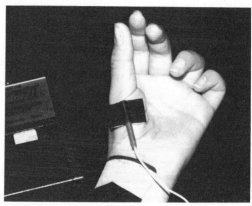

Figure 15–5. Faradic stimulation of the reinnervated thenar muscles to enhance early retraining.

40 pulses per second.[59] Often a few sessions of faradic stimulation suffice for initial muscle strengthening and regained awareness of the function of the muscle. Functional stimulation should not be confused with functional exercise.

Electromyographic (EMG) biofeedback is also used to enable patients to regain motor function (Figs. 15–6 and 15–7). This type of biofeedback has two advantages: (1) quantitative measurement of improvement, and (2) continuous feedback to the patient concerning muscle use. Muscle recovery can be a slow process, leading to patient frustration and boredom during exercise sessions. Electromyographic biofeedback is helpful during the sessions, since it provides patients with a quantitative means of monitoring the smallest amount of progress.[5, 16, 55] Small flickers of movement are characteristic of the early re-education period, and electrodes should be placed far apart for greater pickup. Later, electrodes may be moved closer together to help the patient regain fine motor control. Electrode size is also important; large electrodes cannot pick up small muscle contractions, whereas individual Beckmann-sized electrodes can detect minute muscle activity.

Initial treatment sessions should be brief because of rapid onset of fatigue and should alternate with rest periods of a 20-second minimum.

FUNCTIONAL EXERCISES/WORK CAPACITY

Functional exercises are a part of the entire rehabilitation process. Prior to muscle rein-

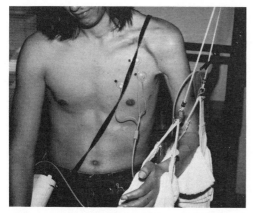

Figure 15–6. Early EMG biofeedback training of the pectoralis major muscle in this patient with a brachial plexus injury. The deltoid sling enhances the small movements and adds additional reinforcement to the patient.

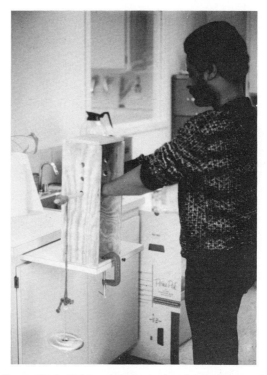

Figure 15–8. Light resistive exercises for both general upper extremity strengthening and specific shoulder strengthening for this patient with a brachial plexus injury, shown 8 months postoperatively.

nervation, these exercises are used to promote circulation and maintain tone in muscles of the arm or hand that are not affected by the injury. Following reinnervation, these exercises, in combination with simulated work tasks, provide sensory input while increasing strength, endurance, and coordination (Fig. 15–8).[10] Simulated work tasks help patients regain the physical capacity to resume familiar activities and gainful employment. The latter is especially important in our clinic, where about 65% of the patients are treated for work-related injuries from heavy labor and industrial jobs.

We usually begin functional exercises 3 to 4 weeks after surgery to decrease edema and

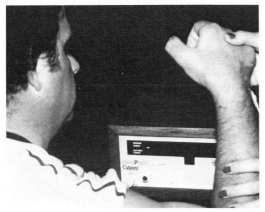

Figure 15–7. The combination of visual EMG biofeedback and the therapist's hands guiding the movement of the flexor carpi ulnaris muscle is shown as the patient undergoes early motor re-education.

encourage motion. Patients start with low resistance exercises to avoid excessive stress on the repair and may wear a dynamic splint during exercise if necessary.

Once reinnervation is underway, patients start muscle strengthening activities. At this stage, biofeedback enables them to monitor specific activities, providing additional reinforcement (Fig. 15–9). Later, during sensory recovery, patients engage in exercises using objects of various sizes, shapes, and textures to reinforce the re-education process (see Chapter 14 for a detailed discussion of sensory re-education).

Bowden and Napier[10] describe hand movement as consisting of two basic patterns—the prehensile grip and the power grip. Use of these patterns is determined by the shape of an object, its function, and the patient's individual habits.[51] Functional exercises are individually designed to retrain each patient in these movement patterns, and patients therefore are more willing to perform meaningful tasks than to carry out mechanical exercises.[52] Specific exercises and activities are discussed in detail in books such as Wynn Parry's *Rehabilitation of the Hand.*[104]

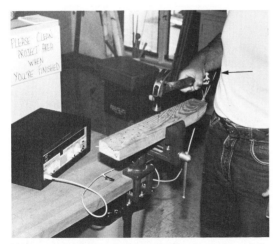

Figure 15–9. This patient sustained a laceration of the ulnar nerve proximally. Now 5 months postoperatively, he is using EMG biofeedback with hammering to reinforce function of the flexor carpi ulnaris muscle.

Ideally, a rehabilitation program should increase the coordination, strength, and physical capacity required for jobs held by patients.[7] A patient's description of work activities (and references such as *The Dictionary of Occupational Titles*[28]) can be very helpful in work simulation and in determining the need for special splints or adaptive devices.[46] The BTE Work Simulator is one device designed for the controlled rehabilitation of upper extremities by means of resistive exercise.[3]

PAIN MANAGEMENT/ DESENSITIZATION

The progress of rehabilitation can be greatly impeded by pain or irritating sensations experienced by the patient. Heat and gentle motion are traditional methods for alleviation of acute pain and causalgia.[91] In addition, there are a number of reports on the use of transcutaneous nerve stimulators (TNS) to relieve both acute and chronic pain.[8, 9, 63, 84] The mechanism involved is unclear. According to Bishop,[8] TNS units may relieve pain via A-fiber stimulation or by interfering with stimuli, as postulated by the gate theory of Malzack and Wall. Mayer and Price[65] also report that the TNS units stimulate the release of enkephalin in the brain.

According to studies of postoperative pain management with TNS units, patients using these devices required less pain medication and recovered more quickly.[9, 84] Mannheimer and Carlsson[63] found that rheumatoid arthritis patients receiving TNS therapy experienced up to 18 hours of relief from wrist pain and were able to increase their grip strength. Both acupuncture-like TNS and traditional TNS are currently used for pain relief.[8]

TNS units are used at our clinic to relieve acute pain following injury and pain associated with postoperative edema and joint stiffness. The method is more effective when electrodes with a high frequency pulse pattern are placed at the pain site or along the nerve pathway. The causalgia-like pain associated with brachial plexus injury has been described in detail by Wynn Parry.[103] However, our experience with this clinical entity is limited, and we have had reasonable success with a combination of heat and high frequency TNS at Erb's point and at the mid-axilla. TNS can also be used as a preliminary measure before initiating a formal desensitization program.

Patients are often troubled and alarmed by the hyperesthesias and paresthesias that accompany nerve regeneration. In the past it was recommended that the patient simply tap the affected area.[37, 64, 73, 88] We now begin progressive desensitization as soon as a patient reports these sensations, moving from simple to complex stimuli.[42] Patients begin with massage and vibration, progressing as soon as these are tolerated to working with various textures and immersion media (sawdust, beans, macaroni) (Fig. 15–10). Patients with fingertip hypersensitivity also apply graded constant pressure to their fingertips. The purpose of these exercises is to reacquaint the hypersensitive part, as well as the patient's brain, with normal stimuli that the cortex has been interpreting as painful. When

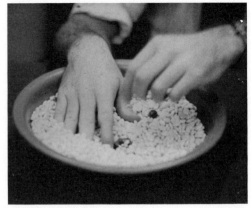

Figure 15–10. This patient uses the immersion technique to desensitize his hypersensitive index digit following nerve grafting and regeneration.

desensitization is complete, the patient is ready to begin sensory re-education.

SENSORY TESTING

More than 30 different tests are available to monitor progress of return of sensation.[2, 19, 22, 25–27, 33, 35, 38, 39, 49, 58, 61, 71, 74, 79, 80, 83, 92, 95, 96, 99–102] Although we are not convinced that these tests are entirely objective and quantitative, they do provide information about the progress of individual patients. Twelve tests and testing devices are used at our clinic: the Ninhydrin test, directional touch test, two-point discrimination test, moving two-point discrimination test, Sensiometer, Semmes-Weinstein Anesthesiometer, braille pattern, point localization, pick-up test, object identification, tuning fork vibration, and Biothesiometer.

The distal progression of the regenerating nerve in the immediate postoperative period can be plotted by eliciting Tinel's sign.[92] Both Tinel's sign and the Ninhydrin test are used to monitor nerve regeneration in the hand; once nerve regeneration reaches the hand, we assess the patient's improving sensory function (on the fingertip pulp only) with the help of the battery of tests mentioned in the preceding paragraph. This is in agreement with findings that the assessment of sensibility changes is achieved more easily by testing the digital pulp rather than the whole hand.[72] Progress during sensory re-education exercises is monitored by testing the entire length of the finger—a technique that has proved successful in documenting changes in point localization (Fig. 15–11).

All sensory testing is conducted in a room with temperature and noise control.[24] A screen is placed between the patient and the examiner to prevent bias. The hand to be tested is cradled on a towel or immobilized in putty. Testing intervals (weekly, monthly, or every 6 months) depend upon the stage of recovery.

SPLINTING

Splints are used throughout postoperative rehabilitation of the patient with an upper extremity peripheral nerve injury. The objectives of splinting are to (1) prevent ankylosis of the joints, (2) maintain joint mobility and tendon glide, (3) correct joint or soft tissue deformity, and (4) encourage functional use of the hand throughout the period of reinnervation. Splints have been used frequently for rehabilitation purposes, but specific biomechanical effects of splinting have not been researched. Effective use of the splints requires a thorough understanding of the pathologic conditions, the objectives of splinting, and the desired biomechanical effects. Two types of splints, static and dynamic, are used in the management of patients with upper extremity peripheral nerve injuries (Figs. 15–12 and 15–13).

Protection of the nerve repairs in the early postoperative period requires static splinting. Static splints are also used later to stress scars, most often in the case of median and ulnar nerve lesions at the wrist. Tendon glide in this area is frequently restricted by heavy volar scarring with associated dermotenodesis, and patients may develop compensatory patterns of wrist use. Dorsal static splints can gradually increase the range of wrist extension during exercise, exposing the volar scar to additional stress.

Cylinder casting is another method of static splinting used to increase small joint motion. This method is used most often in dealing with proximal interphalangeal joint contractures, an area where, according to Kolumban,[54] proved cylinder casting significantly more successful than dynamic splinting.[54]

Capener[17, 18] developed and advocated the use of "lively" or dynamic splints for the treatment of peripheral nerve injuries. These splints allow controlled movement of innervated muscles, thereby promoting venous return, maintaining muscle tone, and preventing soft tissue shortening. Dynamic splints allow patients more efficient use of their hands than static splints; their use, according to Fess,[34] leads to increased patient compliance (Fig. 15–14). Wynn Parry[103] found that 70% of the 50 patients with brachial plexus injuries who were studied considered dynamic splints worthwhile and wore them regularly.

Although a wide array of static and dynamic splints are available for patients with upper extremity peripheral nerve injuries, the choice of splint in each case depends on how the patient will use his or her hand during a particular phase of rehabilitation. The primary objectives of splinting are to prevent deformity and improve function.[34, 77] Reinnervation and sensory re-education take a long time and consequently patient com-

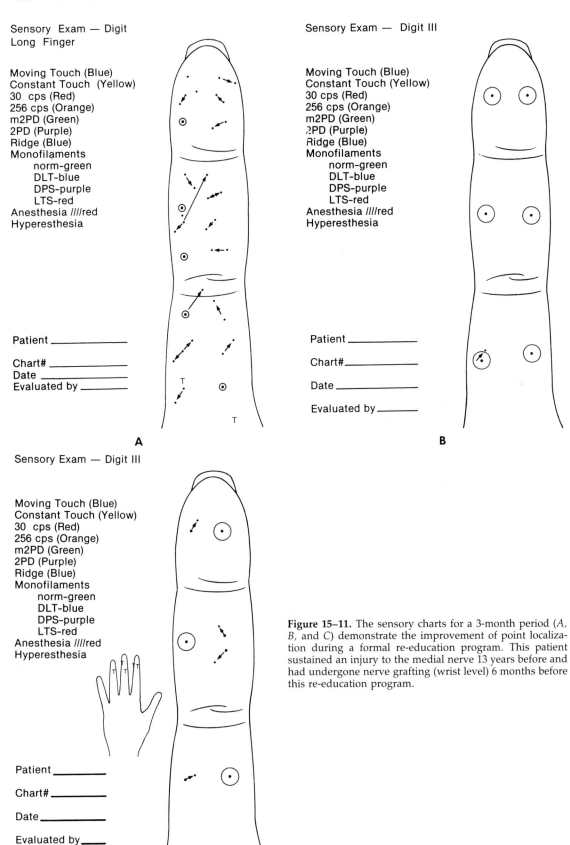

Sensory Exam — Digit
Long Finger

Moving Touch (Blue)
Constant Touch (Yellow)
30 cps (Red)
256 cps (Orange)
m2PD (Green)
2PD (Purple)
Ridge (Blue)
Monofilaments
    norm-green
    DLT-blue
    DPS-purple
    LTS-red
Anesthesia ////red
Hyperesthesia

Patient _____

Chart# _____
Date _____
Evaluated by _____

A

Sensory Exam — Digit III

Moving Touch (Blue)
Constant Touch (Yellow)
30 cps (Red)
256 cps (Orange)
m2PD (Green)
2PD (Purple)
Ridge (Blue)
Monofilaments
    norm-green
    DLT-blue
    DPS-purple
    LTS-red
Anesthesia ////red
Hyperesthesia

Patient _____

Chart# _____

Date _____

Evaluated by _____

B

Sensory Exam — Digit III

Moving Touch (Blue)
Constant Touch (Yellow)
30 cps (Red)
256 cps (Orange)
m2PD (Green)
2PD (Purple)
Ridge (Blue)
Monofilaments
    norm-green
    DLT-blue
    DPS-purple
    LTS-red
Anesthesia ////red
Hyperesthesia

Patient _____

Chart# _____

Date _____

Evaluated by ____

C

Figure 15–11. The sensory charts for a 3-month period (*A, B,* and *C*) demonstrate the improvement of point localization during a formal re-education program. This patient sustained an injury to the medial nerve 13 years before and had undergone nerve grafting (wrist level) 6 months before this re-education program.

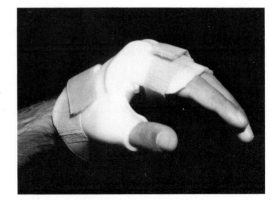

Figure 15–12. Example of a static splint for low median/ulnar nerve injury.

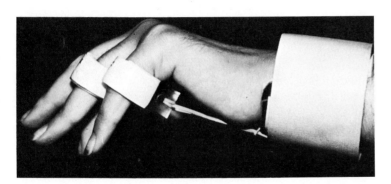

Figure 15–13. Example of a dynamic splint for low median nerve injury.

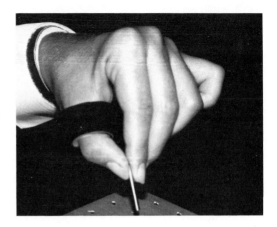

Figure 15–14. The use of a dynamic splint in a patient with low median nerve injury to encourage functional use of the hand.

Table 15–1. SPLINTING OBJECTIVES AND SPLINT EXAMPLES FOR MANAGING THE PERIPHERAL NERVE INJURED–HAND

Nerve	Splinting Objective	Splint Component(s)
Median (low)	Maintain thumb web space	C-bar Dynamic thumb opponens Cuff
Median (high)	MP flexion to I and III digits	MP static or dynamic splint
Ulnar	MP flexion to IV and V digits	MP static or dynamic flexion splint
Combined median and ulnar	Same as median and ulnar nerves	Same as median and ulnar nerves
Radial (high)	Wrist extension Thumb extension	Dynamic wrist extension or static wrist cock-up Thumb IP extension outrigger

pliance becomes a major problem—one that must be considered in deciding on the appropriate splint. Table 15–1 provides examples of splints and their objectives.

SUMMARY

This chapter has outlined a treatment approach to the management of the patient with an upper extremity peripheral nerve injury. It is very important to understand that the total process begins immediately following evaluation and continues until the patient achieves maximum functional independence and, hopefully, returns to work.

References

1. Arem, A., and Madden, J.: Effects of stress on healing wounds: intermittent noncyclical tension. J. Surg. Res., 20:93, 1976.
2. Arezzo, J., and Schaumburg, H.: The use of the Optacon as a screening device. J. Occup. Med., 22:461, 1980.
3. Arezzo, J., and Schaumburg, H.: BTE Work Simulator. Baltimore, Therapeutic Equipment Company, 1981.
4. Baker, L.: Handbook of Functional Muscle Stimulation. Los Angeles, Rancho Los Amigos, 1980.
5. Baker, M., Regenos, E., Wolf, S., et al.: Developing strategies for biofeedback. Phys. Ther., 57:402, 1977.
6. Barr, N.: The Hand: Principles and Techniques of Simple Splint Making in Rehabilitation. London, Butterworths, 1975.
7. Baxter, P.: Physical capacity evaluation and work therapy. In Hunter, J., Schneider, L., Mackin, E., et al. (eds.): Rehabilitation of the Hand, 1st Ed. St. Louis, The C. V. Mosby Company, 1978.
8. Bishop, B.: Pain: Its physiology and rationale for management: Parts II and III. Phys. Ther., 60:21, 1980.
9. Bohm, E.: Transcutaneous electrical nerve stimulation in chronic pain after peripheral nerve injuries. Acta Neurochir., 40:277, 1978.
10. Bowden, R., and Napier, J.: The assessment of hand function after peripheral nerve injuries. J. Bone Joint Surg., 43B:481, 1961.
11. Brand, P.: Rehabilitation of the hand with motor and sensory impairment. Orthop. Clin., 4:1135, 1973.
12. Brand, P., and Wood, H.: Hand Volunteer Instruction Sheet. Carville, Louisiana, U.S. Public Health Service Hospital.
13. Braum, R.: Epineural nerve repair. In Omer, G., and Spinner, M. (eds.): Management of Peripheral Nerve Disorders. Philadelphia, W. B. Saunders Company, 1980.
14. Brown, D., DeBacher, G., and Basmajian, J.: Feedback Goniometers for Hand Rehabilitation. J. Occup. Ther., 33:458, 1979.
15. Brown, D.: Current concepts and capabilities of EMG and electrokinesiologic feedback in the total management of traumatic hand injuries. In Hunter, J., Schneider, L., Mackin, E., et al. (eds.): Rehabilitation of the Hand, 1st Ed. St. Louis, The C. V. Mosby Company, 1978.
16. Brudny, J., Karein, J., Grynbaum, B., et al.: EMG feedback therapy: A review of treatment of 114 patients. Arch. Phys. Med. Rehab., 57:55, 1976.
17. Capener, N.: Lively splints. Physiotherapy, 53:371, 1967.
18. Capener, N.: Physiological rest with special reference to arthritis and nerve injuries. Br. Med. J., 2:761, 1946.
19. Carlson, W., Shlomo, S., Taylor, W., et al.: Instrumentation for measurement of sensory loss in the fingertips. J. Occup. Med., 21:260, 1974.
20. Chou, H., Cleveland, D., and Davenport, H.: Atrophy and regeneration of the gastrocnemius-soleus muscles. J.A.M.A., 113:1029, 1939.
21. Clarke, G., and Stenner, L.: Use of therapeutic ultrasound. Physiotherapy, 62:185, 1976.
22. Craig, J.: Vibrotactile letter recognition: The effect of a masking stimulus. Percept. Psychophys., 20:317, 1976.
23. Cugola, L., and Tarolli, G.: Auto-electrotherapy in nerve lesions. Hand, 10:279, 1978.
24. deJesus, P., Hausmanow, I., and Barchi, R.: The effect of cold on nerve conduction of human slow and fast nerve fibers. Neurology, 23:1182, 1973.
25. DeMichelis, F., Giaretti, W., Barbaeris, W., et al.: Biomedical instrumentation for measurements of skin sensitivity. IEEE Trans. Biomed. Engr., 26:326, 1979.
26. Dellon, A.: Clinical use of vibratory stimulus to

evaluate peripheral nerve injury and compression neuropathy. Plast. Reconstr. Surg., 65:466, 1980.

27. Dellon, A.: The Moving 2PD Test. J. Hand Surg., 3:474, 1978.
28. Dictionary of Occupational Titles, 4th Ed. Washington, D.C., U.S. Department of Labor, 1977.
29. Donatelli, R., Owen, B., and Burkhart, H.: Effects of immobilization on the extensibility of periarticular connective tissue. J. Orth. Sports Phys. Ther., 3:67, 1981.
30. Dyson, M., and Pond, J.: The effects of ultrasound in circulation. Physiotherapy, 59:284, 1973.
31. Dyson, M., and Suckling, J.: Stimulation of tissue repair by ultrasound: A survey of mechanisms involved. Physiotherapy, 64:105, 1978.
32. Eccles, M.: Hand volumetrics. Br. J. Phys. Med., 19:5, 1956.
33. Edshage, S.: Experience with clinical methods of testing sensation after peripheral nerve surgery. In Jewett, D., and McCarroll, H. (eds.): Nerve Repair and Regeneration. St. Louis, The C. V. Mosby Company, 1980.
34. Fess, E.: Hand Splinting, Principles and Methods. St. Louis, The C. V. Mosby Company, 1981.
35. Flynn, J., and Flynn, W.: Median and ulnar nerve injury: Long-range study with evaluation of Ninhydrin test, sensory and motor returns. Ann. Surg., 156:1002, 1962.
36. Gersten, J.: Thermal and non-thermal changes in isometric tension, contractile protein and injury potential produced in frog muscle by ultrasound energy. Arch. Phys. Med. Rehab., 34:675, 1953.
37. Grant, G.: Methods of treatment of neuromata of the hand. J. Bone Joint Surg., 33A:841, 1951.
38. Gregarson, G.: Vibratory perception threshold and motor conduction velocity in diabetics and non-diabetics. Acta Med. Scand., 183:61, 1968.
39. Gregg, E.: Absolute measurement of vibratory threshold. Arch. Neurol. Psychiatry, 66:403, 1951.
40. Griffin, J., Echternach, J., and Bowmaker, K.: Results of frequency differences in ultrasonic therapy. Phys. Ther., 50:481, 1970.
41. Griffin, J.: Nerve and muscle stimulation. In Griffin, J., and Karselis, T. (eds.): Physical Agents for Physical Therapists. Springfield, Illinois, Charles C Thomas, Publisher, 1978.
42. Hardy, M., Moran, C., and Merritt, W.: Desensitization of the traumatized hand. Virg. Med. J., 109:134, 1982.
43. Herbison, G., Teng, C., Reyes, T., et al.: Effect of electrical stimulation on denervated muscle of rat. Arch. Phys. Med. Rehab., 52:516, 1971.
44. Hills, W., and Byrd, R.: Effects of immobilization in the human forearm. Arch. Phys. Med. Rehab., 54:87, 1973.
45. Hines, H., Melville, E., and Wehrmacher, W.: The effect of electrical stimulation on neuromuscular regeneration. Am. J. Phys., 144:278, 1945.
46. Inglis, J., Campbell, D., and Donald, M.: EMG biofeedback and neuromuscular rehabilitation. Can. J. Behav. Sci., 8:299, 1976.
47. Jackson, E., and Seddon, H.: Influences of galvanic stimulation on muscle atrophy resulting from denervation. Br. Med. J., 3:485, 1945.
48. Jackson, S.: The role of galvanism in the treatment of denervated voluntary muscle in man. Brain, 68:300, 1945.
49. Jaminson, D.: Sensitivity training as a means for differentiating the various forms of leprosy found in Nigeria. Int. J. Leprosy, 39:504, 1972.

50. Johnson, D., Thurston, P., and Ashcroft, P.: The Russian technique in the treatment of chondromalacia patellae. Physiother. Can., 29:2, 1977.
51. Kamakaura, N., Matsuo, M., Ishii, H., et al.: Patterns of static prehension in normal hands. Am. J. Occup. Ther., 34:445, 1980.
52. Kidner, T.: Occupational therapy: its development, scope and possibilities. Occup. Ther. Rehab., 10:1, 1931.
53. Kischer, C., and Shetlar, M.: Microvasculature in hypertrophic scars and the effects of pressure. J. Trauma, 19:757, 1979.
54. Kolumban, S.: The role of static and dynamic splints, physiotherapy techniques, and time in straightening contracted interphalangeal joints. Leprosy India, 2:323, 1969.
55. Kukula, C., Brown, D., and Basmajian, J.: Biofeedback training. A preliminary report for early joint mobilization. Am. J. Occup. Ther., 29:469, 1975.
56. Lehmann, J., Masock, A., Warren, G., et al.: Effect of therapeutic temperature on tendon extensibility. Arch. Phys. Med. Rehab., 51:481, 1970.
57. Lehmann, J., DeLateur, B., Warren, G., et al.: Heating joint structures by ultrasound. Arch. Phys. Med. Rehab., 49:28, 1968.
58. Levin, S., Pearsall, G., and Ruderman, R.: Von Frey's method of measuring pressure sensitivity in the hand: An engineering analysis of Semmes-Weinstein pressure anesthesiometer. J. Hand Surg., 3:211, 1978.
59. Liberson, W. T.: Electrotherapy. In Ruskin, A. P. (ed.): Current Therapy in Physiatry. Philadelphia, W. B. Saunders Co., 1984, pp. 161–191.
60. Lomo, T., Westgaard, R., and Dahl, H.: Contractile properties of muscle: Control by pattern of muscle activity in the rat. Proc. Roy. Soc. (B)., 187:99, 1974.
61. McQuillan, W., Nelson, J., Boardman, A., et al.: Sensory evaluation after median nerve repair. Hand, 3:101, 1971.
62. Macowiak, P.: The Effect of Continuous and Pulsed Ultrasound on the Physical Characteristics of Scar Tissue. Unpublished Master's Thesis, Medical College of Virginia, 1981.
63. Mannheimer, C., and Carlsson, C.: The analgesic effect of transcutaneous nerve stimulation in patients with rheumatoid arthritis. Pain, 6:329, 1979.
64. Matthews, G., and Osterholm, J.: Painful traumatic neuromas. Surg. Clin., 51:1313, 1972.
65. Mayer, D., and Price, D.: Central nervous system mechanisms of analgesia. Pain, 2:379, 1976.
66. Mennell, J.: Joint Pain. Boston, Little, Brown & Company, 1964.
67. Middlemast, S., and Chatterjee, D.: Comparison of ultrasound and thermotherapy for soft tissue injury. Physiotherapy, 64:331, 1978.
68. Miehlke, A., Stennert, E., and Chilla, R.: Postoperative management of facial paresis. Clin. Plast. Surg., 6:465, 1979.
69. Millesi, H., Meissl, G., and Berger, A.: Further experience in interfascicular grafting of the median, ulnar, and radial nerves. J. Bone Joint Surg., 58A:209, 1976.
70. Millesi, H., Meissl, G., and Berger, A.: The interfascicular nerve grafting of the median and ulnar nerves. J. Bone Joint Surg., 54A:727, 1972.
71. Moberg, E.: Objective method of determining the functional value of sensibility in the hand. J. Bone Joint Surg., 40B:454, 1958.
72. Moran, C.: Comparison of Sensory Testing Methods Using Carpal Tunnel Syndrome Patients. Un-

published Master's Thesis, Medical College of Virginia, 1981.

73. Nathan, P.: Improvement in cutaneous sensibility associated with relief of pain. J. Neurol. Neurosurg. Psychiatry, 23:202, 1960.

74. Onne, L.: Recovery of sensibility in sudomotor activity in the hand after nerve suture. Acta Chir. Scand. Suppl., 301:1, 1962.

75. Paaske, W., Hovind, H., and Sejrsen, P.: Influence of therapeutic ultrasonic irradiation on blood flow in human cutaneous, subcutaneous, and muscular tissue. Scand. J. Clin. Lab. Invest., 3:389, 1973.

76. Patrick, M.: Application of therapeutic pulses ultrasound. Physiotherapy, 64:103, 1978.

77. Peacock, E.: Dynamic splinting for the prevention and correction of deformities. J. Bone Joint Surg., 34A:789, 1972.

78. Pollock, L., et al.: The effect of massage and passive movement upon the residual of experimentally produced section of the sciatic nerves of the cat. Arch. Phys. Med., 31:265, 1950.

79. Poppen, N., McCarroll, R., Doyle, J., et al.: Sensibility after suture of digital nerves. J. Hand Surg., 4:212, 1979.

80. Porter, R.: New test for fingertip sensation. Br. Med. J., 2:927, 1966.

81. Pospisilova, J., Samohyl, J., Koprivova, M., et al.: Our experience with use of ultrasound in the rehabilitation of the hand. Acta Chir. Plast., 22:191, 1980.

82. Post, B.: Value of galvanic muscle stimulation immediately after paresis. In Rubin, L. (ed.): Reanimation of the Paralyzed Face. St. Louis, The C. V. Mosby Company, 1977.

83. Renfrew, S.: The fingertip sensation. Lancet, 2:396, 1969.

84. Rosenberg, M., Curtis, L., and Bourke, D.: Transcutaneous nerve stimulation for relief of postoperative pain. Pain, 5:129, 1978.

85. Rosselle, N., DeMeinar, J., DeKeyser, C., et al.: Electromyographic evaluation of therapeutic methods in complete peripheral paralysis. Electromyog. Clin. Neurophys., 17:179, 1977.

86. Shamberger, R., Talbot, T., Tipton, A., et al.: The effect of ultrasonic and thermal treatment on wounds. Plast. Reconst. Surg., 68:860, 1981.

87. Sherman, R., Sherman, C., and Gall, N.: A survey of current phantom limb pain treatments in the US. Pain, 8:85, 1980.

88. Stayman, J.: Care of the nerve-injured extremity. Surg. Clin., 52:1337, 1972.

89. Stillwell, G., and Wakim, K.: Effects of varying intervals between sessions of electric stimulation of denervated rat muscle. Arch. Phys. Med. Rehab., 43:95, 1962.

90. Stillwell, C.: Physiatric management of postmastectomy lymphedema. Med. Clin., 46:1051, 1973.

91. Sunderland, S.: Pain mechanisms in causalgia. J. Neurol. Neurosurg. Psychiatry, 39:471, 1976.

92. Tinel, J.: The tingling sign in peripheral nerve lesions—1915. Translated by Kaplan, E.: In Spinner, M. (ed.): Injuries to Major Branches of Peripheral Nerves in the Forearm. 2nd Ed. Philadelphia, W. B. Saunders Company, 1978.

93. Tupper, J.: Fascicular nerve repair. In Omer, G., and Spinner, M. (eds.): Management of Peripheral Nerve Problems. Philadelphia, W. B. Saunders Company, 1980.

94. Vasudevan, D., and Melvin, J.: Upper extremity edema control: Rationale of the techniques. Am. J. Occup. Ther., 33:520, 1979.

95. Vierck, C., and Jones, M.: Size discrimination on the skin. Science, 163:488, 1969.

96. VonPrince, K., and Butler, B.: Measuring sensory function of the hand after peripheral nerve injury. Am. J. Occup. Ther., 21:385, 1967.

97. Wakim, K., and Krusen, F.: The influence of electrical stimulation on work output and endurance of denervated muscle. Arch. Phys. Med. Rehab., 36:370, 1955.

98. Warren, C., Lehmann, J., and Koblank, J.: Elongation of rat tail tendon: Effect of load and temperature. Arch. Phys. Med. Rehab., 52:465, 1971.

99. Weber, E.: The Sense of Touch. Translated by Ross, H., and Murray, D. New York, Academic Press, 1978.

100. Weinstein, S., and Sersen, E.: Tactual sensitivity as a function of handedness and laterality. J. Comp. Physiopsychol., 54:665, 1961.

101. Weinstein, S.: Tactile sensitivity in the phalanges. Percept. Motor Skills, 14:351, 1962.

102. Werner, J., and Omer, G.: Evaluating cutaneous pressure sensation of the hand. Am. J. Occup. Ther., 24:347, 1970.

103. Wynn Parry, C.: The management of traction lesions of the brachial plexus and peripheral nerve injuries in the upper limb. The Ruskoe Clarke Memorial Lecture, 1979.

104. Wynne Parry, C.: Rehabilitation of the Hand. 2nd Ed. London, Butterworths, 1973.

105. Zeissler, R., Rose, G., and Nelson, P.: Postmastectomy lymphedema: Late results of treatment in 385 patients. Arch. Phys. Med. Rehab., 53:159, 1972.

16

Clinical Application of Electrophysiologic Recordings

■

Julia K. Terzis, M.D., Ph.D.
Nelson G. Publicover, Ph.D.

One of the main reasons why microsurgical reconstruction of peripheral nerves cannot yet claim to restore normal function is that peripheral nerves are complex functionally but appear anatomically homogeneous even under the highest power of the operating microscope. The functional evaluation of the peripheral nerve and the pursuit of *objective* means of intraoperative assessment of the degree of nerve activity in lesions in continuity constitute the present areas of intense investigation. Investigators in various specialties, including histochemistry, biochemistry, and immunochemistry, are attempting to decipher the sensory-motor components of peripheral nerve trunks. Furthermore, sequential computerized appraisals of the intraneural topography of peripheral nerves have recently added a new dimension to our understanding of fascicular organization.[22]

Invasive electrophysiologic analysis has been recently introduced in peripheral nerve surgery[20, 23] and constitutes perhaps one of the few objective tools we have for intraoperative diagnosis prior to fascicular repair procedures.

The action potential of a single nerve (see Fig. 6–1) is a fixed-amplitude voltage change less than 1-msec in duration, the shape of which alone provides little diagnostic information. However, the compound action potential (CAP), which is the total potential recorded from a nerve trunk as a result of many simultaneously excited nerve fibers, can be used as a diagnostic tool for nerve repair procedures (see chapter on Physiologic Assessment of Nerve Injuries).

The disadvantage of the CAP is that it requires the simultaneous production of action potentials in many fibers. Activity in a few fibers does not produce sufficient voltage at the surface of the nerve to be detected by conventional recording apparatus. Thus, a large number of fibers must be activated simultaneously. It is difficult to produce simultaneous action potentials in a large number of fibers using natural stimuli. Electrical stimuli must therefore be used. Since electrical stimuli bypass the receptors and activate fibers on the basis of their diameters, the resulting pattern of neural activity traveling along the nerve is one not found when the nerve is stimulated naturally. Nevertheless, despite these shortcomings, the electrically elicited CAP can provide a great deal of clinically useful information.

TYPES OF RECORDINGS

The term "voltage" always refers to the potential *difference* between two points. It is related to the amount of energy required to move a charged particle from one point to another. Therefore, any measurement of potential involves at least two recording contacts.

Most interpretations of the CAP are based on *monopolar* recordings (Fig. 16–1). In this

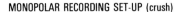

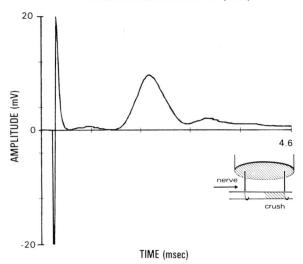

Figure 16–1. Monopolar recording setup. This figure illustrates the monopolar recording arrangement using a region of crushed nerve for the location of the indifferent electrode. The resultant CAP is principally monophasic. The CAP has been recorded from the sciatic nerve of a frog. (From Terzis, J. K., and Publicover, N.: Clin. Plast. Surg., *11*:48, 1984.)

case a single, "active" electrode is placed on or near the nerve under investigation. A second "reference" electrode is placed in neutral or inactive tissue that is in electrical contact with the nerve. A recording consists of measuring the potential difference between these two points.

Any process that generates an electrical gradient between the two contacts will cause a deflection in the signal. This can be generated internally (e.g., from a nerve or muscle) or result from the flow of current due to an externally applied field (e.g., 50- or 60-cycle interference from room lights). Since any signal other than the one generated by the nerve is undesirable, the reference electrode should be placed in an inactive region as close to the active electrode as possible.

Experimentally this can be achieved by blocking conduction to a segment of the nerve itself. Common methods include crushing the nerve or using chemical means to block conduction and placing the reference electrode in this inactive region. It is important to block conduction along a sufficient portion of the nerve so that the reference electrode is not able to detect any of the CAP via volume conduction. In the case of the isolated frog sciatic nerve, this distance can be several millimeters when using 26-gauge platinum hook electrodes.

The major advantage of a monopolar recording situation is the principally monophasic response that can be obtained. (All events causes a deflection in the same direction.) The responses from individual fibers

or bundles *sum* constructively, regardless of the phase of the responses. The total area under the CAP is related to the total number of active fibers (also being aware of the numerous other factors that affect the shape of the CAP). Thus, the signal is more readily interpreted.

Clinical applications of the CAP do not permit segments of nerve to be crushed to obtain a better reference electrode. Therefore, a reference electrode placed in nearby inactive tissue (at the expense of increased noise) (Fig. 16–2) or *bipolar* recordings can be introduced. Bipolar recordings (Fig. 16–3) consist of two electrodes in contact with the nerve under investigation. (There may be a third "reference" electrode to ensure that the signals from the two active electrodes stay within the operational range of the input stage of the amplifier.) The signal recorded by one electrode is subtracted from the signal recorded by the other electrode. In this way, any signals that are common to both electrodes (such as muscle noise or any other non-neural source distant from the electrodes) generate no *net* response. This is called common mode rejection.

The propagating CAP generated by the nerve passes by the first electrode, causing a deflection in one direction. It then passes by the second electrode, causing a deflection in the opposite direction. The result is a principally biphasic response, as shown in Figure 16–3. The major advantage of this technique is a significantly reduced noise level owing to common mode rejection.

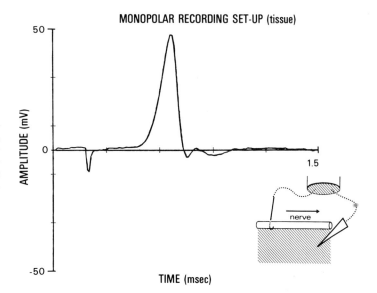

Figure 16–2. Monopolar recording in tissue. If the surrounding tissue is inactive, it is feasible to obtain a monopolar recording using an indifferent needle electrode placed in the nearby tissue. (From Terzis, J. K., and Publicover, N.: Clin. Plast. Surg., *11*:49, 1984.)

If a population of fibers is active near one electrode at the same time that another population of fibers is active near the second electrode, the two responses will tend to cancel each other. This simple example shows that the contributions by two populations of fibers are not necessarily additive. The total magnitude of the bipolar response depends on both the magnitude and the phase (with respect to the distance between the recording electrodes) of the responses that make up the CAP. Although less discernible than the monopolar CAP, the bipolar CAP does indicate the presence or absence of conduction and gives some indication of the magnitude (due to the dominant contribution by the rapid large myelinated fibers).

A variety of other electrode configurations utilizing three or more contacts have been used experimentally.[18] With their associated electronics, they are designed to enhance signals in certain directions or at specified conduction velocities. However, at present, they are not in wide use clinically.

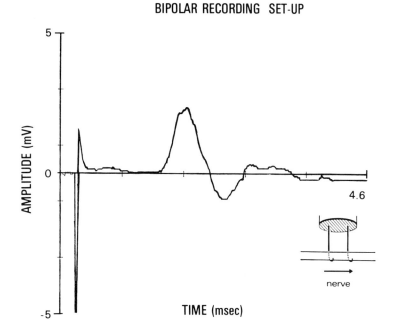

Figure 16–3. Bipolar recording setup. During bipolar recordings, the signal in one electrode is subtracted from the response recorded in the other. Distant signals, common to both electrodes, result in no net response. (From Terzis, J. K., and Publicover, N.: Clin. Plast. Surg., *11*:49, 1984.)

CLINICAL USE OF THE CAP

Of course, the primary concern in the clinical application of the CAP is the safety of the patient. Recent advances in semiconductor technology have continued to minimize any risk to the patient and have improved the quality of the signals that can be recorded.

With regard to electrophysiologic recordings, the greatest potential risk to the patient arises from the possibility of the flow of current between two or more instruments (including the operating table itself) in contact with the patient. This risk is minimized by the use of stimulus isolation units (SIUs) and isolation amplifiers, which provide no electrical pathway between the electrode contacts and either the "ground" or the power lines of the instrument. There are two general types of SIU in common use: (1) a (radiofrequency) isolation transformer that can transfer power to stimulating electrodes, and (2) a separate circuit run by a high voltage battery controlled via an optical link.

By completely isolating both the stimulating and the recording electrodes, no pathway to "ground" or to the building power source is possible. In addition, isolating the patient will diminish leakage currents, thereby reducing the artefactual responses caused by the stimulus. Only in the event of a catastrophic component failure can current flow from one instrument (e.g., heart monitor) to another through the patient. Thus, all instruments should be securely connected to the same power source. Then, even if component failure occurs in such a way as to "ground" the patient, the potential difference between instruments should be small.

Another consideration in the clinical use of the CAP is the toxicity of the electrodes. This is especially important in the case of stimulating electrodes because of the passage of current. A number of interactions are possible at the electrode-tissue interface in the presence of current. Platinum wire (22 to 26 gauge) is generally preferred for electrodes.

If stimulation causes muscle contraction, the force must be restrained in order not to injure the patient or interfere with the recording. This can usually be done by weights or by securely immobilizing the extremity. Muscle relaxants may be useful in patients in whom only nerve recordings are to be conducted and assessment using muscle stimulation is not needed. Indeed, one of the common misinterpretations of the CAP is due to the signal generated by synchronous muscle contractions. Curare will abort signal transmission across the neuromuscular interface but will not affect the CAP.

In addition, inadvertent movement of the electrodes due to displacement of the wire leads must be controlled. Our laboratory has successfully employed a connector that slips apart if too much force is applied. In the future, it may be possible to use small FM transmitters confined to the operative field with no wire connections to the recording apparatus. This will also avoid problems associated with patient isolation.

INSTRUMENTATION FOR INTRAOPERATIVE RECORDING OF CAPS

There are a variety of instruments available to assess neural responses preoperatively or postoperatively using either percutaneous or surface electrodes. Examples include models manufactured by Cadwell, Disa, Grass, Neurodiagnostics, Teca, and Tracor Northern. Most of these units contain features such as multichannel signal averaging and are capable of a variety of clinical applications (somatosensory, auditory, visual-evoked responses, etc.).

One area that has not been pursued as vigorously is the field of invasive intraoperative electrodiagnosis based on signals obtained using microsurgical isolation of individual nerve fascicles or groups of nerve bundles whose functional integrity is questionable.[13, 20, 23] This approach permits a more precise verification and localization of the injury site in partial lesions in continuity and a clearer definition of the degree of injury on an intraneural basis. The criteria for such an instrument, which differ from criteria for noninvasive methods, include:

1. The instrument must be compact and controlled in a concise manner in whole or in part by a surgeon working with sterile technique. It must also provide rapid diagnostic results to minimize the overall time that the patient is kept under anesthesia.

2. The total sampling time must be flexible and include durations as short as 1 msec. The length of nerve to be exposed is generally minimal and is governed by other surgical criteria. Keep in mind that rapidly conducting fibers can travel up to 10 cm within 1 msec.

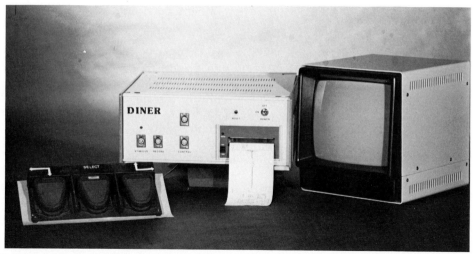

Figure 16–4. Photograph of DINER. DINER (center) is a self-contained computer that can be brought directly into the operating room. The television set (right) can be located anywhere and all of the operations of DINER (except for turning on the power) can be controlled by a cluster of three foot/hand switches (left). The foot switches allow it to be operated by the surgeon.

3. The event produced by rapidly conducting fibers is a fraction of a millisecond in duration. Thus, a frequency response greater than 20 kHz is desired (high in comparison with evoked-response recorders).

The existing commercial models meet only some of the needs of an instrument for intraoperative use. Over the past several years, our laboratory has developed an instrument specifically designed for intraoperative use. This device has been given the acronym DINER (a *d*evice for *i*ntraoperative *n*eural *e*lectrophysiologic *r*ecordings).

DINER

DINER (Figs. 16–4 and 16–5) is a self-contained microprocessor-based instrument capable of performing neural stimulation and recording the elicited CAPs. Responses are displayed on large television screens that are often present in modern operating rooms designed for microsurgery. Graphics and printed results can be viewed at some distance from the site of surgery to avoid clutter around the operating table. All of the functions of DINER can be controlled via three foot-operated (and/or hand-operated) switches. Except for the sterilized electrodes used for stimulation and recording, there is no invasion of the sterile field, even if DINER is operated directly by the surgeon.

The heart of DINER is a microprocessor-based computer that is able to perform rapid

calculations and assist in the decision-making processes of the surgeon. A schematic block diagram of the flow of information within DINER is shown in Figure 16–5. The major hardware components of DINER are a central processing unit, various types of memory, a television interface, circuitry to control stimulation and recording, and a hard-copy plotter.

Several categories of information can be stored and displayed (Fig. 16–6). These in-

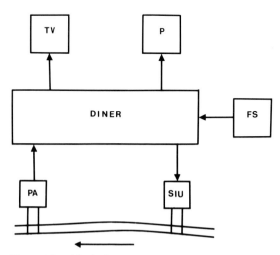

Figure 16–5. Block diagram of DINER. This diagram is a schematic representation of the major components of DINER, a device for intraoperative neural electrophysiologic recordings. Symbols represent the following components: SIU = stimulus isolation unit, PA = preamplifier, TV = video monitor, P = printer-plotter, FS = foot switch.

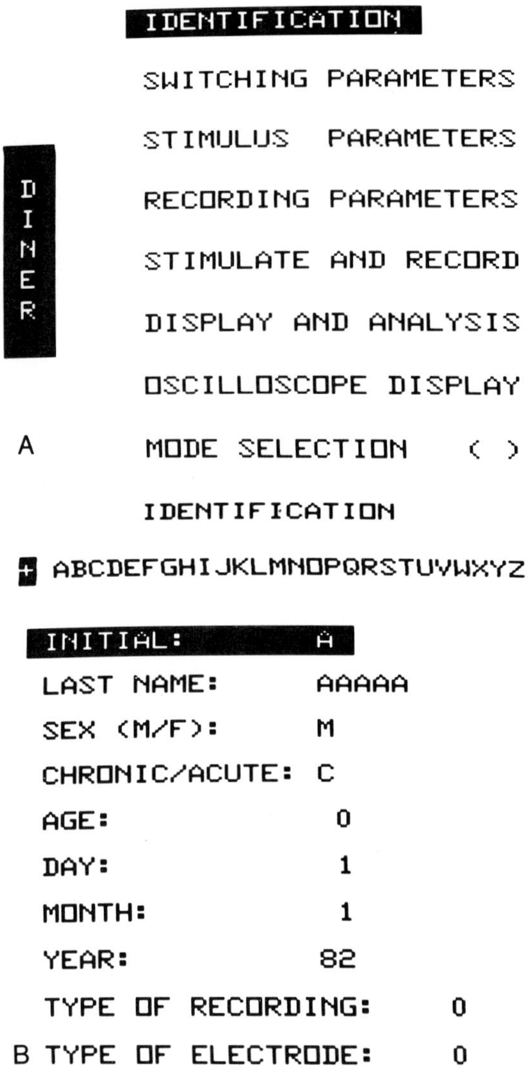

IDENTIFICATION

SWITCHING PARAMETERS

STIMULUS PARAMETERS

RECORDING PARAMETERS

STIMULATE AND RECORD

DISPLAY AND ANALYSIS

OSCILLOSCOPE DISPLAY

A   MODE SELECTION   < >

IDENTIFICATION

■ ABCDEFGHIJKLMNOPQRSTUVWXYZ

INITIAL: A

LAST NAME: AAAAA

SEX (M/F):   M

CHRONIC/ACUTE: C

AGE: 0

DAY: 1

MONTH: 1

YEAR: 82

TYPE OF RECORDING: 0

B TYPE OF ELECTRODE: 0

Figure 16–6. *A*, DINER provides the surgeon with several options for choosing various parameters by simply pressing on the foot switch. *B*, Identification parameters are requested for entry of pertinent information regarding each patient prior to CAP recordings.

clude patient identification, stimulating parameters, recording parameters, and the type of display. DINER can also be operated in much the same way as an oscilloscope to help isolate sources of electrical noise. In addition, previously stored blocks of parameters can be recalled to assist during common recording situations. Each of these categories can be selected from a central menu at any time during the operation of DINER (Fig. 16–6).

All of the various recording and stimulating parameters, including amplifier gains and sampling durations, are under the direct control of the computer. This has two important consequences: (1) There is *no* array of knobs that need to be set for each recording situation (in fact, the only switch other than the foot/hand controls is a single power-reset button). (2) The computer can record each parameter with every CAP trace, avoiding the possibility of human error.

Depending on the type of isolation unit used, stimulation can be controlled as either constant current or constant voltage. The computer employs an 8-bit digital-to-analog converter to control magnitude, providing a stimulus resolution of 0.05%. The duration of the stimulus can be selected in increments of 0.02 msec, and, during averaging, up to 10 stimuli/second can be presented.

Two stages are employed to control the magnitude of the response. The first is an isolation preamplifier with a fixed voltage gain of 100. This is located in a small unit close to the recording electrodes in order to reduce electrical noise. The CAP is then fed to a software programmable–gain amplifier,

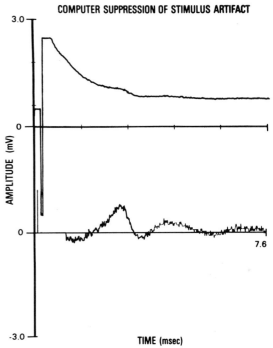

COMPUTER SUPPRESSION OF STIMULUS ARTIFACT

Figure 16–7. Computer-assisted assessment of the CAP. When recording in a confined space from a fascicular bundle, it is often difficult to obtain a large signal and to reduce the effects of the stimulus artifact. The computer can assist in the diagnosis by digitally subtracting the artifact to enhance the response.

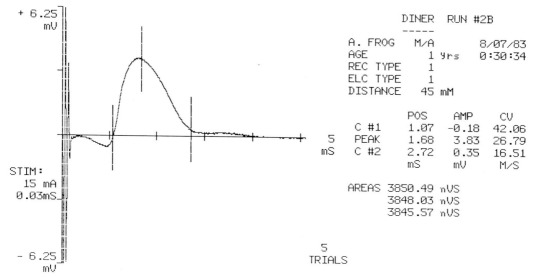

Figure 16–8. Sample of DINER printout. The results generated by DINER can be plotted at any time. Shown here is a copy of one such printout recorded in the laboratory from the sciatic nerve of a frog. Actual results are printed on heat-sensitive paper, which requires few moving parts and contributes almost no noise to the operating room environment.

where it is further amplified by a factor of up to 1000. Finally, the signal is directed to an 8-bit (0.05% resolution) analog-to-digital converter that is capable of gathering up to 200,000 samples/second. Adequate temporal resolution is available even with total sampling durations as short as 0.05 msec.

Results are displayed immediately on the television screen. Two cursors are available to denote the onset and termination of the CAP. If desired, these can be moved to any portion of the response. As cursors are moved, the amplitude of the response, the latency, and the conduction velocity are continuously updated. After the second cursor is moved, the computer also calculates the area under the trace between the cursors and automatically assigns a third cursor to the peak of the response between the two denoted locations.

Selected traces can be stored in the computer for comparison with future recordings. In addition, a paper trace, including the waveform, all measurements, and identification information, can be plotted at any time. Examples of such a recording are shown in Figures 16–7 and 16–8.

To date these procedures have been applied in only a handful of patients. However, as software and hardware improve, there appears to be a great potential in the future for far more widespread clinical use.

References

1. Aminoff, M. J.: Electrodiagnosis in Clinical Neurology. New York. Churchill Livingstone, 1980.
2. Brazier, M. A. B.: The Electrical Activity of the Nervous System. London, Pitman Medical Publishing Company, Ltd., 1968.
3. Buchthal, F., and Rosenfalck, A.: Evoked action potentials and conduction velocity in human sensory nerves. Brain Res., 3:1–122, 1966.
4. Butikofer, R., and Lawrence, P. D.: Electrocutaneous nerve stimulation. 1: Model and experiment. IEEE Trans. Biomed. Engineering, *BME-25*:526–531, No. 6, 1978.
5. Dorfman, L. J., Cummins, K. L., and Leifer, L. J.: Conduction Velocity Distributions. New York, Alan R. Liss, Inc., 1981.
6. Erlanger, J., and Gasser, H. S.: The compound nature of the action current of nerve as disclosed by the cathode ray oscillograph. Am. J. Physiol., 70:624–666, 1924.
7. Gassel, M. M., and Trojaborg, W.: Clinical and electrophysiological study of the pattern of conduction times in the distribution of the sciatic nerve. J. Neurol. Neurosurg. Psychiatry, 27:351–357, 1964.
8. von Haller, A: Elements Physiologiae Corporis Humani. Lausanne, Grasset, 1762, No. 4, p. 596.
9. von Helmholtz, H: Mossungën uber den zeitlichen Verlauf der Zuckung animalischer Muskeln und die Fortpflanzungsgeschwindigkeit der Reizung in den Nerven. Joh. Muller's Arch. Anat. Physiol., 1850, pp. 276–364.
10. Hodgkin, A. L., Huxley, A. F., and Katz, B.: Ionic currents underlying activity in the giant axon of the squid. Arch. Sci. Physiol., 3:129–150, 1949.
11. Jack, J. J. B., Nobel, D., and Tsien, R. W.: Electric Current Flow in Excitable Cells. London, Oxford University Press, 1975, pp. 5–260.

12. Katz, B., and Miledi, R.: Propagation of electric activity in motor nerve terminals. Proc. Roy. Soc., *161*:453–482, 1965.

13. Kline, D. C., and Nulsen, F.E.: The neuroma in continuity. Its preoperative and operative management. Surg. Clin. North Am., *52*:1189–1209, 1972.

14. Lascelles, R. C., and Thomas, P. K.: Changes due to age in internodal length in the sural nerve in man. J. Neurol. Neurosurg. Psychiatry, *20*:40–44, 1966.

15. Ranck, J. B., Jr.: Which elements are excited in electrical stimulation of mammalian central nervous system: a review. Br. Res., *98*:417–440, 1975.

16. Smorto, M. P., and Basmajian, J.V.: Clinical Electroneurography: An Introduction to Nerve Conduction Tests. Baltimore, The Williams & Wilkins Company, 1972.

17. Smorto, N. P., and Basmajian, J.V.: Electrodiagnosis: A Handbook for Neurologists. New York, Harper & Row, 1977.

18. Stein, R. B., Charles, D., Davis, J., Jhamandas, J., Mannard, A., and Nichols, T. R.: Principles underlying new methods for chronic neural recording. J. Can. Sci. Neurol., August, 1975, pp. 235–244.

19. Swallow, M.: Fibre size and content of the anterior tibia nerve of the foot. J. Neurol. Neurosurg. Psychiatry, *29*:205–213, 1966.

20. Terzis, J. K., Dykes, R. W., and Hakstian, R. W.: Electrophysiological recordings in peripheral nerve surgery: a review. J. Hand Surg., *1*:52–66, 1976.

21. Terzis, J. K.: Sensory mappings. Clin. Plast. Surg., *3*:59–64, 1976.

22. Terzis, J. K., and Felker, B.: A computerized study of the intraneural organization of the median nerve. J. Hand Surg. (submitted).

23. Williams, H. B., and Terzis, J. K.: Single fascicular recordings: an intraoperative diagnostic tool for the management of peripheral nerve lesions. Plast. Reconst. Surg., *57*:562–569, 1976.

17

Electrical Assessment of Muscle Denervation
■

Jean Raimbault, M.D.

The primary aim of electrical investigation of a neuromuscular system is to verify the intactness of the system and, in the event of any deficit being discovered, to determine the site of the lesions, their nature, and their extent. In this manner the investigation can confirm and define the diagnosis suggested by the clinical examination and, to a certain degree, can establish a prognosis.

There are two main aspects to electrology:

1. *Electrodiagnosis by stimulation.* This was introduced by the French neurologist Duchenne (1806–1875) and, until World War II, was the only electrical technique of neuromuscular investigation. It involves the visual or tactile assessment of the form and amplitude of the muscle contraction elicited by an electrical current applied to the nerve or directly to the muscle. Electrodiagnosis by stimulation is a purely qualitative method, although at the turn of the century it gained a quantitative element by Lapicque's contribution of chronaximetry.

2. *Electrodiagnosis by detection.* This is represented by electromyography, a relatively recent technique, whose development corresponded to that of electronics: its purpose is to detect and record the electrical activity produced by a muscle during physiologic contraction or in response to an electrical stimulus applied to the nerve or to the muscle bundles. This latter technique will be discussed in this chapter.

MATERIALS AND METHODS

The signals emitted by muscle contraction are detected by means of electrodes, which pick up the differences in potential produced within the muscle and direct them to the amplifiers of the apparatus designed to translate and record them, i.e., the electromyograph. These signals reflect the condition of the muscle and indirectly that of the nerve which supplies it.

Detection Materials

Detection electrodes are always arranged in pairs—one being the active electrode, the other the reference electrode—and are coupled to a third electrode linking the subject to the ground. There are two types of electrodes:

1. *Needle electrodes.* These electrodes are implanted in the muscle bundles themselves and come in the form of narrow-bore hypodermic needles (0.4 to 0.6 mm). The needle lumen contains two insulated conducting wires representing the active and the reference electrodes, with the insulating sheath replacing the ground electrode.

2. *Surface electrodes.* Three surface electrodes are used: the active and reference electrodes, which are applied to the integument covering the muscle body, and the ground electrode, which is applied to another part of the body. These electrodes come in the form of cupulas or small plates of conducting metal and have a relatively wide surface that cannot be less than 25 mm^2.

Needle and surface electrodes cannot be used interchangeably. They have a specific and complementary role in defining muscle activity, and the meanings of the signals they transmit are not identical. Thus, needle electrodes are inserted directly into the middle of the muscle bundles and their bevel edge is in contact with only a few motor units; they pick up localized activity and provide an electromyogram of motor units. In contrast, surface electrodes pick up the sum of muscle activity and provide an electromyogram of overall contraction.

The two modes of detection are not applicable to all muscles or to all individuals. Muscle activity can be detected by surface electrodes only when the muscle is in proximity to these electrodes and is separated from the electrodes by skin and subcutaneous tissue that are not too thick. Even under these conditions, the muscle to be tested must still have a surface area that is large enough to apply the electrodes. Thus, a study that is possible for an adult muscle, even a small one in the hand or foot, is not possible for the same muscle in a newborn child. It is also difficult to gain access to some muscles (e.g., the subscapularis or muscles lying beneath a layer of superficial muscles, such as the posterior tibialis or brachialis). For these reasons, it is preferable to use needle electrodes on a semi-systematic basis. In addition, needle electrodes are often better tolerated and are always more selective than surface electrodes.

Detection Techniques

A healthy muscle at rest shows no detectable activity on electromyography, and all that is seen on the oscilloscope screen is a flat and totally silent tracing. In order to assess the functional quality of such a muscle, it must be investigated while it is contracting. Two methods of achieving this are available:

1. The detection method. This is a physiologic method that records the activity of a muscle undergoing voluntary contraction.

2. The stimulo-detection method. This is a nonphysiologic process that records the muscle response elicited by an electrical stimulus applied either to the nerve at some point along its path or to the motor point of the muscle or else directly to the muscle bundles. After proper application of the electrodes, the *simple detection method* involves obtaining a gradually increasing voluntary contraction, which will be translated onto the electromyograph screen as a natural physiologic activity, the appearance of which varies according

to the force of muscle movement. This method obviously requires total cooperation of the patient. However, this is not always achieved, and voluntary contraction of a particular muscle is often poorly executed despite the patient's best efforts. For the handicapped patient, voluntary muscle contraction can be painful and difficult to control. Investigation is even more difficult in children, particularly the newborn or the very young child, who cannot usually carry out the desired movement on request or do so in a controlled fashion and who may even refuse to cooperate.

The *stimulo-detection method* helps to compensate for the insufficiencies and drawbacks of voluntary contraction method. It is used less often than the simple detection method, and its many advantages are less well known.

Electrical current is applied to the nerve by two stimulation electrodes of opposite polarity, negative cathode and positive anode. For a certain level, known as the threshold intensity, an excitation occurs under the cathode for which the parameters can be precisely determined. In practice, in a healthy subject, this consists of a square wave lasting 0.2 to 1.0 msec, with an intensity varying according to the nerve from 20 to 90 mA and delivered at the rate of one stimulus every 2 seconds. In patients with pathologic disorders, in order to obtain any response from the muscle, it may be necessary to increase the duration of the stimulus up to 5 msec or even longer and to increase the intensity of the current.

Electrical stimulation of a nerve along its length or at the motor point of a muscle is followed after a short interval by a muscle contraction. This is shown on the electromyograph screen as a response that is defined by precise parameters such as *morphology, threshold, duration, amplitude,* and *latency,* all of which are completely independent of the subject's conscious control. The values of these different parameters obviously vary according to the nerve and muscle concerned and also, for the same nerve, according to the distance separating the point of stimulation from its spread through the muscle.

In certain circumstances (to be discussed later), in particular when no further response or no response at all is being obtained by electrical stimulation of the nerve at any point along its path or at the motor point of the muscle, it becomes necessary to test the striated muscle fibers directly to determine the degree and extent to which they are denervated. Such disconnected muscle fibers, which have lost the ability to respond to nerve signals, can no longer be excited except by prolonged and high intensity stimuli. The technique used is known as *direct long pulse stimulation*, which was conceived and perfected approximately 25 years ago by Humbert, but which remained little known for a long time. The method consists of applying a galvanic current to the muscle body through the integument. The current usually lasts at least 50 msec, but, if necessary, can last 100, 150, or even 200 msec by placing the cathode at the farthest point possible from the motor point and placing the anode at the other end. The detection electrode, which is necessarily a needle electrode, is implanted in the middle of the muscle bundles between the two stimulation electrodes, at a point approximately equidistant from both (Fig. 17–1). The cathode-to-anode current runs longitudinally through the muscle fibers, along their entire length, and excites them directly, without requiring the intermediary of a nerve.

However, this technique cannot be used with every kind of electromyograph, but only with those that have a stimulation system that is telecommanded by a long-duration current. This is because such a disproportion exists between the strength of current required to excite the muscle through the skin and subcutaneous tissue and the intensity of the phenomena to be detected (i.e., individual muscle fiber potentials) that the artifact created by stimulation using ordinary equipment reaches a high amplitude. This makes the recording uninterpretable or even drives the spot right off the oscilloscope in some cases. Humbert and his group have developed a device that is now used with most modern electromyographs but that will not be described in detail here. Its basic concept is that of using hertzian waves to telecommand an independently driven stimulator that is insulated from the ground and therefore has no direct or secondary link to the recording apparatus, either via the ground or via the electrical power supply system. The Humbert device reduces the stimulation artifact to two small peaks that are of short duration and of opposite polarities; these

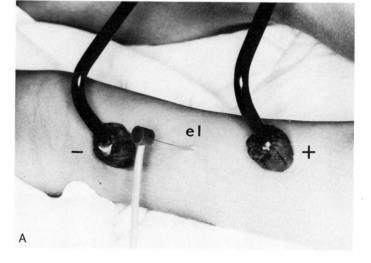

Figure 17–1. *A* and *B*, Technique of eliciting fibrillation in the biceps muscle by direct longitudinal stimulation with a long-acting current. Positioning of stimulatory electrodes and position of needle electrode are shown.

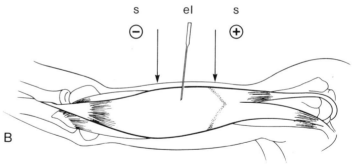

peaks correspond to the switching off and on of the current and thus represent time signals (see Fig. 17–5).

ELECTROMYOGRAPHY OF NORMAL MUSCLE

Before describing the electrical signs of denervated muscle, it may be useful to recall briefly the classic findings of healthy muscle activity.

Simple Detection

Three types of electromyographic patterns can be recorded during gradual voluntary contraction (Fig. 17–2):

1. *Single motor unit potential pattern.* This is provided by contractions of the lowest intensity and represents the rhythmic activity of one or two motor units in the form of individual muscle action potentials, varying in amplitude from 300 μV to 1 mV and standing out from a flat and regular baseline.

2. *Partial interference pattern.* This is caused by a more powerful contraction, character-

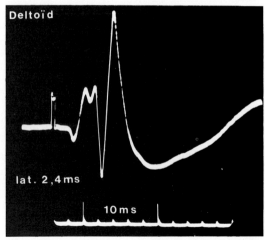

Figure 17–3. Normal response of the deltoid muscle to short (0.5 msec) electrical stimulation of the brachial plexus at Erb's point. (From Raimbault, J.: Clin. Plast. Surg., *11*:54, 1984.)

ized by the deployment of a greater number of motor units and providing action potentials that are closer together but between which a baseline can still be seen.

3. *Interference Pattern.* This results from maximum contraction and consists of densely packed, high-peaked motor unit potentials that obliterate the baseline.

These different patterns help in assessing the morphology, amplitude, duration, and frequency of the muscle action potentials obtained by voluntary contraction. They can be used as standards for comparison with pathologic patterns.

Stimulo-detection

The response of normal muscle to electrical stimulation of its nerve or motor point may be diphasic, triphasic, or sometimes quadriphasic, at least as far as the limb muscles are concerned (Fig. 17–3). The response has an average amplitude of 1 to 2 mV and lasts from 3 to 8 msec.

Of greater interest is the length of the latency period, because it shows only slight variation in normal subjects and also because it is the parameter that is most affected by motor neuron lesions.

The latency of a muscle response is defined by the time that elapses between applying the electrical stimulus to the nerve and the beginning of the muscle response. It is expressed in milliseconds. This response rep-

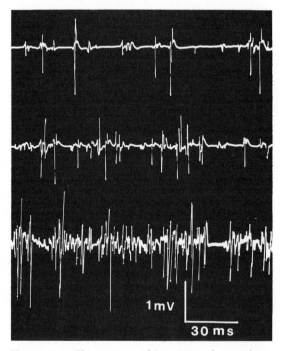

Figure 17–2. Electromyographic activity of normal peripheral muscle of the limbs during progressive voluntary contraction, with the three types of tracing from above downward. (From Raimbault, J.: Clin. Plast. Surg., *11*:54, 1984.)

Table 17–1. LATENCIES OF THE MAIN NERVES IN THE UPPER LIMB

Nerve	Reference Muscle	Site of Stimulation	Latency Period (msec.)		Limits–Values (msec.)
			Mean	*S.D.*	
Axillary	Deltoid	Brachial plexus	2.62	0.35	2.1–3.9
Musculocutaneous	Biceps	Brachial plexus	3.18	0.46	2.3–4.5
Radial	Extensor digitorum	Brachial plexus	5.85	1.22	4.4–8.3
Radial	Extensor digitorum	Sulcus radialis	2.78	1.00	1.8–4.9
Median	Abductor pollicis brevis	Elbow	5.10	0.76	3.2–8.5
Median	Abductor pollicis brevis	Wrist	2.39	0.33	1.3–4.7
Ulnar	Abductor digiti minimi	Elbow	4.81	0.78	3.1–8.4
Ulnar	Abductor digiti minimi	Wrist	2.08	0.35	1.2–4.2

resents the time taken for the nerve signal to be transmitted from the point of excitation to the activated muscle bundles. It is therefore a reflection of the state of nerve conductibility.

The latency of a nerve appears to be remarkably constant for the same muscle when the stimulation point is kept fixed, i.e., always at the same distance from the muscle. It is constant in the same subject and remains at the same level from one subject to another. Furthermore, the latency of a given nerve shows no significant age-related variation, in contrast to observations of nerve conduction speeds, which rise rapidly during the first months of life to reach adult levels only gradually by the age of 10 years. This concept of the stability of nerve latency in healthy subjects is extremely useful for calculating the extent of denervation and monitoring nerve regeneration. As will be discussed, in lesions of peripheral nerves, alterations in the latency period (sometimes of striking proportions) have a high diagnostic value and, to some degree, a prognostic value.

It is thus useful for the clinician to have a normal reference standard available as a basis for the comparison of pathologic lesions. Tables 17–1 and 17–2 give the average latency values for the main nerves of the upper and lower limbs, calculated in normal subjects without breakdown according to age.

ELECTROMYOGRAPHIC SIGNS OF DENERVATION

A preliminary remark is necessary before considering the results of electromyographic investigations in patients with surgical pathology. Not infrequently, there is a discrepancy between the conclusions of the electrologist and those reached by the clinician. The latter, in concluding his examination of a patient with a peripheral nerve lesion, may note that a given muscle was incapable of voluntary contraction and therefore was considered totally paralyzed, whereas the electrologist, using a needle electrode implanted in the muscle body, may obtain a response

Table 17–2. LATENCIES OF THE MAIN NERVES IN THE LOWER LIMB

Nerve	Reference Muscle	Site of Stimulation	Latency Period (msec.)		Limits–Values (msec.)
			Mean	*S.D.*	
Femoralis	Rectus femoris	Ligamentum unguinale	3.00	0.57	1.3–4.4
Obturatorius	Gracilis	Canalis obturatorius	2.64	0.42	2.0–3.56
Peroneus communis	Extensor digitorum brevis	Caput fibulae	6.92	1.84	4.1–13.0
Peroneus profundus	Extensor digitorum brevis	Articulatio talocruralis	3.38	1.22	1.6–7.2
Tibialis	Flexor hallucis brevis	Fossa poplitea	8.03	2.12	4.6–15.7
Tibialis	Flexor hallucis brevis	Sulcus malleolaris	3.98	0.95	2.0–9.9

to electrical stimulation of the motor neuron that is often quite considerable. The explanation for this discrepancy is that the electrode has picked up some motor units in an apparently inert muscle that are still active and able to respond to excitation of the nerve, but that are too few overall to alter the dimensions of the muscle.

The opposite situation may also occur. The clinician perceives muscle that is still capable of some movement, whereas the electrologist fails to detect any activity or any response to nerve stimulation because the tip of his electrode is not in contact with active motor units and is lying in an inert zone of muscle.

Such discrepancies occur particularly in longstanding neuromuscular deficiency states, in which the patient loses his ability to use one particular muscle and uses another more appropriate one instead. Awareness of such a situation allows the investigator to perform a painstaking exploration of several areas of any muscle that fails to show electrical activity at the outset, since his ability to show evidence of muscle bundles that are still active in an apparently inert muscle has great importance for decisions to be made by the surgeon.

Total Denervation

A muscle that is completely denervated can no longer be activated voluntarily and has no response to electrical stimulation of its nerve. However, the muscle fibers continue to live for some time (several weeks to several years) if their nutritional requirements are maintained by an adequate blood supply. During this period they are the site of a special activity, termed *fibrillation*, which has great diagnostic and prognostic importance. Fibrillation is a potential from an individual muscle fiber that has become self- and hyperexcitatory because it is no longer governed by the motor neuron and is therefore no longer synchronized with its neighboring fibers in the motor unit. Under these special circumstances, the resting muscle, which normally is electrically silent, becomes the site of spontaneous activity.

Fibrillatory activity appears after a time interval that varies according to the specific muscle. It is longer for limb muscles than for muscles of the face, but generally first appears more than 2 weeks after the nerve lesion. Its distinguishing features are single, biphasic, very short action potentials that do not exceed 2 msec, are of low amplitude (always less than 200 μV), and occur rhythmically at a low frequency, approximately 1 to 10 beats/second (Fig. 17–4). Fibrillation is most often associated with axon degeneration.

However, fibrillatory activity remains a relatively rare and temporary phenomenon. It is not easy to detect, even when care has been taken to warm the muscle body, and it is difficult to demonstrate in the young child. For these reasons, while the presence of fibrillatory activity in a muscle is evidence of motor unit desynchronization, its absence cannot be taken as conclusive proof of muscle intactness.

The technique of longitudinal direct stimulation with a long-duration current is used in this situation, since it makes detection of denervated muscle fiber activity much easier by eliciting the autoexcitability and desynchronization of the fibers electrically. The recording obtained is that of *elicited fibrilla-*

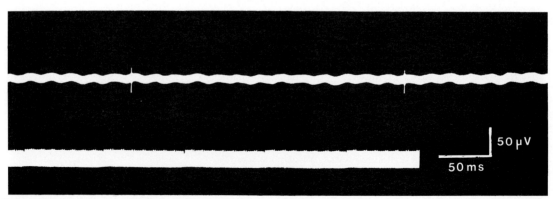

Figure 17–4. Spontaneous fibrillation of resting deltoid muscle after traumatic avulsion of the brachial plexus: two distinct fiber potentials can be seen. (From Raimbault, J.: Clin. Plast Surg., *11*:56, 1984.)

tions, in contrast to spontaneous fibrillatory activity. By placing the stimulation electrodes directly on the muscle under investigation (according to the method detailed earlier) and starting at a certain threshold that is always very low, fiber potentials are obtained at the end of the stimulation artifact and may even be found after the electrical current has been turned on. Increasing the stimulus intensity causes an increase in the frequency and amplitude of these potentials until they invade the greater part of the artifact (Fig. 17–5).

Individually observed potentials from elicited fibrillation have many of the same features as those from fibrillatory activity. They occur only after the same time interval of 2 weeks and they are very short and of low voltage; however, they are much more plentiful, bunched up, and out of rhythm, since they no longer correspond to a single depolarized fiber but to a group of depolarized fibers. In fact, this is why the elicited fibrillation method for diagnosing denervation is much more reliable than looking for fibrilla-

tory activity. The results of elicited fibrillation are positive in virtually all patients with nerve lesions.

Demonstrating fibrillatory activity by whatever method in a denervated muscle is of cardinal importance for prognosis. In the absence of any voluntary activity or response to electrical stimulation of the nerve, i.e., given a muscle that is physiologically unexcitable, such a demonstration shows that the muscle fibers are still alive and that consequently they are, in principle, able to be reinnervated.

A muscle that is no longer stimulated must undergo atrophy, and the fibrillatory activity will eventually die down. However, such activity will persist for much longer (in fact for more than 1 year) if the muscle is made to work mechanically by physiotherapy or electrotherapy.

Partial Denervation

A muscle that remains linked to its nerve, even by a limited number of nerve fibers, remains capable of a degree of activity and continues to respond to electrical stimulation of the nerve trunk. Obviously these possibilities vary according to the extent of the nerve lesions, and every degree of activity can be seen, from activity that is limited to a few action potentials and a minimum response to reactions that are almost those of normal muscle. Whatever the case, a certain number of electromyographic signs make possible a reasonably precise assessment of the extent of the neuromuscular deficit.

In the days following the nerve lesion, *voluntary contraction* shows poor activity. Contraction is of lower voltage than that of normal muscle and is generally quite different from the standard pattern; i.e., a maximum contraction effort results in only a single motor unit potential pattern, occasionally causes a partial interference pattern, but has no interference pattern. However, a number of denervated muscle fibers are quickly taken over by healthy motor neurons, which considerably increases their motor unit territory—by 100% or more. The electrical activity of voluntary contraction alters very rapidly and gives rise to what is known as "neurogenic" activity, consisting of large, high amplitude potentials, separated from one another and running at a rhythm of 20 to 30

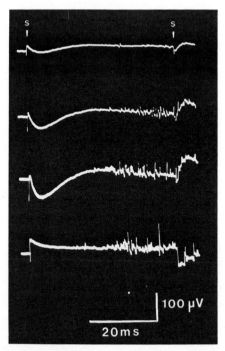

Figure 17–5. Fibrillation elicited by direct galvanic stimulation of the muscle body (flexor pollicis brevis after accidental division of the median nerve). From top to bottom there is a gradual increase in the density and amplitude of the fiber potentials, matching the increase in strength of the electrical current. The arrowheads on the upper recording mark the beginning and end of the stimulation artifact (50 msec), i.e., the switching off and on of the current.

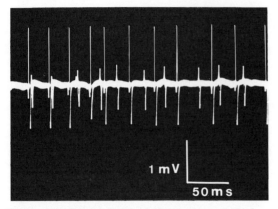

Figure 17–6. Fixed and chronic neurogenic activity during voluntary contraction in long-standing muscle atrophy. Note the simplified pattern of the action potentials and their great amplitude (2.5 mV) and regular rhythm. (From Raimbault, J.: Clin. Plast. Surg., *11*:56, 1984.)

cps or more rapidly, depending on the number of reconstituted motor units.

At this stage, electromyographic follow-up should be performed regularly to monitor the course of the muscle deficit. If the atrophy becomes chronic, neurogenic activity becomes definitive and replaces all other forms of activity by giving an uninterrupted succession of individual, highly simplified, large potentials, biphasic in form, of high voltage, and running at a particularly regular and unchanging rhythm (Fig. 17–6). If, however, neuromuscular regeneration takes place, the neurogenic potentials multiply and take on a particular polyphasic morphologic appearance, which represents gradual muscle fiber reinnervation (Fig. 17–7).

However, no matter what the extent and course of muscle atrophy observed clinically, it is always most important to look for fibril-

lation at this stage. This allows the presence of individual muscle fibers to be detected, i.e., fibers not involved by axon regeneration, and thus makes possible a more or less long-term prognosis. Several eventualities are possible:

1. A neurogenic-like activity may be present that already has a simpler appearance, a high amplitude, and a rhythm that does not seem to alter. If fibrillation is still occurring, nerve regeneration is not complete. If, however, no individual fiber potential can be demonstrated, the atrophy is chronic and becomes irreversible.

2. Electromyographic activity may be present that is normal in appearance and relatively plentiful, but remains intermediary in type. The absence of fibrillation means that rupture of nerve fibers is not likely to have occurred, but rather that simple contusion (neurapraxia) took place with the integrity of axon continuity maintained. Demonstration of fibrillation, on the other hand, often indicates a break in axon continuity (axonotmesis).

Nerve trunk stimulation also provides valuable information about the degree, extent, and nature of a nerve lesion. However, it should be emphasized that during the first days after trauma, electrical stimulation of the distal part of the nerve, i.e., beyond the lesion, always gives a near-normal response. This is because even when a nerve is completely divided, there is a certain time lapse before the signs of degeneration occur in the divided axons. Most physiologists agree that histologic changes begin to be seen about 12 hours after division of the nerve and that the conducting properties of nerve fibers alter by 24 hours and disappear completely after 3 days. Electrical examination of the neuro-

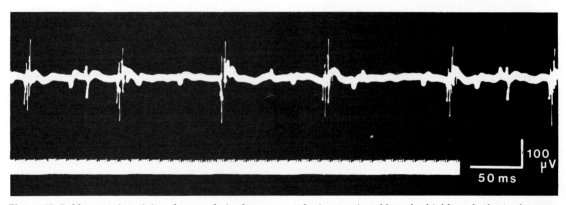

Figure 17–7. Neurogenic activity of a muscle in the process of reinnervation. Note the highly polyphasic character of the action potentials. (From Raimbault, J.: Clin. Plast. Surg., *11*:57, 1984.)

muscular system should therefore not be carried out too soon after the trauma, i.e., not before at least 3 days have elapsed.

If partial denervation occurs, electrical stimulation of the nerve trunk proximal to the lesion always evokes a muscle response, the pattern and levels of which obviously vary with the degree of the deficit:

1. If the nerve lesion is considerable and thus transmission of the impulse occurs only via the intermediary of a small number of intact fibers, the muscle response is highly simplified, monophasic, and low in amplitude, often being less than 100 μV (Fig. 17–8).

2. If the nerve lesion is benign and only a few axons have been divided, the muscle response preserves a near-normal pattern, but demonstration of fibrillation by direct galvanic stimulation betrays the presence of degenerating motor units.

3. If the nerve lesion is fairly extensive but irregular and associated with different and unequal alterations in the axons, the response to nerve stimulation appears polyphasic (often extremely so). The nerve fibers transmitting the impulse at naturally differing speeds do not respond in unison, and this series of gaps causes a prolongation of the muscle response.

In these different eventualities, there is always one parameter that is altered to a greater or lesser degree—the length of the latency period. When a nerve is injured, its latency period is always increased (sometimes considerably so) as a result of difficulties in the transmission of the nerve impulse.

A polyphasic muscle response and a lengthening of the latency period are two important factors in diagnosis and prognosis. Together they provide an assessment of neuromuscular deficit and a means of following its course.

THE MONITORING OF REINNERVATION

Nerve regneration is expressed differently according to the type of original lesion. As a basis for our description, the type of gradual regeneration that occurs after surgical repair by neurotization or graft for complete division of a nerve will be discussed.

The signs of reinnervation detectable by the stimulo-detection method usually precede those evidenced by simple detection, although this is not an absolute rule.

Using the technique of electrical nerve stimulation, it can be seen that electromyographic recuperation takes place in several stages. During the first stage, after several weeks' or months' silence, a highly simplified, monophasic, and low amplitude response occurs (Fig. 17–8) with a markedly long latency period, sometimes as long as 20 msec. This response corresponds to the regeneration of a minimum number of nerve fibers.

In the next stage, which can occur at almost any time from the first stage, depending on the particular cases, "perfectioning" of the response occurs: it becomes polyphasic, sometimes extremely so (Fig. 17–9A and B), and is spread over 10 to 15 msec or even longer. It increases gradually in amplitude, but the latency period remains lengthened for a long time. The polyphasic pattern is an important sign heralding the process of reinnervation; it corresponds to the taking over of multiple muscle fibers by nerve fibers with differing conduction speeds. As repair takes place, there is a gradual reduction in polyphasic pattern and in the length of the latency period until they reach normal levels, while attempts to demonstrate fibrillation are negative.

Once the pattern and latency of the response have returned to normal, the process of muscle reinnervation can be considered complete. This does not mean, however, that the damaged nerve has totally recovered; the number of axons that have regrown can be less than the total number of axons in the normal nerve. This accounts for the discrepancies that are sometimes observed between

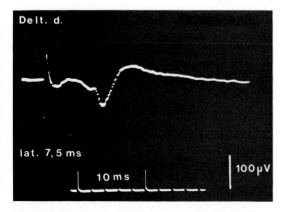

Figure 17–8. Very simplified monophasic muscle response at the stage of the onset of reinnervation.

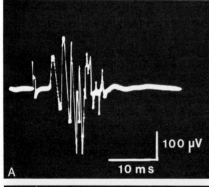

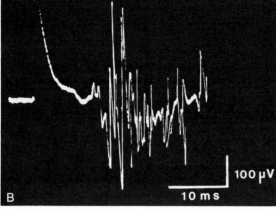

Figure 17–9. *A* and *B*, Muscles at different stages of reinnervation. Nerve responses to brief stimulation are shown. Note the highly polyphasic nature and lengthening of the latency period.

the results of electromyography and the functional power of the reinnervated muscle. It also explains what is often noted during the examination of a patient with an untreated longstanding nerve lesion; i.e., the nerve fibers that have spontaneously regenerated give muscle responses to the needle electrode that are near normal in pattern and latency, whereas the actual muscle being tested may have remained functionally almost completely impotent.

Approximately the same electromyographic signs are observed after spontaneous reinnervation as after surgical repair. In the case of simple nerve contusion, the successive stages of regeneration take place at an accelerated rate, and the first of these stages is so short that it may well pass unnoticed if there is a sufficient gap between electromyographic examinations.

Simple detection electromyography also shows signs of nerve regeneration in the form of large neurogenic potentials. These are also polyphasic, separate from one another, rhythmical, and high in amplitude (see Fig. 17–7). Their number and density gradually increase up to a certain level that corre-sponds to the degree of functional recuperation. However, the data from simple detection are less precise than those obtained by stimulo-detection.

CONCLUSIONS

Electromyography provides the clinician with two techniques, simple detection and stimulo-detection. The advantage of stimulo-detection is that it is essentially objective:

1. It makes precision testing of the nerve-muscle complex possible by studying the parameters of duration, amplitude, and latency in the muscle response.

2. It also allows direct testing at the level of the striated muscle fibers by the technique of longitudinal stimulation by long-acting current, demonstrating the denervated fibers that have become self-excitatory.

When summarizing the results of the clinical investigation of the lesions and when an apparently inert muscle is being examined, demonstration of muscle fibrillation provides proof of a nerve lesion. It is also evidence of the continuing vitality of the desynchronized muscle fibers, suggesting that these fibers are, in principle, in a suitable state for reinnervation.

Later, when monitoring the course of a neuromuscular deficit and nerve regeneration, the aim of repeated follow-up investigations is to track the two factors that are essential for the prognosis—the pattern and latency of the muscle response:

1. A polyphasic pattern to the response is a sign of muscle reinnervation that should normally progress toward gradual simplification until it reaches the classic pattern of a normal response.

2. Similarly, the latency period, which at the outset is greatly increased, should gradually fall toward normal levels, and this is a sign of progress toward the return of normal functional activity.

In some cases, however, in particular those patients with longstanding and stable neuromuscular deficits, there may be discrepancies between the electromyographic results and the degree of clinical recovery. Such discrepancies underscore the need for regular follow-up and early treatment of any nerve lesion.

References

1. Dumoulin, J.: La Stimulo-Détection par Courants de Longue Durée: Etude Clinique et Expérimentale. Paris, Maloine, 1963, p. 248.
2. Humbert, R.: La Stimulo-détection. Actualités Neurophysiologiques. Paris, Masson, 1963.
3. Humbert, R.: L'électrodiagnostic de stimulo-détection. J. Radiol. Electrol., 45:89–93, 1964.
4. Humbert, R., Dehouve, A., and Laget, P.: Recherche sur l'électromyogramme du muscle sain et pathologique de l'homme stimulé électriquement. Rev. Neurol., 95:473–478, 1956.
5. Raimbault, J.: Contribution of clinical neurophysiology in the studies of lesions and regeneration of peripheral nerves. Int. J. Microsurg., 3:161–169, 1981.
6. Raimbault, J.: Les conductions nerveuses chez l'enfant normal. Etude électromyographique (in press).

18

Nerve Grafting

∎

Hanno Millesi, M.D.

In the 1870s Philipeaux and Vulpian[58] reported on experiments in which they grafted a segment of the lingual nerve between the two stumps of the transected hypoglossal nerve. In 1876 Albert[6] bridged defects in human peripheral nerves by nerve grafts. Already in this very early phase of peripheral nerve surgery the role of tension at the suture site was recognized. Nerve grafting seemed to be an acceptable solution to managing peripheral nerve defects. However, with the clinical use of nerve grafts many problems arose that prevented nerve grafting from becoming a standard procedure.

WHAT TO EXPECT FROM A WELL-FUNCTIONING NERVE GRAFT

A nerve graft bridges the defect between the two stumps of a transected peripheral nerve. Since the nerve fibers within the nerve graft undergo Wallerian degeneration, the graft serves as a guiding structure to allow axon sprouts to grow from the proximal stump along the graft into the distal stump. The degree and quality of neurotization of the graft are two of the conditions necessary for useful regeneration across the graft. The fact that the graft serves only as a guiding structure led to the belief that surviving neural structures are not important for this function. Although it is true that a graft serves only as a guiding structure, there is a difference if the graft helps to guide the direction of the axon sprouts or if it serves to guide a neuroma that is proceeding along the graft. Consequently, we can distinguish two types of neurotization of a graft:

1. Neurotization of the graft by axon sprouts from the proximal stump occurs in the same way as a distal stump is neurotized in an end-to-end neurorrhaphy. The axon sprouts cross the gap between the proximal stump and the proximal end of the graft. They meet Schwann cells in the graft and neurotize the graft as they would do with the distal stump of a peripheral nerve after neurorrhaphy. They then cross the gap between the distal end of the graft and the distal stump and neurotize the distal stump in the same way as they would after neurorrhaphy. In this case the nerve graft is equivalent to a distal peripheral nerve stump. It serves as a guiding structure for axons.

2. If the nerve graft does not contain Schwann cells, the axon sprouts cannot proceed easily along the graft. They have to bring their own Schwann cells with them in the form of mini-fascicles. A neuroma is then formed, which proceeds slowly along the graft. If it reaches the distal stump, neurotization of this stump is possible. Schröder and Seiffert[62] called this type of neurotization "neuromatöse Neurotisation." In this case the nerve graft serves as a guiding structure for a neuroma. This form of neurotization occurs if the nerve graft did not function well, if it became fibrotic, or if it consisted of a preserved, cell-free allograft.

For neurotization to be successful, the following conditions should be fulfilled:

1. Complete survival of the connective tissue framework of the nerve graft must take place without necrosis.

2. There should be no fibrosis within the nerve graft. Fibrosis occurs if areas, especially the central part of a thick nerve graft, suffer ischemic damage.

3. Wallerian degeneration should proceed in the graft in the same way as in a distal stump after transection.

4. Only if the Schwann cells survive within the endoneurial tubes (as they do in a distal stump) is the graft able to serve as a guiding structure for axons and to function like a distal stump after transection. For a long time the survival of Schwann cells following transplantation was questioned. We were quite sure that Schwann cells survive a successful grafting procedure, but final proof of this was provided only by the elegant experiments of Aguayo et al.[2-4] using the Trembler mouse. The Schwann cells of the Trembler mouse are not able to produce myelin. In a nerve graft from a normal mouse to an immunosuppressed Trembler mouse the Schwann cells from the normal mouse produce normal myelin sheaths within the graft. This means that the normal Schwann cells had survived grafting. In the reversed experiments, the Schwann cells of a graft from the Trembler mouse do not produce a myelin sheath after being grafted into a peripheral nerve defect of a normal mouse. This means again the Trembler mouse Schwann cells had survived grafting.

PROBLEMS CONNECTED WITH NERVE GRAFTING

Graft Survival and Revascularization of the Graft

Revascularization occurs by spontaneous anastomosis of small vessels of the recipient bed with small vessels of the graft or by ingrowth of vessels from the recipient site into the graft. Circulation has to be re-established before the cells of the graft suffer ischemic damage. It is reasonable to assume that the cells in the center of a graft are exposed to ischemia longer than are cells in the periphery. Consequently, a thin graft has a better chance of full survival because of the favorable relationship between its surface and its diameter. A thick graft has a relatively small surface in relation to its diameter, and revascularization therefore takes a longer time to reach the center.

Based on these considerations, Foerster[31] utilized cutaneous nerve grafts as free grafts to bridge defects in peripheral nerves. Bielschowsky and Unger[13] performed experiments that proved that fibrosis developed in

the center of a thick nerve trunk after free grafting. In contrast, cutaneous nerve grafts survive without fibrosis. Single cutaneous nerve grafts have been used successfully by Ballance and Duel,[10] Bunnell,[22] and Bunnell and Boyes.[23]

To ensure graft survival, Strange[72] developed the technique of pedicled nerve grafting. This technique was used to some degree by Brooks[18] and others, but it never really did become popular. The most elegant way to ensure full graft survival is re-establishing circulation by microvascular anastomosis, as suggested by Taylor and Ham[75] in 1976. The value of this technique for graft survival is unquestioned if the microvascular anastomoses remain open. However, whether this way of grafting, with the possibility of reducing ischemia to a minimum, facilitates the quality and rapidity of neurotization is still unproved.[34, 35]

Pre-Degeneration

To facilitate neurotization of a nerve graft, use of pre-degenerated nerve grafts has been suggested. It was assumed that if Wallerian degeneration has already occurred within the nerve graft before actual grafting, neurotization might be enhanced. To test this theory, prospective nerve grafts were transected 3 weeks before the grafting procedure. Use of pre-degenerated nerve grafts was studied by different authors, but the results of experimental investigations were contradictory and significant advantage of pre-degeneration could not be proved. Our own experiments[50, 52] demonstrated a quick neurotization of fresh nerve grafts without any impairment by the simultaneously ongoing Wallerian degeneration.

Intraneural Structure of a Graft

At first glance it would seem ideal if a defect in a median nerve at a certain level could be bridged by a graft derived from exactly the same level of another median nerve. The graft would be similar in diameter and correspond well to the lost segment. However, based on our knowledge of intraneural topography, we have to conclude that corresponding median nerve segments of different individuals do *not* correspond in intraneural structure. Even if we could provide a nerve graft at exactly the same level from another individual and use it as an allograft to bridge a defect in the median nerve, we could not be sure that the corresponding fascicles were united. Because of the changing fascicular pattern, the possibility that nerve fibers of a specific type from the proximal stump would meet fascicles having a corresponding function in the distal stump would be a random occurrence.

If we are able to define the distribution of nerve fibers having a certain function in the proximal and distal stumps, it is better to unite these areas directly by cutaneous nerve grafts because we know exactly which fascicle groups we are connecting. If a trunk graft is used, the intraneural structure of the graft determines the pathway of nerve fibers that enter the graft in a certain location of the proximal cross section and leave the graft at the peripheral end. Therefore, which fascicle groups are actually united occurs at random.

Caliber Difference

Each peripheral nerve contains a certain number of nerve fibers. When bridging a defect between two nerve stumps, a nerve graft (or nerve grafts) consisting of a similar number of endoneurial tubes is attempted.

In the early phases of nerve grafting, surgeons did not pay much attention to the intraneural structures. A nerve graft of the same caliber as the two nerve stumps to be repaired, i.e., a trunk graft, was regarded as ideal. However, such a graft is not available for routine clinical use because sacrificing a well-functioning peripheral nerve in order to use it as a graft is not justified. Nerve trunks without function are available for use as trunk grafts only if the patient has had an amputation of an upper or lower extremity. If two parallel running peripheral nerves were defective, using one of them as a graft donor to repair the more important one was suggested. This principle was applied by Strange[72, 73] to repair the median nerve by a pedicled nerve graft derived from the ulnar nerve. It is evident that a lack of a graft donor of the same caliber as the nerve to be repaired was one of the reasons for the attempts to use allografts.

Another attempt to solve the problem of the caliber difference was the development of the so-called cable graft. Several cutaneous nerves were packed together by stitches[63, 64]

or by fibrin.[82] Successful use of the cable graft was reported by Seddon[63, 64] and Brooks.[18] In this technique a trunk graft is simulated by the use of several nerve grafts. However, the survival of the cutaneous nerve grafts is endangered by this method because each nerve graft is in contact with another graft and a part of its surface is not in contact with the recipient bed. As no efforts were made to unite corresponding fascicles or fascicle groups, these cable grafts shared the disadvantages of trunk grafts as far as the problem of intraneural structure was concerned. In fact, the cable grafts never did become very popular and were abandoned in the 1960s. (If the reports of Seddon[63–66] over the years are analyzed, it can be noted that cable grafts were no longer performed after 1963.)

Many surgeons apply the term cable graft in a more general way to mean all cases in which cutaneous nerve grafts were utilized. To avoid misunderstanding, the term cable graft should be restricted to its original meaning, i.e., the formation of a graft of the same caliber of the nerve to be repaired by combining several cutaneous nerves (cables).

The alternative to using a trunk graft or a cable graft of the same caliber as the nerve to be repaired is preparing the two stumps by interfascicular dissection and splitting the stumps into minor units that have a caliber similar to the caliber of the grafts.[49] Use of this technique means that large fascicles, having a caliber similar to the cutaneous nerve grafts, are isolated and united individually by one segment of a cutaneous nerve graft (i.e., fascicular nerve grafting) or that groups of fascicles of a size similar to the cutaneous nerve grafts are united by one segment of a cutaneous nerve (i.e., interfascicular or fascicular group nerve grafting). Theoretically it is possible to isolate all the fascicles, even in a polyfascicular nerve consisting of many small fascicles, and to attempt to unite these small fascicles by individual nerve grafting (i.e., fascicular nerve grafting of small fascicles, using single fascicles as grafts). However, this implies splitting of a cutaneous nerve graft into minor units of the same size as the small fascicles. Such a technique was suggested by Tupper.[77] In the case of a polyfascicular nerve stump without group arrangement in which interfascicular dissection is not advisable, the sectors of a cross section of the nerve stumps are defined and united by individual nerve grafts (i.e., sectoral nerve grafting). The point to emphasize is that in all these cases the segments of cutaneous nerves that are used as grafts are applied individually without major contact with each other along their course and have optimal contact with the recipient site (for details see Chapter 1).

The number of nerve fibers that can be reconstituted by all grafts after neurotization presents no problems if the defect to be bridged is not too large. Many segments of cutaneous nerve grafts can be used in order to achieve an optimal covering of the fascicles of the two stumps. Problems do arise in very long defects because even by utilizing all available donor nerves it might not be possible to apply a sufficient number of grafts. In this situation, allografts, as well as autografts, would be desirable.

Length of the Graft

In the past surgeons used all available means to make a defect as short as possible (flexion of adjacent joints, vast mobilization, transposition) and applied nerve grafts to bridge the remaining defect. It was thought that the graft should be as short as possible, and this view seemed to be supported by published figures showing the degree of recovery in relation to the length of the grafts. Geldmacher and Albers[33] reported that the functional result decreases with the length of the graft. This, of course, is true, but a long graft was used mainly because the nerve tissue defect was also long. There is good evidence that the length of the *defect* of a peripheral nerve is the decisive factor rather than the length of the nerve grafts. It is our experience that the result following repair of a given defect is not influenced by the length of the graft. To the contrary, if a longer graft is used to bridge a given defect of a peripheral nerve without tension at the two sites of coaptation, the result is better than if a given defect is bridged by a rather short graft with tension at the sites of coaptation (for details see Chapter 1).

Two Suture Sites

The great disadvantage of any grafting procedure is the fact that the axon sprouts have to cross two sites of coaptation. For this reason a graft, by definition, has to be inferior to an end-to-end neurorrhaphy performed under similar conditions. However, with an increasing defect the problems in achieving an end-to-end neurorrhaphy become more significant, and the conditions for axon sprouts crossing the one site of coaptation become more unfavorable. By utilizing a sufficiently long nerve graft, the two coaptations can be performed under ideal conditions, offering optimal chances for functional recovery of a graft on either an upper or a lower extremity. Beyond a certain point the chances of functional recovery become better for a graft than for a neurorrhaphy under tension. However, there is still a possibility that scar tissue had already formed at the distal site of coaptation by the time the axon sprouts reached this site. Stookey,[71] Lewis,[42] Bsteh and Millesi,[20] and others suggested resecting the distal site of coaptation if the advancement of the axon sprouts was stopped at this level and performing another end-to-end coaptation between the distal end of the graft and the distal stump. In the past, when using classic techniques of nerve grafting, this procedure was necessary in all our grafts measuring over 3 cm in length.

With the use of microsurgical grafting techniques,[49, 50, 52, 53] the need to do something to avoid a block at the distal site of coaptation decreased significantly. A block at the distal site of coaptation occurred only in 7 (14%) of the first 50 patients with interfascicular nerve grafts. With increasing experience, the number dropped to 1 to 2%. However, even with this low percentage, we should not neglect the possibility of a block at the distal suture site. The surgeon has to follow his patients and make sure that regeneration advances beyond the distal site of coaptation. One gets some idea about neurotization of the graft and the distal stump by observing advancement of the Tinel-Hoffmann sign. If the Tinel-Hoffmann sign stops at the distal site of coaptation for a period of 2 or 3 months, surgical exploration should be considered. Bosse[16, 17] suggested planning nerve grafting as a two-stage procedure. In the first stage, the nerve graft is transplanted and connected only with the proximal stump. In the second stage, if the nerve graft has already become neurotized, the connection between the distal end of the graft and the distal stump is carried out. This principle had already been used successfully by other surgeons for cross-face grafting in order to perform a nerve transfer between the normal and the paralyzed facial nerve.[8] Since our records show that problems at the distal site of coaptation occur in only a low percentage of cases, we still prefer to perform nerve grafting in one stage. In addition, this offers a better chance to unite the corresponding fascicles, fascicle groups, or sectors because the two coaptations are performed at the same time.

Availability of Donor Grafts

If the patient has suffered an amputation, several nerve trunks are available as donor grafts. They can be used as vascularized nerve grafts or split in a longitudinal direction to be divided into smaller units with a smaller diameter and utilized as free grafts.

In cases of brachial plexus lesions with avulsion of roots C8 and T1, the ulnar nerve will be used as a vascularized nerve graft or may be split in a longitudinal direction and its components used as free grafts. In all other cases trunk grafts are not available, and in no instance is sacrifice of a functioning nerve trunk ever justified.

In the vast majority of cases only cutaneous nerve grafts are available as donor grafts. According to my experience a sural nerve is the first choice as a donor graft. The nerve is easily accessible, has a long course without branches, consists of one or a limited number of fascicles in its proximal portion, and becomes a polyfascicular nerve in its distal portion. Thus, one can select the proper segment according to the fascicle groups to be united. The nerve can be harvested easily by a small number of transverse incisions along its course. By applying atraumatic techniques, damage to the nerve can be prevented. Brunelli[19] believes that excision of the nerve under direct vision, utilizing a long skin incision along the course of the nerve, is preferable in order to reduce eventual surgical trauma. This technique can be recommended for all surgeons who are not familiar with atraumatic techniques. In about 10% of cases the sural nerve develops from two sources, one coming from the tibial and the other from the peroneal nerve. This is easily recognized by palpation of the nerve along its course after the distal segment behind the lateral malleolus is exposed and traction is exerted. If a nerve stripper is used, one of the sources may be destroyed; therefore, we do not recommend use of this instrument.

Another nerve that can be used for grafting is the lateral femorocutaneous nerve, which is located underneath the anterior iliac spine. The nerve leaves the pelvis at this point underneath the inguinal ligament and lies underneath the fascia. A nerve graft of about 20 cm may be obtained. The lateral femorocutaneous nerve divides into two branches and, if only a thin nerve graft is needed, one of the two branches may be selected. The nerve can be followed across the abdominal wall into the pelvis and transected at this level in order to have the proximal stump disappear within the pelvis. At this length the nerve is a suitable donor graft for treatment of a painful neuroma.

The saphenous nerve may be used successfully, but we do not recommend the simultaneous excision of the saphenous and the sural nerve in the same extremity.

The medial antebrachial nerve is a very good donor nerve and may provide a graft of about 30 cm in length. It can also be excised by several transverse incisions. Its distal half is divided into two branches. This nerve should not be used if the ulnar nerve of the same extremity has a lesion because of a certain overlapping of these two nerves. Branches of the medial antebrachial nerve in the forearm are suitable donors to repair defects of very thin nerves, such as the palmar branch of the median nerve for treatment of a painful neuroma.

The lateral antebrachial nerve, which is derived from the radial nerve, is also an excellent donor nerve. We do not recommend its use simultaneously with the medial cutaneous nerve.

The superficial branch of the radial nerve was used occasionally as a donor graft, especially in brachial plexus lesions, when many nerve grafts were required. This nerve may also be used as a vascularized nerve graft. Because of its small diameter, it cannot bridge a defect of a nerve trunk without additional use of free grafts.

Intercostal nerves have been recommended as free grafts with the provision that they contain motor fibers and may therefore be more suitable for reconstruction of mixed nerve trunks. However, clinical experience demonstrates that satisfactory motor recovery can be achieved by the use of cutaneous nerve grafts, which contain only sensory fibers. I therefore do not believe that nerve grafts using motor nerves give significantly better results. The intercostal nerves have a great disadvantage in that they have many branches that innervate the intercostal muscles along their course; thus, many fibers are lost if these nerves are used as grafts.

To avoid loss of axon sprouts by free-ending branches of nerve grafts, using the nerve grafts in a reversed way was recommended. Since the nerve grafts have to be neurotized from the proximal stump, it is not necessary to place the nerve grafts into the defect in an orthodromic direction. The grafts are neurotized just as well if they are applied in a reversed way. If nerve grafts with minimal branching are used, this problem is unimportant.

Any nerve trunk may be used as a vascularized nerve graft after studying its segmental blood supply. Reports are available about the use of the peroneal nerve and the median and ulnar nerves. In addition, the superficial branch of the radial nerve has been used as a vascularized nerve graft, and techniques have been developed to utilize the sural nerve in this way as well.[29, 76]

Autografts

Everything that has been said thus far about graft survival, neurotization, etc. refers to autografts, which are not exposed to immunologic problems. To date, autografts have proved to be the only reliable source of nerve grafts. With a few exceptions, autografting can meet all clinical requirements in a satisfactory way.

Allografts

Some surgeons have attempted to use allografts for nerve grafting. To my knowledge, Albert[6] was the first to report on allografting in human patients in 1878.

The use of allografts would avoid a second site of operation in order to harvest the graft. Any functional loss could be prevented and grafts would be available in unlimited quantities. Corresponding segments of peripheral nerves could be used, which, of course, is not possible with autografts. This last advantage, however, did not prove too important (at least for peripheral portions of peripheral nerves) in light of the knowledge of intraneural topography and the changing fascicular pattern (see earlier discussion).

The use of isografts (between identical twins) is without complications, but allografts between immunologically different individuals do cause problems. Two basically different allograft types have to be distinguished: (1) living allografts, and (2) the stroma of allografts without living cells.

Living Allografts. At the time of grafting, living allografts behave like autografts. Wallerian degeneration occurs, and axon sprouts cross the proximal side of the coaptation and commence to neurotize the graft. The axon sprouts come in contact with living Schwann cells, as in an autograft or a distal stump. After a certain period of time, an allograft reaction occurs, and the graft becomes more or less replaced by fibrous tissue.[11, 14, 27, 43, 57, 67, 70]

Das Gupta[26] and Edidin[28] held the view that antibody formation is mainly caused by the myelin of the allograft. Levinthal et al.[40, 41] observed a strong reaction against the epineurium but no reaction or a much diminished response against isolated fascicles. They believed that the epineurium was the main factor for antibody formation.

Nigst[56] used cortisone medication to retard the rejection of nerve grafts in rabbits in the hope that the allograft reaction would occur only after the graft had been neurotized. Attempts to prevent cellular allograft reaction by immunosuppressive treatment were not successful.[25, 47, 59, 78]

Mackinnon et al.[44] investigated the cellular and humoral response to peripheral nerve allografting. By using the ^{51}Cr release test, Bainbridge et al.[12] and Rotstein et al.[61] determined that the humoral response could be quantitated. The cellular and humoral response against nerve tissue grafts was less pronounced compared with the reaction against skin allografts. If donor and host had only minor histocompatibility differences, the humoral response was significantly retarded. There was no difference in the cellular response, which consisted mainly of fibrosis of the epineurium and ingrowth of lymphocytes and macrophages into the fascicles.

In animals with major histocompatibility differences, the cellular reaction started on day 5 and consisted of cellular infiltration of the epineurium. The perineurium seemed to act as a barrier. There was swelling of the endothelium of endoneural vessels, which were full of white blood cells. By day 8 infiltration of the endoneurium by lymphocytes also occurred. By day 40 the epineurium was transformed to a scar, and there were only a few immunologically active cells within the fascicles.

If histocompatibility differences were only minor (e.g., between Fisher rats and Lewis rats), the immunologic reaction lasted much longer (up to day 80). Considering the late onset and longer duration of the humoral response, based on the ^{51}Cr release test, the authors suggested the following: With minor differences in histocompatibility, the early cellular response in these animals (which occurs at the same time as in animals with major histocompatibility differences) is produced by immunologically less active cells and "immunocompetent cells" occur later. According to Mackinnon et al.,[44] this response in matched donor-host situations provides the chance of neurotization of a graft before the retarded immunologic reaction occurs, even without immunosuppressive treatment.

Clinical use of living allografts would be justified if:

1. The chance of immediate graft survival was equal to that of autografts.

2. The risk of fibrosis was low.

3. The allograft response could be prevented or retarded by treatment that did not involve any general risk for the patient.

Strong immunosuppressive treatment may involve some general risk for the patient. Such a risk is justified in heart or kidney transplantation, but certainly not in peripheral nerve grafting. If immunosuppression without *any risk* for the patient were available and if the allograft response could be retarded by selection of matched donors and hosts, a new era of nerve grafting would commence.

Allograft Stroma Without Living Cells. The majority of allografts in clinical use in the past were preserved allografts, which contained only stroma and no cells. For this reason these allografts are less immunogenic. Immediately after grafting they become populated by fibroblasts from the host. Since they contain no Schwann cells, neurotization develops by neuromatous neurotization (see earlier discussion).[62]

Deep-frozen allografts, wrapped in a Millipore membrane to avoid ingrowth of cells, have been utilized by Campbell et al.[24] and Böhler.[15] Lyophilized allografts were used by Weiss and Taylor[79] in 1943. Jacoby et al.[38] reported a successful series of allografts in which the lyophilized grafts were additionally wrapped with lyophilized dura. Kuhlendahl et al.[39] had the opportunity to study patients operated on by Jacoby et al. They were not able to prove nerve conduction in one of the grafts investigated. Fischler et al.[30] detected regeneration in only one of eight grafts. The results reported by Wilhelm[80] were also disappointing.

Cialite-Preserved Allografts. Afanasieff[1] introduced this technique of preserving nerve grafts in 1:5000 cialite solution. This method was utilized by several workers, especially in France. A follow-up study by Iselin[36] of patients of different authors was disappointing, in that some sensibility returned in only a few patients.

Irradiated Allografts. Marmor et al.[45-47] recommended allografts preserved by irradiation. Similar attempts were made by Roberts[60] (use of freezing plus irradiation), Ashley et al.,[9] and Snyder.[69] All these attempts were unsuccessful.

In summary, the use of preserved allografts without living Schwann cells, by definition, must give inferior results as compared with autografts because nerve regeneration develops by neuromatous neurotization.

New Developments. Progress in tissue culture techniques holds forth the prospect of constructing nerve grafts. Schwann cells of the host are provided, extended in tissue culture, and introduced into an allograft stroma, thus forming a graft that is completely populated by host cells.[5, 21] Aguayo[5] showed experimentally that even a xenograft is accepted following immunosuppressive therapy and that the Schwann cells survive grafting. Axons grow across the graft under the guidance of xenogenic Schwann cells. If immunosuppressive therapy stops, the Schwann cells die, but axons and basal lamina, which seem to be less antigenic, survive until new Schwann cells of the host are produced.

PERSONAL EXPERIENCE

In the years before 1963 a series of nerve grafts had been performed.[14] Cutaneous nerves were used as cable grafts or nerve trunks as trunk grafts. A 14-cm-long defect of the median nerve was bridged by a free trunk graft with satisfactory return of protective sensibility.[48] All these patients had some recovery, but the results remained far below the results expected with end-to-end neuror-rhaphy. In all nerve grafts longer than 3 cm, a block at the distal suture site occurred and a resection with new coaptation of the distal end of the graft with the distal stump was performed.

A new technique of nerve grafting, de-signed on the basis of animal experiments,[50–52] was first applied in 1963. This technique is based on the following considerations:

Tension at the suture site is a very unfavorable factor, as the advantages of an atraumatic microsurgical technique cannot be exploited if a neurorrhaphy is performed under tension. Even if the neurorrhaphy is performed without tension by marked flexion of the adjacent joints, the unfavorable consequences are manifested when the limb is mobilized. Under these circumstances, a higher degree of fibrosis develops at the suture site, and axon sprouts that have already crossed the suture line may suffer new damage and undergo axonolysis.[51, 53, 68]

The epineurial connective tissue is the main source for connective tissue proliferation at the site of coaptation. The presence of a high percentage of interfascicular connective tissue in the cross section (as in a polyfascicular nerve) increases the chances of malalignment during surgery. Resection of the epifascicular epineurium and separation of large fascicles or fascicle groups reduce the connective tissue proliferation and the danger of malalignment.

Under these conditions it is not necessary to simulate a trunk graft by packing together several cutaneous nerve grafts, as was done with the cable graft techniques. Instead, the segments of the cutaneous nerves can be transplanted individually between large fascicles (fascicular nerve grafting) or fascicle groups (interfascicular nerve grafting). The main step in this procedure is the resection of the epifascicular epineurium and the separation of fascicles or fascicle groups by interfascicular dissection. This technique was of course possible only after the microscope and microsurgical instruments were available to perform this dissection in an atraumatic way.

The fascicles in the peripheral portion of peripheral nerves are very often arranged in fascicle groups (polyfascicular pattern with group arrangement, see Chapter 1), and these groups are constant over a long distance.[49, 52–54] The concept of group arrangement was confirmed more recently by

Williams[81] and Jabaley et al.[37] Fascicle groups are isolated by dissection in the preformed spaces between them. They are not artificially created, as quoted in Sunderland's textbook.[74]

Since the lengths of the cutaneous nerve grafts were selected with the adjacent joints in neutral position and without other efforts to shorten the distance between the two nerve stumps (see Chapter 1), only minimal surgical maneuvers were necessary to achieve and maintain coaptation between grafts and fascicles or fascicle groups. Usually, one stitch was sufficient to obtain approximation and maintain the coaptation. I do not hesitate to use a second or third stitch if optimal coaptation is not achieved by one stitch but the aim remains to manipulate as little as necessary. The stitches are anchored in the epineurium of a cutaneous nerve graft and in the perineurium of large fascicles or in the remaining interfascicular epineurium of fascicle groups. Different suture techniques were used in the same procedure and even in the same stitch. If the nerve graft was placed in optimal coaptation without a stitch, we did not use any stitches at all. This was especially true if the interfascicular dissection of the nerve stumps and the resection of the neuroma were performed in such a way that the individual fascicle groups that protruded out of the nerve stumps were of different lengths. In this case an interdentation between grafts and fascicle groups is achieved, contributing significantly to the stability by side-to-side contact between grafts and fascicles or fascicle groups (Fig. 18–1).

The coaptation is maintained merely by normal fibrin clotting and by the few stitches necessary for approximation. For this reason, shearing forces must be avoided during wound closure. Immobilization is obtained by applying a plaster cast in exactly the position that the limb was in during the operation. One important point in using this technique is to avoid dislocation of the grafts during wound closure and during the period prior to immobilization. If these two steps are performed carelessly, the grafts are dislocated and the coaptations may rupture.

Immobilization is maintained for 8 to 10 days. After that period of time the coaptations are strong enough and the patient is allowed to move the limb freely.

One of the crucial points is the identification of corresponding fascicles or fascicle

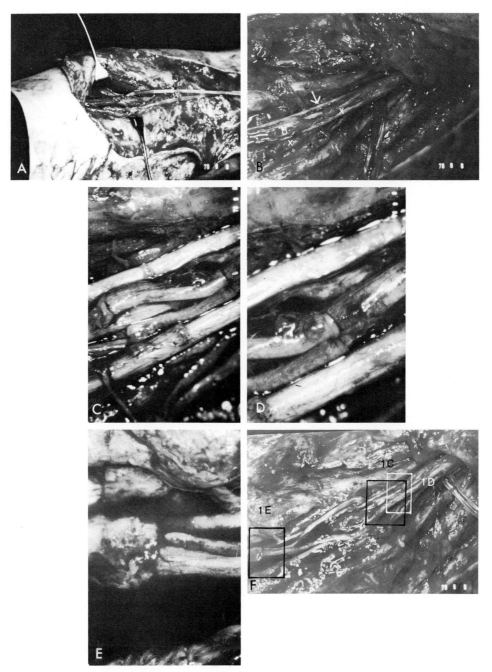

Figure 18–1. Partial lesion of the median nerve at the cubital fovea along with a lesion of the cubital artery in a 25-year-old male patient 17 months after the injury. The primary repair had been performed but more details are not known. The patient has fairly good motor function but severe loss of sensibility. Is the good motor function the result of the primary repair, is there an anomaly of innervation, or was only a partial transection performed? The poor sensibility is the decisive indication for surgery. At the exploration, the nerve was adherent to the surrounding tissue. An external neurolysis was performed. *A,* The nerve is fibrotic, and some stitches are at the surface. *B,* After epifascicular epineurectomy the individual fascicle groups are clearly seen. Some do not show any changes (*arrow*); others are interrupted and have formed a neuroma (X) or they are enveloped in fibrotic tissue (O). After resection of the neuroma, the fascicle is repaired (to establish continuity) by a short cutaneous nerve graft, which is simply put into the defect without requiring any stitches or glue. *C,* A close-up view demonstrates the optimal coaptation between one large fascicle group and two (*D*) or even three grafts (*E*). In spite of an exact coaptation, it is impossible to line up the fascicles perfectly because of the different numbers and different sizes of the fascicles. *F,* An overall view after internal neurolysis and completion of the grafting.

Table 18–1. FUNCTIONAL RESULTS OF RADIAL NERVE REPAIR BY NERVE GRAFTING
IN 30 PATIENTS*

Functional Level	Defect (cm)	N	Age (yrs)	Interval (months)
M5	6.8 ± 6.8 (1–15)	13	32.3 ± 16.0 (11–64)	5.7 ± 4.6 (1–18)
M4	8.5 ± 2.4 (4–12)	12	28.8 ± 18.0 (8–69)	8.2 ± 8.3 (0–29)
M3	10.3 ± 3.5 (6–14)	4	22.2 ± 15.0 (8–42)	12.7 ± 11.0 (3–29)
M2	10	1	62	3

*Numbers in parentheses indicate standard deviation. (From Millesi, H.: Clin. Plast. Surg., *11*:108, 1984.)

Table 18–2. FUNCTIONAL RESULTS OF MEDIAN NERVE REPAIR BY NERVE GRAFTING
IN 39 PATIENTS

	Mixed Innervation*			M4–5			M3			M2		
	Age (Yrs)	Interval (Months)	Defect (cm)	Age (Yrs)	Interval (Months)	Defect (cm)	Age (Yrs)	Interval (Months)	Defect (cm)	Age (Yrs)	Interval (Months)	Defect (cm)
S3+ −4	21	4	5.0	19	6	2.5				23	4	7.0
	20	1	2.0	22	8	8.0						
	25	2	3.5	18	7	7.0						
	40	2	2.0	21	2	6.0						
	27	2	3.5	10	9	5.0						
	49	1	6.5	9	2	5.0						
	44	8	5.0	20	3	5.0						
	7	2	2.0	46	5	3.5						
	13	4	4.0	50	2	2.0						
				10	4	4.0						
S3	21	4	4.5	35	6	2.0	43	8	5.0	41	28	15.0
	21	2	6.0	19	2	4.0	44	36	12.0			
	46	4	2.0	50	2	3.0	48	18	7.0			
	24	4	5.0				25	2	5.0			
	27	2	4.0				6	5	4.0			
	52	12	4.5									
	30	9	10.0									
	23	5	4.0									
	61	3	4.0									
S2	26	11	16.0									

*These patients had an innervation anomaly in which the thenar muscles were innervated by the ulnar nerve as well as by the median nerve. (From Millesi, H.: Clin. Plast. Surg., *11*:108, 1985.)

groups. This is achieved by retrograde tracing. The peripheral portion of the nerve is exposed up to its division, and the individual fascicle groups are traced back to the cross section of the distal stump, following their course on the surface of the nerve. An exact sketch is made of the fascicular structure of the distal stump. Consequently, the fiber quality for each of the fascicle groups is well known by retrograde tracing. A sketch of the fascicular pattern of the proximal stump is made, and by comparing the two sketches, the corresponding fascicles or fascicle groups are defined in the proximal stump. This can easily be achieved in patients with short defects, but it becomes more and more difficult in patients with longer defects. This is the reason why the length of the defect is a decisive factor in determining functional recovery after nerve grafting. However, this fact is applicable to all techniques that may be used to manage a nerve defect.

If the nerve segment involved consists of many fascicles without group arrangement (polyfascicular pattern without group arrangement), separation of groups by interfascicular dissection is not possible. In this situation the separation would be artificial. Polyfascicular pattern without group arrangement is mainly found in proximal segments of peripheral nerves and in the brachial plexus. General knowledge about nerve fiber distribution is applicable in the situation. We know, for instance, that the dorsal sector of the radial nerve contains relatively more fibers, which finally will form the posterior interosseous nerve. In the case of a long defect, the nerve grafts (which are connected with the posterior interosseous nerve) are coapted with fascicles within the dorsal sector of the radial nerve in the proximal stump. This type of coaptation between grafts and stumps is called sectoral nerve grafting. It is evident that the chances for recovery are decreased in such a long defect, in which the distal end is connected with a segment that already has a group arrangement and the proximal portion is connected with a nerve segment without group arrangement. However, useful recovery was achieved in several patients with defects of 15 or 20 cm.

The results obtained by this technique are shown in Tables 18–1 to 18–4. The evaluation of results was performed by use of the M0 to M5 and S0 to S4 schema, as applied by Nicholson and Seddon.[55] All these cases involved secondary repairs. Only a few of the patients for whom we did secondary repairs had their initial treatment performed by our service as well. The vast majority were treated in other hospitals and were admitted to our unit only after failure of other techniques. In many patients the time interval between injury and repair was more than 12 months (up to 36 months). We still attempted a nerve repair in these cases, with the hope that protective sensibility might at least return. In spite of the fact that these patients evidently have a much poorer prognosis, the results of all of them are included in the tables. This fact must be considered if these results are compared with results of other series, in which only patients selected for primary repair were evaluated.

Table 18–1 lists the functional results in 30 of 38 patients with a radial nerve defect who were operated upon between 1964 and 1974. Six patients could not be followed, and two patients with radial nerve repair were excluded from the study because the repair had been performed following limb replantation. This involves different factors because eventual ischemic damage to the muscles must be considered. In one patient, a 60-year-old male, the result was less than M3. Two patients of the M3 group needed tendon transfer to increase muscle power. In all other cases the functional result was satisfactory to excellent.

Median nerve repair by nerve grafting was performed in 47 patients between 1964 and 1974 (Table 18–2). Six patients could not be followed, and two patients were excluded because the repair was performed following limb replantation. Nineteen of the remaining 39 patients had partial innervation of the thenar muscles by the ulnar nerve. These individuals were not evaluated as far as motor function was concerned. Therefore, only 20 patients remained for evaluation of motor function, but 39 were evaluated for sensory function.

Nerve grafts were performed between 1964 and 1974 in 49 patients with isolated ulnar nerve lesions. One patient had nerve grafts after limb replantation, and four patients could not be followed. The results of the remaining 44 patients are listed in Table 18–3.

In Tables 18–2 and 18–3 each patient is represented by three numbers indicating the age in years, the interval in months, and the defect in centimeters. In Table 18–3 high lesions are marked with a triangle.

Table 18–3. FUNCTIONAL RESULTS OF ULNAR NERVE REPAIR USING NERVE GRAFTING IN 44 PATIENTS

Each motor-recovery group (Mixed Innervation, M4–5, M3, M2+, M2, M1, M0) lists patients by: Age | (Months) | Interval Defect (cm) | ▲ (high lesion). Rows are grouped by sensory grade (S3+–4, S3, S2, S1, S0).

Sensory	Mixed Innervation	M4–5	M3	M2+	M2	M1	M0
S3+–4	4 5 2.0 18 10 6.0	11 2 5.0 11 3 6.0 12 2 5.0 ▲ 12 3 3.0 ▲ 7 4 4.5 20 36 7.0 23 2 5.0 28 9 5.0 40 6 3.0	13 6 5.0 55 4 2.0				
S3		11 12 5.0 12 3 10.0 ▲ 17 5 7.0 16 6 4.0 21 4 6.0 22 7 2.0 ▲ 19 1 3.0 ▲ 49 2 4.0 ▲ 63 13 3.0 ▲ 64 1 2.0 ▲ 67 13 3.0 ▲ 25 2 3.0 ▲ 27 10 4.0	18 3 2.0 34 31 20.0 ▲ 39 11 18.0 ▲ 40 8 5.0 ▲ 48 3 6.0 49 4 4.0 45 5 4.0 54 8 3.0 56 2 3.0	27 7 10.0 ▲▲ 18 7 13.0 ▲▲ 37 6 3.0 ▲	31 48 20.0 ▲▲ 17 6 6.0 ▲▲		
S2				25 8 6.0 ▲		28 ▲	5 15.0 ▲
S1				64 2 16.0 ▲	44 7 11.0 ▲	16 ▲	−4 6.0 ▲
S0						33 ▲	6 19.0 ▲

▲ = high lesion. (From Millesi, H.: Clin. Plast. Surg., 11:109, 1984.)

Table 18–4. FUNCTIONAL RESULTS OF MEDIAN AND ULNAR NERVE REPAIR IN 29 PATIENTS

		M4–5 S3+−4	M4–5 S3	M3 S3+−4	M3 S3	M3 S2	M2+ S3	M2 S3+−4	M2 S3	M2 S2	M1 S3	M0 S3+−4	M0 S3	M0 S2
Median Nerve $n_1 = 30*$														
	n	4	3 + 1 NS	2	7			2	3	3	2	2		1 NL
Interval	<6	4	1	1	6				1					
(months)	6–12		2		1			1		2	2			
	12<		1 NS	1				1	2	1		2		1 NL
Ulnar Nerve $n_1 = 28*$														
	n	2	8	1	5 + 1 NS	2	6		1		1		1	
Interval	<6	2	5		2	1	3							
(months)	6–12		2	1	2		2		1		1		1	
	12<		1		1 + 1 NS	1	1							

*NS = nerve suture; NL = neurolysis. (From Millesi, H.: Clin. Plast. Surg., 11:110, 1984.)

Table 18–4 lists the functional results of 30 median and 28 ulnar nerve repairs in 29 patients with combined lesions of the median and ulnar nerves. One patient had bilateral lesions, bringing the number of involved extremities to 30. Additional patients with combined lesions could not be followed and are not represented in the table. The median nerve was repaired in all 30 extremities. In 28 patients the median nerve was bridged by a nerve graft, in one patient an end-to-end neurorrhaphy was performed, and in one patient the continuity was preserved and a neurolysis was carried out. The ulnar nerve in the two extremities of the patient with bilateral lesions was not repaired. In this patient the nerve damage was due to a severe electrical burn of both extremities. The nerve repair was performed only to achieve some protective sensibility several years after the accident, and, consequently, no motor recovery could be expected. In 27 out of the 28 ulnar nerve repairs, nerve grafts were employed, and in one instance an end-to-end neurorrhaphy was performed. The functional results are shown in Table 18–4.

SUMMARY

For a long time nerve grafting was used as a last resort if all other means of managing a nerve defect were unsuccessful. All attempts to use allografts were disappointing. With the development of a new technique based on microsurgery, free nerve grafting has become a reliable procedure. The results are close to the results achieved by neurorrhaphy under favorable conditions and are better than the results achieved by neurorrhaphy under tension. Today this fact is recognized by nearly all surgeons. Disagreement is limited only to the length of defect, i.e., for which defects can neurorrhaphy still be used and which defects represent an indication for nerve grafting? It is logical that in this regard different surgeons have different results, according to their training, their background, and the number of patients they have treated. If the caseload includes primary repairs, neurorrhaphy will be favored; if it includes more late secondary repairs, nerve grafts will be used more often. The vascularized nerve graft represents a new technique that certainly will have its indication in selected cases. If the immunologic problems associated with nerve grafting can be solved, a new era in nerve grafting will commence.

References

1. Afanasieff, A.: Premières résultats de 20 homogreffes de nerfs conservés par le cialit (main et avant-bras). Presse Méd., 27:65, 1409, 1967.
2. Aguayo, A. J., Attiwell, M., Trecarten, J., Perkins, S., and Bray, G.M.: Abnormal myelination in transplanted Trembler mouse Schwann cells. Nature, 265:73, 1977.
3. Aguayo, A.J., and Bray, G.M.: Experimental nerve grafts. In Jewett, D.L., and McCarroll, H.R., Jr. (eds.): Nerve Repair and Regeneration. Its Clinical and Experimental Basis. St. Louis, The C.V. Mosby Company, 1980, p. 68.
4. Aguayo, A.J., Bray, G.M., and Perkins, S.C.: Axon-Schwann cell relationship. Ann. N.Y. Acad. Sci., 317:512, 1979.
5. Aguayo, A.J.: Construction of grafts. In Gorio, A., Mellesi, S., and Mengrino, S. (eds.): Posttraumatic Peripheral Nerve Regeneration. Experimental Basis and Clinical Implications. New York, Raven Press, 1981, p. 365.
6. Albert, E.: Berichte der Naturwissenschaftlich-Medizinischen in Innsbruck. Vol. 9, Innsbruck, 1878, p. 97.
7. Albert, E.: Einige Operationen am Nerven. Wien Med. Presse, 26:1285, 1885.
8. Anderl, H.: Reconstruction of the face through cross face nerve transplantation in facial paralysis. Chir. Plast., 2:17, 1973.

9. Ashley, F.L., Murphy, J.E., Morgan, S.C., Balch, C.R., Conover, W.A., Galloway, D.V., and Cross, L.: Axon growth through irradiated median and ulnar nerve homografts in primates. Plast. Reconstr. Surg., 42:313, 1968.

10. Ballance, C., and Duel, A.B.: Operative treatment of facial palsy by the introduction of nerve grafts into fallopian canal and by other intratemporal methods. Arch. Otol., 15:1, 1932.

11. Barnes, R., Bacsich, P., Wyburn, G.M., et al.: A study of the fate of nerve homografts in man. Br. J. Surg., 34:34, 1946.

12. Bainbridge, D.R., and Gowland, G.: Detection of homograft sensitivity in mice by the elimination of chromium-51 labeled lymph node cells. Ann. N.Y. Acad. Sci., 129:257, 1966.

13. Bielschowsky, M., and Unger, E.: Überbrückung grosser Nervenlücken. Beiträge zur Kenntnis der Degeneration und Regeneration peripherer Nerven. J. Physiol. Neurol., 22:267, 1916–1918.

14. Blackwood, W., and Holmes, W.: Histopathology of nerve injury. In: Seddon, H.J. (ed.): Medical Research Council on Peripheral Nerve Injuries. London, Her Majesty's Stationary Office, Special Report No. 88, 1955, p. 155.

15. Böhler, J.: Nervennaht und homoioplastische Nerventransplantation mit Milliporeumscheidung. Langenbeck's Arch. Chir., 301:900, 1962.

16. Bosse, J.P.: Personal communication at the 5th International Symposium on Microsurgery, Guaruja, Brazil, May 15–18, 1979.

17. Bosse, H.J.: Discussion. In Gorio, A., Millesi, H., and Mingrino, S. (eds.): Posttraumatic Peripheral Nerve Regeneration. Experimental Basis and Clinical Implications. New York, Raven Press, 1981, p. 347.

18. Brooks, D.: The place of nerve grafting in orthopaedic surgery. J. Bone Joint Surg., 37A:299, 1955.

19. Brunelli, G.: Graft preparation: Sural Nerve withdrawal. In Gorio, A., Millesi, H., and Mingrino, S. (eds.): Posttraumatic Peripheral Nerve Surgery. Experimental Basis and Clinical Implications. New York, Raven Press, 1981, p. 337.

20. Bsteh, F.X., and Millesi, H.: Zur Kenntnis der zweizeitigen Nerveninterplantation bei ausgedehnten peripheren Nervendefekten. Klin. Med., 12:571, 1960.

21. Bunge, R.P.: Construction of grafts. In Gorio, A., Millesi, H., Mingrino, S. (eds.): Posttraumatic Peripheral Nerve Regeneration. Experimental Basis and Clinical Implications. New York, Raven Press, 1981, p. 366.

22. Bunnell, S.: Surgery of nerves of the hand. Surg. Gynecol. Obstet., 44:145, 1927.

23. Bunnell, S., and Boyes, H.J.: Nerve grafts. Am. J. Surg. 45:54, 1939.

24. Campbell, J.B., Andrews, C.L., Husby, J., Thulin, C., and Feringa, E.: Microfilter sheathing peripheral nerve surgery. J. Trauma, 1:139, 1961.

25. Chung, P.K.C., and Chung, S.K.Y.: Evaluation of Imuram and Locke's solution in peripheral nerve homografts. Exp. Neurol., 42:141, 1974.

26. Das Gupta, T.K.: Mechanism of rejection of peripheral nerve allografts. Surg. Gynecol. Obstet., 125:1058, 1967.

27. Davis, L., and Ruge, D.: Functional recovery following the use of homogenous nerve grafts. Surgery, 27:102, 1950.

28. Edidin, M.: The tissue distribution and cellular location of transplantation antigens. In Kahan, B.D., and Reisfeld, R.A. (eds.): Transplantation Antigens, Markers of Biological Individuality. New York, Academic Press, 1971, p. 125.

29. Fachinelli, A., Masquelet, A., Restrepo, J., and Gilbert, A.: The vascularized sural nerve. Anatomy and surgical approach. Int. J. Microsurg., 3:57, 1981.

30. Fischler, M., Hoehne, O., Sindermann, F., and Sollmann, H.: Klinische und elektromyographische Verlaufsuntersuchungen bei Patienten mit homologen lyophilisierten Nerveninterponaten. Arch. Psychiatr. Nervenkr., 219:223, 1974.

31. Foerster, O.: Communication held at the ausserordentliche Tagung der Deutschen Orthopädischen Gesellschaft, Berlin, February 8–9, 1916. Münchener Med. Wschr., 63:283, 1916.

32. Foerster, O.: Die Leitungsbahnen des Schmerzgefühls und die chirurgische Behandlung der Schmerzzustände. Berlin-Vienna, Urban & Schwarzenberg, 1927.

33. Geldmacher, J., and Albers, W.: Personal communication at the 4th Congress of the European Section of the International Confederation for Plastic and Reconstructive Surgery, Athens, May 10–14, 1981.

34. Gilbert, A.: Personal communication at the International Symposium on Clinical Frontiers and Reconstructive Microsurgery, Anaheim, California, June 25–28, 1981.

35. Gilbert, A.: Personal communication at the Intensive Course on Microsurgery, Oklahoma City, Oklahoma, May, 1982.

36. Iselin, F.: Discussion: Les problèmes d'évaluation pre- et postopérative des nerves périferiques. Résultats de questionnaire. Groupe d'Etude de la Main Meeting, Montpellier, 1975.

37. Jabaley, M.E., Wallace, W.H., and Heckler, F.R.: Internal topography of major nerves of the forearm and hand: A current review. J. Hand Surg., 5:1, 1980.

38. Jacoby, W., Fahlbusch, R., and Mackert, B.: Indikation und Technik der Überbrückung von Nervendefekten mit homologen lyophilisierten Nerven. Melsunger Med. Mitteilungen, 46:116, 209, 1972.

39. Kuhlendahl, H., Mumenthaler, M., Penzholz, H., Röttgen, P., Schliack, H., and Struppler, A.: Behanlung peripherer Nervenverletzungen mit homologen Nervenimplantaten. Z. Neurol., p. 202, 1972.

40. Levinthal, R., Brown, W.J., and Rand, R.W.: Fascicular nerve allograft evaluation. Part 1: Comparison with autografts by light microscopy. J. Neurosurg., 48:423, 1978.

41. Levinthal, R., Brown, W.J., and Rand, R.W.: Fascicular nerve allograft evaluation. Part 2: Comparison with whole-nerve allograft by light microscopy. J. Neurosurg., 48:428, 1978.

42. Lewis, D.: Some peripheral nerve problems. Boston Med. Surg. J., p. 188, 1923.

43. Lyons, W.R., and Woodall, B.: Atlas of Peripheral Nerve Injuries. Philadelphia, W.B. Saunders Company, 1949, p. 339.

44. Mackinnon, S., Hudson, A., Falk, R., Bilbao, J., Kline, D., and Hunter, R.T.: Nerve allograft response: A quantitative immunologic study. Neurosurgery, 10:1, 1982.

45. Marmor, L.: Regeneration of peripheral nerve defects by irradiated homografts. Lancet, 1:1911, 1963.

46. Marmor, L., Foster, J.M., Carlson, G.J., and Arpels, J.C.: Experimental irradiated nerve homografts. J. Neurosurg., 24:656, 1966.

47. Marmor, L., and Hirasawa, Y.: Further studies of irradiated nerve heterografts in animals with Immuran immunosuppression. J. Trauma, 8:32, 1968.

48. Millesi, H.: Klinische und experimentelle Erfahrungen bei der Wiederherstellung peripherer Nervenläsionen. Langenbecks Arch. Dtsch. Z. Chir., *301*:893, 1962.
49. Millesi, H.: Zum Problem der Überbückung von defekten peripheren Nerven. Wien. Med. Wschr., *118*:182, 1968.
50. Millesi, H., Ganglberger, J., and Berger, A.: Erfahrungen mit der Mikrochirurgie peripherer Nerven. Chir. Plast. Reconstr., *3*:47, 1967.
51. Millesi, H., Berger, A., and Meissl, G.: Razvoj reparatorno operativnih postupaka kod ozijeda periferinih zivaca. Drugi Simpozij I Bolestima Ozljedama Sake. Zagreb, 1970, p. 161.
52. Millesi, H., Berger, A., and Meissl, G.: Experimentelle Untersuchung zur Heilung durchtrennter petripherer Nerven. Chir. Plast., *1*:174, 1972.
53. Millesi, H., Berger, A., and Meissl, G.: The interfascicular nerve grafting of the median and ulnar nerves. J. Bone Joint Surg., *54A*:717, 1972.
54. Millesi, H., Meissl, G., and Berger, A.: Further experience with interfascicular grafting of the median, ulnar and radial nerves. J. Bone Joint Surg., *58A*:2, 209, 1976.
55. Nicholson, O.R., and Seddon, H.J.: Nerve repair in civil practice. Results of treatment of median and ulnar nerve lesions. Br. Med. J., *2*:1065, 1957.
56. Nigst, H.: Freie Nerventransplantation und Cortison. Basel, Stuttgart, Benno Schwabe & Company, 1957.
57. Nulsen, F.E., Lewey, F.H., van Wagner, W.P.: Peripheral nerve grafts in the medical department, US Army, for surgery in World War II. *In* Spurling, R.G., and Woodall, B. (eds.): Neurosurgery, Vol. II. Washington, D.C., US Printing Office, 1959, p. 493.
58. Philipeaux, J.M., and Vulpian, A.: Note sur les essais de greffe d'un troncon de nerf lingual entre les deux bouts de thypoglose. Arch. Phys. Norm. Pathol., *3*:618, 1870.
59. Pollard, J.D., Gye, R.S., and McLeod, J.G.: An assessment of immunosuppressive agents in experimental peripheral nerve transplantation. Surg. Gynecol. Obstet., *132*:839, 1971.
60. Roberts, T.S.: Fate of the frozen irradiated allogeneic nerve graft. Surg. Forum, *18*:445, 1967.
61. Rotstein, L.E., Makowka, L., Falk, R.E., Kirby, T.J., Nossal, N., and Falk, J.A.: Selective immune stimulation during induction of allograft tolerance in the rat by radical immunosuppression. Transplantation, *30*:417, 1980.
62. Schröder, J. M., and Seifert, K.E.: Die Feinstruktur der neuromatösen Neurotisation von Nerventransplantaten. Virchow's Arch. (Cell Pathol.), *5*:219, 1970.
63. Seddon, H.J.: The use of autogenous grafts for the repair of large gaps in peripheral nerves. Br. J. Surg., *35*:151, 1947.
64. Seddon, H.J.: Restoration of function in peripheral nerve injuries. Lancet, *1*:148, 1947.
65. Seddon, H.J.: Nerve grafting. J. Bone Joint Surg., *45B*:447, 1963.
66. Seddon, H.J.: Surgical Disorders of Peripheral Nerves. Edinburgh, Churchill Livingstone, 1972.
67. Seddon, H.J., and Holmes, W.: The late condition of nerve homografts in man. Surg. Gynecol. Obstet., *79*:342, 1944.
68. Seitelberger, F., Sluga, E., Meissl, G., and Millesi, H.: Morphologische Untersuchungen an Nähten und Transplantaten nach Nervenläsionen. Lecture held at the Gesellschaft d. Ärzte, Vienna, November, 21, 1969.
69. Snyder, C.G.: Alternative methods of nerve repair. Lecture held at the Microsurgery Workshop Symposium, New York, October 14–18, 1974.
70. Spurling, R.G., Lyons, W.R., Whitcomb, B.B., et al.: The failure of the whole fresh homogenous nerve grafts in man. J. Neurosurg., *2*:79, 1945.
71. Stookey, B.: The futility of bridging nerve defects by means of nerve flaps. Surg. Gynecol. Obstet., *29*:287, 1919.
72. Strange, F.G. St. C.: An operation for nerve pedicle grafting. Preliminary communication. Br. J. Surg., *34*:423, 1947.
73. Strange, F. G. St. C.: Case report on pedicle nerve graft. Br. J. Surg., *37*:331, 1950.
74. Sunderland, S.: Nerves and Nerve Injuries, 2nd Ed. Baltimore: The Williams and Wilkins Company, 1978.
75. Taylor, G.I., and Ham, F.J.: The free vascularized nerve graft. Plast. Reconstr. Surg., *57*:413, 1976.
76. Townsend, P.: Microvascular nerve grafts. Communication at the 4th Congress of the European Section of the International Confederation for Plastic and Reconstructive Surgery, Athens, May 10–15, 1981.
77. Tupper, J.: Fascicular nerve repair. *In* Jewett, D.L., and McCarroll, H.R., Jr. (eds.): Nerve Repair and Regeneration. Its Clinical and Experimental Basis. St. Louis, The C.V. Mosby Company, 1980, p. 320.
78. Verhoog, B.D., and van Bekkum, D.W.: Peripheral nerve allografts. Modifications of allograft reaction using experimental model in rats. Transplant. Proc., *3*:591, 1971.
79. Weiss, P., and Taylor, A.C.: Repair of peripheral nerves by grafts of frozen dried nerves. Proc. Soc. Exp. Biol. Med., *52*:326, 1943.
80. Wilhelm, K.: Ergebnisse nach Nerven Rekonstruktion mit homologen Lyo-Nerven. Paper read at the Congress of the International College of Surgeons, Amsterdam, 1975.
81. Williams, H.B.: Communication at the 5th International Symposium on Microsurgery, Guaruja, Brazil, May 15–18, 1979.
82. Williams, H.B.: Peripheral nerve injuries in children. *In* Kernahan, D.A., and Thomson, H.G. (eds.): Pediatric Plastic Surgery. St. Louis, The C. V. Mosby Company, 1982.
83. Young, J.Z., and Medawar, P.B.: Cable grafts with fibrin. Lancet 2:126, 1940.

19

Lower Extremity Nerve Lesions

■

Hanno Millesi, M.D.

LUMBOSACRAL PLEXUS

The peripheral nerves of the lower extremity originate from the lumbosacral plexus. Unlike the brachial plexus, the lumbosacral plexus is well protected within the pelvis and is therefore exposed to injury in only rare instances. In our case material involving 136 patients with lower extremity nerve lesions, the lumbosacral plexus was involved in only four patients. In two patients the lesion was due to a gunshot wound. In these patients the individual parts of the lumbosacral plexus were not interrupted but were compressed by scar tissue formation, and neurolysis was performed with good recovery. In one of these patients the return of peroneal nerve innervation to muscles was not satisfactory, and a tibialis posterior transfer had to be carried out.

One patient suffered an injury when skiing. A foreign body entered the perineum and damaged the upper portions of the lumbar plexus; roots L3, L4, and L5 were especially involved. Continuity was restored by nerve grafts measuring 9 cm in length. The remaining segments of the lumbosacral plexus were neurolyzed.

In a fourth patient the lesion was due to fracture of the pelvis and a luxation of the hip joint. The lower roots S1 to S3, forming the sciatic nerve, were involved. Nerve grafts were performed between the roots and the sciatic nerve, and partial recovery occurred.

The exposure of the lumbosacral plexus is performed with the patient in the dorsal position, using a long lateral incision and an extraperitoneal approach to the lumbar and sacral areas.

In the case of involvement of the sciatic nerve, two types of access were used. With the patient in the lateral position, the sciatic nerve was exposed by an extrapelvic approach and the lumbosacral plexus by an extraperitoneal approach from above (as described in the preceding paragraph).

ILIOHYPOGASTRIC NERVE

This nerve is sometimes damaged by surgical incisions. The symptoms are hypesthesia in the inguinal area and at the symphysis or at the lateral surface of the pelvis if the lateral branch is involved. Two cases have been observed in which the symptoms occurred after urologic surgery. In both cases there was spontaneous improvement and no additional surgery was required.

ILIOINGUINAL AND GENITOFEMORAL NERVES

Loss of function of the ilioinguinal nerve leads to hypesthesia in the inguinal area and inner side of the thigh as well as in the scrotum in the male and the labia majora in the female.

The *ilioinguinal syndrome* is associated with pain in the sacral and inguinal areas. Internal rotation of the hip joint is also painful. The syndrome is caused by constriction of the nerve when traversing the abdominal wall.

Damage to the genitofemoral nerve produces hypesthesia in the trigonum scarpae at the scrotum in the male or at the labia majora in the female and at the opposing

239

skin of the thigh. In addition, the cremaster muscle is paralyzed.

Four patients with symptoms of damage to the ilioinguinal nerve were studied. Two patients also had a lesion of the genitofemoral nerve. In these two patients, as well as in one of the remaining two, the lesion was due to damage during surgery for inguinal hernia. In one patient the ilioinguinal nerve was caught in a stitch. This patient had a true ilioinguinal syndrome. In all four patients the nerves were explored and their proximal stumps were followed across the abdominal wall far into the pelvis and transected at a very high level. Three patients are now free of pain after several years. In one patient the symptoms recurred after 2 years, but to a much lesser and more tolerable degree.

LATERAL FEMOROCUTANEOUS NERVE

One patient suffered from burning pain and paresthesias in the lateral aspect of the thigh; these symptoms were aggravated when walking. This corresponds to the syndrome of meralgia paresthetica, as described in the older literature.[1, 2, 10] In this patient the lateral femorocutaneous nerve was compressed at its exit from the pelvis by a double layer of the inguinal ligament.[4] After the nerve was explored and transected high in the pelvis, the symptoms disappeared.

OBTURATOR NERVE

Damage to this nerve causes paralysis of the adductor muscles and loss of sensibility at the inner side of the thigh. Irritation of the nerve may be produced by an obturator hernia, by inflammatory processes at the os pubis, and by scars on the inner side of the thigh. Nerve damage may extend to the knee joint, and chronic irritation may cause an adduction contracture.[3] However, we could not observe such a lesion in our case material.

FEMORAL NERVE

A lesion of the femoral nerve leads to paralysis of the quadriceps femoris muscle with lack of active extension of the knee joint. The area of sensory loss includes the anterior aspect of the thigh and the supply zone of the saphenous nerve down to the medial aspect of the foot. The nerve leaves the pelvis in the lacuna musculorum and splits into many branches. Extrapelvic damage usually causes only a partial lesion.

In two patients the femoral nerve was resected within the pelvis during an operation for a malignant neoplasm (hypernephroma) or a semimalignant tumor (recurrent fibroma with increased cell activity). A 15-cm-long gap was bridged by four cutaneous nerve grafts. Both patients were over 50 years of age. One had an excellent recovery (grade M4); the other had only moderate improvement (grade M2).

In three patients the femoral nerve was damaged during surgical procedures. There was loss of continuity or damage of 4th degree (loss of fascicular structure but continuity preserved by connective tissue), which required resection. In all three patients continuity was restored by nerve grafts. Two patients had an excellent recovery; the third could not be followed. In three other patients the nerve was also damaged by trauma during surgery (hernia repair or vascular surgery). In these patients, however, continuity was preserved, and neurolysis resulted in full recovery.

In summary, seven of eight patients with femoral nerve lesions could be followed; six had full and one had partial recovery.

SAPHENOUS NERVE

In one patient a painful neuroma that occurred after a lipectomy of the thigh was treated by resection with good results.

SUPERIOR GLUTEAL NERVE

A spontaneous compression syndrome caused marked muscle atrophy in one patient. The compression was located at the site of the exit of the superior gluteal nerve from the pelvis. Decompression and neurolysis were followed by full recovery.

INFERIOR GLUTEAL NERVE

Following a gunshot wound, one patient had loss of continuity of this nerve associated with a simultaneous lesion of the sciatic nerve. Neurorrhaphy was followed by full recovery.

SCIATIC NERVE

The sciatic nerve supplies all muscles of the dorsal and ventral aspects of the calf and of the foot. The sensory nerves for the sole of the foot are also provided by the sciatic nerve. In spite of these important functions, it is interesting to note how well patients do even following complete transection of the sciatic nerve. The main complication is loss of sensibility in the sole, which sooner or later leads to trophic ulcer formation due to anesthesia. The patient still has control of the knee joint but cannot move the foot or toes. If the foot is stabilized by an orthopedic device, the patient is able to walk quite well. Consequently, the most important function to be restored is protective sensibility of the sole. The second important function is plantar flexion, which can be actively performed if the gastrocnemius and soleus muscles are reinnervated. If after loss of sciatic nerve function the patient has regained protective sensibility and active plantar flexion, the result can be regarded as *satisfactory*. Under these circumstances, the patient has to wear an orthopedic device to avoid equinovarus deformity of the foot. If function is restored to the other muscles of the calf innervated by the tibial nerve, especially the tibialis posterior muscle, useful active motility of the foot can be obtained by a tibialis posterior tendon transfer. Such a result can be regarded as *good*. In complete lesions of the sciatic nerve, it is very rare that muscles innervated by the peroneal nerve are actively reinnervated (Table 19–1).

Vasomotor function plays an important role in sciatic nerve lesions, as the vasomotor response is retarded and the patient develops cyanosis and discomfort when the leg is in the vertical position. The return of a satisfactory vasomotor response is also an important factor for evaluation of the functional result.

Thirty-nine patients had sciatic nerve lesions due to various causes (Table 19–2). The results of treatment were as follows:

High Lesions at the Foramen Infrapiriforme. Of 10 patients with a lesion at this level, 9 had suffered a fracture of the pelvis with central luxation of the hip joint. The functional loss was induced by traction and maintained by pressure of bone fragments or

Table 19–1. EVALUATION OF FUNCTIONAL RECOVERY AFTER SCIATIC NERVE LESIONS

Level	Result

3	Good result:
	Good vasomotor function
	Protective sensibility
	Active plantar flexion
	Active dorsal flexion—two possibilities must be distinguished:
	  3 (T + P): Dorsal flexion due to useful recovery of the muscles innervated by the common peroneal nerve
	  3 (T): Dorsal flexion due to functioning tibialis posterior tendon transfer; in this case there must be useful recovery not only in the gastrocnemius and soleus but in the other muscles innervated by the tibial nerve as well

2	Satisfactory result: Good vasomotor function Protective sensibility Active plantar flexion due to reinnervation of the gastrocnemius (M3 or better) An orthopedic device is required
1	Poor result: Good vasomotor function Protective sensibility No useful motor recovery An orthopedic device is required
0	Nil: No nerve regeneration

T + P = tibial and peroneal nerves; T = tibial nerve only.

osteosynthetic material. In none of these patients was the sciatic nerve completely transected. The treatment was exposure, intraneural neurolysis, and nerve grafting of fascicle groups that were severely damaged. Results are summarized in Table 19–3. In one patient the damage was due to a gunshot wound, and neurolysis was performed with full recovery.

Lesions Caused by Injection. In six patients the sciatic nerve lesion was due to an

Table 19–2. CAUSES OF SCIATIC NERVE INJURY (39 PATIENTS)

Cause	Number
Gunshot wound	5
Fracture of the pelvis and luxation of the hip joint	9
Injection	6
Soft tissue wound at the thigh with or without fracture	19
Total	39

Table 19–3. FUNCTIONAL RESULT IN 39 PATIENTS WITH A POST-TRAUMATIC SCIATIC NERVE LESION

| | | | According to Site of Lesion and Type of Operation | | | | |
| | | | Foramen Infrapiriforme | Gluteal Area | Thigh | | |
Level	Results	All Cases	NL + NG	NL (Injection Lesion)	NG	NG + NL	NL
3	Good	28	9	5	7	2	5
3 (T + P)	Tibial and peroneal nerves	6	2	1	2	1	—
3 (T)	Tibial nerve only	22	7	4	5	1	5
2	Satisfactory	6	1	1	3	1	—
1	Poor	5	—	—	4	—	1
0	Nil	—	—	—	—	—	—
Total		39	10	6	14	3	6

NL = neurolysis; NG = nerve graft.

injection and was associated with severe fibrosis. Neurolysis was subsequently performed. In five there was good recovery of the muscles innervated by the tibial nerve. In two patients a tibialis posterior tendon transfer had to be performed because the muscles innervated by the peroneal nerve did not regain sufficient strength.

Lesions Along the Femoral Shaft. Four patients had gunshot wounds and 19 others had soft tissue injuries with or without fracture of the femur. In 14 patients continuity was restored by nerve grafts. In three patients about 90% of the nerve was transected, with some fascicles in continuity. In these cases nerve grafting was combined with neurolysis. Six patients had neurolysis only. (For results see Table 19–3.)

Lesions Caused by Tumor Surgery. Two patients were operated upon because of involvement of the sciatic nerve by a tumor. The nerve was resected and the continuity was restored by nerve grafts (not included in Tables 19–2 and 19–3).

Surgical Exploration. Exploration of the sciatic nerve was done by a curved incision on the lateral border of the gluteal area, crossing the dorsal aspect of the thigh along the groove between the gluteal region and the thigh and going along the dorsal aspect of the thigh in a zig-zag fashion. The sciatic nerve was first explored underneath the lower border of the gluteus maximus muscle. The gluteus maximus muscle was completely exposed by lifting the medially based skin flap. By dissection along the nerve the gluteal muscles were elevated as far proximally as

possible. According to the level of the lesion, one or two incisions were made parallel to the fibers of the gluteus maximus muscle, in order to create windows into this muscle for direct visualization. By this technique it is possible to explore the foramen infrapiriforme without disinsertion or transection of the gluteus maximus muscle. If the foramen suprapiriforme has to be explored, a third window is necessary. Creation of windows causes minimal muscle damage. The exposure of the course of the sciatic nerve along the dorsal aspect of the thigh to the popliteal fossa does not cause damage. Because of the size of the sciatic nerve, it may be difficult to provide a sufficient number of nerve grafts if a longer defect has to be bridged. This is the situation in which allografts are desirable. Since the chance of motor recovery in the peroneal nerve area is minimal with a complete lesion and a longer defect, the peroneal nerve was used as a graft with good success in two patients.

TIBIAL NERVE

Ten patients with tibial nerve lesions were treated. The damage was due to direct trauma (two cases), gunshot wounds (two cases), fracture (two cases), and compression in the form of a compartment syndrome after trauma (two cases). In two other patients the tibial nerve was excised as a tendon graft. In eight patients continuity was restored by nerve grafts, and neurolysis was performed in two patients. The chances for return of useful motor function and protective sensibility are good following treatment of these lesions.

In the two patients in whom the nerve was excised as a tendon graft, defects of 30 and 42 cm, respectively, were bridged by grafts. Both patients regained protective sensibility at the sole; one of them regained motor function of the flexor hallucis longus and flexor digitorum longus muscles (grade M2).

TARSAL TUNNEL SYNDROME

The final branches of the tibial nerve (ramus plantaris tibialis and ramus plantaris fibularis) are occasionally compressed in the tarsal tunnel.[5, 6] Patients have burning pain and hypesthesia in the plantar pedis. Very often pain occurs at night and is improved by movement or by suspending the leg over the bed. Sometimes the course of the tibial nerve along the calf is painful. Two patients were operated upon by opening the tarsal tunnel and performing neurolysis. Symptoms disappeared in both patients following surgery.

SURAL NERVE

One patient was operated upon because of a painful neuroma of the sural nerve after transection of this nerve during operation for varicose veins. The neuroma was resected and the proximal stump was covered with a polyethylene cylinder. The patient has subsequently remained free of pain.

MORTON'S METATARSALGIA

In one patient the symptoms of Morton's metatarsalgia[9] were caused by a neuroma in continuity of the common digital nerve between the third and fourth metatarsal bones. Resection of this area was performed, and the patient remained free of symptoms.

PERONEAL NERVE

The results following peroneal nerve repair are poorer than results following repair of other peripheral nerves. The symptoms of a peroneal palsy (lack of dorsiflexion, lack of extension of the toes, and lack of eversion)

cause much discomfort for the patient. The loss of sensibility is not an important factor. Within a relatively short time, the foot becomes fixed in the equinovarus position by shortening of the nonparalyzed muscles, which now do not work against an antagonist. Although foot drop can be corrected by a peroneal splint, allowing the patient to walk nearly normally, most patients do not easily accept a splint as a permanent solution because they feel that, with the exception of the peroneal palsy, the leg has full strength and motility, and they anticipate return of full function.

No data are available to explain the poor prognosis following peroneal nerve lesions. There is no reason to believe that nerve regeneration develops in a different way in the peroneal nerve, compared with the tibial nerve. On the other hand, it is well known that muscles innervated by the peroneal nerve are much weaker than their opponents. This leads to a spontaneous foot drop with inactivity if patients must stay in bed for an extended period and are not encouraged to do exercises. There is a tendency for the muscles innervated by the peroneal nerve to become overstretched, and even when regeneration does occur, it does not lead to useful function.

Etiology

The following concept of treatment of peroneal nerve lesions is based on 72 cases. Fifty-eight patients had post-traumatic lesions (80%), seven developed peroneal nerve symptoms because of a tumor or tumor surgery (10%), and seven had iatrogenic peroneal nerve palsy (10%). The majority of post-traumatic lesions were caused by traffic or sports accidents. Domestic injuries and gunshot wounds played a minor role. Two patients were lost to follow-up and are therefore excluded from the study. In eleven patients the time of follow-up is too short to evaluate the results. Fifty-nine patients can therefore be evaluated (Table 19–4).

Applied Surgical Techniques[7]

The exposure is usually performed by an excision starting at the lateral border of the popliteal fossa and extending to the calf (far below the course of the peroneal nerve un-

Table 19–4. CAUSES OF PERONEAL NERVE
LESIONS (59 PATIENTS)

Cause	Number
Clean cut (knife, glass, metal sheath)	10
Extensive soft tissue wounds	6
Gunshot wounds	3
Knee injury with rupture of the lateral ligament	9
Closed injuries	4
Fracture of tibia and fibula	1
Fracture of fibula	2
Fracture of tibia and fibula with ischemic muscle damage	1
Varia	2
Long-term peroneal nerve palsies	7
Peroneal nerve palsy due to external pressure (plaster of Paris cast, 4; elastic bandage, 1)	5
Peroneal nerve palsy after surgery	2
Resection of the peroneal nerve during tumor surgery	1
Pressure due to neurinoma of the peroneal nerve	1
Pressure due to cystic tumor of the peroneal nerve	5
Total	59

derneath the head of the fibula) in order to provide a skin flap that covers the nerve after surgery. The incision is continued along the anterolateral aspect in zig-zag fashion, as far as necessary. If a scar is already present along the course of the nerve, the scar is used for the primary incision. After nerve repair, a bipedicled flap is formed to cover the entire course of the nerve, with secondary free split-thickness skin grafts at the dorsal aspect of the calf. The nerve is explored proximal to the lesion along the lateral border of the popliteal fossa. If this portion of the nerve is also damaged, which usually is the case in peroneal nerve lesions associated with an injury to the lateral ligament of the knee joint, the sciatic nerve is explored in the distal third of the thigh and the peroneal nerve portion of the sciatic nerve is defined. Distally, the superficial branch of the peroneal nerve is explored and followed in order to easily locate the main trunk distal to the lesion. The canal for a peroneal nerve is opened and left open after nerve repair. The nerve repair itself is performed according to the guidelines for neurorrhaphy or nerve grafting. In the vast majority of cases, nerve grafts were used.

Achilles Tendon Tenotomy. In all patients in whom a tendency for contracture of the gastrocnemius and soleus muscles were ob-

served, a frontal Z-incision was performed in the Achilles tendon for lengthening.

Tibialis Posterior Tendon Transfer. This is used to correct the equinovarus position and to strengthen the paralyzed peroneal-innervated muscles or protect them against overstretching. By an oblique incision, following the tension line of the skin above the tuberositas ossis navicularis, the insertion of the tibialis posterior tendon is exposed and the tendon is disinserted. The tibialis posterior tendon is defined by an independent incision dorsal to the internal malleolus. The tendon sheath is opened and the tendon is retracted. The same incision is used for Achilles tendon tenotomy and a Z-plasty, if necessary.

A longitudinal incision is made along the medial aspect of the calf from the middle downwards. After transection of the fascia, the gastrocnemius muscle is identified, and the dissection enters the space between the gastrocnemius and soleus, and the deep muscles. At the same time the deep muscles are disinserted from the tibia and the interosseous membrane. A long incision along the fascia is necessary to provide sufficient space to define the tibialis posterior muscle. The tibialis posterior tendon is then retracted from the incision behind the internal malleolus to the incision of the calf.

Another longitudinal incision is made at the ventral aspect of the calf. After incision of the fascia, the dissection enters between the tibialis anterior muscle and the tibial bone, exposing the interosseous membrane. The interosseous membrane is next split longitudinally for about 6 to 8 cm, carefully saving the interosseous vessels. The tibialis posterior tendon is now transferred to the anterior aspect of the calf.

Using two more transverse incisions (at the talo-crural joint and at the dorsum of the foot) the tibialis posterior tendon is brought to the dorsum of the foot lateral to the tibialis anterior tendon and subcutaneous to the crucial ligaments. It is anchored at the cuboid bone by a pull-out wire, which crosses the bone through a drill hole and is fixed externally at the skin of the lateral sole, using a small metal plate and a lead ball.

The crucial factor is to estimate the correct length of the tendon. The tendon should touch the surface of the bone in extreme dorsiflexion. This position is maintained by using a split plaster of Paris cast for 6 days and a plaster of Paris boot for 6 weeks.

This procedure is used as the only operation in patients with long-term peroneal nerve palsies. It is performed as a secondary operation after peroneal nerve repair if no useful functional recovery was achieved, or it is done simultaneously with peroneal nerve repair. In the latter case, with the patient in the lateral position, the peroneal nerve is explored first, the diagnosis and the treatment plan are established, and everything is prepared for grafting. As a second step, the tibialis posterior tendon transfer is performed, except for the insertion of the tendon to the cuboid bone. The nerve grafting procedure is then accomplished, all wounds are closed, and, as a last step, the insertion to the cuboid bone is carried out.

This sequence of steps is followed in order to avoid dislocation of the nerve grafts during the tibialis posterior tendon transfer. After the tendon transfer has been done, the nerve grafting itself can be performed with ease because it is no longer necessary to maintain the foot in the dorsiflexed position, as the bone insertion is not yet accomplished. Finally, after the nerve grafting is completed and all the other incisions are closed, the tendon is inserted into the bone in maximal dorsiflexion, the final wound is closed, and plaster cast immobilization is begun.

Evaluation of Results

The operation is a failure and the result is *poor* if the patient is not able to bring his foot into at least a 90° dorsiflexion and maintain it at that degree. If the patient is able to do this, if lateral stability of the foot is secured, and if there is no tendency for inversion, the result can be regarded as *fair*. This result can be achieved by tibialis posterior tendon transfer alone, with the tibialis posterior tendon performing dorsiflexion and providing active eversion by its eccentric insertion. In a *satisfactory* result, the patient is able to achieve dorsiflexion of more than 90° and has no problems when walking or running. In a *good* result, the function of the foot is nearly normal, and the patient is able to resume all prior activities, including sports. Satisfactory and good results can be achieved by nerve regeneration after neurolysis and in some cases after early nerve repair. In many patients with positive nerve regeneration, proved by electromyography, the functional result remains poor because of overstretching of the muscles.

If nerve repair and tibialis posterior tendon transfer have been performed in the same patient, either secondarily or simultaneously, three levels of results can be distinguished:

1. *Good* result with good nerve regeneration: In this case the tibialis posterior transfer provides active dorsiflexion of over 90°, and all the muscles innervated by the peroneal nerve have recovered full strength. In this situation the tibialis posterior tendon can be transected and relocated again, as was actually done in a few cases.

2. *Satisfactory* result with partial nerve regeneration: In this case the tibialis posterior tendon transfer provides dorsiflexion. All the peroneal-innervated muscles are functioning again and the patient is able to move all his toes, but the strength of the recovery of the tibialis anterior muscle is not sufficient to provide dorsiflexion alone.

3. *Fair* result: In this case the tibialis posterior tendon is responsible for dorsiflexion and the peroneal-innervated muscles have not resumed useful function.

Sensibility does not play an important role in peroneal nerve lesions. It is usually not completely lost, and return of sensibility helps to control the degree of nerve recovery.

Clean Transection of the Peroneal Nerve (Table 19–5)

Ten patients were evaluated because of a clean transection of the peroneal nerve. Two patients were treated by *primary neurorrhaphies*. In both cases the results were unsatisfactory. One patient showed no response, and the other had only nonuseful return of motor function. Both were treated secondarily with tibialis posterior tendon transfers and one also underwent neurolysis. The latter patient had a satisfactory result with partial nerve regeneration; the former had only a fair result without nerve regeneration.

Two patients were treated primarily or within 1 month of the original injury by restoring the continuity with nerve grafts. Both showed good function with full nerve regeneration. A third patient (an 11-year-old boy who had restoration of continuity by nerve grafts within 4 months of injury) had good recovery as well (Fig. 19–1). Two other patients were treated with nerve grafts after

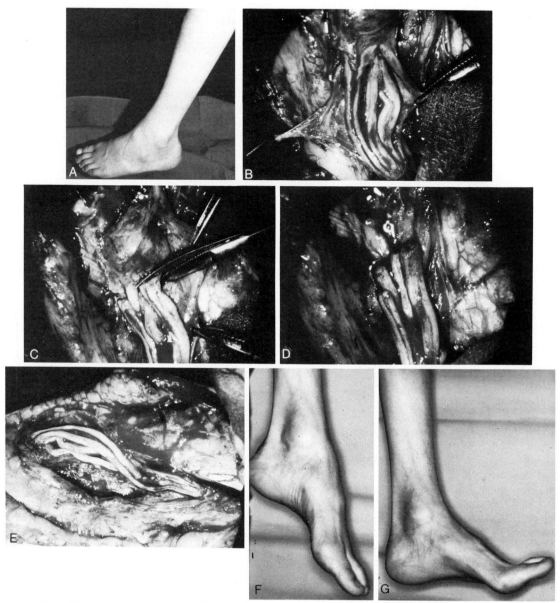

Figure 19–1. Complete paralysis of the left peroneal nerve in an 11-year-old boy due to a clean transection 4 months after injury (see text) (*A*). After longitudinal incision, the epifascicular epineurium is reflected (*B*). Note the different layers. The fascicle groups are exposed. Each one is transected where it merges into the neuroma (*C*). Four fascicle groups are isolated (*D*) and not created (as is sometimes described in textbooks). Each fascicle group is connected with the corresponding one of the distal stump (*E*). Full motor and sensory recovery occurred (*F* and *G*).

Table 19–5. FUNCTIONAL RESULTS AFTER CLEAN TRANSECTION OF THE PERONEAL NERVE
(10 PATIENTS)

Result	Neurorrhaphy	NG Within 4 Months	NG After 4 Months	NG More Than 4 Months After Injury + Simult. TPTT
Good result:				
With good nerve regeneration		3		3
Satisfactory result:				
With partial nerve regeneration				
Fair result:				
With partial nerve regeneration				
Without nerve regeneration				
Poor result:				
With partial nerve regeneration	1*		2‡	
Without nerve regeneration	1†			

*Improved to fair result after NL.
†Improved to fair result after TPTT.
‡One patient improved to a fair result and the other to a good result after secondary TPTT.
NG = nerve graft; TPTT = tibialis posterior tendon transfer.

a time interval of more than 4 months and had only partial, nonuseful nerve regeneration. Secondary tibialis posterior tendon transfer led to a fair result in one patient and to a good result with good nerve regeneration in the other.

The next three patients, who underwent surgery during a time interval between 3 and 7 months after the original injury, were treated by restoring the continuity with nerve grafts and simultaneous tibialis posterior tendon transfers. All three patients had a good result with good nerve regeneration. After 2 years the tibialis posterior tendon was not important for providing functional results.

Loss of Nerve Substance (Table 19–6)

Twenty-one patients suffered a severe loss of nerve substance. These patients can be divided into three groups:

1. Five patients (four with injuries to the knee joint and rupture of the lateral ligament and one with surgical complications) were treated by bridging the long defects by nerve grafts in the usual way. All had less than useful functional recovery. At the time that these patients were treated, tibialis posterior tendon transfers were not being performed.

2. Seven patients (four with nerve defects after extensive loss of soft tissue, one with a pressure sore, one following resection for tumor, and one with a nerve defect associ-

ated with a fracture of the fibula) were also treated by nerve grafts. Five patients had partial nerve regeneration without useful function (Fig. 19–2); in the other two the paralyzed muscles did not respond. A tibialis posterior tendon transfer was performed in all seven patients. Five patients developed good function with good nerve regeneration; one had satisfactory function with partial nerve regeneration; and one had a fair result without nerve regeneration.

3. Nine patients (two with defects due to extensive loss of soft tissue, four with injuries to the knee joint with rupture of the lateral ligament, one with surgical complications, one with a fracture of the fibula, and one with other injuries) were treated by restoring continuity with nerve grafts and simultaneous tibialis posterior tendon transfer. All patients responded well. Five patients had a good result with good nerve regeneration, and four had a satisfactory result with partial nerve regeneration (Fig. 19–3).

An analysis of these cases allows one to conclude that restoring better muscle balance as a result of tibialis posterior tendon transfer has a positive influence on nerve regeneration after nerve grafting.

Lesion in Continuity

Thirteen patients were treated because of a lesion in continuity (Table 19–7). All these

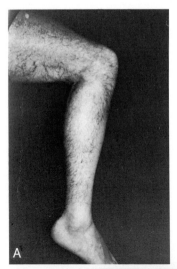

Figure 19–2. Complete paralysis of the peroneus-innervated muscles in a 26-year-old man following an accident (*A*). Exploration revealed a defect within the peroneal nerve of 6 cm, requiring bridging of the defect by cutaneous nerve grafts (*B*). At the lower extremity skin closure is sometimes difficult but should not be forced. Compression and shearing forces must be avoided (*C*). It is better to protect nerve and nerve grafts by a flap (*D*) with a secondary split-thickness skin graft cover (*E*). Nerve regeneration produced a level 2 result (*F* and *G*), which was improved to level 3 by a tibialis posterior tendon transfer.

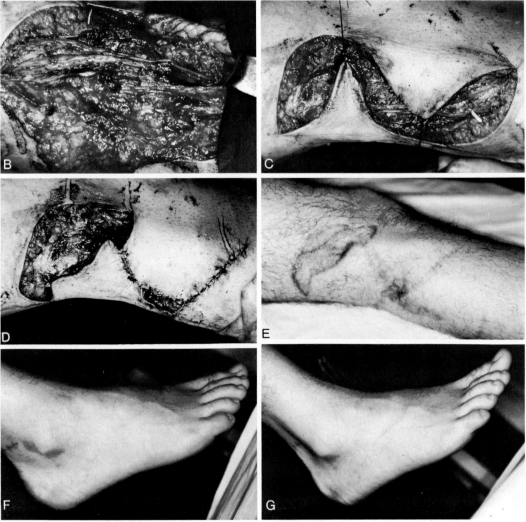

Table 19–6. FUNCTIONAL RESULTS AFTER PERONEAL NERVE LESIONS WITH SEVERE LOSS OF NERVE SUBSTANCE (21 PATIENTS)*

Result	NG Only (1st Series)	NG Only (2nd Series)	Same Patients (2nd Series) After TPTT	NG + Simult TPTT (3rd Series)
Good result: With good nerve regeneration			5	5
Satisfactory result: With partial nerve regeneration			1	4
Fair result: With partial nerve regeneration				
Without nerve regeneration			1	
Poor result: With partial nerve regeneration	5	5		
Without nerve regeneration		2		
Total	5	7	—	9 (= 21)

*All were treated by secondary nerve grafts at more than 4 months after injury.
NG = nerve graft; TPTT = tibialis posterior tendon transfer.

patients had a complete loss of peroneal nerve function clinically. Some remanent innervation could be detected by electromyography in several patients, indicating that some fibers in continuity were still present.

In all these patients the initial operation was a neurolysis. If the nerve looked good, if the patient was young, and if the injury occurred only a few months ago, neurolysis alone was performed. Neurolysis alone was also used for patients whose injuries occurred over a longer time interval but who had only partial nerve lesions without complete denervation. Seven patients fell within this group. If the time interval was longer (more than 6 months), if the patient was older, and if the nerve appeared more damaged, a tibialis posterior tendon transfer was performed simultaneously (see Table 19–7). Six patients fell within this group (marked with a + in Table 19–7). In some patients neurolysis was combined with nerve grafting if partial interruption occurred. All 13 patients responded well and developed good function with good nerve regeneration.

Peroneal Nerve Lesion Due to Pressure by Nerve Tumors

One patient had a peroneal neurinoma that was resected. At the same time the nerve was decompressed, and the continuity of the involved fascicle was restored by a nerve graft. Five patients had varying degrees of palsy and irritation of the peroneal nerve due to a tumor within the nerve underneath the head of the fibula. The symptoms were caused by a cystic tumor (ganglion), which was removed by intraneural neurolysis.[8] All these patients developed good function, and the symptoms of irritation disappeared.

Table 19–7. CAUSES OF PERONEAL NERVE LESIONS IN CONTINUITY (FOR RESULTS, SEE TEXT)

Cause	Neurolysis
Closed injury	4[+]
Gunshot wound	2[+]
Injuries to the knee joint with rupture of the lateral ligament	1
Fracture	1[+]
Other	1
Pressure	4[+++]

[+]Indicates one patient in each group ([+++] means three patients) in whom, in addition to the neurolysis, a tibialis posterior transfer was performed.

Chronic Cases

In seven patients in whom the peroneal nerve lesion occurred 2 to 5 years earlier, no attempt was made to repair the nerve and a

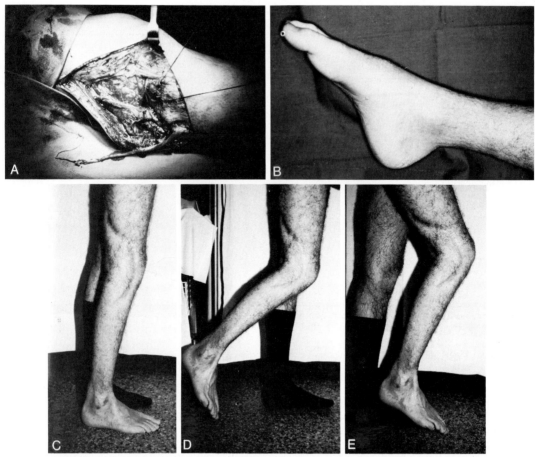

Figure 19–3. Lesion of the lateral ligament of the right knee joint with avulsion of the peroneal nerve following a motorcycle accident involving a 26-year-old man on April 5, 1980. (*A*). Complete paralysis of the peroneal nerve with equino-varus position (*B*) in June 1980. Exploration on June 12, 1980 revealed an 18-cm defect of the peroneal nerve, which was bridged by two cutaneous nerves (sural nerve). Simultaneously, the Achilles tendon was lengthened by Z-plasty and the tibialis posterior tendon was transferred across the interosseous membrane to the dorsum of the foot and anchored in the cuboid bone. Seven months later (*C*) the patient was able to walk normally (*D* and *E*). Note the innervation of the extensor digitorum longus (*D*) when walking.

tibialis posterior tendon transfer alone was performed. Another patient, who had suffered an injury 10 months before, received the same treatment. As a fracture was combined with ischemic damage to the muscles, no reinnervation of the damaged muscles could be expected. All these patients had a fair result.

Postoperative Complications

The above-mentioned results were the final results. Not all patients achieved the final result immediately. In one case fibrosis developed at the site of nerve grafting, and no advancement of the Tinel sign could be observed. The patient underwent surgery again, based on the assumption of a block at the distal side of the graft. The exploration demonstrated complete fibrosis of the entire graft. The graft was resected, and the grafting procedure was repeated along with a tibialis posterior tendon transfer. This was followed by a good result. In several patients the transferred tibialis posterior tendon was too long, and the early functional result was not satisfactory. In these cases the tendon was shortened and reinserted. To avoid a pes planus after tibialis posterior tendon transfer, a mold was prescribed for all patients.

To date, only one patient developed symptoms as a consequence of a tibialis posterior tendon transfer. In this patient the continuity of the nerve was restored by nerve grafts, and a tibialis posterior tendon transfer was performed simultaneously. When symptoms occurred 5 years after this operation, the patient had had a good functional result with full nerve recovery. The tibialis posterior tendon was therefore disinserted, relocated, and reinserted into its original insertion, using a tendon graft.

In summary, in a clean transection of a peroneal nerve, restoration of continuity by nerve grafting has a good chance of achieving a good functional result if the procedure is performed in a young patient very early after injury. In older patients, in patients with longer defects, and in patients in whom the time interval since the original injury was longer than 3 or 4 months, the chances of achieving good nerve and muscle regeneration are increased significantly if a tibialis posterior tendon transfer is carried out simultaneously or as a second step. If continuity is preserved, there is a good chance of recovery in young patients, in patients with partial lesions, and in those with minor degrees of nerve damage (first or second degree, according to Sunderland[11]). If the damage is more severe, if there is a longer time interval since the original injury, and if the patient is older, neurolysis is performed at the same time as the tibialis posterior tendon transfer.

Superficial Branch of the Peroneal Nerve

Two patients were operated upon because of a pain syndrome of the superficial branch of the peroneal nerve. In one patient the nerve was damaged during an osteosynthesis because of a fracture of the fibula. The painful neuroma was resected and the continuity restored by fascicle group neurorrhaphy.

The second patient had an injury of the dorsum pedis caused by glass and associated with a lesion of the superficial branch of the peroneal nerve. A painful neuroma developed. The patient had been operated upon four times before, always with resection of the neuroma. After the fourth operation the painful neuroma was located in the middle of the calf. The neuroma was explored and resected, and the continuity between the proximal stump in the calf and the distal stump at the dorsum pedis was restored by two cutaneous 20-cm nerve grafts. Three years after the operation, the patient is still free of pain.

References

1. Bernhardt, M.: Über isoliert im Gebiete des Nervus cutaneus femoralis externus vorkommende Paraesthesien. Neuro. Zantralbl., *14*:242, 1895.
2. Zollinger, A.: Die Meralgia paraesthetica. Klinisches Bild und Pathogenes anhand von 158 eigenen Fällen. Schweiz. Arch. Neurol. Neurochir. Psychiatry, *87*:58, 1961.
3. Fettweis, E.: Kniegelenk- und Hüftgelenkskontrakturen bei narbiger Irritation des sensiblen Astes des Nervus obturatorius. Dtsch. Med. Wschr., *91*:313, 1966.
4. Gore, D., and Larson, S.: Medial epicondylectomy for subluxing ulnar nerve. Am. J. Surg., 3:851, 1966.
5. Keck, C.: The tarsal tunnel syndrome. J. Bone Joint Surg., *44A*:180, 1962.
6. Lam, S.J.S.: A tarsal tunnel syndrome. Lancet, 2:1354, 1962.
7. Millesi, H.: Unfallschäden peripherer Nerven. *In* Zenker, R., Deucher, F., and Schink, W. (eds.): Chirurgie der Gegenwart, 4th Ed. Munich, Berlin, Vienna, Urban & Schwarzenberg, 1975, pp. 1–75.
8. Millesi, H.: Chirurgische Erkrankungen der peripheren Nerven. *In* Zenker, R., Deucher, F., and Schink, W. (eds.): Chirurgie der Gegenwart, 5th Ed. Munich, Berlin, Vienna, Urban & Schwarzenberg, 1978, pp. 1–38.
9. Morton, T.G.: A peculiar and painful affection of the fourth metatarsophalangeal articulation. Am. J. Med. Sci., *71*:37, 1876.
10. Roth, W. K.: Meralgia paraesthetica. Medskoe Obozr. Sprimona, *43*:678, 1895.
11. Sunderland, S.: A classification of peripheral nerve injuries producing loss of function. Brain, *74*:491, 1951.

20

Surgical Management of Lower Extremity Nerve Lesions (Clinical Evaluation, Surgical Technique, Results)

■

Laurent Sedel, M.D.

Many authors have insisted on the poor prognosis for lower extremity nerve lesion repair. Seddon[6] reported his experience based on 365 lower extremity nerve lesions. Few patients were operated upon, and the results were fair after surgical exploration. He concluded that there was no need to repair severe lower extremity nerve lesions with loss of substance. Major arguments were the risk of increased pain after operation and the fact that lower extremity paralysis, especially involving the sciatic nerve and its branches, can result in an acceptable return of function (64% of patients had a satisfactory result after total sciatic nerve paralysis, 89% after common peroneal nerve paralysis, and 87% after tibial nerve paralysis).

In fact satisfactory cases include the patients "able to walk with special shoes or apparatus with little or no pain, no disabling overreaction to cutaneous stimuli, able to follow up his occupation."[6]

It is true that complete tibial nerve paralysis is compatible with a very good functional result.[2] The only problems are overreaction and hypesthesia, which is sometimes very difficult to control; contact sores are rather rare. Surgical exploration in certain circumstances is then indicated. However, common

peroneal nerve paralysis or sciatic nerve paralysis is responsible for foot drop, and in the case of sciatic nerve paralysis, hypesthesia and contact sores are frequent and may develop many years after injury. Special shoes are not always sufficient and can lead to psychological problems, especially in young adults. Therefore, the best results can come only from nerve recovery.

Microsurgical techniques such as nerve grafting have provided new hope for nerve repair. However, lower extremity nerve lesions still have a poorer prognosis than upper extremity lesions. In fact, it is very difficult to determine results because few series have been published. Millesi presented 16 cases of lower extremity nerve repair with 10 neurotizations but said nothing about the quality of recovery.[4]*

We could not find any large series on lower extremity nerve repair after a search of the recent literature. Therefore, we looked at our own cases. Since 1972 we have operated on 50 lower extremity nerve lesions and have done 23 microsurgical nerve grafts. We will present the indications for surgery, which depend mainly on the etiology, and then the results following our 23 major repairs.

---

*See, however, this volume. *Editor*

MATERIAL AND METHODS

We have seen many patients with lower extremity nerve palsies in whom surgical exploration was not indicated. In some of these patients we did a palliative tendon transfer (i.e., the tibialis posterior on the tibialis anterior tendon) or a talar or subtalar fusion. They included patients with chronic nerve palsy (lasting more than 2 years), patients with partially recovered palsies, or those with pain problems in whom surgical exploration was not recommended. Other patients for whom surgical exploration of the nerve lesions was not indicated are those who recovered spontaneously after acute compression (hip or knee surgery, knee splinting, hip dislocation).

The remaining patients underwent surgical exploration because of various etiologic circumstances (Table 20–1). They are all referred patients except for a few who were treated for acute compression.

We will first present the management of nerve lesions based on the etiology and clinical features and then will analyze separately the involving nerve grafts to better understand the functional results that can be expected at the time of microsurgery.

CLINICAL FEATURES OF DIFFERENT LESIONS

Traumatic Lesions

Clean Wounds (Table 20–2). We have operated on six patients with clean nerve wounds: two patients with wounds involving the sciatic nerve, three with common peroneal nerve wounds, and one with a tibial nerve wound.

Two cases were iatrogenic, involving the common peroneal nerve: one section during stripping of the lateral sural vein and one section during a fibula transfer as a bone graft for anterior spinal fusion. In all cases, the nerve lesion was noted after the original accident, and the nerve was never explored as part of the emergency procedure. In one case the diagnosis was made 6 months later.

At examination, the paralysis was complete in at least one neurologic region in all six patients: complete paralysis of the common peroneal nerve in two patients, complete paralysis of the anterior tibial nerve in one, complete paralysis of the sciatic nerve in one, complete common peroneal and partial tibial nerve paralysis in one, and complete paralysis of the gastrocnemius muscle in one.

Three of these patients were children (7, 9, and 10 years old). The result is very good in two patients (case 6 [Fig. 20–1] and case 5), good in one (case 2), and unknown in three patients for whom the follow-up is insufficient.

Missile Injuries. Missile injuries are responsible for more or less complete immediate paralyses that sometimes recover spontaneously. The anatomic lesion can result in a section or in transient vascular damage due to the blast injury. A section can be partial because of the large size of the sciatic nerve,

Table 20–1. SURGICAL EXPLORATION OF LOWER EXTREMITY NERVE LESIONS

Etiology	No.	Emergency	Referred Case	Sciatic Nerve	Common Peroneal Nerve	Tibial Nerve	Graft	Neurolysis
Clean wound	6		5	2	3	1	6	
Missile wound	4		4	3		1	2	2
Traction injuries	9		9	1	8		8	1
Crush injury	3		3	2		1	2	1
Ischemia	2		2		2		2	
Acute compression	5	5		4 + (1 femoral)				5
Chronic compression	5		3	1	2	2		5
Tumor	6		6	1 + (1 femoral)	1	3	3	2 + (1 excision without repair)
Leprosy	10		10		10			10
Total	50		42	14 + (2 femoral)	26	8	23	26 + (1 excision of tumor)

Table 20–2. CLEAN WOUND LESIONS

| Patient (Case No.) | Age (years) | Sex | Palsy | Nerve Involved | Repair | | | | | Prede- gener- ated | Results | | | | |
					Delay	Graft	Length	No. of Cables			Follow-up	Motor	Sensory	Comments
ANB (1)	7	M	CPN + partial TN	Sciatic	45 days	Partial	3 cm	5		Yes	4 months			
CAC (2)*	9	M	Sciatic	Sciatic	2 months	Complete	6 cm	8		Yes	3 years	Grade 5 Grade 0	S3 S0	TN CPN good
CAR (3)	50	M	CPN	CPN	2 months	Complete	4 cm	5		Yes	None			
GUI (4)	19	M	CPN	CPN	8 months	Complete	2 cm	4		No	None			
HOU (5)	24	M	Triceps surae	TN	11 months	Partial	4 cm	3		Yes	16 months	Grade 4	S2	Very good
KOW (6)	10	M	Deep pero- neal	CPN	6 months	Partial	2 cm	2		No	24 months	Grade 5	S3	Very good

*This patient was operated on by Dr. J. Witvoet.
CPN = common peroneal nerve; TN = tibial nerve.

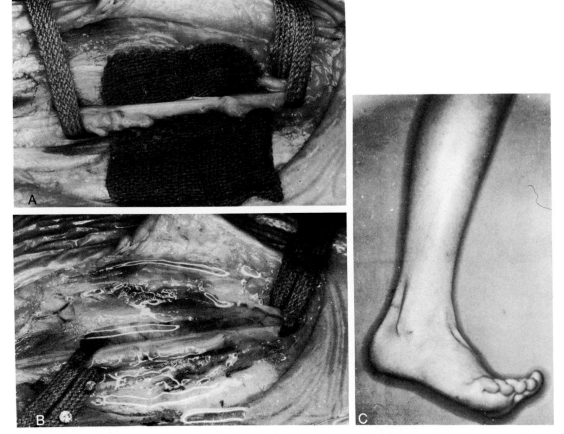

Figure 20–1. Case 6 (see text and Table 20–2). A 10-year-old child presented with a complete deep peroneal nerve paralysis 6 months after a scissors point injury. *A,* At exploration, we found a partial section of the common peroneal nerve involving the fascicles for the deep peroneal nerve. *B,* Graft: aspect of the two cables. *C,* Results after 12 months: motor and sensory recovery is nearly complete.

and it is always difficult to appreciate the extent and the severity of the nerve damage during emergency exploration. In addition, debris from clothes increases the risk of sepsis after repair. For all reasons, we prefer not to explore missile injuries of nerves as an emergency procedure. We choose to wait for 3 to 5 weeks, as the clinical features are generally clearer. In many instances the paralysis recovers spontaneously, which can be documented by clinical and electrical examinations. The Tinel-Hoffmann sign progresses and there is no need for nerve exploration. On the other hand, in some instances the palsy remains unchanged, the Tinel-Hoffmann sign does not progress, and the electromyogram confirms the absence of recovery. If nothing changes after 2 months (even in one partial area), surgical exploration is indicated. The procedure consists of a wide exposure of the nerve at the Tinel-Hoffmann

site, dissection of the nerve in a noninjured area, and then fine dissection carried out under a microscope. Electrical stimulation is very useful during the operation. Thus, it is possible to differentiate noninjured fascicles from injured ones with neuroma formation. The neuromas are excised, and the injured fascicles are repaired by interfascicular grafting.

We have operated on four patients with missile injuries of lower extremity nerves (Table 20–3), two for persistent paralysis after a few months and two for persistent severe pain. Two partial grafts of the sciatic nerve were done: one had a good result (Fig. 20–2), the other is unknown. The two patients operated on for persisting pain were satisfied with the degree of relief obtained, although they continue to have some pain.

Traction Injuries. Traction injuries of the common peroneal nerve due to adduction of

Table 20–3. MISSILE INJURIES

| Patient (Case No.) | Age (years) | Sex | Palsy | Pain | Delay | Repair | | | | Neurolysis | Follow-up | Results | Comments |
						Graft	Length	No. of Cables	Prede-generated				
DAU (7)	31	F	Sciatic (triceps 2, flexor digito-rum 2)	0	8 months	Partial of the sciatic	6 cm	6	Yes		Insufficient		
DEOL (8)	24	M	CPN	0	2 months	Partial of the sciatic	3.5 cm	4	Yes		20 months	T.A. 4+ per-oneus L et B 5 ext. H.L. ext. D.L. 4	Good results
TES (9)	28	F	TP	+++	8 months	Partial of the TP				Excision of the neuroma	10 months	Pain +	Good result
ROUV (10)	30	M	Sciatic (partial triceps, 3)	+++	3 years					External neu-rolysis	2 years	Pain + palsy unchanged	

CPN = common peroneal nerve; TP = posterior tibial nerve.

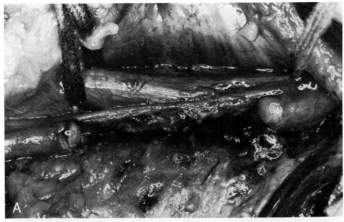

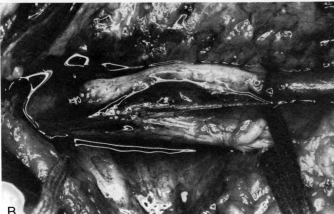

Figure 20–2. Case 8 (see text and Table 20–2). A 24-year-old man sustained a bullet injury of the thigh with an immediate common peroneal nerve (CPN) palsy. Two months later we operated and found a neuroma of the common peroneal nerve and the sural nerve. After resection (*A*) we performed a 3.5 cm graft with four cables (*B*). Good function of the tibialis anterior and all muscles innervated by the CPN was restored, but the ankle is stiff and we plan to perform a tendo-Achilles lengthening.

the knee were first described by Platt.[5] Seddon considered that repair is impractical in these injuries because of the extent of the lesion and the associated vascular damage to the leg.[1]

We must emphasize that spontaneous recovery is frequent and that surgical repair must never be carried out as an emergency procedure, even if the nerve appears badly damaged at the time of exploration for ligament suture. Proper management is to repair the ligaments, vessels, and muscles. During rehabilitation, regular clinical and electrical examinations are carried out, and if there is no clinical or electrical recovery associated with a nonmigrating Tinel-Hoffmann sign, surgical exploration is indicated.

The exploration must be carried out using a very long incision. Palpation and dissection of the nerve determine whether a rupture is present and, if so, where to transect the nerve in a healthy zone. Generally the traction injury involves the common peroneal nerve from the sciatic division to the neck of the fibula; thus, the loss of substance is very

extensive (7 to 20 cm with a mean of 15 cm in our experience) (Fig. 20–3).

We have repaired nine traction injuries, eight of the common peroneal nerve and one of both distal branches of the sciatic nerve. One neurolysis and eight grafts were done (Table 20–4 and Fig. 20–4).

The result after neurolysis was very good; however, we must note that exploration after 6 months discovered a very badly damaged nerve that did not recover after neurolysis. Of the four patients with sufficient follow-up, two had a satisfactory result, one fair, and one poor. This last patient had a nerve rupture and compartmental syndrome associated with popliteal artery rupture. We had to perform a tibialis posterior transfer in one patient who recovered in whom dorsiflexion was strong but control insufficient. The transfer permitted return of full function. Actually we think it is possible to obtain a good result even in these patients if the nerve resection is large enough to enable the suture to be made in an uninjured zone. We try to use the upper part of the sural nerve with its

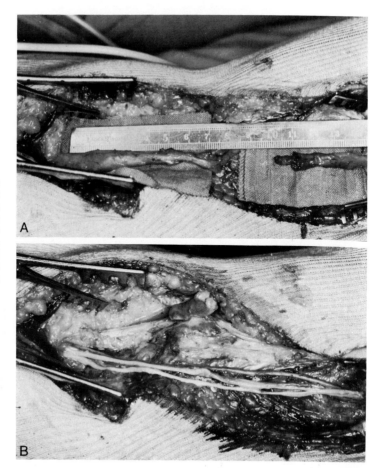

Figure 20–3. Case 15 (see text and Table 20–2). A 33-year-old man sustained a ligament tear of his right knee with a complete paralysis of the CPN. Six months later, we explored the nerve and found a severe traction lesion (*A*). After resection the loss of substance was 15 cm long. We performed a graft with four cables (*B*). The follow-up has been too short to evaluate results.

vessels, similar to a vascularized graft. This was possible in our last two patients.

Two patients in whom follow-up is insufficient showed electrical signs of regeneration.

Other Traumatic Injuries (Table 20–5). Sciatic nerve palsies can occur after hip fracture, posterior hip dislocation, or hip surgery, e.g., total hip replacement. Generally, palsy is due to neurapraxia, which will recover spontaneously. Rarely, it is due to a section or traction lesion of the lumbosacral plexus. To establish the diagnosis, a sacroradiculogram has been proposed in some instances. This shows a meningeal pouch in cases of lower root avulsion. The prognosis is not always poor, as Harris et al. have shown that recovery can be expected even when these pouches are present.[3]

Indications for nerve exploration at the buttock are very rare. We attempted this procedure once in order to repair the inferior gluteal nerve, but were not successful. We have explored the sciatic nerve after severe femoral shaft fracture, in one case when all the soft tissue of the posterior thigh had been avulsed and there was a 22-cm loss of substance of the sciatic nerve. We used the common peroneal nerve to graft the posterior tibial nerve. The patient recovered a very slight protective sensibility of the sole of the foot.

Another patient had a complete sciatic nerve paralysis after a femoral shaft fracture. Seven months later we found a large neuroma in continuity at exploration and performed an internal neurolysis. Some months later the patient recovered completely. Another patient had contact sores and hypesthesia complicating a severe tibial fracture with a complete lesion of the posterior tibial nerve. We performed a graft of this nerve 5 years later, with a fair result.

Two other patients presented with severe ischemic lesions, one of whom had a complete paralysis of the deep peroneal nerve as a result of severe compression. We performed a partial graft of this nerve. The result

Table 20–4. TRACTION INJURIES

Patient (Case No.)	Age (years)	Sex	Injury	Palsy	Delay	Repair Graft or Neurolysis	Length	No. of Cables	Vascularized	Predegenerated	Results Follow-up	Motor	Sensory	Palliative Transfer	Comment
SOL (11)	20	F	Knee, ligament tears	CPN	3 months	G	15 cm	2	No	Yes	26 months	4 +	S2	0	Very good
LER (12)	21	F	Ligament tears	CPN	6 months	G	7 cm	4	No	No	3 years	4	S2	+	Good
GUY (13)	17	F	Knee dislocation	CPN	11 months	G	15 cm	4	No	No	21 months	0	0	+	Compartmental syndrome
DOS (14)	18	M	Ligament tears	CPN	6 months	G	7 cm	3	No	No	21 months	TA: 2 PL: 4 Ext. HL: 2	0	0	Fair
LEP (15)	33	M	Ligament tears	CPN	6 months	G	15 cm	4	No	No	None				
LAG (16)	16	M	Ligament tears	CPN	12 months	G	16 cm	4	One	No	None				
BOU (17)	30	M	Ligament tears	CPN	3 months	G	20 cm	5	Two	No	None				
DUD (18)	17	M	Fracture of femur	Sciatic	7 months	G Partial	13 cm	1	CP on PT	Yes	None				
CHE (19)	18	M	Ligament tears	CPN	6 months	N					24 months	5	4		Complete recovery

CPN = common peroneal nerve; TA = tibialis anterior; PL = peroneus longus; Ext. HL = extensor hallicis longus; CP = common peroneal; PT = posterior tibial.

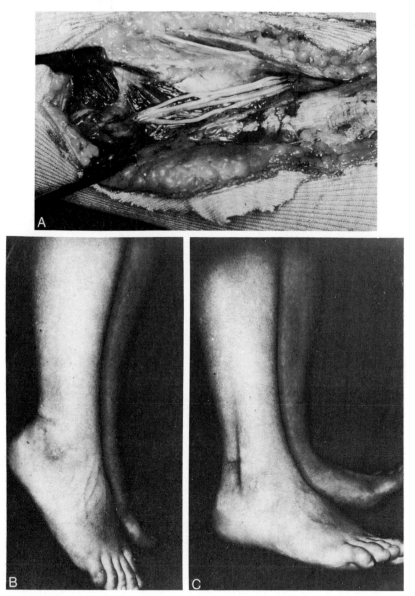

Figure 20–4. Case 12 (see text and Table 20–2). A 21-year-old woman sustained a severe ligament tear of her right knee with complete CPN palsy. Six months later, we explored the nerve and found a severely damaged nerve. We did a 7 cm graft with four cables (*A*). After 3 years, the result is good and powerful (*B* and *C*). However, the harmony was only fair, so we had to perform a tibialis posterior transfer on the tibialis anterior to achieve an excellent result. She can now run easily and participate in many sports.

Table 20–5. MISCELLANEOUS TRAUMATIC INJURIES

Patient (Case No.)	Age (years)	Sex	Type of Injury	Palsy	Delay	Repair				Follow-up	Results		Comment
						Graft	Neurolysis	Length	No. of Cables		Motor	Sensory	
CAL (20)	17	M	Femoral fracture + avulsion	Sciatic complete	28 months	TP		22 cm	1 (CPN)	19 months	0	S1	
THE (21)	20	M	Femoral fracture	Sciatic complete	7 months		+			12 months	M5	S4	Complete recovery
SÂK (22)	26	M	Tibial fracture	TP pain	5 years	+		8 cm	3	33 months	0	S1	Fair
YAK (23)	20	M	Compression lesion	Deep peroneal	6 months	+ TA		24 cm	1	5 years	M4	S2	Had a palliative transfer
AUG (24)	63	F	Knee fracture, splint compression	CPN	10 months	+		5 cm	3	34 months	0	0	Skin badly damaged

CPN = common peroneal nerve; TP = tibialis posterior; TA = tibialis anterior.

was very good clinically and electrically, but another surgeon performed a tibialis posterior tendon transfer six months later.

The other patient had a complete common peroneal paralysis due to a compressive splint and a contact sore. The skin was badly damaged, and the nerve underneath was completely fibrotic. We performed a graft that was applied in a healthy muscular bed; however, there was no recovery.

Acute or Chronic Nerve Compression

Acute Compressions Due to Plaster Casts, Splints, or Hematoma. The common peroneal nerve paralysis due to a tight splint or plaster cast is generally reversible if the compression is relieved quickly after the first signs. Recovery is longer if the compression has been maintained for more than 6 hours. In this event, the paralysis can remain for a few months or even permanently.

Acute Compression of the Sciatic Nerve by a Hematoma. This is a rather frequent complication of anticoagulation therapy. We have operated on six patients with lesions of this type. Three were due to anticoagulation therapy alone without any associated surgical procedure. The sciatic nerve was involved in two patients, the femoral nerve in one. In three other patients the lesions developed a few days after major hip surgery (repair of acetabulum fracture, total hip replacement, cup arthroplasty). In all these patients an emergency procedure was carried out, but the procedure was delayed in two patients because of the hazards associated with anticoagulation therapy.

The results were good and recovery was rapid if the compression was released within 6 hours. Within 12 hours, surgical release may still be helpful, but the results are less convincing. If the patient cannot be operated on within 12 hours, it is better not to attempt surgery. Generally, recovery will take place within 1 or 2 years. If there are any remaining complications, such as hypesthesia, it is possible to perform an intraneural neurolysis at that time. We did one such procedure at 2 years, with a rather good result as far as reducing pain was concerned.

Chronic Compression or Entrapment Neuropathy. Entrapment neuropathy of the leg is less frequent than of the arm. We have operated on four patients with entrapment lesions at two locations.

Two lesions involved the common peroneal nerve at the neck of the fibula. The associated clinical features were pain, muscle atrophy and disability, a positive Tinel-Hoffmann sign, and slow electrical conduction rates at this level. The patients were 19 and 62 years old, respectively. After operation one recovered within 3 months, the other one had only partial recovery.

Two lesions involved the posterior tibial nerve at the tarsal tunnel. Both were late consequences of tibial fracture treated by a plaster cast. Release of the tarsal tunnel was followed by complete recovery and disappearance of pain.

These chronic compressions can also be located on the posterior tibial nerve at the soleus arcade. The problem is to differentiate nerve entrapment and compartmental syndromes, especially when the lateral compartment of the leg is involved.

Lower Extremity Nerve Tumors

We have operated on six nerve tumors of the leg. The predominating clinical feature can be a progressive palsy, a tumor, or progressive pain. In the case of pain the diagnosis can be difficult if a sciatic radiculalgia is present, and the tumor is therefore diagnosed late.

Four tumors were benign schwannomas, three of which were excised. Two of these involved the posterior tibial nerve, which was kept intact after intraneural neurolysis. The third excised tumor involved the femoral nerve and was a giant intra- and extramedullary neurinoma. We excised this tumor completely, and there has been no recurrence after 4 years. Another schwannoma, in a 45-year-old woman, was of the plexiform type and developed in the common peroneal nerve branch. It was not possible to salvage the nerve. After excision, we performed an 18-cm graft using three cables. The patient was lost to follow-up.

Two tumors were classified as malignant. One occurred in a 25-year-old man who developed a large tumor of the sciatic nerve at the thigh. We did a large en bloc resection and then a graft with two cables 20 cm long. Four years later there was no recovery but rather a tumor recurrence at the distal part of the graft. We then did another en bloc resection. This patient has now been followed for 3 years.

Another malignant tumor developed in a 67-year-old woman on the tibial nerve at the popliteal level. We excised the tumor and the nerve completely, using an en bloc excision (Fig. 20–5). We then did a graft 10 cm long with seven cables. This patient has been followed for over 2 years. There has been no recurrence of tumor. Recovery of the gastrocnemius and return of some protective sensibility of the foot have occurred.

Lower Extremity Leprosy Palsies

Leprosy involving the nerves of the leg is less frequent than that of the arm. However, it is not uncommon. We have seen numerous patients with old lesions in whom we did palliative procedures.

We have operated on ten patients. Indications are recurring pain or recent palsy (less than 2 years). It is very important to begin medical treatment before surgery, as in some cases this will eliminate the need for surgery.

The surgical exposure must be very long, extending from the thigh to the neck of the fibula. The common peroneal nerve is generally involved; sometimes the posterior tibial nerve is also involved. We do not use microsurgical techniques but only do an epineurotomy without intrafascicular dissection. Re-

sults are known for ten patients. Pain disappeared in five of six patients. Motor recovery was good in six of seven patients, and sensory recovery occurred in four of seven patients. It seems that a poor prognosis is related to the extent of the lesion and to limited epineuriectomy.

DISCUSSION

Repair of lower extremity nerve lesions was not recommended previously because of the unimpressive results noted by Seddon (only 30% classified as good). However, by using microsurgical techniques and nerve grafting and by waiting more than 18 months after surgical repair, the result is apparently good enough in many instances to provide strong evidence that these nerves must be repaired.

Some authors have pointed out that nerve repair can lead to increase in pain, particularly of the sole of the foot. This is true for posterior tibial nerve repair, and for this nerve alone not doing a repair may be better in some instances. Nonetheless, we prefer to repair this nerve and to tell the patient that pain can increase during the recovery period, which lasts 1 to 2 years. Then the pain diminishes.

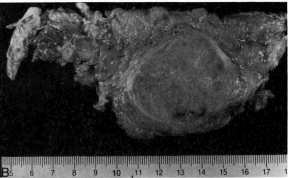

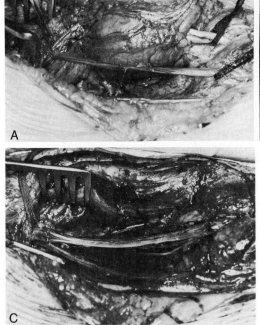

Figure 20–5. A 67-year-old woman presented with a mass in the inferior part of the thigh. Biopsy revealed a shwannosarcoma and she was referred to us. One month after the biopsy we performed an en bloc resection of the tumor, which had developed on the tibial nerve (*A* and *B*). After resection there was a 10 cm loss of substance. We performed a graft with five cables (*C*). The follow-up is now 2 years without recurrence and with partial recovery of sensation.

Pain can also be a problem after sciatic nerve repair. However, there are now many ways to treat nerve pain (e.g., drugs, stimulation), and we prefer to restore nerve function even if some pain develops and to tell the patient of this eventuality. In fact, pain can be a major problem without nerve repair, and one of the best ways to cure it is to approximate the nerve ends or even use a graft.

Results. It is true that the patient with a foot drop or a complete sciatic nerve paralysis is able to walk. However, the disability may interfere with sports or the patient's social life or affect the esthetic appearance of the leg.

We think that the best solution is to repair the nerve. If the result is very good, there will be no need for a further operation. If the result is partial, contact sores are still avoided, and even with a limited palliative procedure the result can be very good. If nerve repair fails, the patient has lost nothing.

The overall results for 23 grafts of lower extremity nerve lesions are known for 12 patients. We must wait 18 months for a distal branch common peroneal or posterior tibial nerve repair and 2 years for a sciatic trunk repair before evaluating results. They were classified as very good (nearly full recovery) in four patients, good (full recovery even with one transfer) in two patients, fair in two patients, and a failure in four patients. The four failures involved very severe defects (two grafts more than 20 cm in length, one associated with a compartmental ischemic syndrome and the other with skin and nerve necrosis).

Even after large loss of nerve substance caused by traction injuries, good results (one good and one very good) were obtained in this series.

CONCLUSIONS

The management of lower extremity nerve lesions is not very different from management of upper extremity lesions when microsurgical techniques are used. The different points to be emphasized are:

1. Many lower extremity nerve palsies recover without surgery. The indications for surgery must therefore be very accurate.

2. All complete lower extremity nerve lesions need to be repaired.

3. Very fine surgery is needed, and the nerve must be transected in a healthy zone, especially for traction injuries, which are very frequent.

4. Local vascularized grafts should be done using the sural nerve or its accessory branch by rerouting its ends.

5. A compressing hematoma must be evacuated as an emergency procedure within the first hours after injury to achieve quick and complete recovery.

6. Diagnosis may be difficult in nerve tumors, chronic nerve entrapment, upper sciatic lesions or roots, and after major hip surgery or hip trauma. In these cases, electromyograms may be of great assistance.

7. This type of procedure is rather easy surgery, with the patient lying in the prone position and the donor nerve being in the same area as the injured nerve.

References

1. Clawson, D. K., and Seddon, H. J.: The results of repair of the sciatic nerves. J. Bone Joint Surg., 42B:205, 1960.
2. Clawson, D. K., and Seddon, H. J.: The late consequences of sciatic nerve injury. J. Bone Joint Surg., 42B:213, 1960.
3. Harris, W. R., Rathbun, J. B., Wortzman, G., and Humphrey, J. G.: Avulsion of lumbar roots complicating fracture of the pelvis. J. Bone Joint Surg., 55A:1436, 1973.
4. Millesi, H.: Traitement des lésions nerveuses par greffes libres fasciculaires. In Michon, J., and Moberg, E. (eds.): Les Lésions Traumatiques des Nerfs Périphériques. Monographies du G. E. M., 2nd Ed. Paris, Expansion Scient., 1980.
5. Platt, H.: On the peripheral nerve complications of certain fractures. J. Bone Joint Surg., 10:403, 1928.
6. Seddon, H.: Surgical Disorders of the Peripheral Nerves, 2nd Ed. London, Churchill Livingstone, 1975.
7. Sedel, L.: Résultats des greffes nerveuses du sciatiques Communication à la journée d'hiver de la Société Française de Chirurgie Orthopédique et Traumatologique, January 10, 1981.
8. Sedel, L., and Bricout, N.: Résultats des greffes de gros troncs nerveux. Ann. Chir. Plast., 26:341, 1981.

21

Functioning Muscle Transplantation to the Arm

■

Ralph T. Manktelow, M.D., F.R.C.S.(C)

Successful transplantation of functioning muscle is an improbable procedure. The many factors that should affect both survival and useful function could be expected to make the results of this procedure unreliable. The requirement that a transplanted muscle not only survive, but duplicate the precise function of the missing muscle, may be unrealistic. Nevertheless, there have been a few muscle transplantations that have come close to simulating this requirement.

Free muscle transplantation is a procedure that involves the transfer of a skeletal muscle from one site to another with complete sep-

aration of the muscle from its normal location. Circulation is maintained by microvascular anastomosis of artery and vein of the transplanted muscle to a suitable artery and vein in the recipient site. Reinnervation and active muscle contraction are produced by suturing an undamaged motor nerve in the recipient site to the motor nerve of the transplanted muscle. When muscle transplantation is used in the forearm to replace missing finger flexor musculature, the muscle is fixed to the medial epicondyle and to the flexor digitorum profundus tendons in the forearm or wrist. With reinnervation, voluntary mus-

Figure 21–1. Case M. T. Four-year-old boy with severe Volkmann's ischemic contracture, shown with gracilis muscle prior to transplantation to forearm.

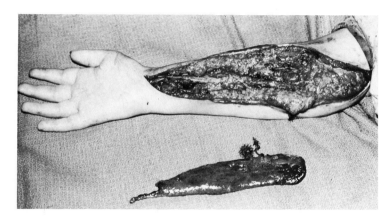

cle contraction produces finger flexion. Muscle transplantation by microvascular anastomosis, without reinnervation, has been used to provide soft tissue coverage and bulk. In functioning muscle transplantation, the muscle is reinnervated and is capable of active contraction.

In 1970, Tamai et al.[12] reported successful muscle transplantation by microneurovascular techniques in the dog. Histologic and electromyographic studies established that the muscles survived and underwent satisfactory reinnervation. In 1973, a portion of the pectoralis major muscle was transplanted to the human forearm by surgeons at the Sixth People's Hospital in Shanghai.[11] The principal author examined this patient 3 years later and observed good muscle bulk, range of finger flexion, and grip strength. In 1973, Harii et al.[3] did the first successful functioning muscle transplantation for reanimation of facial paralysis. Subsequently, Ikuta et al.,[4, 5] Schenck,[10] O'Brien,[9] and Manktelow and McKee[6, 7] reported clinical cases. Ikuta et al.[5] described eight cases of muscle transplantation to the arm. Although six were described as successful, a functional evaluation of the cases was not reported. Schenck[10] described a single case of rectus femoris transplantation without any follow-up. In 1978, Terzis et al.[13] studied muscle transplantation in rabbits. Their quantitative assessment of the function of transplanted muscle provided a new understanding of the factors that govern success. Gordon and Buncke[1] employed nerve grafts to reinnervate the transplanted gastrocnemius muscle in monkeys. Four of the six muscles survived and two had functional capability.

In 1978, we described two cases of muscle transplantation with partial functional evaluation[6] (Fig. 21–2). The gracilis muscle was used in one case to replace the long flexors of the fingers. The patient developed a grip strength of 35 lb and a nearly full range of finger motion. The other patient, who had a pectoralis major transplantation to the forearm, had nearly full finger flexion and increasing grip strength at the time of reporting. After observing these two patients for over 1 year, we were sufficiently encouraged by the functional results to do an additional 21 muscle transplantations. In total, 15 transplantations were done to replace forearm

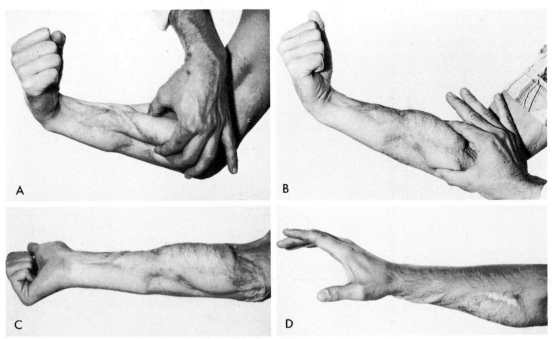

Figure 21–2. Case R. G. Gracilis muscle transplantation to forearm attached to flexor digitorum profundus and innervated by anterior interosseous nerve. (Preliminary report in J. Hand Surg., 3:416–426, 1978.) Long-term follow-up demonstrates increase in muscle bulk from (A) 10 months postoperatively to (B) 30 months postoperatively. Gracilis muscle palpated between examiner's fingers is 6 cm wide. Muscle provides full finger flexion in wrist flexion. C, wrist extension–grip strength is 42 pounds. D, Muscle allows finger extension with wrist extended, indicating the excellent excursion of the transplanted muscle. (From Manktelow, R. T.: Clin. Plast. Surg., 11:61, 1984.)

musclature. One muscle transplantation was used to replace the anterior compartment muscle of the lower leg and seven transplantations were used for facial reanimation.

This chapter will discuss muscle transplantation to the extremity, with emphasis on patient selection and operative technique. Twelve patients with forearm transplantations have been followed for a mean period of 3 years and form the basis for a detailed review of functional results.

INDICATIONS FOR MUSCLE TRANSPLANTATION

This procedure should be used for patients who have sustained a major loss of skeletal musculature that results in a significant functional deficit that cannot be adequately replaced by a simpler procedure, such as tendon transfer.

The usual causes of muscle loss are direct trauma to the muscle compartments, Volkmann's ischemic paralysis, major electrical burns, post-replantation, and gas gangrene. Muscle transplantation has also been tried in the treatment of brachial palsy. Gilbert and Narakas have transplanted the gracilis to replace the biceps in patients with brachial plexus injuries. Nerve grafts connected uninjured proximal nerves to the muscle. The muscles did not develop a functional range of contraction.

The type of patient who is suitable for this operation is one who has sustained a major injury to the forearm with loss of all flexor musculature and some damage to the extensor musculature. The median and ulnar nerves are undamaged, leaving good sensibility and intrinsic function to an uninjured hand. The primary functional problem is lack of grip capability. Local tendon transfers have been ruled out as a result of muscle injury.

Proper patient selection is important. If the extremity will become significantly more functional by the addition of a single functioning muscle, it is worth considering muscle transplantation. The rules that govern successful tendon transfers must be followed. There must be a good range of passive joint motion, adequate muscles for proximal joint stability and balance, good skin cover and bed for tendon gliding, and adequate hand sensibility. If the muscle is to be used to provide good finger flexion, there must be

a mechanism for finger and thumb extension, intrinsic muscle balance, and wrist stabilization. In this situation, the addition of a functioning muscle can create a functioning hand.

The personality, work requirements, and motivation of the patient are important in determining the suitability for operation. The patient must be well motivated to pursue the prolonged postoperative course of resisted exercises that must precede useful hand function.

OPERATIVE TECHNIQUE

The description of operative technique will apply to the forearm, as this is the most common site of transplantation. However, the principles of technique are the same for any site of extremity transplantation.

Assessment of Recipient Site

All structures that will be involved in the transplantation must be evaluated. This includes an assessment of the likely location of the arterial and venous vasculature, available motor nerves, and the expected location of the flexor tendon stumps in the forearm or wrist. If the vasculature of the forearm is not clearly established, a preoperative arteriogram is required to select a suitable artery for anastomosis. Either end-to-side or end-to-end anastomoses are suitable. Adequate veins may be found either as venae comitantes or as superficial veins in the forearm. The history and physical examination should indicate which motor nerve branches are likely to be present in the forearm. In two of our patients, a preliminary exploration was done to establish the status of the motor nerve. Histologic examination indicated that the anterior interosseous nerve was virtually normal in both patients and the transplantation was considered feasible. The anterior interosseous nerve is protected from injury by its deep position and is frequently available for transplantation despite severe forearm trauma. In some cases, the nerves used were other motor branches of the median or ulnar nerves. The sine qua non for proceedings with a muscle transplantation is the presence of an undamaged motor nerve that can be used to reinnervate the transplanted muscle. The presence and location of tendons can usually be determined from the physical examination. It is important that good skin flap coverage be available over the distal half of the forearm to allow tendon gliding at the junction between the muscle and the flexor tendons. This may require application of a skin flap prior to the muscle transplantation to provide good coverage, or the muscle may be taken as a myocutaneous flap.

The anticipated positions of the muscle must be outlined on the forearm, and the probable location of each of the vascular, nerve, and tendon structures is marked on the forearm (Fig. 21–3). A pattern of the desired muscle is taken from the forearm. This outlines the shape and size of the muscle and the location of structures to be repaired. This pattern is then matched to the muscles that are available for transfer and the most suitable one is selected.

Preparation of the Forearm

The forearm incision should be designed to allow adequate exposure of all structures and to create suitable skin flaps for coverage of the distal portion of the muscle and muscle-tendon junction. If the muscle to be transplanted will carry a cutaneous flap with it, the design of this flap should be incorporated in the forearm incision. Frequently, a split-thickness skin graft over the proximal portion of the muscle will provide adequate muscle coverage.

Vessels, nerves, and tendons are then prepared for the transplantation. In the scarred forearm, this preparation requires meticulous dissection under tourniquet control. A dissection from proximal to distal, beginning in an undamaged area, will provide the safest exposure of the desired vessels and nerves. Of necessity, the dissection is tedious if vital

structures are to be prepared without damage. Exposure of the anterior interosseous artery or nerve is facilitated by temporarily separating remnants of the pronator teres from its insertion. As the dissection and freeing up of venae comitantes to the anterior interosseous artery can be frustrating because of the many cross connections, the availability of a superficial vein will simplify the preparation. If an end-to-end anastomosis is planned, the artery should be divided and the forcefulness of the spurt of blood evaluated. If this is not normal, a more proximal position must be tried on the artery or another artery selected. This is a valuable test of the adequacy of blood flow in a damaged artery. Unfortunately, this is not a reliable test when doing an end-to-side anastomosis.

The selection of the motor nerve requires a detailed understanding of the pattern of motor branches of the median and ulnar nerves. There is considerable variation in the number of motor branches to each muscle in the forearm.[3] If there are remnants of functioning muscle, a nerve stimulator may be helpful. When nerves have been selected, they should be divided under the microscope and the funicular pattern observed. If intraneural fibrosis is present, additional slices of nerve must be removed until an undamaged area of nerve is identified. Quick section evaluation by a neuropathologist will provide confirmation of the presence of undamaged axons.

The medial epicondyle and fascia of common flexor origin are exposed and prepared for fixation of the muscle's origin. The flexor digitorum profundus tendons and flexor pollicis longus are identified in the distal wrist, and their gliding ability is assessed by traction on their ends. If inadequate, a tenolysis may be required as a secondary procedure.

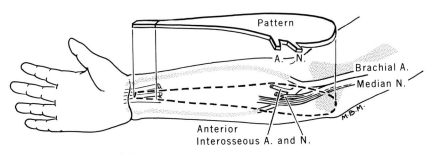

Figure 21–3. The expected location of all tendons, vessels, and nerves to be used in the transplantation is marked on the forearm. A pattern can then be taken from the arm with the required location on the muscle of all structures to be repaired. In practice, the anatomy of the gracilis muscle has been suitable for most injured forearms.

Preparation of the Muscle

In order to minimize operating time, a two-team approach is advisable. Many muscles can be used for neurovascular transplantation. These include the gracilis, latissimus dorsi, pectoralis major and minor, extensor digitorum brevis, brachioradialis, semitendinosus, serratus anterior, gastrocnemius, and tensor fasciae latae. The first three are most likely to be considered for use in the forearm, and the gracilis has been the most popular choice to date. Not only do its anatomic and microvascular qualifications make it suitable for transplantation, but its functional capability is adequate to replace forearm flexor musclature.

The gracilis is a superficial muscle that lies on the medial side of the thigh (Fig. 21–4). It is a broad strap muscle that takes its origin from the body of the pubis and its inferior ramus and the adjacent ramus of the ischium. The gracilis lies posterior to the adductor longus and sartorius muscles immediately deep to the superficial fascia. It terminates in a well-defined tendon that passes posterior and medial to the condyle of the femur. The insertion is into the shaft of the tibia just below the tibial tubercle. The tendon can be isolated distally where it lies posterior to the sartorius and anterior to the semitendinosus. There is a single motor nerve, which is a branch of the obturator and enters the muscle 6 to 12 cm from its orgin. The nerve is usually composed of two to four fascicles, but occasionally more. There are two or three vascular pedicles to the muscle. The pedicle, which lies between 8 and 12 cm from the muscle's origin, is always dominant. The artery is 1 to 2 mm in diameter and 4 to 6 cm in length and is derived from the profunda femoris artery. There are two venae comitantes that measure 1 to 2.5 mm in diameter. Including some cases on which the gracilis was used for cover only, 28 clinical free gracilis transplants have been completely perfused by this single dominant pedicle. However, Narakas has had one case in which a second artery needed to be anastomosed in order to perfuse the distal portion of the muscle. All pedicles enter the muscle on the deep aspect of its anterior margin. The muscle can be removed with no apparent functional deficit.

The gracilis is removed with the leg abducted and externally rotated and with the knee flexed. The procedure may be done either with the legs in stirrups or from the opposite side of the operating table. With the leg in this position, a straight line is drawn between the adductor longus tendon and the tibial tubercle. The gracilis muscle lies posterior to this reference line. Although a musculocutaneous flap can be taken, the most reliable portion of the cutaneous flap is over the proximal half of the muscle. The distal portion of the muscle will not reliably support a cutaneous flap, and this is the area in which flap coverage is usually required to provide good distal gliding and cover for the tendon suture. If the cutaneous flap is taken, it can be used as a monitor of the circulation to the muscle. However, vascular insufficiency may occur within the cutaneous flap while the muscle's circulation remains intact. As the cutaneous flap is neither a good monitor nor a cosmetic asset, our present practice is to take the gracilis muscle without a skin flap and to apply a skin graft to the muscle belly if necessary. A skin graft on the muscle provides a smooth contour to the forearm and, when placed on only the proximal muscle belly, does not limit movement.

An incision is placed along the reference line over its proximal half and carried down through the superficial fascia. The anterior border of the gracilis and posterior border of the adductor longus are identified. The adductor is elevated to expose the neurovascular bundles entering the gracilis. The motor

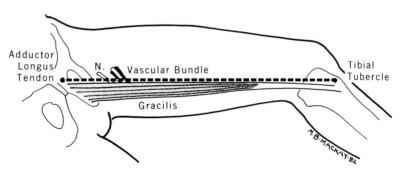

Figure 21–4. The gracilis muscle lies posterior to a line drawn from the adductor longus tendon to the tibial tubercle.

Adductor Longus Tendon — N. — Vascular Bundle — Gracilis — Tibial Tubercle nerve enters just proximal to the major vascular bundle. With elevation of the adductor, multiple side branches on the vascular bundle can be ligated with fine nylon ties or occluded with metal clips. When the pedicle has been dissected, the dissection is then carried over the superficial surface of the gracilis to identify the inferior border. The muscle can then be freed up with blunt dissection. Vascular attachments to the distal portion of the muscle should have a short pedicle left intact if doubt exists about the adequacy of the proximal pedicle. The tendon is divided through a transverse incision in the distal thigh. Prior to tendon division, markers are placed on the muscle, as described under the section on Muscle Tension. When the muscle has been completely separated from its origin and insertion and remains attached by a single vascular pedicle, its circulation should be observed. Color, contractility, and, if necessary, bleeding are adequate signs of muscle viability.

Muscle Transplantation

The muscle is removed from the thigh and placed on the forearm. Its position is evaluated for repair of all structures. The muscle should be positioned so that the repair of the motor nerve can be placed as close to the neuromuscular junction as possible in order to minimize reinnervation time. This requirement dictates the preferred position of the muscle on the forearm. With the muscle in place, the likely position of the vascular anastomosis and tendon repair is assessed. If this position is satisfactory, the muscle should be lightly tacked to the medial epicondyle and to other surrounding structures so that it will not move during the nerve and vessel repairs.

The anesthetist can promote successful revascularization by maintaining good peripheral perfusion throughout the lengthy operative procedure. The most important factors are adequate intravenous fluid replacement and the maintenance of body temperature. The patient should be placed upon a heating blanket and a double-thickness O.R. table cushion to prevent pressure problems. Muscle relaxants should not be administered during the time of identification of motor nerve branches in the forearm in order that a nerve stimulator may be used during the assessment.

In order to develop good muscle function, five important technical considerations must be satisfied. These are good revascularization, an excellent nerve repair, balanced tendon adjustment, positioning of the muscle at optimum tension, and adequate flap coverage.

Revascularization. Microvascular repairs are done between the muscle's dominant artery and the largest venae comitantes and a suitable artery and vein within the forearm. Although the ischemia time should be minimized, ischemic damage is unlikely unless there are operative complications. The ischemia time in most of our cases has been 2 hours or less. Although a single artery was suitable in all gracilis muscle transplantations, it may be necessary to anastomose two veins if the venae comitantes are smaller than the muscle's artery. Technically perfect anastomoses are important, as revisions of thrombosed anastomoses are particularly undesirable in this procedure. The muscle should become pink and bleed from the perimysium promptly upon completion of the anastomoses. The distal few centimeters of the gracilis will take a few minutes to become pink.

Nerve Repair. The nerve repair should be placed as close to the neuromusclar junction as possible. Usually this will be 2 to 3 cm from the junction. The gracilis motor nerve contains considerable fatty connective tissue. If an epineural repair is done, many of the fascicles may not be lined up with the fascicles of the motor nerve from the forearm. It is therefore necessary to separate the individual fascicles from their connective tissue and do a fascicular repair with interrupted 11–0 nylon suture (Fig. 21–5).

Balanced Tendon Fixation. Following revascularization and nerve repair, the origin of the muscle is attached in the region of the medial epicondyle and common flexor origin, and the distal attachment of the tendon is planned. In order to produce a balanced grip, all fingers must flex in unison. The profundus tendons are first sewn side to side to each other in this balanced position. If the muscle is also going to provide flexor pollicis longus function, this muscle must be carefully sewn to the profundus tendons in such a way that the thumb will be brought into opposition against the fingers after the fingers have started to form a fist. If the flexor pollicis longus is too tight, the thumb will be brought into the palm before the fingers,

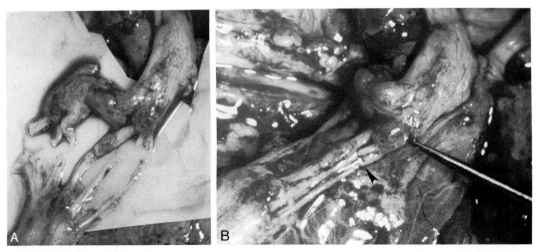

Figure 21–5. Fascicular nerve repair. *A,* Anterior interosseous nerve above and gracilis motor nerve below, with fascicles dissected prior to suture. Note large volume of fatty connective tissue throughout gracilis nerve. *B,* Fascicular nerve repair with 11–0 nylon.

interfering with their grip. Tendon fixation is accomplished by weaving the flexor tendons into the gracilis tendon and muscle and fixing with multiple mattress sutures. To prevent tendon dehiscence, the hand is splinted for 3 weeks with the wrist and fingers flexed.

Positioning Muscle at Optimum Tension. The tension at which the tendons are sewn into the gracilis must be carefully estimated in order to provide good muscle balance and optimal grip strength. If the hand has intact extensor tendons and intrinsic musculature, the fingers will sit in the position of function when the tendon repair is completed. However, in many patients with damaged extensor tendons and musculature, this position of balance may not be evident and another method is required to select the optimum muscle tension. This method is predicated upon two assumptions. (1) The most powerful contraction occurs when the muscle is almost fully stretched. (2) If the muscle selected has a range of excursion greater than that required in the arm, a full range of finger flexion will be possible. The objective of this method is to fix the muscle so that when stretched to its maximum physiologic length, it allows full finger and wrist extension. Full flexion should then be possible within the most powerful range of contraction of the muscle. Prior to removal of the muscle from its normal site, it is placed at its maximum physiologic stretch by abducting and externally rotating the thigh and extending the knee. Sutures and a vital dye are then placed along the surface of the muscle every 5 cm as markers (Fig. 21–6). When placed in the forearm and revascularized, the muscle is fixed proximally to the medial epicondyle and stretched until the distance between each of the markers is once again 5 cm and the fingers and wrist are fully extended. The

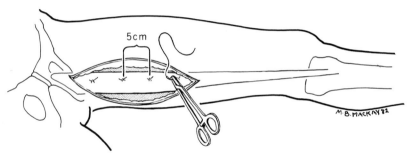

Figure 21–6. Prior to removing the gracilis muscle, it is extended to its maximum by abducting the thigh and extending the knee. Suture markers are placed on the muscle's surface at 5-cm intervals.

position of the flexor tendon stumps on the stretched gracilis tendon is noted. Adjacent positions are marked on the flexor tendons and the gracilis tendon (Fig. 21–7A). The wrist and fingers are then brought back into flexion, and profundus to gracilis tendon fixation is done at the points marked (Fig. 21–7B).

This procedure ensures that full finger and wrist extension will be possible. As the muscle selected has a range of contraction in excess of 8 cm, a full range of finger flexion can be expected, not only in wrist extension but in wrist flexion as well. In the relaxed position of finger and wrist flexion, the tension at the muscle-tendon junction is mild to moderate. Clark and McKee have investigated muscle blood flow in dogs in our laboratory. They found that the blood flow immediately after detachment of the muscle's origin and insertion was only slightly increased from the undetached state. Some authors[5] have recommended caution in applying tension to the muscle, as they fear that this may produce ischemia. We do not believe that this is a problem. However, we are very concerned that enough tension is applied so that the muscle realizes its functional potential. Skeletal muscles are normally under significant tension at rest, and they are well perfused.

Flap Coverage. Our present technique for housing the muscle is to cover the proximal portion of the muscle with a split-thickness skin graft. However, the distal forearm, in the region of the distal third of the muscle and tendon, must have good flap coverage to allow tendon gliding (Fig. 21–8). If a secondary tenolysis becomes necessary, this procedure will be difficult if the distal forearm is not covered by a flap.

Postoperative Care

Antiplatelet agents are unnecessary. The vital signs and urine output are carefully monitord in the first 24 hours, and an adequate volume of intravenous fluids is given to maintain good peripheral perfusion. The wrist and fingers are splinted in moderate flexion to relax the muscle-tendon junction. As the muscle is denervated, there is not an undue amount of tension at the site. Separation of the muscle-tendon junction has not occurred.

At 3 weeks postoperatively, a program of passive stretching of the wrist and fingers is commenced. Within a few weeks or months, a full range of wrist extension and finger extension will be obtained. Perhaps passive stretching develops the gliding mechanism at the muscle-tendon junction, which will be necessary when active contraction occurs following reinnervation.

The first clinical signs of reinnervation will

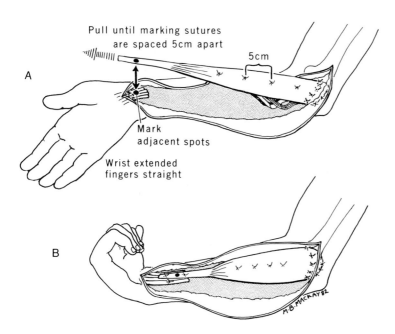

Figure 21–7. *A*, Following microneurovascular repair and proximal fixation, the muscle is pulled distally until the marking sutures are 5 cm apart. With the wrist and fingers extended, adjacent points are marked on the gracilis and flexor digitorum profundus tendons. *B*, The wrist and fingers are then flexed and the muscle allowed to retract to facilitate easy tendon repair at the points marked.

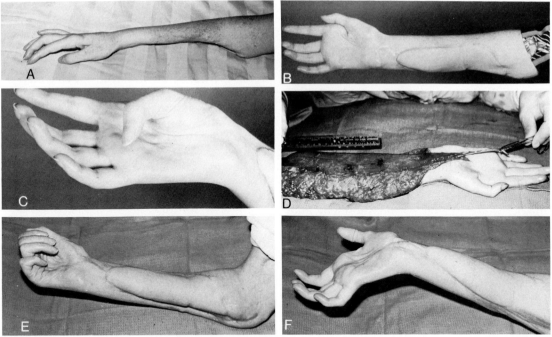

Figure 21–8. Case P. K. *A,* Thirty-one-year-old female following shotgun injury to forearm with loss of the FDP and FDS and weakening of extensor muscle mass. *B,* Preliminary abdominal flap applied to distal forearm to replace extensive scar tissue and provide cover for muscle transplant. *C,* Only flexor function in the hand was of the medial innervated thenar musculature and flexor pollicis longus. *D,* Transplantation of gracilis muscle. Following revascularization and fixation of origin to medial epicondyle, the muscle is stretched until markings are 5 cm apart to determine position for suturing to flexor tendons. *E,* Range of flexion at 10 months postoperatively. *F,* Range of extension allowed by muscle 10 months postoperatively. Note clawing tendency due to ulnar nerve loss.

occur 2 to 4 months postoperatively. With increasing reinnervation, the patient will develop an increasing range of muscle excursion. When a full range of excursion has occurred, usually between 6 and 12 months, the patient is placed on a program of resisted exercise. Our best results have occurred in those patients who were well motivated and accepted their exercise program with the seriousness of an athlete who was preparing for a major sporting event. This exercise program should be continued until the grip strength has reached a plateau, usually 2 years following surgery.

RESULTS

The success of the transplantation is measured in terms of the patient's increased functional capabilities and objective criteria that the examiner can evaluate. Although criteria have been established for many procedures, such as tendon repair and joint replacement, none are established for muscle transplanta-

tion. Criteria that would assess a muscle transplantation must be applicable to different anatomic locations and relate to the capability of the transplanted muscle to replace the function of the missing muscle. A completely successful muscle transplantation would provide a contractile excursion that moves the involved joints through their full range of motion. It would also supply a contractile force equal to that which has been lost, and this movement would be under precise and volitional control. In addition, the muscle may need to supply independent contractile units to provide independent finger and thumb movements. These are goals that may be achieved at some time in the future. However, at this time, functioning muscle transplantation is still in its infancy and just beyond the stage at which the surgeon is delighted that the muscle will actually live through the transplantation. At this time, our criteria for success are a muscle transplantation that supplies a useful range of motion, provides adequate grip strength for the patient's functional activities, and is under volitional control.

Detailed Assessment of Results

Eleven of twelve transplantations survived completely and one survived partially. By the criteria outlined, 11 out of 12 were successful (Table 12–1).

A detailed follow-up of these 12 patients is difficult because of the distance they live from our center. Eight of the twelve live outside the province of Ontario.

The range of muscle contraction was related as full if the fingers could be fully extended and fully flexed to touch the palm with the wrist in the neutral position. Twelve muscles were available for measurement, and nine provided a full range of finger motion with the wrist stationary. Five of these also provided a full range of finger flexion in both wrist flexion and extension.

Only five patients with transplantations were available for reliable measurement of their grip strength. The other seven patients, who live thousands of miles from Toronto, could not be measured by the author. The grip strength in four adults ranged from 18 to 60 lb with the Jaymar Dynamometer. For the 4-year-old child, grip strength was 4.5 lb. The maximum grip strength was 50% of the strength of the patient's normal arm. In two patients who returned to heavy manual work, the muscle appeared to have the same stamina as that of the normal arm.

All muscles were under precise volitional control, as was anticipated in view of the selection of the motor nerves. The nerves used were motor branches of the median nerve (including the anterior interosseous), motor branches of the ulnar nerve, and, for the extensor muscle, a motor branch of the radial nerve.

The onset of muscle contraction varied from 2 to 4 months following transplantation. A full range of muscle contraction was obtained within 6 to 9 months of transplantation. Grip strength gradually increased over a period of 2 years and then slowly increased for an additional year or more (see Fig. 21–10E). In most cases, the muscle's bulk was easily visible and palpable on contraction. This allowed the width of the contracting muscle to be measured and compared with its recorded pretransplantation bulk. In most cases the muscle returned to its pretransplantation bulk, and in two cases it appeared to get larger than it had been at transplantation. These two cases involved patients who were particularly well motivated to pursue a vigorous exercise program, as indicated by their overall increase in muscle strength.

The patient with partial muscle survival had a pectoralis major transplant for Volkmann's ischemic paralysis. The muscle survived the transplantation and showed clinical and electromyographic evidence of reinnervation at 4 months postoperatively. Shortly thereafter, it abruptly lost almost all contractility. The arteriogram demonstrated that occlusion of the anterior interosseous artery had occurred. A small portion of the muscle that was attached to the flexor pollicis longus remained functional and the remainder underwent atrophy.

DISCUSSION

When selecting a muscle for transplantation, there are anatomic, microvascular, and dynamic factors that must be considered. Based upon the pattern that the surgeon can derive from the forearm, it is possible to outline the *anatomic requirements* that will be necessary for the muscle to fit into the defect in the forearm. These will include the length of the muscle required, the need for a tendon at its distal insertion, the location of the neurovascular structures on the muscle, and the need for skin coverage in the forearm. The presence of motor nerves in the forearm and their location may govern the selection of a muscle for transplantation. The gracilis muscle has a single nerve composed of two to six fascicles. The latissimus dorsi has a similar innervation. However, nerves to the sternocostal portion of the pectoralis major vary from four to ten motor branches, each supplying a separate portion of the muscle.[8] All fascicles or branches must be supplied by appropriate nerves in the forearm, or portions of the muscle will not reinnervate adequately. This may be a problem in a traumatized arm with a shortage of available motor nerves.

The feasibility of a muscle's insertion in a particular site depends not only on the muscle's length and bulk and on its transferability by microvascular anastomoses, but upon the location of the muscle's neurovascular structures with respect to those in the recipient area. A short vascular pedicle can be augmented by grafts without concern for muscle survival. However, the distance of the nerve anastomosis from the neuromuscular junction should be minimized and preferably should be kept to 2 cm or less.

The *microvascular requirements* relate primarily to the vascular pedicle(s), which allow the muscle to be transferred on microvascular anastomoses. The muscle must be supplied by vessels of a size and configuration that allow anastomosis. Only a single artery and one or two veins should supply the entire muscle, or revascularization becomes unduly complicated.

The *dynamic requirements* of a transplanted muscle are that it provide adequate strength of contraction and adequate range of motion to provide the desired function. In order to replace the long flexors of the finger, a range of motion following transplantation of 6 to 7 cm must be obtained. This will provide full finger flexion in either wrist extension or wrist flexion. Since the total amount of muscle contraction is proportional to the length of the individual muscle fibers, a strap muscle will shorten more than a pennate muscle. Following transplantation, if the muscle is positioned at a tension that is slightly too tight or too loose, a portion of the useful range of contraction will be outside the range of motion of the joints. For this reason, a muscle should be chosen that has a greater range of motion in its normal site than will be desired in the transplantation location. For example, a strap muscle that normally has a range of motion of 10 cm has the potential for providing full finger flexion and extension in any wrist position. Strap muscles such as the gracilis, pectoralis major, and latissimus dorsi have more than an adequate range of contraction to provide full finger flexion throughout normal wrist excursion.

The strength of the muscle is proportional to the cross-sectional area of its fibers. Therefore, if the muscle is a strap muscle, its maximum contractile force is proportional to the cross-sectional area of the entire muscle. Six months after our first gracilis muscle transplantation, the patient had developed a full range of finger motion but very little grip strength. We believed that we had transplanted a muscle with insufficient cross-sectional area and elected to use the lower four-fifths of the pectoralis major in our second patient, as this muscle has a greater cross-sectional area and therefore has a contractile strength that is two to three times that of the gracilis. The pectoralis major was expected to provide a much better grip strength than the gracilis. We observed both patients for an additional year before doing further transplantations. Eventually, at 30 months post-

operatively, the gracilis transplant patient had a grip strength of 42 lb and the pectoralis major transplant patient had an even more powerful grip of 60 lb. We decided to employ this simpler gracilis muscle for most of our future patients. However, the pectoralis major is indicated when a patient requires a muscle with independent functioning territories to supply separate thumb and finger flexion. When an exceptionally powerful grip is required or when a reliable cutaneous flap is required over the distal muscle-tendon junction, the pectoralis is also a good choice. The pectoralis could probably be even stronger than that of patient GW (see Table 21–1) if a more satisfactory muscle to tendon junction had been achieved (Fig. 21–9). As seen in the sequence of photographs between the second and fifth year after transplantation (Fig. 21–10A and B), portions of the muscle pulled proximally from the tendons, as evidenced by the increased balling-up effect seen in the late postoperative picture. The latissimus dorsi muscle has a functional potential similar to that of the pectoralis major. In addition, it has a simpler innervation, longer muscle length, and a capability of carrying a reliable cutaneous flap over its entire length.

After an erudite experimental investigation of function following muscle transplantation, Terzis concluded that work capacity is only 25% of normal after transplantation.[13] In her experimental study, she also observed that prior tenotomy followed by repair produced an even greater decrease in the force of contraction than prior neurovascular division and repair. This illustrates the severe functional insult that occurs when a muscle is forced to function at a shortened length, as likely occurred following her tenotomy study. We feel that one of the major reasons for the excellent grip strength that our patients developed is the relatively large amount of tension at which our muscles are fixed.

One of the disadvantages of this procedure is the prolonged period until useful function is obtained. This is due to the slow return of muscle contractility that is seen with reinnervation. Although a good range of active contraction will occur early, usually within 6 months of surgery, very minimal functional capability will be present at that time. Light activities will become possible between 6 and 12 months, but it will take another year before full muscle strength is obtained. Thus, a person doing heavy labor may be unable

Table 21–1. FUNCTIONING FREE MUSCLE TRANSPLANTATION

		Pathology			Operation					Results			
Case	Sex	Date of Injury	Etiology of Muscle Deficit	Date	Age of Patient (years)	Muscle Transplanted	Recipient Site	Functional Objective	Muscle Contraction	Range of Finger Movement	Max. Grip Strength (lb)	Muscle Bulk as Fraction of Preop Width	Additional Functional Operations
RG	M	1974	Crush injury in a machine	10/5/1976	17	Gracilis	Forearm	Finger flexion	Yes	Full	42	1	Flexor tenolysis
GW	M	6/1974	Crush injury in a machine	11/1976	24	Pectoralis major	Forearm	Finger & thumb flexion	Yes	Full	60	1	FPL tendon lengthening to balance fingers and thumb
MP	M	12/1975	Crush injury, motor vehicle	1/1978	43	Gracilis	Forearm	Finger flexion	Yes	Full	29	1	
MP	M	12/1975	Crush injury, motor vehicle	1/1979	44	Gracilis	Forearm	Finger & thumb extension	Yes	Full	NA*	1	Extensor tenolysis

RM	M	3/1979	Electrical burn	5/1979	20	Gracilis	Forearm	Finger flexion	Yes	Full	18	⅔	
LR	M	5/1965	Volkmann's contracture	10/1978	18	Pectoralis major	Forearm	Finger & thumb flexion	Partial, to thumb only	0	0	⅓	ECRL to FDP due to failure of muscle
KH	M	5/1976	Gas gangrene	6/1978	35	Gracilis	Forearm	Finger flexion	Yes	Full	NA	NA	
MT	M	1977	Volkmann's contracture	4/1979	4	Gracilis	Forearm	Finger flexion	Yes	Full	4.5	1	Flexor tendon shortening and tenolysis
EH	M	1978	Trauma	6/1979	11	Gracilis	Forearm	Finger flexion	Yes	Full	NA	NA	
TT	M	6/1976	Electrical burn	3/1978	19	Gracilis	Forearm	Finger flexion	Yes	4/5 full	NA	NA	Fl. tenolysis
EP	F	1952	Volkmann's contracture	9/1979	33	Gracilis	Forearm	Finger & thumb flexion	Yes	⅔ full	NA	⅔	
PK	F	5/1977	Shotgun injury	7/1980	31	Gracilis	Forearm	Finger flexion	Yes	Full	NA	NA	Tendon transfers for claw hand secondary to ulnar nerve paralysis

*NA = not available.

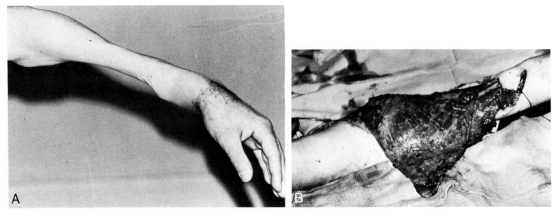

Figure 21–9. Case G. W. *A,* Twenty-four-year-old man with an hourglass deformity of the forearm due to traumatic loss of flexor and extensor musculature. (Preliminary report in J. Hand Surg., 3:416–426, 1978.) *B,* Patient received transplantation of four fifths of sternal head of pectoralis major muscle. Innervated by anterior interosseous nerve and shown here prior to insertion of sternal margin into FDP and FPL.

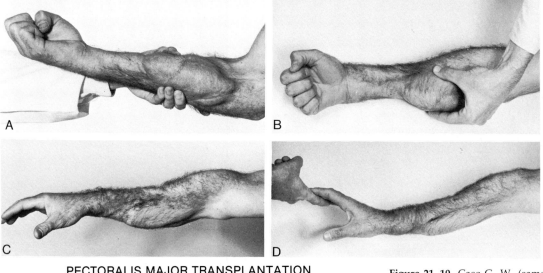

PECTORALIS MAJOR TRANSPLANTATION

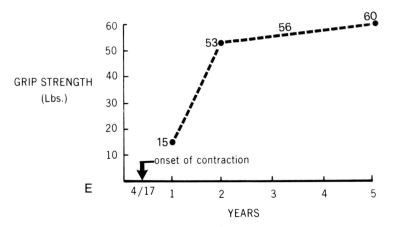

Figure 21–10. Case G. W. (same patient as in Figure 21–9). *A,* At 14 months postoperatively, a full range of excursion and considerable muscle bulk has returned, as demonstrated between the examiner's fingers and thumb; grip strength 15 lbs. *B,* Four years postoperatively, the muscle no longer tapers down to attach to the flexor tendons, but is more ball-shaped and has more bulk on contraction. Some muscle fibers appear to have pulled out of the flexor tendons. Grip strength is 60 pounds. *C,* Active finger and thumb extension is provided by brachioradialis transfer. *D,* With muscle relaxation, nearly full passive finger and wrist extension is possible. *E,* Grip strength increased rapidly up to 2 years postoperatively, and then increased more slowly until the present. This patient worked at heavy construction and practiced weight lifting.

to return to work for 2 years from the time of the muscle transplantation. In contrast, a transfer of a radial wrist extensor to the profundus tendons may not give as good an excursion as a muscle transplantation, but it will provide a useful range of motion that is available for light to heavy work between 2 and 6 months postoperatively.

The concept that a myocutaneous flap is necessary in order to use the skin as an indicator of continued patency of the vessel anastomosis and survival of the underlying muscle may provide a false sense of security. It is likely that by the time an anastomosis has thrombosed and produced sufficient clinically apparent signs in a skin flap, the return to the operating room and successful revision of the anastomosis would exceed the 4 hours beyond which an ischemic insult to the muscle can be predicted. Initially, we were concerned that the split-thickness skin graft would restrict the increase in muscle bulk that occurs following reinnervation, but this has not been the case.

CONCLUSIONS

Functioning muscle transplantation to the upper extremity is technically feasible based upon microvascular anastomosis and fascicular nerve repair. It is now possible to transplant a muscle from one location to another and obtain a good range of powerful muscle contraction.

Muscle transplantation is a prolonged and complicated procedure with many pitfalls to trap the unwary. In addition to the rules that govern tendon transfers, there are a number of rules that are specific for functioning muscle transplantation. These rules govern selection of the patient and muscle selection, the operative technique, and the postoperative care.

A muscle must be selected that has the required anatomic, microvascular, and dynamic characteristics to suit the recipient site. Placement of the muscle at optimum tension, a precise fascicular nerve repair, and adequate flap coverage of the distal muscle-tendon junction are critical operative details. An aggressive postoperative exercise program begins with passive extension exercises and concludes with a long period of active resistance exercises. If these rules are satisfied, transplantation of the gracilis muscle to the forearm for finger flexion can provide a grip strength that is 50% of normal with a full range of finger motion.

The indication for muscle transplantation to the forearm is a major functional deficit due to loss of musculature when the simpler techniques such as tendon transfer are unavailable. The disadvantages of the procedure are the long operative time and the long time to return of function.*

---

*These cases were done as two-team procedures with either Dr. R. M. Zuker or Dr. N. H. McKee. The author recognizes their assistance and contributions to the development and success of the operative procedures.

References

1. Gordon, L., and Buncke, H. J.: Heterotopic free skeletal muscle autotransplantation with utilization of a long nerve graft and microsurgical techniques. A study in the primate. J. Hand Surg., 4:103–108, 1979.
2. Harii, K., Ohmori, K., and Torii, S.: Free gracilis muscle transplantation with microvascular anastomoses for the treatment of facial paralysis. Plast. Reconstr. Surg., 57:133–143, 1976.
3. Hollingshead, W. H.: In Anatomy for Surgeons, Vol. 3. New York, Harper & Row, 1969, pp. 418–422.
4. Ikuta, Y., Kubo, T., and Tsuge, K.: Free muscle transplantation by microsurgical technique to treat severe Volkmann's contracture. Plast. Reconstr. Surg., 58:407–411, 1976.
5. Ikuta, Y., Yoshioka, K., and Tsuge, K.: Free muscle transfer. Aust. N.Z. J. Surg., 50:401–405, 1980.
6. Manktelow, R. T., and McKee, N. H.: Free muscle transplantation to provide active finger flexion. J. Hand Surg., 3:416–426, 1978.
7. Manktelow, R. T.: Microsurgical composite tissue transplantation. In Serafin, D., Buncke, H. J. (eds.): Muscle Transplantation. St. Louis, The C. V. Mosby Company, 1979, pp. 369–390.
8. Manktelow, R. T., McKee, N. H., and Vettese, T.: An anatomical study of the pectoralis major muscle as related to functioning free muscle transplantation. Plast. Reconstr. Surg., 65:610–615, 1980.
9. O'Brien, B. Mc.C.: In Microvascular Reconstructive Surgery. Edinburgh, Churchill Livingstone, 1977, pp. 290–305.
10. Schenck, R. R.: Free muscle and composite skin transplantation by microneurovascular anastomoses. Orthop. Clin. North Am., 8:367–375, 1977.
11. Shanghai Sixth People's Hospital: Free muscle transplantation by microsurgical neurovascular anastomoses. Chinese Med. J., 2:47–50, 1976.
12. Tamai, S., Komatsu, S., Sakamoto, H., et al.: Free muscle transplants in dogs with microsurgical neurovascular anastomoses. Plast. Reconstr. Surg., 46:219–225, 1970.
13. Terzis, J. K., Dykos, R. W., and Williams, H. B.: Recovery of function in free muscle transplants using microneurovascular anastomoses. J. Hand Surg., 3:37–59, 1978.

MICRORECONSTRUCTION OF BRACHIAL PLEXUS INJURIES

PART
3

22

The Quantitative Microanatomy of the Brachial Plexus in Man: Reconstructive Relevance

■

Craig L. Slingluff, Jr., M.D.
Julia K. Terzis, M.D., Ph.D.
Milton T. Edgerton, M.D.

When you can measure what you are speaking about, and express it in numbers, you know something about it; but when you cannot measure it, when you cannot express it in numbers, your knowledge is of a meager and unsatisfactory kind: it may be the beginning of knowledge, but you have scarcely, in your thoughts, advanced to the stage of science.

Popular Lectures and Addresses
William Thomson, Lord Kelvin (1824–1907)

This study was undertaken to provide detailed quantitative information on brachial plexus anatomy at the fascicle level that might assist the surgeon operating on the brachial plexus in better understanding this structure.

During the past few decades, with increased use of the operating microscope, advancement of microsurgical techniques, and better understanding of neurophysiology, repair of peripheral nerve lesions has become widely accepted as feasible in restoring function after traumatic injuries.

In 1984, Millesi[32] reported 90% satisfactory to excellent functional results in nerve graft repairs of radial nerve lesions. In contrast, when he reported results of surgical intervention in 158 patients with total brachial plexus lesions, only 64.5% had useful recovery.[33]

Brachial plexus injuries can be severely disabling and frequently occur in younger age groups. Microsurgical reconstruction of these lesions, while offering some hope of restored function, historically has often been unsatisfactory.

Existing literature on brachial plexus anatomy is voluminous but is nonetheless insufficient for the surgeon who seeks to advance the state of the art of repair of plexus lesions. Narakas[37] comments on the difficulty of establishing a precise and valid understanding of plexus topography, but contends that such knowledge would have "much importance to surgical reconstruction of the plexus" (translated).

BACKGROUND

On both gross and microscopic levels, the anatomy of the brachial plexus has been studied by a number of workers during the past 100 years. Some remarkable work was done early in this period with only the limited technology available. The primary method of studying peripheral nerves has been interfascicular (longitudinal) dissection, i.e., meticulous removal of connective tissue and subsequent identification and tracing of fascicles. More recently, this work has been augmented by the use of microinstruments and higher quality microscopes, but with few significant advances in understanding the anatomy.

In 1877, Walsh reported dissection of 350 human brachial plexuses. His technique employed nitric acid to macerate connective tissue, thereby simplifying interfascicular dissection. His was one of the early works to report the spinal nerve supply to the various branches of the plexus. He argued that variations in plexus gross anatomy were essentially artefactual effects of connective tissue. Aside from these effects, Walsh concluded that "there is only one arrangement, which the nerves follow without much deviation,"[65] suggesting that there might be some order in plexus structure.

In 1887, Herringham[17] produced a work of such magnitude that it continues to be cited frequently in recent literature. Herringham dissected 55 plexuses and recorded observations about both the peripheral distribution of each spinal nerve and the proximal derivation of each peripheral nerve. However, his work, like that of Walsh, was only qualitative in nature. He identifies the spinal nerves contributing to each peripheral nerve, but does not quantify the contribution of each, except in referring occasionally to a "large fiber" as opposed to a "tiny fiber."

Perhaps Herringham's single most important contribution was his first law (one of two) that

Any given fibre may alter its position relative to the vertebral column, but will maintain its position relative to the other fibres.[17]

In 1903, Harris[16] reported results of 27 plexus dissections and observed that 85% of plexuses contain a lateral head of the ulnar nerve, i.e., a contribution to the ulnar nerve from the lateral cord or directly from the C7 spinal nerve. According to Kerr,[23] Walsh also noted this formation, but had "entirely overlooked this branch in the first 60 (plexuses) but once his attention was directed to it he found it absent in only 25 of the remaining 290." That Walsh failed to observe this formation in his first 60 plexuses points out the failure of interfascicular dissection in discerning some anatomic subtleties.

In 1918, Kerr[23] presented another major work, second only to Herringham's. Kerr and his co-workers dissected 175 embalmed plexuses. They assessed variations in gross anatomy and variability between sexes, races, and opposite sides of the body. They assessed, as well, the distribution of fibers from proximal to distal and discussed the complexity of the interfascicular anatomy of the plexus in qualitative terms. Kerr, like Walsh, used a nitric acid solution to facilitate removal of epineurium, and his work was limited to longitudinal interfascicular dissection and nonquantitative methods.

Since Kerr's work, there have been few serious advances in the understanding of plexus anatomy other than observations accorded by clinical experience with plexus lesions. The peripheral nerves of the arm and forearm, however, have been studied extensively since the 1940s, most notably by Sunderland. He and his colleagues studied the nerves distal to the plexus itself by thin serial cross sections of one specimen each of the radial and median nerves and two specimens of the ulnar nerve as well as one fetal arm.[50, 52, 54] He also studied specimens of the musculocutaneous and axillary nerves.[49, 50, 52] His work and the subsequent work of Jabaley et al.,[20] who serially sectioned three median nerves at intervals of 5 to 10 mm, suggested the value of serial section techniques for quantitation and for an appreciation of the relationship of connective tissue and fascicles without disruption of cross-sectional localization. Based on their work, it was apparent that sectioning more frequently than every centimeter would be important for an understanding of fascicle topography.

Additional works in the elucidation of plexus anatomy have included studies of sympathetic supply to the spinal nerves by Harman[15] and Sunderland[51, 53] and reports on plexus embryology by Bardeen and Lewis,[3] Fenart,[13] and Lewis.[27]

In 1972, Narakas[37] published in Spanish a hypothetical schema for the cross-sectional localization (within each spinal nerve, trunk, and cord) of those axons destined for each of the various peripheral nerves. He reported the schema as hypothetical, based on several microdissections by Martonini and on a number of generalizations, specifically including the first law of Herringham. In 1978, Narakas[35] republished a similar schema in English.

Alnot and Huten[2] have also published a schema of intraneural topography resembling that of Narakas but limited to the root level and based on longitudinal microdissection.

Bonnel[5-7] published work based on cross sections of the plexus, which appear to have been taken about 10 mm apart. His findings include axonal counts and several salient findings regarding fascicular numbers, sizes, and arrangement, including the observation of monofascicular spinal nerves in some cases. He also provides partial documentation of the percentage of plexus elements composed of connective tissue, as opposed to neural tissue, but his data are limited by the large distance between sections. Quantitation of plexus neural tissue is not reported, and his conclusions do not offer means of systematizing the plexus.

In summary, a century of longitudinal dissection studies has made substantial contributions toward elucidating plexus anatomy. Many questions, however, have remained unanswered.

OBJECTIVES

The following questions about plexus anatomy seemed particularly relevant to reconstruction, and this study was begun in hopes of answering them.

1. What is the neural tissue content of each plexus element and of each peripheral nerve formed from the plexus?

2. How far can fascicles and fascicle groups be traced in the plexus without interaction with other fascicles?

3. Are there quantitative bases for systematizing the plexus, with its myriad variations?

4 What is the clinical relevance of pre- and post-fixation of brachial plexuses?

5. Are there any consistent patterns in the number and arrangement of fascicles in the various elements of the plexus?

6. Does the intraneural topography of the plexus follow anatomic rules similar to those governing the nerves of the arm and forearm or does it follow different rules?

7. Where in the cross section of each plexus element is the greatest number of motor and sensory fibers?

METHODS

Twenty-one brachial plexuses were meticulously dissected and removed from 11 fresh adult human cadavers, and branches were identified by identifying their end-organs. Branches were labeled before removal, and 6–0 silk was used to mark the anterior aspect of the various elements of the plexus. Epi-

neural tissue was preserved. Measurements of the plexuses and of the cadavers were recorded, and photographs and drawings of each plexus specimen were made. After fixation in 10% formalin, seven plexuses were serially sectioned by hand, reducing each of these specimens entirely to sections 0.5 to 1 mm in thickness. Both fixation and use of a histologic fluorocarbon freezing spray were helpful in stiffening the nerve tissue, permitting thin, good quality sections. Each section was stained with 0.083% methylene blue and examined under a Zeiss Opmi operating microscope, fascicles stained dark blue, and connective tissue stained very pale yellowish-green. Changes in fascicular pattern were noted. Fascicles and their interactions could thereby be evaluated along the full length of each element of each plexus. By using a light source transmitted from below the specimen, in the rare case in which a fascicle was formed and subsequently merged with another fascicle all within the distance between the proximal and distal faces of a single section, its shadow could be appreciated through the section. Any remaining questions were answered by microdissection of this section. Using this method of serial sectioning (Fig. 22–1), changes through the full length of the plexus could be identified. In staining and studying sections, particular care was directed toward both obtaining good quality staining and preventing any dehydration. A photomicrograph (Fig. 22–2) and a sketch were made of each serial section, providing a permanent record of each plexus. A total of 4089 serial sections were cut and studied on the fascicle level, using the operating microscope and computer-assisted quantitative methods.

Of the specimens not studied by serial section, one was microdissected in a longitudinal fashion with detailed assessments of fascicular topography. The remainder of the 21 specimens were studied for gross anomalies, configuration, and exit points of branches.

Quantitative Data

The cross-sectional areas of each fascicle were measured every 3 to 4 mm at all levels for all serially sectioned plexuses. The cross-sectional areas of fascicles are referred to as neural tissue areas for the purpose of this study, but it must be understood that this

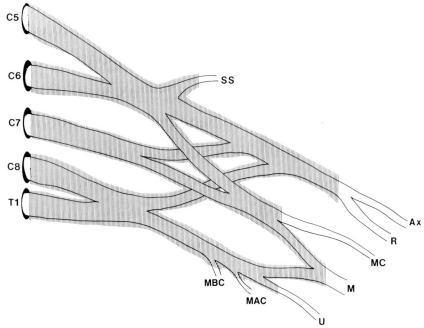

Figure 22–1. The plexus was studied by serial cross-section throughout its length. This figure demonstrates the distance between sections. Cuts were perpendicular to the nerve elements, not oblique as shown here.

tissue actually contains Schwann cells and endoneurium as well as axons. We refer to epineurium and perineurium together as connective tissue.

These areas were measured on a Talos digitizing tablet interfaced to a Cromemco computer, and extensive analysis of the obtained data was performed with computer assistance. Approximately 20,000 fascicle cross-sectional neural tissue areas were recorded and studied.

The standard error for digitizing cross-sectional areas of fascicles at least 0.5 mm in diameter was less than 1% This is shown in Figure 22–3. Shrinkage of neural tissue due to fixation was not statistically significant compared with that of fresh tissue, but had an absolute value of 2%.

The determination of the difference between a single fascicle with a septation and two truly distinct fascicles was considered of crucial importance in counting fascicles correctly. Carefully studying individual sections under the operating microscope, considerable time was invested in determining proper identification by strict adherence to the accepted definition of a fascicle adopted by the Committee of the International Society of Reconstructive Microsurgery.[34] Modified staining procedures for perineurium were particularly helpful as well.

GROSS ANATOMY: OVERVIEW AND ANOMALIES

C4 Contribution to the Plexus

Of seven serially sectioned plexuses, two had definite C4 contributions to C5, measuring 1.0060 mm^2 and 0.2713 mm^2 and making up 3% and 1% of the total plexus neural tissue, respectively. In three plexuses there was no C4 contribution to C5. In one, C4 interacted with the plexus only insignificantly via the phrenic nerve where it crossed the upper trunk. In one specimen, C4 and C5 interacted via small connections in a plexiform fashion.

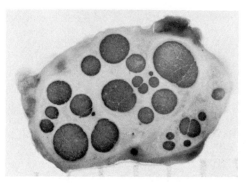

Figure 22–2. This is one of the cross-sections studied and photographed. It is from the medial cord.

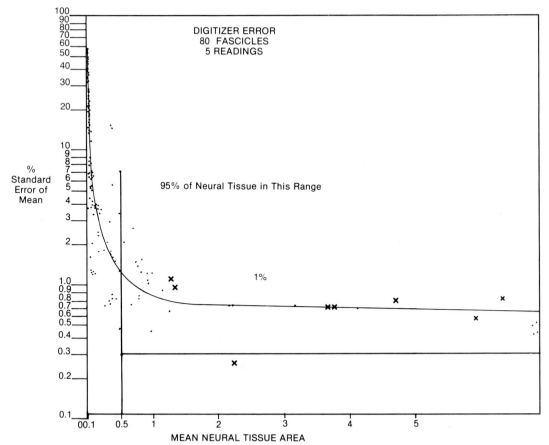

Figure 22–3. The standard error of the mean is plotted against the mean of five measures, for each fascicle in a single section. The resultant curve of digitizer error shows that most neural tissue can be measured within a 1% standard of error and 95% within a 5% standard of error.

For the purpose of calculations, C4 is not discussed as a separate spinal nerve contributing to the plexus, but as a contributing branch to C5. Reference to C5 is made with the understanding that part of the spinal nerve may actually be supplied by C4.

When present, C4 was often found to send most of its neural tissue to the dorsal scapular nerve, as was also noted by Walsh.[65]

T2 Contribution

No direct contributions from T2 to T1 were observed, but in many cases cutaneous innervation to the intercostobrachial and medial arm regions was supplied in part by T2, often via communications with T1 branches. Thus, overlap of T2 and the brachial plexus was not by direct contributions to the lower trunk and was difficult to quantitate reliably.

C8 Contribution to the Lateral Cord

In three of the seven specimens studied by serial section, C8 contributed to the lateral cord. In the specimens not dissected in detail and in the plexus studied by microdissection, this contribution was not grossly apparent but could not be ruled out in three of the specimens without serial sectioning or detailed dissection. Therefore, the incidence of C8 contributions to the lateral cord was 3 to 6 of 21 specimens, or between 14 and 29%. In the cases in which it was observed, this branch exited C8 at the same level as the divisions to the medial and posterior cords. The cross-sectional areas in these three cases were 3.84, 1.83, and 2.59 mm^2, representing 12.8, 6.1, and 9.6% of plexus neural tissue in plexuses 1, 5, and 12, respectively. A negative correlation was observed between the size of C5 neural tissue and the size of the

C8 contribution to the lateral cord. When C5 contributed over 12.5% (one eighth) of the neural tissue of the plexus, this formation was absent.

Transfers Between the Musculocutaneous and Median Nerves

In 24% of 21 specimens, the musculocutaneous nerve sent a branch to the median nerve in a proximodistal direction. This transfer of neural tissue was measured in two cases as being 0.5183 and 0.7702 mm^2, representing 22.7 and 31.0% of the musculocutaneous nerve in plexuses 9 and 12, respectively. The transferred neural tissue increased the neural tissue area of the median nerve by 10.4 and 19.6%, respectively, in these cases. The observed transfers occurred 10, 13, and 17 cm distal to the origin of the median nerve for three specimens.

The median and musculocutaneous nerves were not dissected to their full lengths in most cases; therefore, transfers occurring more distally may have been missed. In no case was transfer from the median to the musculocutaneous nerve observed.

In each of the three cases observed in serially sectioned specimens, C7 contributed to the musculocutaneous nerve. However, in at least two other plexuses, C7 contributed to musculocutaneous nerve but musculocutaneous/median transfers were absent.

Transfers Between Anterior and Posterior Elements of the Plexus

In 4 of 21 plexuses (19%), small communications between the radial and ulnar nerves were observed. In two of these (plexuses 10 and 17), the communication was a direct transfer from the radial nerve proximally to the ulnar nerve distally. In the other two cases, a direct transfer, if present, was not well defined, the principal interaction being between branches of the ulnar and radial nerves jointly supplying the same muscle groups. In one of these, there was a loop, or ansa, supplied by both the radial and the ulnar nerves and from which two terminal branches to muscle were formed.

In plexus 14, in addition to the radial-ulnar anastomosis, there was a direct transfer from the medial cord to the proximal radial nerve.

This branch was exceedingly small, with a measured neural tissue area of 0.1036 mm^2, representing 0.89% of the radial nerve and only 0.30% of the plexus neural tissue. Such a formation was unique, in that it appeared in no other plexus; thus, its observed incidence was 5% (1 of 21).

Variability in the Spinal Nerves Supplying the Lateral and Medial Cords

Of the seven serially sectioned specimens, the lateral cord was formed in three cases (43%) from C5, C6, and C7; in three cases (43%) from C5, C6, C7, and C8; and in one case (14%) from C5 and C6 alone. In none of the remaining 14 specimens was C7 absent from the lateral cord; therefore, a better estimate of the incidence of this formation is 5% (1 of 21). As noted previously, C8 probably contributed to the lateral cord in no more than 3 of the 14 specimens not studied by cross section. We therefore estimate the incidence of this formation as between 14 and 29%, leaving 66 to 81% of specimens following the classic pattern.

The medial cord was supplied by C8 and T1 alone in 86% of the serially sectioned plexuses and by C7, C8, and T1 in 14% (one case). The presence of C7 contributions to the medial cord in at least one or two additional specimens is in agreement with these frequencies.

Attachments of C7 to the Upper and Lower Trunks

It was not uncommon for the middle trunk to lack distinct identity because of significant connective tissue attachments with the upper trunk (5%) or lower trunk (29%). As a rule, mixing of fascicles between middle and upper or lower trunks did not occur, even in these cases, until distal to the divisions.

Plexus Length and Correlation with Arm Length

Measuring the length of a plexus from the C5 foramen to the origin of the median nerve, the average plexus length was 15.3 cm, with a standard deviation of 3.4 cm, 22.2% of mean length (n = 20). The arm lengths were more constant, with a mean of 29.4 cm (n = 15) from the lateral edge of the acromion to the medial humeral epicondyle. The standard deviation of these lengths was only 2.3 cm (15.7% of mean length). The variations observed in adult arm lengths did not seem to bear on the relatively greater variability in plexus lengths. Correcting lengths measured along the plexus for their respective arm lengths did not reduce variability of the values and was therefore not considered helpful in this group of similar adult plexuses. Such corrections are reported only in brief.

The distance from C5 to the origin of the median nerve was 0.53 times the distance from the acromion to the medial epicondyle, to the musculocutaneous nerve 0.48, to the lateral pectoral nerve 0.28, and to the suprascapular nerve 0.22. Similarly, the distance from the C8 foramen to the ulnar nerve was 0.38, and the distance to the medial pectoral nerve 0.23 times the distance from the acromion to the medial epicondyle, averaged over 15 plexuses. On average, trunks separated into divisions 6.5 cm from the foramina.

Sample Population

Of the 21 plexuses studied, 11 were from males and 10 from females; 11 were right sided and 10 were left sided. Of the seven studied by serial section, four were right sided and three were left sided; six were from females and one from a male. Interestingly, the male specimen has the least number of fascicles of the group.

FASCICLE ORGANIZATION

Size of Fascicles: New Parameter—F90

The plexus was found to have a wide range of fascicle sizes at most levels. Adequate description of the fascicular arrangement must take into account both the variability and the sheer numbers. Because some fascicles are too small to repair reliably and are insignificant in their contribution to the total amount of neural tissue, when comparing numbers of fascicles, it is important to use a parameter selective for fascicles of significant size, as well as a parameter that has conceptual relevance. Additionally, it is useful to exclude fascicles so small that some investigators might not visualize them, whereas others would. We have developed a parameter termed F90, which is the minimum number of fascicles required to constitute at least 90% of the total neural tissue cross-sectional areas of a given nerve or fascicle group. A demonstration of its relevance is provided in Figure 22–4.

Although total fascicle numbers and other parameters were also recorded, our reports focus on the F90 values. An example of calculation of F90 is given below:

For a section with a total neural tissue cross-sectional area of 4.3725 mm^2 and seven fascicles with the following areas, the first three fascicles (indicated by an asterisk) sum to 93.9% of the total, so the F90 = 3:

$$
\begin{array}{lll}
1 & 2.1691 \text{ mm}^2 & = 49.6\%^* \\
2 & 1.5227 \text{ mm}^2 & = 34.8\%^* \\
3 & 0.4121 \text{ mm}^2 & = 9.4\%^*
\end{array}
$$

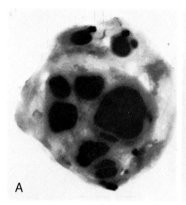
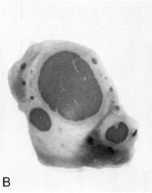
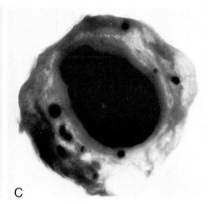

A   B   C

Figure 22–4. The total fascicle counts of (A) and (B) are both 13, but the F90 values of 7 and 3, respectively, more appropriately differentiate them, in accord with their cross-sectional appearance. In (C) a single fascicle predominates; therefore, despite several very small peripheral fascicles, its F90 equals 1, and the nerve is considered monofascicular at this level.

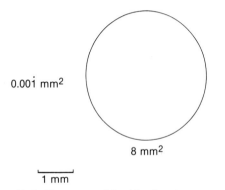

Figure 22–5. The range of fascicle sizes is represented schematically. Scale: 1 mm of fascicle is equal to 7 mm in real measurements.

4	0.1729 mm² =	4.0%
5	0.0922 mm² =	2.1%
6	0.0019 mm² =	< 0.1%
7	0.0016 mm² =	< 0.1%

To be complete, our data included both the total numbers of fascicles and the num-

bers of fascicles larger than 0.1 mm in diameter (diameter is calculated from measured area), in addition to the F90 values.

Fascicle sizes varied markedly within individual sections, their cross-sectional areas ranging over four orders of magnitude from less than 0.001 to 8 mm² (Fig. 22–5). These largest fascicles were present almost exclusively at the spinal nerve level, where a single large fascicle commonly carried over 90% of the neural tissue of a given spinal nerve. Also, in one (plexus 1; see Fig. 22–9A), unique for the small number of fascicles at all levels, similar large fascicles were present at many regions of the plexus, even at the cords. In general, however, the range of fascicle sizes decreased when moving distally from spinal nerves to cords.

A consistent pattern was the wide range of sizes at the spinal nerve level, intermediate range at the trunk level, and narrow range at the cord level.

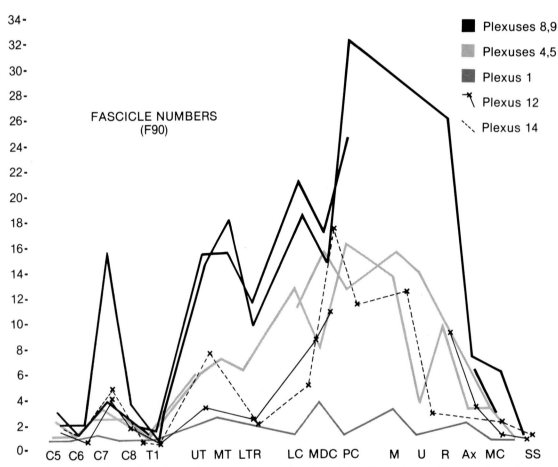

Figure 22–6. Mean F90 values for each plexus element are plotted for all specimens. Plexuses from the same individual have very similar values. Plexuses with many number of fascicles at any given level tend to have many fascicles at all levels. The trend to increased fascicle numbers at the cord level is evident.

Variability from Level to Level: Correlation of Fascicle Number with Plexus Level

Figure 22–6 and Tables 22–1 to 22–3 show that the cords contain the largest number of fascicles, that trunks contain an intermediate number, and that spinal nerves are generally oligo- or monofascicular. From the specimens examined, it was also apparent that the major peripheral nerves of the arm and forearm (ulnar, median, radial) have fascicle numbers in the more intermediate range. The more proximal peripheral nerves of the shoulder (axillary, musculocutaneous, suprascapular) were often at the lower end of the scale.

The fascicle numbers of the divisions are not specifically included in Figure 22–6, but several are listed in Table 22–3. The divisions were often very short in length and variable in their separation from each other, blending gradually into cords, e.g., the anterior division of the lower trunk was simply the prox-imal end of the medial cord in most cases, and spinal nerves sometimes formed divisions before forming trunks or vice versa. Both divisions of the upper trunk were each typically monofascicular during part, although not all, of their length, the anterior division usually more consistently so and at a more proximal level (see Table 22–7). Otherwise, the divisions were not particularly remarkable and were simply intermediate between the spinal nerves and the trunks.

A correlation of fascicle numbers with proximity to branch points is demonstrated in Figure 22–7 and Table 22–4, in which the average number of branches per plexus element correlated in about a 1:3 ratio with the average F90 for all spans at a given level. Branch count included all the named branches as well as the divisions. The correlation coefficient for the number of fascicles and for the number of branches per cord, per trunk, or per spinal nerve is significant to $p < 0.05$.

Table 22–1. F90 VALUES FOR INDIVIDUAL FREE SEGMENT

Plexus	1	4	5	8	9	12	14	Mean ± SD
Free segment								
C5	1.1	1.3	2.3	3.0	2.0	1.7	1.8	1.9
C6	1.0	1.3	1.3	1.3	2.0	1.0	4.0	1.7
C7	1.3	2.8	3.3	4.0	15.7	3.8	5.0	5.1
C8	1.1	2.8	2.0	2.7	3.5	2.0	1.3	2.2
T1	1.0	1.3	1.0	1.5	1.0	1.0	1.0	1.1
UT	2.3	6.1	6.2	15.3	14.0	3.5	7.8	7.9
MT	2.8	7.3	—	15.6	18.3	—	—	11.0
LTR	—	6.4	—	11.5	9.6	2.5	2.2	6.4
LC†	3.0§	12.9	11.2	21.4	18.6	7.5	5.4	11.4
MDC‡	4.1	8.4	15.7	17.1	14.7	11.0	17.2	12.6
PC	3.1‖	16.4	12.8	24.5	32.3	—	11.6	16.8
Median*	3.4	13.7	15.7	—	—	—	12.5	11.3
Ulnar*	1.5	3.8	14.0	—	—	—	3.0	5.6
Radial*	—	10.0	9.7	—	26.0	8.3	—	13.5
Axillary*	2.2	7.0	3.3	6.4	7.3	3.3	—	4.9
Spinal nerve								
mean =	1.1	1.9	2.0	2.5	4.8	1.9	2.6	2.4 ± 2.2
Trunks								
mean =	2.6	6.6	6.2	14.1	14.0	3.0	5.0	7.4 ± 8.9
Cords								
mean =	3.4	12.6	13.2	21.0	21.9	9.3	11.4	13.3 ± 12.0
Peripheral nerve								
mean =	2.0	8.6	8.2	6.4	16.7	5.8	8.8	8.1 ± 8.2

*The proximal 2 cm of these peripheral nerves were sectioned and measured in several specimens.
†The lateral cord values represent the portion proximal to the exit of the musculocutaneous nerve.
‡The medial cord values represent the portion proximal to the exit of the ulnar nerve.
§‖The lateral and posterior cords of the plexus 1 are each composed of two spans of nerve that ultimately merge together. The fascicle numbers recorded here are the sums of the two parts.
UT = upper trunk, MT = middle trunk, LTR = lower trunk, LC = lateral cord, MDC = medial cord, PC = posterior cord.

Table 22–2. MEAN NUMBERS OF FASCICLES FOR EACH REGION OF THE BRACHIAL PLEXUS*

	Total No. Fascicles	Fascicles > 0.1 mm Diameter	F90
Spinal nerve (mean)	8.0	5.5	2.4
Trunks (mean)	16.9	13.6	7.4
Cords (mean)	24.6	21.9	13.3
Peripheral nerve (mean)	15.4	13.4	8.1

*Averaged for seven plexuses.

Figure 22–8 plots F90 data points for individual sections in representative plexus segments. There is a gradual increase in fascicle numbers with increasing distance from the vertebral foramina, approaching the axilla. Aberrations exist in the upper trunk, but the trend is typical.

Variability Among Individuals

The mean F90 values for each plexus ranged from 2 to 12, a 6-fold range of variability, but most of the plexuses were similar in numbers of fascicles at the various levels, generally staying within a 2-fold range. Except for the single example of each extreme, the mean spinal nerve F90 values ranged from 1.9 to 2.6 fascicles, the mean trunk F90 values ranged from 3.0 to 14.0, and the mean cord F90 values ranged from 11.4 to 21.0. Although the range of trunk values was high, the three middle values were similar: 5.0, 6.2, and 6.6.

Individual F90 values ranged from 1.0 in the spinal nerves of some plexuses to over 30.0 in cords of some plexuses. Table 22–1 presents the individual fascicle counts for the free segment of each plexus element. Figure 22–6 shows the average F90 values for each element of all seven plexuses in such a way that they can be compared plexus by plexus. In the two sets of bilateral plexuses studied

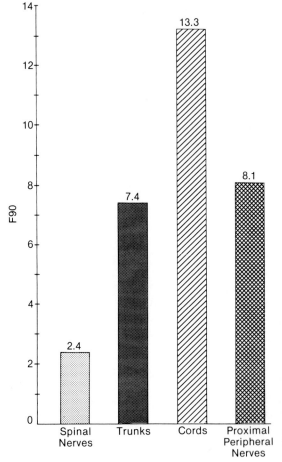

Figure 22–7. The average F90 per spinal nerve, trunk, or cord, for all plexuses.

by serial section (plexuses 4 and 5, plexuses 8 and 9), F90 values for corresponding levels were almost identical in most cases. Variability was more marked among different individuals than between opposite sides of the same body.

Also apparent was that a plexus with more fascicles than another plexus at one level had

Table 22–3. F90 VALUES FOR SEVERAL DIVISIONS

Plexus Division	1	4	9	12	14	Mean
Anterior division, upper trunk	—	1.6	5.5	1.0	—	2.7
Posterior division, upper trunk	1.3	3.4	10.4	2.0	6.0	4.6
Posterior division, lower trunk	—	1.9	3.9	2.0	2.0	2.5

Table 22–4. CORRELATION OF FASCICLES TO BRANCHES

	Spinal Nerves	Trunks	Cords
F90 (mean)	2.4	7.4	13.3
No. branches (mean)	4.2	6.9	12.7
No. elements	5	3	3
Branches/elements	0.8	2.3	4.2
$\dfrac{F90}{\text{branches/element}} =$	3.0	3.2	3.2
$=$	3.1 (mean)		

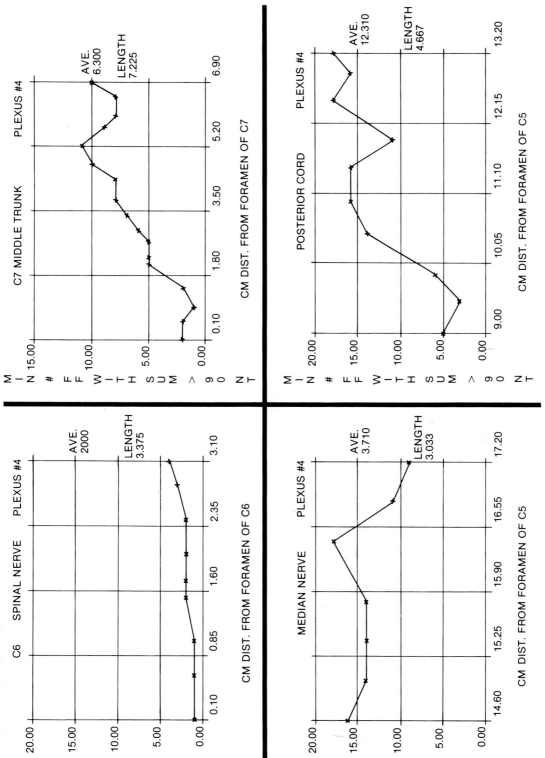

Figure 22–8. F90 values for individual sections of parts of plexus #4, demonstrating the increase in F90 moving distally, the presence of monofascicularity at the spinal nerves, and the decrease in F90 in the median nerve distal to its origin from the medial and lateral cords.

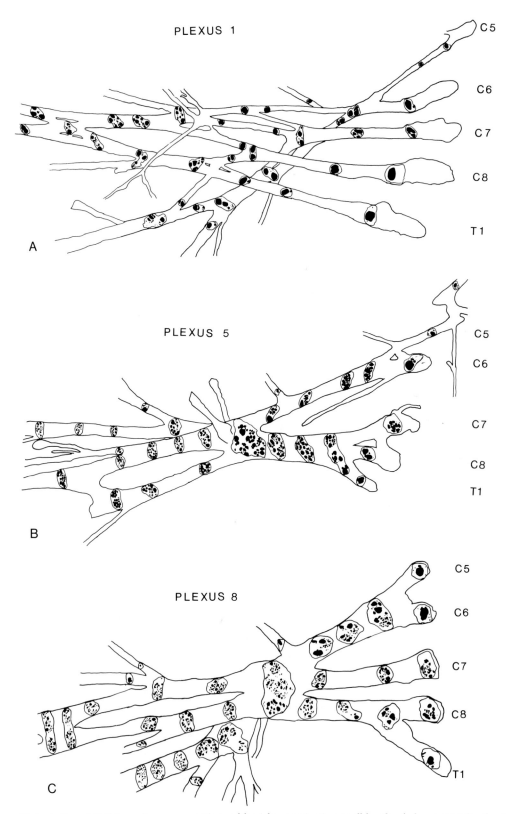

Figure 22–9. *A, B,* and *C,* Schematic representations of fascicle organization at all levels of plexus #1 (oligofascicular), plexus #5 (exemplary), and plexus #8 (polyfascicular).

a strong tendency to have more fascicles at all levels. The converse is true for plexuses with few fascicles.

Certain plexus regions demonstrated characteristic topography that was repeated in most or all specimens, and fascicle numbers consistently increased from proximal to distal (Fig. 22–9).

CHANGES IN TOPOGRAPHY

Changes in topography were assessed in terms of fascicles, fascicle groups, and plexus elements.

TOPOGRAPHY: FASCICLE

Fascicles merged with each other and branched over distance. There was frequent mixing of fascicles, and they could be traced individually rarely more than 1 cm without interaction. Often, two fascicles traveling together merged within a single perineurial sheath, with their axons mingling to an unknown degree, and then branched again into two similar-sized fascicles. Without reliable axonal tracer methods for tracking the course of axons in each such fascicle during such a merger, there was no basis for deducing anything about the consequent rearrangement of axons, except to recognize the range of possibilities, i.e., from the one extreme of no rearrangement to the other of total rearrangement. Calculations took this uncertainty into account.

The anterior and posterior roots of each spinal nerve invariably fused very proximally, rendering indistinguishable the motor and sensory components. In no more than six specimens among the 35 spinal nerves studied by serial section had the ventral and dorsal roots not merged proximal to their exit from the intervertebral foramina. In these, all but one merged within 7 mm, and one merged at 2.1 cm. In C7, although merger into a single fascicle was not the rule, clearly distinct contributions from the ventral and dorsal roots distal to the foramen were identifiable in only one specimen.

Length of a Fascicle. The fascicular topography of the elements of the brachial plexus is, in itself, plexiform in nature. Intraneural topography changed approximately every millimeter. To provide a rough idea of the distance that a fascicle may travel in the

Table 22–5. FASCICLE LENGTHS—SUMMARY

Random Section From	Plexus No.	Mean Fascicle Length (cm)	No. Fascicles
Spinal nerve	4	0.67	10
Trunk	8	0.40	28
Cord	12	0.40	22

Average fascicle length (average of means) = 0.49 cm

Average fascicle length (mean of fascicles sampled) = 0.45 cm

plexus free of other interactions, one section from each of three plexus specimens was selected randomly, representing the spinal nerves, trunks, and cords. Each of the fascicles was then traced proximally and distally through serial sections until it branched or merged with another fascicle or, in the case of three fascicles, exited the nerve element. A total of 60 fascicles were traced to supply these data. Plexus specimens were both normal and multifascicular.

Results in Table 22–5 demonstrate that fascicles in the brachial plexus may be thought of as having a certain length, the limits of which are the result of their merging or branching. In addition, the fascicles that result from the merger or branching have, in turn, certain lengths of their own.

The fascicle lengths for 60 fascicles averaged approximately 5 mm, ranging from approximately 2 to 10 mm in the spinal nerve, 1 to 13 mm in the trunk, and 1 to 12 mm in the cord. For cord, trunk, and spinal nerve , and for each of these plexuses, the length of a fascicle was consistently less than 1.5 cm, averaging approximately 5 mm.

Topography: Fascicle Group

The fascicle groups destined for each peripheral nerve branch were traced proximally from the point of exit to each of three levels: (1) level of segregation, (2) level of purity, and (3) level of localization.

The point of exit is the most proximal section in which the fascicle group is not included in the main plexus element. The level of segregation is the most proximal section in which the fascicle group appears on cross section to be physically separate or distinct from the rest of the fascicles, while still included in the same epineurium. This is the level that is most subjectively assessed.

Table 22–6. DISTANCE BRANCH FASCICLE GROUPS MAY BE TRACED PROXIMALLY*
FROM POINT OF EXIT TO:

	Point of Localization of Fascicle Group (cm)	Point of Purity of Fascicle Group (cm)	Point of Segregation of Fascicle Group (cm)
Dorsal scapular	1.0 (0.4–2.0)	0.7 (0.4–1.2)	0.5 (0.4–0.7)
Long thoracic	1.2 (0.6–2.3)	1.1 (0.4–2.1)	0.9 (0.4–1.6)
Suprascapular	2.0 (1.4–4.5)	1.8 (0.9–4.5)	1.4 (0.6–3.9)
Subscapular	2.2 (1.2–4.0)	1.9 (0.6–4.0)	1.5 (0.6–3.2)
Pectoral	1.9 (0.5–3.6)	1.7 (0.5–3.6)	1.4 (0.4–3.7)
Intercostobrachial	2.7 (1.5–4.1)	2.5 (1.5–4.0)	1.5 (0.4–3.6)
Medial antebrachial cutaneous	2.5 (1.3–3.5)	1.8 (0.7–2.9)	1.0 (0.4–2.1)
Thoracodorsal	1.8 (1.0–2.9)	1.3 (0.6–2.2)	0.9 (0.1–2.1)
Musculocutaneous	4.1 (1.3–8.3)	1.7 (0.7–2.5)	1.6 (0.4–3.0)
Median	4.3 (2.9–5.5)	1.5 (0.2–3.4)	1.0 (0.1–1.6)
Axillary	1.5 (1.0–2.6)	0.9 (0.1–2.0)	1.0 (0.3–1.9)
Radial	2.5 (0.4–5.5)	1.3 (0.1–2.0)	0.9 (0.1–1.5)
Ulnar	4.4 (1.2 –6.4)	1.0 (0.2–2.0)	0.9 (0.1–2.3)
Upper trunk, posterior div.	2.8 (2.0–3.7)	2.3 (0.8–4.6)	2.0 (1.2–3.0)
Upper trunk, anterior div.	2.4 (1.1–3.1)	1.6 (0.8–2.8)	1.7 (0.5–2.6)
Mean (exclude upper trunk divisions)	2.5 (1.0–4.4)	1.5 (0.7–2.5)	1.1 (0.9–1.6)

*Six of seven plexuses included.

The level of purity is the most proximal section beyond (distal to) all significant interactions of fascicles destined for the given branch, i.e., the first section, going proximal to distal, where all the neural tissue of the given branch is contained in fascicles that have no further interaction with fascicles destined for other branches. Very minor interactions were occasionally observed near the exit point of a branch, but when they were isolated and very small, they were not used to determine the level of purity.

The level of localization is the most proximal section in which at least 50% of the neural tissue of the branch is contained in pure fascicles localized to one cross-sectional region of the element.

The results of these data are summarized in Table 22–6 and Figure 22–10. The mean distances from the exit point to the level of localization, level of purity, and level of segregation are 2.5 cm, 1.5 cm, and 1.1 cm, respectively, equivalent to 16%, 10%, and 7% of the mean distance to the crotch of the

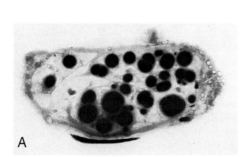
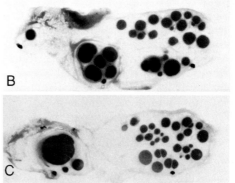

Figure 22–10. Fascicle groups representing each branch were traced proximally from point of exit to *A*, the most proximal point where at least 50% of the neural tissue for the branch was *localized* in pure fascicles; *B*, the most proximal point where all the neural tissue for the branch was localized in *pure* fascicles; and *C*, the most proximal point where the fascicle group was *segregated* for the rest of the plexus element.

The cross-sections *A*, *B*, and *C*, demonstrate these levels. In *A*, the group of fascicles clumped just to the left of center and along the anterior (bottom) will exit as the musculocutaneous nerve. These fascicles are all pure, and the fascicle group is considered *pure*. In *B*, which is more distal, the group of fascicles noted above has moved more superiorly (to the viewer's left) and is clearly *segregated* from the rest of the lateral cord. The single fascicle far to the left will supply the coracobrachialis muscle and will exit the lateral cord proximal to the exit of the musculocutaneous. Even more distally, in *C*, the musculocutaneous has just *exited* the lateral cord.

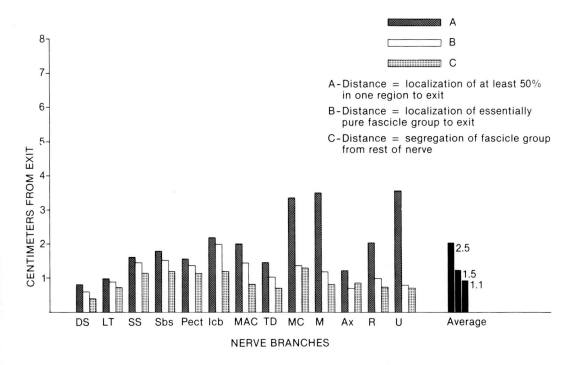

AVERAGE TRACEABLE DISTANCES:
BRANCH FASCICLE GROUPS

A - Distance = localization of at least 50%
in one region to exit

B - Distance = localization of essentially
pure fascicle group to exit

C - Distance = segregation of fascicle group
from rest of nerve

median nerve from the C5 intervertebral foramen.

Figures 22–11 and 22–12 represent the cross-sectional localization of fascicle groups in certain quadrants in a serially sectioned specimen and in an average plexus.

Topography: Plexus Element

There is generally some change in cross-sectional fascicular arrangement every millimeter as a result of merger or branching of at least one fascicle. This varies, but minor changes certainly are frequent. Assuming random distribution of fascicle branch and merger points and knowing that an average fascicle travels 5 mm without interaction, an average plexus element with ten fascicles has almost a 99% chance of change in at least one fascicle over each millimeter.

Although minor changes occur frequently, those changes often involve very small fascicles or are within fascicle groups rather than between them and therefore are of little reconstructive significance. Whereas sections 10 mm apart often seem vastly dissimilar in appearance, tracing fascicles every 0.5 to 1 mm (as we have done) clarifies the exact progression of changes and often reveals

minimal net rearrangement between fascicle groups over 1 to 2 cm.

The sequence of slides shown in Figure 22–13 demonstrates gradual changes in the lateral cord over 2 cm. The sequence of slides of the upper trunk (Fig. 22–14) demonstrates a counterexample, with rapid, important changes as C5 and C6 merge to form the upper trunk and then trifurcate into the suprascapular nerve and the anterior and posterior divisions of the trunk.

Monofascicularity. In the plexus, monofascicularity (F90 = 1) was found consistently in several locations, as outlined in Table 22–7 and shown in Figure 22–15. These locations are in the divisions of the upper trunk, in the spinal nerves, and in the origins of the suprascapular and musculocutaneous nerves. The average lengths of each monofascicular segment are also noted. The posterior division of the lower trunk also had a consistent fascicular pattern, that of bifascicularity.

NEURAL TISSUE QUANTITATION

The quantity of neural tissue is best described as the cross-sectional area of fascicle

Text continued on page 306

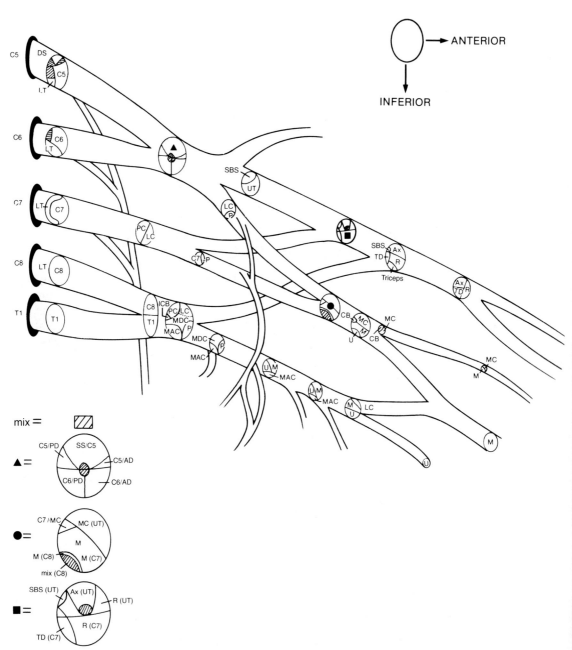

Figure 22–11. Schematic drawing of the localization of fascicle groups within plexus elements as determined by tracing these groups proximally or distally with serial cross sections—average for all plexuses.

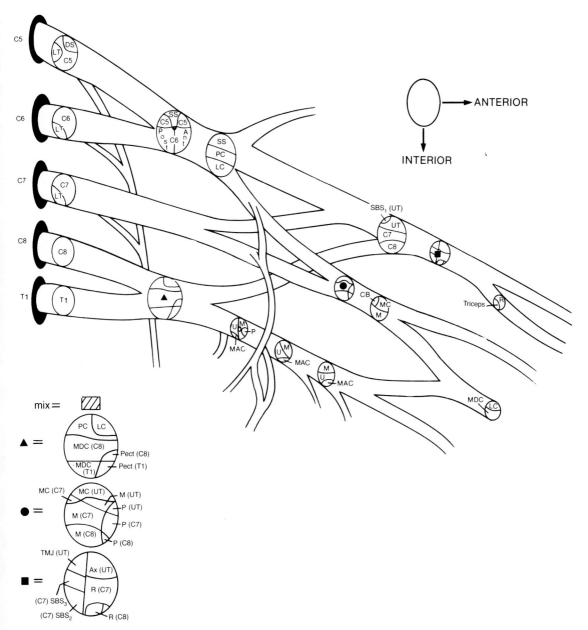

Figure 22–12. Schematic drawing of the localization of fascicle groups within plexus elements as determined by tracing these groups proximally or distally with serial cross sections—example of a single plexus (#5).

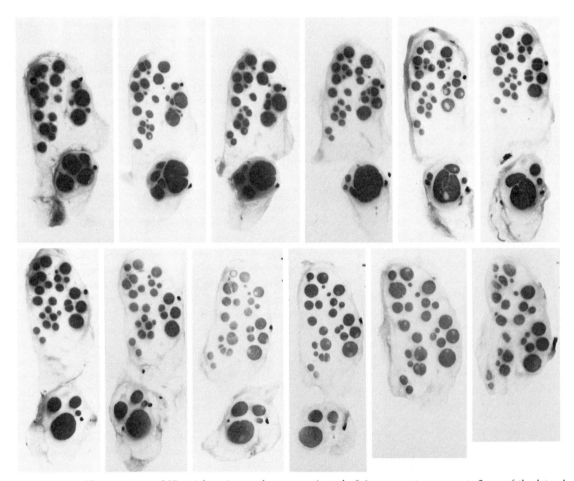

Figure 22–13. This sequence of 27 serial sections, taken approximately 0.6 mm apart, represents 2 cm of the lateral cord in plexus #8 and demonstrates the details of intraneural topography typical through most of the plexus, where gross differences 1 or 2 cm apart can be well traced through gradual changes over each millimeter. The branch that exits superiorly is the musculocutaneous. Note that it coalesces into a single dominant fascicle, while the rest of the lateral cord has about 20 fascicles.

Illustration continued on opposite page

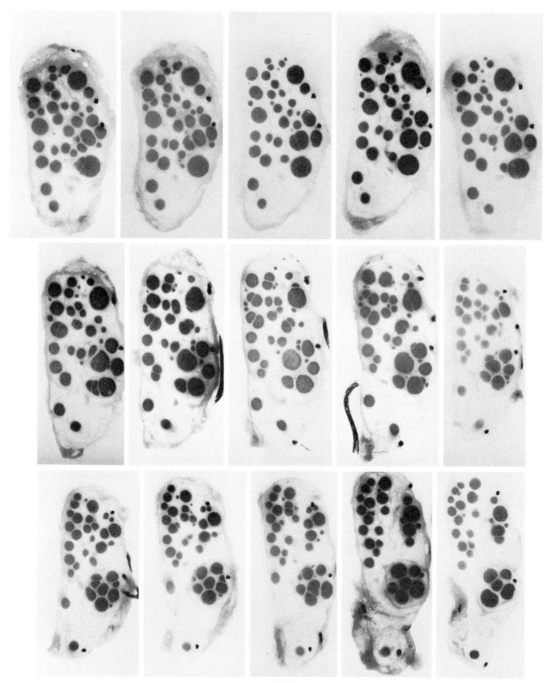

Figure 22–13 *Continued*

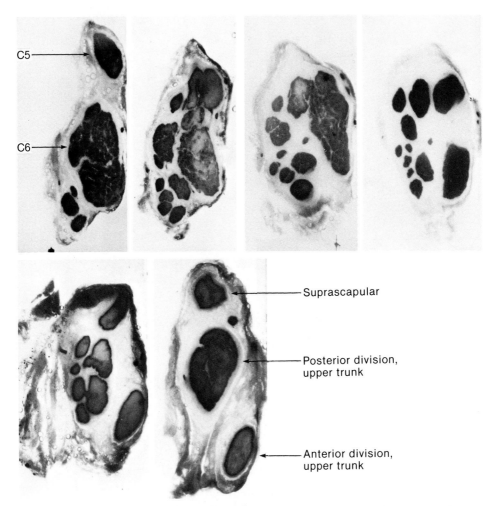

Figure 22–14. This sequence of six sections samples a 3-cm span of the upper trunk from the initial merging of C5 and C6 spinal nerves, through the gross mixing of fascicles, to the rearrangement into three monofascicular components, the anterior and posterior divisions of the upper trunk, and the suprascapular nerve.

Table 22-7. MONOFASCICULARITY IN THE BRACHIAL PLEXUS

Plexus Element	No. and % with F90 = 1		Average Length (cm)	Distance from Foramen (cm)		
				Prox.	*Mid.*	*Distal*
C5	7	100%	1.6	0.3	1.3	2.1
C6	5	71	1.0	0.2	0.9	1.6
C7	3	42	0.5	0.6	1.2	1.7
C8	6	86	1.6	0.4	1.5	2.5
T1	7	100	2.0	0.1	1.1	2.1
UT/AD	5	71	1.7	5.8	7.0	8.1
UT/PD	4	57	0.9	7.9	8.9	9.8
MC	4	57	0.8	10.3	11.1	11.8
SS	7	100	1.8	5.1	6.0	6.9
C8/LC	3*	100	3.1	5.1	6.6	8.1

*In all three cases where C8 contributes to the lateral cord, that plexus element has a segment of monofascicularity. Seven plexuses were examined.

Length of monofascicular segment is averaged over all seven specimens. Proximal and distal ends of monofascicular segment were averaged over those specimens where monofascicularity seen.

All distances are measured from the C5 foramen, except that each spinal nerve is measured from its respective foramen.

UT/AD = upper trunk, anterior division, UT/PD = upper trunk, posterior division, MC = musculocutaneous nerve, SS = suprascapular nerve, LC = lateral cord.

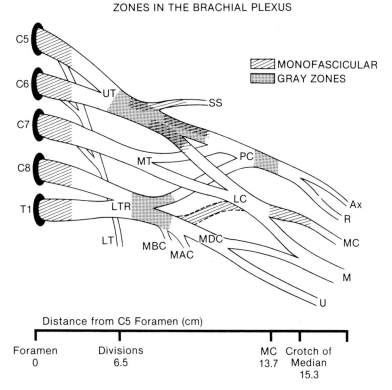

ZONES IN THE BRACHIAL PLEXUS

Figure 22-15. Plexus gray zones and regions of monofascicularity are shown, and average distances along the plexus are marked.

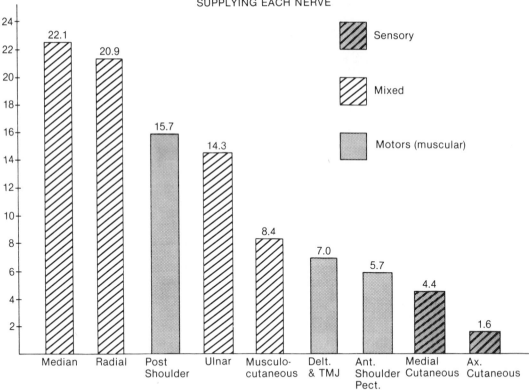

Figure 22–16. Percentage of total plexus neural tissue supplying each major nerve or group of nerves.

contents measured in square millimeters. The neural tissue of the seven plexus specimens has been recorded in several ways. Table 22–8 lists the neural tissue areas for the elements of the plexus (spinal nerves, trunks, and cords). Table 22–9 lists the neural tissue areas of the plexus branches, and Figure 22–16 shows the neural tissue supply in terms of muscle groups. The tables include information from each plexus demonstrating variability. Mean values are also reported.

A high level of conservation of neural tissue from proximal to distal was observed, with the sum of plexus branch areas being 93.1% of the sum of spinal nerve areas (Table 22–10). In describing the percentage of total plexus neural tissue distributed to each of the peripheral nerves, however, the measured area of each branch was divided into the sum of the spinal nerve neural tissue areas, then corrected to sum to 100%.

Noteworthy is that the relative amount of C6, C7, and C8 neural tissue was constant at 24% from plexus to plexus, whereas C5 and T1 tissue varied inversely and widely from plexus to plexus (Fig. 22–17 and Table 22–11). Correlations between the sized C5 and other plexus components are shown in Figure 22–18.

DISTRIBUTION OF NEURAL TISSUE

Fascicle groups were traced from the spinal nerves and trunks distally until localization was lost and from the branches of the plexus proximally until localization was lost. In most cases, there was a level of the plexus at which certain fascicles could be clearly identified as representing a specific spinal nerve proximally and a specific branch distally, so that the neural tissue contribution from the spinal nerves to each peripheral nerve could be determined. In most cases, mixing of fascicle groups produced some ambiguity, so that a certain percentage of a branch's neural tissue could be definitely shown to arise from a certain spinal nerve, but another percentage of that branch's tissue could only be shown to arise from a mixture of two spinal nerves. In these cases, a range of values is provided, so that when 50% of a branch is from C7, 40% is from C8, and 10% is from a mixture of C7 and C8, we report that C7 supplies 50 to 60% and C8 supplies 40 to 50%.

Because the anterior and posterior divisions of the upper trunk were so frequently monofascicular at some level, differentiation of C5 from C6 was lost distal to the divisions in most cases, but knowledge of the size of

Table 22–8. CROSS-SECTIONAL AREAS OF NERVE TISSUE OF EACH ELEMENT OF PLEXUS (mm²)

	1	4	5	8	9	12	14	Average
C5	2.0376	4.0741	3.2700	4.3874	4.2280	2.387	6.1926	3.9767
C6	7.5337	7.2159	7.3673	5.9109	5.9860	5.698	7.8030	6.7878
C7	6.4847	8.2370	7.4871	5.1768	5.9435	6.485	8.3910	6.8864
C8	7.7978	8.3790	7.7700	4.9635	4.2700	5.787	8.2050	6.7389
T1	6.1196	4.5400	3.9990	2.4100	2.2940	6.563	4.3560	4.3259
Sum	29.9734	32.4460	29.8934	22.8486	22.7215	26.920	34.9476	28.5360
UT	10.0460	9.235	8.4594	8.7614	9.551	7.416	13.414	9.555
MT	6.4847	8.157	7.4871	5.2450	5.802	6.378	8.391	6.849
LTR	13.9174	11.934	11.1697	6.5623	7.235	11.460	10.806	10.441
Sum	30.4481	29.326	27.1162	20.5687	22.588	25.254	32.611	26.845
LC	9.8969	6.8612	8.5801	4.7101	6.5764	7.0052	5.1508	6.9687
MDC	5.9933	8.8005	7.2397	5.1750	6.0030	5.4480	12.9340	7.3705
PC	11.1940	9.4890	8.5840	7.2624	7.8893	10.0460	11.8160	9.4687
Sum	27.0842	25.1507	24.4000	17.1475	20.4687	22.4992	29.9008	23.8079

UT = upper trunk, MT = middle trunk, LTR = lower trunk, LC = lateral cord, MDC = medial cord, PC = posterior cord.

Table 22–9. NEURAL TISSUE CROSS-SECTIONAL AREAS FOR ALL BRANCHES, ALL PLEXUSES (mm²)

	1	4	5	8	9	12	14	Mean
DS	0.5383	0.2786	0.4645	0.1791	0.3523	0.2817	—	0.3491
LT	0.9865	0.7207	1.0449	0.6204	0.5517	0.9387	0.9189	0.8260
LT/C5	—	0.3900	0.2985	0.2887	0.0032	0.3136	0.2946	0.2648
LT/C6	0.4694	0.1708 +	0.5740	0.2575	0.4070	0.4112	0.5022	0.3989 +
LT/C7	0.5171	0.1599	0.1724	0.0742	0.1415	0.2139	0.0983	0.1968
LT/C8	—	—	—	—	—	—	0.0238	0.0238
SS	1.3053	1.0806	1.1351	1.1549	1.056	1.227	1.803	1.2517
Subsc + Tmj	—	—	—	—	—	—	—	
1	0.3285	0.0925	0.3594	0.3188	0.2592	0.1614	0.2497	0.2528
2	0.2628	0.4794	0.6193	0.1619	0.2953	—	0.3823	0.3669
3	—	—	—	0.4199	0.0216	—	—	0.2208
Tmj	—	0.735	0.6462	0.2287	0.4683	0.8588	—	0.5874
TD	0.6052	—	—	0.5964	0.4609	0.5127	0.8384	0.6027
AX + Subsc	3.6579	—	—	—	—	—	3.2849	3.4714
AX pure	—	1.734	1.955	2.0317	2.1031	1.9664	—	1.9580
PECTS	1.2597	1.5572	1.6765	1.1522	1.3342	1.5282	2.1177	1.5180
LAT	0.7260	1.2123	1.5202	0.9375	0.4470	1.1636	0.0795	0.8694
LAT	0.4866	—	—	—	0.6204	0.3646	0.8503	0.5804
MED	0.0471	0.3449	0.1563	0.2147	0.2668	—	1.1879	0.3696
MAC	1.4444	0.8530	0.5941	1.0138	1.0160	1.2100	1.1590	1.0415
MBC	—	—	—	—	—	0.1853	—	0.1853
ICB	—	0.1426	—	0.2481	—	0.1720	—	0.1876
MC	2.5912	1.7756	1.7924	1.7953	2.173	2.4810	2.6900	2.1855
Ulnar	3.7823	4.4080	3.8847	3.6683	3.096	2.6660	4.8740	3.7685
Median	6.7782	6.1990	7.3353	5.0481	5.005	3.9392	6.7229	5.8611
Radial	6.2012	5.602	6.3210	4.5104	4.5309	4.8568	6.7794	5.5431
CB	—	—	0.0467	0.1334	0.1137	(0.1224)	—	0.1041

DS = dorsal scapular nerve, LT = lower trunk, SS = suprascapular nerve, Subsc + Tmj = subscapular + teres major, TD = thoracodorsal nerve, AX + Subsc = axillary nerve + some subscapular nerve, AX pure = axillary nerve only, PECTS = pectoral nerves. MAC, medial antebrachial cutaneous nerve, MBC = medial brachial cutaneous nerve, ICB = intercostobrachial nerve, MC = musculocutaneous nerve, CB = coracobrachial nerve.

Table 22–10. PERCENTAGE OF PLEXUS NEURAL TISSUE DISTRIBUTED TO EACH BRANCH

	Neural Tissue Cross-Sectional Area (mm²)	% of Total	Corrected to 100%
MC + CB	2.1855	07.8	08.4
Median	5.8611	20.6	22.1
Ulnar	3.7680	13.3	14.3
Radial	5.5431	19.5	20.9
Scapular girdle	7.3504	26.3	28.2
		87.5	93.9
Axillary sensory	0.4153	1.5	1.6
Medial cutaneous	1.1626	4.1	4.4
		5.6	6.0
Total branch neural tissue		93.1	99.9

With scapular girdle:

Pectoral nerves	1.5180	5.3	5.7
Axillary motor	1.8093	6.5	7.0
Posterior shoulder	4.1040	14.6	15.7
DS	0.2992	1.1	1.2
LT	0.8260	2.9	3.1
Subscapular	1.0745	4.6	4.9
TD	0.6027	1.6	1.7
SS	1.2517	4.4	4.7
Total scapular girdle		26.4	28.4

MC + CB = musculocutaneous + coracobrachial nerves, DS = dorsal scapular nerve, LT = long thoracic nerve of Bell, TD = thoracodorsal nerve, SS = suprascapular nerve.

C5 and C6, as well as knowledge of their contributions to proximal branches, was sufficient to calculate the amount of C5 and C6 still available for more distal branches. When C5 was not large enough to account for all of the mixed fascicles, we recognized that C6 must contribute a minimum portion of the amount in the mixed fascicles, and calculations were revised to account for this information. Calculated distribution of neural tissue for all spinal nerves, trunks, cords, and branches is reported in Tables 22–12 to 22–14. Examples are represented in Figures 22–19 to 22–21.

When a range of values is reported, it does not represent variability among different specimens, but indicates the range of possibilities within one specimen. Specifying where in that range the true value lies has been limited by the amount of fascicle mixing.

PERCENTAGE OF CROSS-SECTIONAL AREA DEVOTED TO NEURAL TISSUE

The percentage of the total cross-sectional area of each element of the plexus devoted to neural tissue is reported in Table 22–15 and is represented graphically for plexus 5 in Figure 22–22. The corresponding connective tissue percentage, including both perineurium and epineurium, is the remainder (100% minus the neural tissue per cent). On average, two thirds of the plexus tissue was connective tissue.

Values for plexus 1 have been excluded because much of the epineurial tissue was dissected off that specimen before sectioning it, thereby falsely increasing the relative neural tissue percentages. In general, however, even in this plexus with few fascicles throughout and with a substantial amount of epineurium removed, the neural tissue was still only approximately 50%. The epineurium on the other specimens was preserved.

An incidental observation is the very low percentage of the distal axillary nerve composed of neural tissue (10 to 20%). Also observed was an increase in connective tissue at branch points, thereby decreasing the relative percentage of the nerve element composed of neural tissue for short intervals.

DISCUSSION

We have studied 21 adult human brachial plexuses with several objectives in mind, the foremost of these being to provide quantitative data about brachial plexus anatomy on the fascicle level, hoping that this might assist the surgeon in better understanding the plexus in a systematic way.

Review of existing work, both at the plexus level and at the level of the major nerves of the arm and forearm, revealed that changes in intraneural topography are frequent. Previous workers used nonquantitative microdissection methods almost exclusively. Cross-sectional data for the brachial plexus are provided only by Bonnel,[5] who showed that marked changes occur in the organization of fascicles every 10-mm. Apparently, his sections were 10 mm apart, and the regions of nerve between these sections were ignored. Sunderland[48] and Terzis et al.[59] found that changes in fascicular topography of the median nerve occurred much more frequently than every 10 mm. We believe that it is important for a surgeon to understand

Text continued on page 314

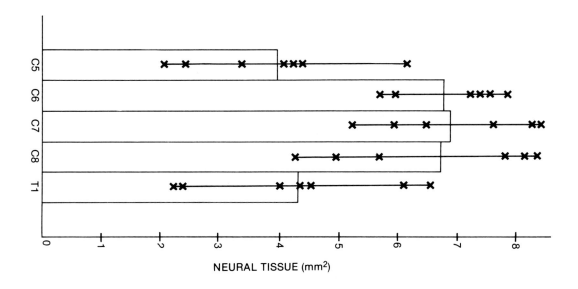

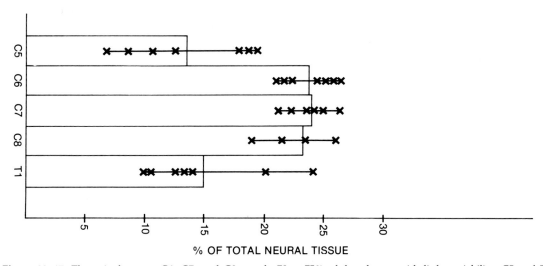

Figure 22–17. The spinal nerves C6, C7, and C8 supply 70 to 75% of the plexus, with little variability. C5 and T1 supply significantly less and vary widely and inversely. The ranges of variability are provided.

Table 22–11. RELATIVE CONTRIBUTION TO THE PLEXUS OF EACH SPINAL NERVE
(PERCENT OF TOTAL)

	1	4	5	8	9	12	14	Mean SD
C5	6.8	12.6	10.9	19.2	18.6	8.9	17.7	13.5 ± 4.6
C6	25.1	21.9	24.6	25.9	26.3	21.2	22.3	23.9 ± 1.9
C7	21.6	25.1	25.0	22.7	26.2	24.1	24.0	24.1 ± 1.4
C8	26.0	25.8	26.0	21.7	18.8	21.5	23.5	23.3 ± 2.6
T1	20.4	14.0	13.4	10.5	10.1	24.4	12.5	15.0 ± 5.0

sum of C5 + T1 means = 28.5%
sum of C6 + C7 + C8 means = 71.3%

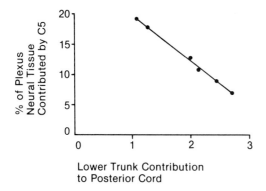

Lower Trunk Contribution
to Posterior Cord

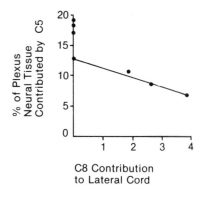

C8 Contribution
to Lateral Cord

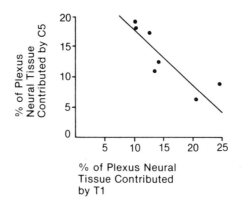

% of Plexus Neural
Tissue Contributed
by T1

Figure 22–18. Correlations between the size of C5 and other aspects of the plexus are demonstrated graphically.

Table 22–12. MEAN PERCENTAGE OF EACH OF THE FOLLOWING NERVES SUPPLIED BY EACH SPINAL NERVE (n = 7)

	Ulnar Nerve	Median Nerve	Musculocutaneous Nerve	Radial Nerve
C5 + C6	0%	11.8–16.6%	83.5–92.0	16.6–41.6
C7	1.3–5.30	34.0–43.1	5.9–16.5	23.9–56.3
C8	31.7–81.7	9.5–45.6	0–2.1	15.9–30.4
T1	17.0–62.8	6.8–39.7	0	2.0–16.9
Lower trunk	94.7–98.7	45.6–53.2		23.5–34.5
Lateral cord	9.9–14.4			

	Pectoral Nerves	Axillary Nerve		Long Thoracic Nerve
C5 + C6	25.8%	64.4–99.9%	C5	27.9%
C7	50.2–50.5	0.1–35.6*	C6	48.6%
C8	12.7–18.6	0	C7	23.3%
T1	5.4–11.3	0	C8	0.4
			T1	0

*In at least four of seven cases, C7 contributed less than 2% of axillary.

Table 22–13. MEAN PROXIMAL AND DISTAL DISTRIBUTION OF EACH CORD (n = 7)

	Posterior Cord	Medial Cord	Lateral Cord
C5 + C6	50.9%	0%	49.4%
C7	30.9	4.8	37.3
C8	14.0–16.7	41.7–55.8	13.3
T1	2.5–5.2	39.3–55.4	0
Lower trunk	19.2	95.2	13.3
Musculocutaneous	0	0	33.8%
Median	0	31.5–37.2%	43.6–45.6
Ulnar	0	42.5–48.2%	4.0–6.0
Radial	58.8	0	0
Axillary	25.1	0	0
Pectoral	0	3.5%	17.2
Medial cutaneous	0	16.5%	0
Thoracodorsal	06.3%	0	0
Subscapular	11.6%	0	0
Unspecified	0	0.2%	0.4

Percentages refer to percentage of each cord distributed to each element listed.

Table 22–14. MEAN PERCENTAGE OF EACH TRUNK AND SPINAL NERVE DESTINED FOR EACH PERIPHERAL NERVE (n = 7)

	Upper Trunk	C7	C8	T1	Lower Trunk
Long thoracic	—	3.0	0.04	0	—
Suprascapular	13.2	—	—	—	—
Pectoral	3.8	10.7–10.8	2.7–4.3	2.5–4.9	3.6
Musculocutaneous	18.7–21.5	2.7–5.2	0–0.9	0	—
Median	7.4–9.9	30.4–37.1	9.6–36.0	8.9–60.0	25.9–28.9
Ulnar	0	0.7–2.8	19.9–50.8	14.2–70.3	35.2–36.5
Radial	14.9–19.0	18.0–40.5	17.5–25.3*	4.9–15.7*	12.6–17.6
Axillary	14.7–25.0	0.1–6.9	0	0	0
Subscapular	4.8–5.2(+)	1.4–4.1	0	0	ø
Thoracodorsal	0.3–0.9	1.6–6.7	*	*	—
Medial Cutaneous	0	ø	0.2–7.7	15.9–26.2	11.2
Intercostobrachial	0	ø	0–0.8	0.8–2.5	0.9
Lateral cord	34.2%	44.0–44.2%	17.3	0	10.2%
Medial cord	0	8.2	53.9–62.1	83.6–93.0	70.7%
Posterior cord	52.6%	44.6–44.8%	20.7–26.5	4.6–13.8	18.1%
	C5 = 32.2%			C8 = 61.6%	
	C6 = 67.8%			T1 = 38.4%	

*Thoracodorsal included with radial.

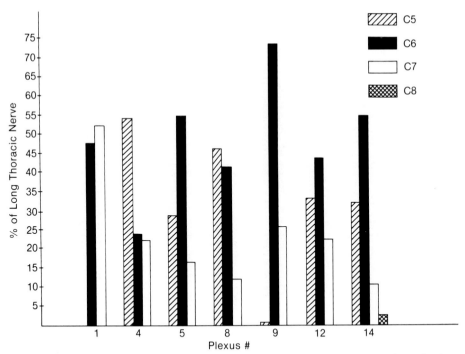

Figure 22–19. The spinal nerve origins of the long thoracic nerve are presented for each plexus.

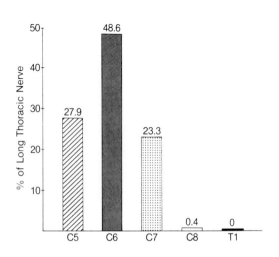

Figure 22–20. The averaged spinal nerve origins of the long thoracic nerve are shown.

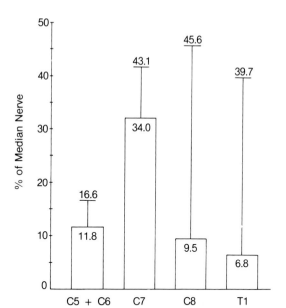

Figure 22–21. The averaged spinal nerve origins of the median nerve are shown, with a range showing the uncertainty due to mixing. Note that C7, C8, and T1 supply the bulk of the nerve, while C5 and C6 together supply very little.

Table 22–15. PERCENTAGE OF CROSS-SECTIONAL AREA DEVOTED TO NEURAL TISSUE

Plexus Element	4	5	8	9	12	14	Mean	SD
C5	47.1	36.4	27.1	29.4	26.3	25.7	32.0	7.6
C6	43.9	37.8	27.4	29.1	38.3	23.8	31.7	7.0
C7/MT	39.9	36.2	21.8	25.6	36.0	37.8	32.9	6.7
C8	31.2	28.6	20.2	23.4	29.9	30.0	27.2	4.0
T1	34.7	38.9	24.6	25.9	27.6	26.5	29.7	5.2
UT	48.7	42.2	26.8	29.9	37.1	31.5	36.0	7.6
LTR	35.4	37.0	21.5	24.9	23.2	37.1	29.9	6.7
MDC	48.9	39.5	29.5	36.6	21.5	26.7	33.8	9.0
PC	39.3	33.3	23.6	20.7	—	24.9	28.4	6.9
LC	44.9	36.3	24.4	27.7	24.7	27.6	30.9	7.4
Median	47.3	39.6					43.5	3.9
Ulnar	58.2	39.7				31.3	43.1	11.2
MC	29.6	24.2		20.6	27.6	—	25.5	3.4
Radial	44.5	31.5	25.4				33.8	8.0
AX prox		28.4	26.6				27.5	0.9
AX dist		18.7	15.5				17.1	1.6
MAC						15.6	15.6	—

Mean of spinal nerves   = 31.0%
Mean of upper, lower trunks   = 33.0
Mean of cords   = 32.5
Mean of prox M, U, R, AX, MC = 34.6

MT = middle trunk, UT = upper trunk, LTR = lower trunk, MDC = medial cord, PC = posterior cord, LC = lateral cord, MC = musculocutaneous nerve, AX = axillary nerve, MAC = medial antebrachial cutaneous nerve.

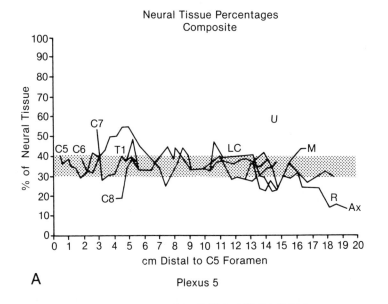

A

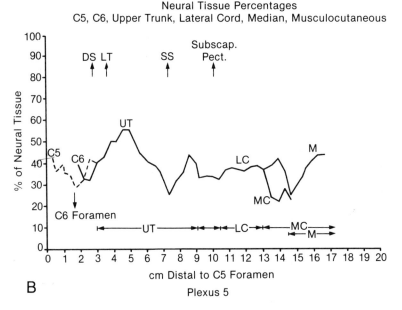

B

Figure 22–22. The percentage of cross-sectional nerve areas composed of neural tissue is shown for individual sections of plexus #5. The average near 40% is typical.

the dynamics of fascicular rearrangement, and we have therefore studied the plexus at 0.5- to 1-mm intervals with added resolution within these intervals achieved by visualization of the sections with transmitted light. We believe that adequate assessment of fascicular topography and certain mechanisms of fascicle group organization could be obtained only at a resolution higher than that previously reported. We found that fascicles in the plexus travel only an average of 5 mm before branching or merging with a neighboring fascicle. Tempering this complexity was the finding that fascicle groups representing the branches of the plexus could generally be localized for approximately five

times that distance, 2.5 cm on average. The objective of assessing intraneural topography was thereby addressed by defining the length of fascicles and fascicle groups as they relate to fascicular reorganization in the various elements of the plexus.

Another significant finding was that fascicle sizes varied widely, i.e., from 0.001 to 8 mm² in cross-sectional area. There were many small fascicles, often less than 0.1 mm in diameter, which were likely of little or no surgical significance but elevated the fascicle counts. We have reported a novel parameter for the description of fascicle numbers, our primary intention being that at those levels at which a single fascicle dominated the nerve, it would be appropriately called monofascicular for the purposes of reconstruction. The parameter is called F90 (refer to the earlier discussion of Fascicle Organization). We believe the range of variability and the regions of consistency can be best appreciated by reference to both the F90 values and the total fascicle counts. These are presented in Table 22–2. The histograms of the frequency of different fascicle sizes reported by Bonnel[5] are descriptive, but complex. Because the F90 value is a simple number that takes into account both the number and the size of fascicles making up the first 90% of the neural tissue, it should tell the surgeon the typical number of fascicles that need to be repaired to provide for at least 90% of the neural tissue.

Although we have found some variability in fascicle numbers, we did find several consistent patterns, in that the numbers of fascicles did increase steadily from spinal nerves to cords and that there were eight regions in the plexus that were most commonly monofascicular.

In addressing the objective of quantifying neural tissue, we have provided neural tissue cross-sectional areas for all branches of the plexus as well as for all spinal nerves, trunks, and cords—for all specimens studied by serial section.

Whereas Kerr[23] deferred judgment on the relevance of pre- and postfixation of the plexus, Dykes and Terzis[11] found that dermatomal and myotomal distributions of the spinal nerves in monkeys varied over a wide range and that they always maintained the same relative cephalo-caudad orientation, supporting the first law of Herringham.[17] These findings were based on single fiber recordings at the spinal nerve roots. We studied our measurements of neural tissue area and found that many aspects of plexus anatomy correlated significantly with prefixation and postfixation and that the relative size of the C5 neural tissue was an excellent index of pre- or postfixation. The arrangements observed in this study suggest that pre- and postfixation are simply two ends of a continuous spectrum of anatomic configurations. More importantly, many aspects of the quantitative anatomy of individual specimens could be predicted from the extent of pre- or postfixation. The development of preoperative means to assess pre- or postfixation would thus presumably be helpful in predicting the relative contributions of certain spinal nerves to the distal muscles in clinical cases, as well as in predicting the size of certain plexus elements and the appearance of certain anomalous configurations that might otherwise delay or mislead the surgeon. Development of preoperative electrophysiologic or radiologic means of assessing pre- or postfixation would enable a more efficient and rational approach to reconstruction.

Assessment of the relative amounts of neural and connective tissue in the plexus is reported in detail and correlates well with values previously reported for the major nerves of the arm and forearm.

Other objectives included determining both the distribution of neural tissue from spinal nerves distally and the derivation of the peripheral nerves from proximal plexus elements. Also of interest was assessing the feasibility of localizing, at the spinal nerve level, neural tissue supplying various branches. Narakas[36, 37] published a schema of such localization, but on an anatomic basis we were unable to localize distinct regions within the spinal nerves that corresponded to his pictorial depiction. Localization was possible at more distal levels, and we were generally in agreement with the schema Narakas reported at those levels; however, we suspect that localization within the spinal nerves of axon groups supplying specific muscles or specific branches of the plexus is not clearly defined. Instead, from our anatomic study, we support the notion that only the most proximal branches have some localization at the spinal nerve level.

Comparison to Axon Counting

Axon counting in the brachial plexus has been reported by Bonnel and Rabischong.[5–7] Correlation of axon counts to neural tissue areas is outlined in Tables 22–16 and 22–17.

Review of the axonal counts revealed that almost 30% of axons counted proximally were not accounted for distally. Bonnel and Rabischong did not report axon counts for the medial cutaneous nerves of the arm and forearm or for the cutaneous branch of the axillary nerve. Even with reasonable assumptions about the contribution of these nerves to the total, almost 25% of the axons were not accounted for by Bonnel and Rabischong's direct axon counting. In comparison,

Table 22–16. TABULATION OF AXON COUNTS AVERAGED FOR 21 PLEXUSES*

	Myelinated Axons	% of Total
C5	16,472	14.0%
C6	27,421	23.2%
C7	23,781	20.1%
C8	30,626	25.9%
T1	19,747	16.7%
Total	118,047	99.9%

	Myelinated Axons	% of Total	% of Total Corrected to 100%
Musculocutaneous	5,023	4.3%	5.7%
Median	15,915	13.5	18.1
Ulnar	14,161	12.0	16.0
Radial	15,964	13.5	18.1
Scapular girdle	31,979	27.1	36.2
Pure cutaneous†	5,301 (est.)	4.5 (est.)	6.0 (est.)
Total	88,343	74.8%	100.1

25.2% of myelinated axons in the spinal nerves are not accounted for

*Reported by Bonnel.[5]
†Bonnel does not report axon counts for the medial brachial and antebrachial cutaneous nerves nor for the cutaneous branch of the axillary nerve. The number of axons was estimated for purposes of comparison, using 6.0% as the proportion of total plexus neural tissue supplying these cutaneous regions.

all but 6.9% of the neural tissue that we measured at the spinal nerve level was accounted for in the peripheral nerves exiting the plexus. Therefore, 93.1% of the neural tissue was conserved, from proximal to distal.

Comparing the relative contribution of spinal nerves to the total plexus axonal counts and to the total plexus neural tissue, both revealed fairly constant values for C6, C7, and C8, (about 23 to 24% of the total), whereas C5 and T1 varied markedly.

Values for the peripheral nerves were com-

pared after correcting each to sum to 100%. When this was done, values showed good correlation, generally within 2 to 4 percentage points. The least consistent was the percentage to the shoulder girdle, but the uncorrected values were remarkably close, at 26.3 and 27.1%.

Laws of Plexus Organization

We have found numerous consistent patterns in plexus organization and offer them as tentative laws of plexus anatomy (Table 22–18). Each is presented with evidence from this study and relevant background information. They are offered as ways of understanding the order of the plexus in the hope that they will stand the tests of time and clinical experience.

Law I: Plexus Anatomy and Anomalies May Be Systematized on the Basis of Prefixation and Postfixation.

The association of many variables with prefixation and postfixation suggests that prefixation may be considered a type of anatomical syndrome. The use of the cross-sectional neural tissue areas of spinal nerves as a basis for defining prefixation and postfixation is novel. Kerr[23] measured spinal nerve diameters but did not find a reliable correlation, did not measure areas, and could not selectively measure the neural tissue.

We propose a definition of a prefixed plexus based on neural tissue cross-sectional areas, as outlined in Table 22–19. A postfixed plexus would be its converse, and the range between them is a continuum.

Variations in the size of certain plexus elements correlated with the size of C5 con-

Table 22–17. COMPARISON OF AXON COUNTING AND NEURAL TISSUE AREAS (CORRECTED TO 100%)

	% of Total Neural Tissue	% of Total Axons	Difference
C5	13.5	14.0	0.5
C6	23.9	23.2	0.7
C7	24.1	20.1	4.0
C8	23.3	25.9	2.6
T1	15.0	16.7	1.7
Musculocutaneous	8.4	5.7	2.7
Median	22.1	18.1	4.0
Ulnar	14.3	16.0	1.7
Radial	20.9	18.1	2.8
Shoulder girdle	28.2	36.2	8.0
Axillary	8.6	7.4	1.2

Table 22–18. LAWS OF PLEXUS ORGANIZATION

   I. Plexus anatomy and anomalies may be systematized on the basis of prefixation and postfixation.

  II. Fascicular topography of the plexus is a summation of varied topographic arrangements of its elements.

 III. Rules systematizing intraneural topography of the plexus are consistent with those governing the major nerves of the arm and forearm.

  IV. Fascicles supplying purely muscular or purely cutaneous branches are less common than mixed fascicles, but they may be found in certain regions near branch points or spinal nerves.

   V. Connective tissue is more abundant than neural tissue throughout the plexus.

Table 22–19. PROPOSED CHARACTERISTICS
OF A PREFIXED PLEXUS

Spinal Nerves
C5 supplies over 15% of the plexus
T1 supplies less that 13% of the plexus

Trunks
The upper trunk supplies over half of the posterior cord
The lower trunk supplies less than 15% of the posterior cord
The upper trunk supplies more than one third of the pectoral nerve supply
The lower trunk supplies less than half of the median nerve
The lower trunk supplies less than 25% of the radial nerve
The upper trunk is larger than the lower trunk

Cords
The lateral cord does not receive a contribution from C8

Peripheral Nerves
Less than 8% of the musculocutaneous nerve is supplied by C7
The ulnar nerve receives a contribution from C7

tribution to the plexus. The statistical significance of these correlations is shown in Table 22–20 and Figure 22–18, demonstrating that when C5 is small, the following are also true: T1 is large, the lower trunk contribution to the posterior cord is large, the upper trunk contribution to the pectoral nerves is small, and C8 contributes to the lateral cord. In addition, the size of the anomalous C8 contribution to the lateral cord, when present, correlates directly with the relative size of C5 in a statistically significant way. The size of the other plexus elements just listed also varies directly with the size of C5.

Many quantitative measures of the proximal derivation of each peripheral nerve are complicated by fascicle mixing; therefore, the values cover a range of possibilities. To assess correlation with prefixation or postfixation, we have put the seven cross-sectioned plex-

uses into three groups, based on the size of C5:

	Group	Plexus
I.	C5 = 0–10% of plexus	(1,12)
II.	C5 = 10–15% of plexus	(4,5)
III.	C5 = 15% or more of plexus	(8,9,14)

The individual measurements of spinal nerve or trunk contributions to several peripheral nerves were averaged for the specimens in each group, taking the mean of the lower end of each range of values and the mean of the higher end as well. These are summarized in Table 22–21, revealing strong trends from prefixed to postfixed.

Among the seven serially sectioned plexuses, only three (8, 9, 14) had a C7 contribution to the ulnar nerve. These are the plexuses of group III, which are the most prefixed. Similarly, the only plexus of the seven in which C7, or the middle trunk, contributes proximally to the formation of the medial cord is plexus 14, also among the most prefixed.

The trends shown here support the concept that when a plexus is more prefixed, it originates from a more cephalad segment of the spinal cord and thereby each of its elements arises from more cephalad portions of the cord.

The spinal nerves C6, C7, and C8 have been shown to be constant in size, allowing only C5 and T1 to vary. In this sample they have varied inversely and linearly. This relationship suggests that the length of the spinal cord segment supplying the plexus is relatively constant and not subject to variability by elongation or contraction, which had otherwise been suggested by Kerr.[23]

By proposing that the nerve supply to each end-organ is located in a certain fixed ce-

Table 22–20. CORRELATION OF PREFIXATION AND THE SIZE OF PLEXUS ELEMENTS

		Correlation Coefficient	No.	p
C5	size of lower trunk posterior division	− .9972	7	p < .001
% of total	size of C8 lateral cord contribution	− .9795	4	p < .05
plexus neural	% of total neural tissue from T1	− .9454	7	p < .02
tissue	% of pectoral from upper trunk	+ .8432	7	p < .02
correlated	% of posterior cord from upper trunk	+ .8621	7	p < .02
with	% of lateral cord from upper trunk	+ .7490	7	p ≈ 0.06
C5	size of lower trunk posterior division	− .8456	7	p < .02
neural	size of C8 lateral cord contribution	− .9769	4	p < .05
tissue	size of upper trunk pectoral contribution	+ .9668	7	p < .001
area (mm²)	T1 neural tissue area	− .5822	7	not significant

Table 22–21. CORRELATION OF C5 SIZE WITH PLEXUS DISTRIBUTION FOR THREE GROUPS

Postfixed	←	I C5 < 10%	II 10% < C5 < 15%	III C5 > 15%	→	Prefixed
% MC < C7 (mean)		8–28.2 (18.1)	6.2–18.8 (12.5)	4.3–7.2 (5.8)		
% M < UT (mean)		4.9–8.8 (6.8)	13.7–17.1 (15.4)	15.2–21.4 (18.3)		
% LT < C7		37.6	19.4	16.1		
% LC < UT		27.0	41.9	69.5		

MC = musculocutaneous nerve, M = median nerve, UT = upper trunk, LT = long thoracic nerve, LC = lateral cord.

phalo-caudad relationship to the others, Herringham's first law suggested that cephalo-caudad shifting of axons supplying one end-organ would be accompanied by a corresponding shift of the others.[17]

Bonnel[5] shows that C6, C7, and C8 are of similar size, based on axonal counts, and Kerr[23] agrees in rank-ordering their gross diameters. Kerr stated: "I feel quite sure that the differences between certain of the nerves especially in the center of the plexus are in many cases so small that under slightly altered conditions two different observers might obtain quite opposite results."

To the best of our knowledge, correlations between prefixation and the size of spinal nerve contributions to more distal plexus elements have not previously been reported.

Law II: Fascicular Topography of the Plexus Is a Summation of Varied Topographic Arrangements of Its Elements.

The mean F90 fascicle counts increase markedly in number from the spinal nerves to the trunks and to the cords. The increase correlates with the number of branches per element and with proximity to the axilla. Bonnel's data support the finding of increased numbers of fascicles from proximal to distal in the plexus.[5] The spinal nerves display a strong tendency to monofascicularity. The divisions of the upper trunk and the posterior division of the lower trunk are characteristically monofascicular and bifascicular, respectively. A wide range of fascicle sizes is typical in the spinal nerves, but the cords have more medium-sized fascicles.

Law III: Rules Systematizing Intraneural Topography of the Plexus Are Consistent with Those Governing the Major Nerves of the Arm and Forearm.

Because of complex topography, it is not reasonable to think of the plexus as a collection of fascicles traveling separate and individual paths along the full length from the spinal nerves distally to the individual nerves of the arm and forearm. The cable concept of nerves is not anatomically accurate in this plexiform structure. Certain rules, however, do govern the fascicular/intraneural topography of the brachial plexus, and these rules correspond well to the rules governing the major peripheral nerves originating from the plexus.

It is not unreasonable to postulate that these rules may be applicable throughout the peripheral nerves of man. Although not supportive of a simplistic concept of fascicular anatomy, these rules should be important to the surgeon who wants to develop a more rational approach to reconstruction of peripheral nerve lesions, in particular, lesions of the brachial plexus. They are as follows:

1. Fascicles in the brachial plexus are arranged in a plexiform manner, the average length of a fascicle being 5 mm without branching or merging with another fascicle.

2. The number of fascicles increases approaching the axilla, which is also the region of greatest branching. This pattern was consistent in all plexuses and, with some limitations, was predictive.

3. Certain regions were characteristically monofascicular.

4. The number of fascicles varied several-fold from plexus to plexus, but most values were within a twofold range at any given level. There was very little difference from right to left in the same individual.

5. Within a given individual, the number of fascicles was high at all levels if it was high at one level and low at all levels if low at one level. The number of fascicles was to some extent a property of the individual.

6. Fascicle groups maintained their identity much longer than individual fascicles, averaging 15 mm without interaction and 25 mm without losing localization. Individual fascicles often merged and subdivided with-

out changing the total neural tissue content of a fascicular group.

7. Fortuitous branching was observed, i.e., the deviation of fascicles or fascicle groups from their classic paths only to return more distally to the same path. An example was the portion of C8 that traveled in the lateral cord in plexuses 1 and 12 but still supplied the ulnar and median nerves via a lateral head of the ulnar nerve.

8. Merging of fascicles was usually accompanied by gradual axonal intermingling. Occasionally, however, rapid transfer of groups of axons across the diameter of the bundle could be appreciated by the appearance of the stained section under light microscopy.

Existing Knowledge of Intraneural Topography. The following discussion is intended to show that there is marked agreement and correspondence between the rules governing the fascicular topography for the major nerves of the arm and forearm and those governing the elements of the brachial plexus. Numbers correspond to each item in the preceding section.

1. Sunderland,[48, 54] Jabaley et al.,[20] and Terzis et al.[59] characterized the intraneural topography of the major nerves of the arm and forearm as plexiform.

2. Terzis et al.[59] reported increased fascicle numbers in those zones of the median nerve with a large number of branches, and Dustin[10] found increased fascicle numbers at branch origins. Sunderland[48] did not confirm those findings, but Terzis et al.[59] did find increased fascicle numbers to be associated with regions of high branching in the median nerve and also found that the regions of high branching were at the elbow and wrist, the two joints of the arm. Sunderland[54] argued that increased fascicle numbers protect against compression injury and stated "funiculi are generally numerous and small where the nerve crosses a joint."[48]

3. Sunderland stated "in general . . . nerves are habitually composed of more bundles at some levels than at others." He also described three regions of monofascicularity in the peripheral nerves of the arm and forearm.[48] These are detailed later in this chapter.

4 and 5. Dustin[10] classified nerves as having either few fascicles or many fascicles. Sunderland[54] found that specimens from opposite sides of the same body were usually of the same classification.

6. Millesi and Terzis[34] discussed fascicle groups as entities different from individual fascicles in their report on terminology in peripheral nerve surgery. Sunderland[54] provided an example, describing the fascicle group of the superficial radial nerve. "Which pursued an independent and localized course for 46 mm over which distance there were 23 changes in the bundle pattern."

7. At the level of the major nerves of the arm and forearm, Sunderland[48] described "those occasions when two funiculi unite to form a common bundle which proceeds without any intermixing of the constituent fibers, and later divides to reproduce the original two bundles." He stated that these formations are not common, but at least suggest some role of random mesenchymal condensation in the definition of fascicular anatomy.

8. Also at the level of the major nerves of the arm and forearm, Sunderland[48] reported occasionally observing fibers or fascicles taking an oblique course "through or over the surface of the nerve."

Monofascicularity. In the arm and forearm, Sunderland[48] identified three sites that are typically monofascicular: (1) the ulnar nerve at the medial humeral epicondyle, (2) the radial nerve in the spiral groove, and (3) the axillary nerve under the shoulder joint (in the axilla).

In the plexus, monofascicularity ($F90 = 1$) was found consistently in several locations as outlined in Table 22–20. The posterior division of the lower trunk was typically bifascicular.

In general, the brachial plexus was typically monofascicular in eight sites, grouped into three anatomic regions: (1) the spinal nerves: C5, C6, C8, T1 (less commonly C7), (2) the upper trunk: anterior and posterior divisions and the origin of the suprascapular nerve, and (3) the musculocutaneous nerve at its origin from the plexus.

Also, in all cases in which there was a C8 contribution to the lateral cord, that branch was monofascicular for an average of 3 cm. We also observed monofascicularity in part of the axillary nerve itself, as noted by Sunderland.

Law IV: Fascicles Supplying Purely Muscular or Purely Cutaneous Branches Are Less Common Than Mixed Fascicles, but They May Be Found in Certain Regions Near Branch Points and Spinal Nerves.

The ventral and dorsal roots of each spinal nerve merged within the intervertebral canal in the large majority of cases. Only six spinal nerves (of 35 nerves studied in 7 plexuses) had an appearance of distinct ventral (motor) and dorsal (sensory) roots. The remaining 29 spinal nerves were, from the level of the intervertebral foramen, either monofascicular or oligofascicular without any clear distinction of ventral and dorsal components. Of the six with ventral and dorsal roots still separate at the level of the foramen, the roots lost their identity by merging with each other within 0.66 cm, on average.

Thus, in over 95% of spinal nerves, motor and sensory differentiation was lost within 1 cm of the intervertebral foramen. This is not to say that mixing of ventral and dorsal elements is immediate. It is not unreasonable to suppose gradual mixing in most cases, so that 2 to 3 cm from the foramen the anterior aspect of the spinal nerve may well have more motor axons than sensory axons, but the distinction must be vague at that level. As is discussed later, the posterior cord is largely motor in composition; therefore, the dorsal roots must send a large proportion of their axons into the posterior divisions of each trunk, which we have found to separate from the anterior division 6.5 cm from their respective foramina, on average. The fascicle groups representing the divisions separate about 1.5 cm proximal to that (see earlier section on Topography: Fascicle Groups); therefore, significant exchange of motor fibers into the posterior aspect of each trunk must occur within 5 cm of the foramen. The same would apply for transfer of sensory fibers to the ulnar, median, and other anterior division nerves from their dorsal position in the spinal nerves.

The nerves of the plexus that are reliably pure muscular or pure cutaneous are listed in Table 22–22. Of course, the muscular nerves include proprioceptive fibers to muscle spindles, and cutaneous nerves innervate skin without supplying skeletal muscle.

Based on data presented earlier in this chapter, we know that on average each fascicular group retains its identity for approximately 2 cm proximally from its point of exit. We can identify areas of muscular or cutaneous supply within those very few centimeters of the proximal end of each spinal nerve and along the path of certain fascicle groups a few centimeters proximal to the exit of each of the proximal branches of the plexus. The relative anterior, posterior, medial (inferior), or lateral (superior) orientations of these fascicular groups within the

Table 22–22. BRANCHES THAT ARE PURELY MUSCULAR OR PURELY CUTANEOUS

	% of Plexus Neural Tissue		Corrected to 100%
Dorsal scapular	1.2%		
Long thoracic	3.1%		
Subscapular	4.1%		
Suprascapular	4.8%		
Pectoralis	5.4%		
Axillary	7.5%		
Thoracodorsal	1.6%		
	27.7%	27.7%	29.8%
Intercostobrachial	0.3%		
Medial cutaneous	4.1%		
	4.4%	4.4%	4.7%
Total		32.1%	34.5%

In reality as much as 18% of the axillary nerve may provide cutaneous innervation, so that it is not pure motor, but nearly so.

nerve elements containing them were presented diagrammatically in Figures 22–11 and 22–12.

Previous work by Sunderland and Bedbrook[50] and by Terzis et al.[59] reveals that the median and ulnar nerves carry mostly cutaneous fibers and that the median nerve is more purely sensory than the ulnar nerve. On the other hand, the radial nerve was found to be mostly motor. Sunderland[50] reported that 77% of the radial nerve, 36% of the median nerve, and 41% of the ulnar nerve supply muscle.

Knowing, from our own work on the plexus, the percentage of the axillary nerve supplying muscle, and knowing, from Sunderland's earlier study,[48] the percentage of the radial nerve supplying muscular fibers, we may calculate that 82% of the entire posterior cord is muscular.

Nerve	% Muscular		Mean Neural Tissue		Motor Neural Tissue
Radial	77%	×	5.5431	=	4.2682
Axillary	82%	×	1.9580	=	1.6056
Subscapularis	100%	×	1.0745	=	1.0745
Thoracodorsal	100%	×	0.6027	=	0.6027
			9.1783		7.5510

$$\frac{7.5510}{9.1783} = 82\% \text{ of posterior cord is motor}$$

This high percentage of muscular fibers in the posterior cord is striking, is much higher than in the medial cord, and may be useful for reconstruction, inasmuch as the posterior divisions as a whole must therefore be of a similar motor composition.

There is good reason to think that, for the most part, fascicles of the plexus contain mixtures of motor and sensory (and cutaneous and muscular) fibers as well as mixtures of fibers supplying separate end-organs. From Sunderland's illustrations in *Nerves and Nerve Injuries*,[48] it is apparent that fascicles in the proximal ends of the median, ulnar, and radial nerves (at their respective origins from the plexus) cannot be identified as supplying only a single muscle, a single dermatome, or skin region. The fibers appear to mix substantially. Sunderland[48] states, "At the axillary outlet, it is usual for the majority of the funiculi to contain representative fibers from most, if not all, of the peripheral branches."

From tracing fascicles in the plexus by serial cross section, we know that mixing of fascicles occurs and at least makes axonal rearrangement possible. From previous nerve degeneration studies in animals, Sterling and Kuypers[45] and Rao et al.[41] have shown that in cats and buffalo the cell bodies supplying each muscle or muscle group are arranged in nuclei within the spinal cord, spanning several vertebrae in most cases and residing in a specific locus within the cord cross-section. Sterling and Kuypers have shown that the nuclei of the flexors tend to be more dorsal in the cord than the nuclei of the extensors. This arrangement may or may not be present in man. If present, it requires in addition that axons in the ventral-most aspect of the spinal cord (and presumably, therefore, the spinal nerve root) must traverse the diameter of the spinal nerves and trunks to enter the posterior divisions.

In response to Narakas' schema of plexus organization,[35, 37] this vast mixing and the columnar arrangement of neuron cell bodies in the spinal cord would seem to make fairly unlikely the discrete localization (and perhaps even the vague localization) of associated groups of axons or fascicles at the spinal nerve or even the trunk level.

It may be best to conceptualize the axonal composition of the trunks and anterior divisions as consisting of well-mixed motor and sensory axons and thereby being less likely to provide good motor-motor coaptation in plexus reconstruction surgery. The high proportion of muscular fibers in the posterior divisions may, on the other hand, offer a reliable source of concentrated muscular fibers to anastomose or graft to distal muscular-predominant branches or fascicle groups.

Law V: Connective Tissue Is More Abundant Than Neural Tissue Throughout the Plexus.

An average of 65 to 70% of plexus cross-sectional area is connective tissue. Only 30 to 35% is neural tissue, on average. Data showing a large percentage of connective tissue in a nerve element can be important in deciding whether to do an epineurial or a perineurial repair; the former may permit substantial blind growth of proximal axonal stumps into connective tissue distally. This significance was pointed out by Sunderland.[48]

Our data correlate well with the percentages reported by Sunderland[53] for the median nerve (25 to 71% neural tissue), ulnar nerve (21 to 78% neural tissue), and radial nerve (16 to 71% neural tissue). They reported an average of approximately 40 to 50% of nerve cross-sectional areas composed of neural tissue at the peripheral nerve level. The additional connective tissue at the plexus level is not surprising, given the active joint, which requires adequate cushioning epineurium, and the large number of branches, which appear to be associated with an increased amount of connective tissue. There may also be a factor of shrinkage, in that the histologic processing used by Sunderland may well have caused more than the 2 to 3% shrinkage observed in our specimens. Bonnel[5-7] also reports connective tissue percentages, but the details of his methods of quantitation are not made clear, and there is more variability than that observed with our methods.

NOVEL CONCLUSIONS REGARDING THE MICROANATOMY OF THE HUMAN BRACHIAL PLEXUS

Specific conclusions, narrower in focus than the proposed laws of plexus organization, follow. All except those marked with an asterisk are novel.

Fascicle Organization

1. Fascicle sizes vary from 0.001 to 8 mm².
2. The number of fascicles (F90) at a given level may vary over a sixfold range from plexus to plexus, but most values are near the middle of the range.

3. Fascicle organization appears to vary less from right to left in the same individual than from individual to individual.

4. The number of fascicles at a given level is dependent both on the level and on the individual.

5. Monofascicularity is typical for the spinal nerves, the anterior and posterior divisions of the upper trunk, and the origins of the suprascapular and musculocutaneous nerves.

6. Bifascicularity is typical for the posterior division of the lower trunk.

7. F90 values increase from a mean of 2.4 at the spinal nerve level to 7.4 at the trunk level to 13.3 at the cord level, whereas total fascicle numbers increase from a mean of 8.0 to 24.6, and the range of fascicle sizes decreases moving from proximal to distal.

8. A more generalized conclusion is that there is a local increase in fascicle numbers at all the joints of the upper extremity.

Fascicle Topography

1. The average distance a fascicle travels without merging or branching is 5 mm. Rarely, a fascicle will travel over 1 cm without interaction.

2. The elements of the brachial plexus have a plexiform intraneural topography.*

3. Fortuitous branching occurs.

Branches

1. Fascicle groups can be traced proximally an average of 1.1 cm from the point of exit to the point of segregation from the rest of the plexus element, 1.5 cm to the level of purity, and 2.5 cm to the level of localization.

2. Fascicle groups of branches generally assumed the same cross-sectional localization in different plexus specimens.*

Quantitation of Neural Tissue

1. C6, C7, and C8 consistently contribute 24% of the plexus neural tissue each, whereas C5 and T1 vary considerably in an inverse fashion to supply the remaining 28% of the plexus neural tissue.

2. The motor supply to the shoulder girdle receives 28.2% of the plexus neural tissue and the cutaneous supply is 1.6%; therefore, the shoulder receives 30% of the plexus neural tissue.

3. Twenty-two per cent of the plexus neural tissue supplies the median nerve.

4. Twenty-one per cent supplies the radial nerve.

5. Fourteen per cent supplies the ulnar nerve.

6. Eight per cent supplies the musculocutaneous nerve.

7. Four per cent supplies the medial cutaneous nerves.

Distribution of Neural Tissue

1. There are several "gray zones," i.e., plexus regions where little or no localization of fascicle groups can be made because of mixing. Although gradual both proximal and distal to these regions, it appears extensive in these gray zones because of a summation of this gradual mixing over distance. These zones are: (a) the upper trunk at the formation of the divisions and the origin of the suprascapular nerve, (b) the lower trunk as it forms the medial cord, and (c) the posterior cord between the posterior divisions and the axillary nerve origin. The monofascicular character of all elements entering the upper trunk (C5, C6, anterior division, posterior division, and suprascapular nerve) often renders impossible the task of differentiating subset fascicle groups.

2. The upper trunk supplies approximately 50% of the posterior cord; T1 supplies less than 10% in all individuals and less than 5% in most persons.

3. C8 may supply as much as 38% of the lateral cord in postfixed plexuses.

4. C7 may supply at least 10 to 15% of the musculocutaneous nerve, although it usually supplies less than 10% and mostly tends to supply the coracobrachialis nerve.

5. C6 is the primary contributor to the long thoracic nerve in most individuals.

6. C5 and C6 together supply only about 15% of the median nerve on average. C7 supplies about 35%, and C8 and T1 supply about 25% each.

7. T1 supplies most of the medial cutaneous nerves as well as the intercostobrachial nerve, but C8 often contributes to these nerves.

8. Nerve supply to the subscapularis muscle is from C5, C6, and C7, with the upper trunk usually supplying 100% of the first subscapular branch.

9. The thoracodorsal nerve may in some cases have no upper trunk supply, but its spinal nerve origins are variable and confused by substantial mixing.

10. At least 40% of the ulnar nerve was supplied by C8 in most cases, the average proportion of ulnar neural tissue supplied by C8 being between 31.7 and 81.7%.

Percentage of Neural Tissue

1. Thirty-two per cent of the plexus consists of neural tissue, the remainder is connective tissue.

Anomalies of the Plexus

1. Anomalous C8 contributions to the lateral cord correlated well with the size of C5. They were measured in three specimens.

2. Anastomoses between the musculocutaneous and median nerves were observed in 24% of cases, and such anastomoses were one third the size of the musculocutaneous nerve.

3. Anastomoses between the anterior and posterior elements of the plexus are unusual and small, but may exist.

Methods

1. The technique of hand-sectioning and staining with methylene blue, as a modification of Sunderland's methods, is shown to be accurate, inexpensive, and reliable for assessment of intraneural topography and quantitative microanatomy.

2. The error of digitizer area measurements is generally less than 1 to 3%.

3. Neural tissue area measurements provided consistent quantitation. Ninety-three per cent of neural tissue area at the spinal nerve level was conserved at the level of the peripheral nerves.

References

1. Alnot, J. Y., Augereau, B., and Frot, B.: Traitement direct des lesions nerveuses dans les paralysies traumatiques par élongation du plexus brachial chez l'adulte. Chirurgie, *103*:935–947, 1977.
2. Alnot, J. Y., and Huten, B.: La systematisation du plexus brachial. Rev. Chir. Orthop., *63*(1):27–34, 1977.
3. Bardeen, C. H., and Lewis, W. H.: Development of the limbs, body-wall and back in man. Am. J. Anat., *1*:1–35, 1901–1902.
4. Birch, R.: Traction lesions of the brachial plexus. Br. J. Hosp. Med., Sept., 1984, pp. 140–143.
5. Bonnel, F.: Microscopic anatomy of the adult human brachial plexus: an anatomical and histological basis for microsurgery. Microsurgery, *5*:107–117, 1984.
6. Bonnel, F., and Rabischong, P.: Anatomy and systematization of the brachial plexus in the adult. Anat. Clin., *2*:289–298, 1981.
7. Bonnel, F.: Configuration interne histo-physiologique. Rev. Chir. Orthop., *63*(1):35–38, 1977.
8. Chetrick, A., and Del Guercio, L. R. M.: An unusual brachial plexus formation. Yale J. Biol. Med., *23*:395–398, 1950–1951.
9. Daniel, R., and Terzis, J. K.: Reconstructive Microsurgery. Boston, Little, Brown & Company. Chapters 7–9, 1977.
10. Dustin, A. P.: La fasciculation des nerfs: son importance dans le diagnostic, le pronostic et le traitement des lesions nerveuses. Ambulance de "l'Ocean," *2*:135–137, 1918.
11. Dykes, R. W., and Terzis, J. K.: Spinal nerve distributions in the upper limb: The organization of the dermatome and afferent myotome. Philosoph. Trans. Roy. Soc. London, Series B, *293*:509–554, 1981.
12. Dykes, R. W., and Terzis, J. K.: Functional anatomy of the deep motor branch of the ulnar nerve. Clin. Orthop. Related Res., *128*:167–179, 1977.
13. Fenart, R.: La morphogenese du plexus brachial, ses rapports avec la formation du cou et du membre supérieur. Acta Anat., *32*:322–360, 1958.
14. Frohse, F., and Frankel, M.: Die Muskeln des Menschlichen Armes. *In* von Bardeleben, K. (ed.): Handbuch der Anatomie des Menschen. Jena, Gustav Fischer, 385–387, 1908.
15. Harman, B.: The anterior limit of the cervico-thoracic visceral efferent nerves in man. J. Anat. Physiol., *34*(N.S. 14):359–380, 1900.
16. Harris, W.: Prefixed and postfixed types of brachial plexus. Brain, *26*:613–615, 1903.
17. Herringham, M. B.: The minute anatomy of the brachial plexus. Proc. Roy. Soc. London, *41*:423–441, 1887.
18. Inouye, Y., and Buchthal, R.: Segmental sensory innervation determined by potentials recorded from cervical spinal nerves. Brain, *100*:731–748, 1977.
19. Jabaley, M. E.: Current concepts of nerve repair. Clin. Plast. Surg., *8*:33–44, 1981.
20. Jabaley, M. E., Wallace, W. H., and Heckler, F. R.: Internal topography of major nerves of the forearm and hand: A current view. J. Hand Surg., *5*:1–18, 1980.
21. Kaplan, E. B., and Spinner, M.: Normal and anomalous innervation patterns in the upper extremity. *In* Omer, G. E., Jr., and Spinner, M. (eds.): Management of Peripheral Nerve Problems. Philadelphia, W. B. Saunders Company, 1980, pp. 75–99.
22. Kendall, H. O., Kendall, R. P., and Wadsworth, G. E.: Muscles, Testing, and Function, 2nd Ed. Baltimore, Williams & Wilkins, 1971, pp. 38–70.
23. Kerr, A. T.: The brachial plexus of nerves in man, the variations in its formation and branches. Am. J. Anat. *23*:285–395, 1918.
24. Koizumi, I.: On the brachial plexus of the gibbon. Acta Anat. Nippon, *55*(2):86–102, 1980.
25. Kreiger, N., Kelsey, J. L., Harris, C., and Pastides, H.: Injuries to the upper extremity: patterns of occurrence. Clin. Plast. Surg., *8*:13–19, 1981.

26. Lang, J., and Spinner, M.: An important variation of the brachial plexus—complete fusion of the median and musculocutaneous nerves. Bull. Hosp. Joint Dis., *31*:7–13, 1970.

27. Lewis, W. H.: The development of the arm in man. Am. J. Anat., *1*:145–183, 1901.

28. Mansat, M.: Anatomie topographique chirurgicale du plexus brachial. Rev. Chir. Orthop., *63*:20–26, 1977.

29. Merle D'Aubigne, R., and Deburge, A.: Etiologie, évolution et pronostic des paralysies traumatiques du plexus brachial. Rev. Chir. Orthop. Repar. Appareil Moteur (Paris), *53*:23–42, 1967.

30. Merle D'Aubigne, R., and Gerard, Y.: Les paralysies obstetricales du membre supérieur. *In* Merle D'Aubigne, R., Benassy, J., and Ramadier, J. O., (eds.): Chirurgie Orthopedique des Paralysies. Paris, Masson et Cie, 1956, pp. 99–139.

31. Miller, R. A., and Detwiler, S. R.: Comparative studies upon the origin and development of the brachial plexus. Anat. Rec., *65*:273–292, 1936.

32. Millesi, H.: Nerve grafting. Clin. Plast. Surg., *11*:105–113, 1984.

33. Millesi, H.: Brachial plexus injuries: management and results. Clin. Plast. Surg., *11*:115–120, 1984.

34. Millesi, H., and Terzis, J. K.: Problems of terminology in peripheral nerve surgery: committee report of the International Society of Reconstructive Microsurgery. Microsurgery, *4*:51–56, 1983.

35. Narakas, A.: Surgical treatment of traction injuries of the brachial plexus. Clin. Orthop. Related Res., *133*:71–90, 1978.

36. Narakas, A.: Paradoxes en chirurgie nerveuse peripherique au niveau du plexus brachial. Med. Hygiene, *354*:833–839, 1977.

37. Narakas, A.: Plexo braquial. Terapeutica quirurgica directa. Tecnica, Indicacion operatoria. Resultados. Rev. Ortoped. Traumatol., *16*:855–920, 1972.

38. Omer, J. E., and Spinner, M.: Management of Peripheral Nerve Problems. Philadelphia, W. B. Saunders Company, 1980.

39. Parry, C. B.: Brachial plexus injuries. Br. J. Hosp. Med., Sept., 1984, pp. 130–139.

40. Perotto, A. O., and Delagi, E. F.: Funicular localization in partial median nerve injury at the wrists. Arch. Phys. Med. Rehabil., *60*:165–169, 1979.

41. Rao, G. S., Sahu, S., and Saigal, R. P.: The somatotopic arrangement of motor neurons in the spinal cord of buffalo. A. Brachial plexus. Acta Anat., *70*:250–254, 1971.

42. Robertson, W. C., Jr., Eichman, P. L., and Clancy, W. G.: Upper trunk brachial plexopathy in football players. J.A.M.A., *241*:1480–1482, 1979.

43. Selig, R.: Die Nervennaht und ihre Erfolge mit besonderer Berucksichtigung der Nervenanatomie und Studien uber den Plexus. Deutsche Z. Chir., *137*:455–456, 1916.

44. Sterling, P., and Kuypers, H. G. J. M.: Anatomical organization of the brachial spinal cord of the cat. I. The distribution of dorsal root fibers. Brain Res., *4*:1–15, 1967.

45. Sterling, P., and Kuypers, H. G. J. M.: Anatomical organization of the brachial spinal cord of the cat. II. The motoneuron plexus. Brain Res., *4*:16–32, 1967.

46. Sunderland, S.: Founder's lecture—American Society for Surgery of the Hand. J. Hand Surg., *4*:210–211, 1979.

47. Sunderland, S.: Advances in diagnosis and treatment of root and peripheral nerve injury. Adv. Neurol., *22*:271–305, 1979.

48. Sunderland, S.: Nerves and Nerve Injuries. Edinburgh, Churchill Livingstone, 1968.

49. Sunderland, S., Marshall, R. D., and Swaney, W. E.: The intraneural topography of the circumflex, musculocutaneous and obturator nerves. Brain, *82*:116–129, 1959.

50. Sunderland, S., and Bedbrook, G. M.: The cross-sectional area of peripheral nerve trunks occupied by the fibres representing individual muscular and cutaneous branches. Brain, *72*:612–615, 1949.

51. Sunderland, S., and Bedbrook, G. M.: The relative sympathetic contribution to individual roots of the brachial plexus in man. Brain, *72*:297–301, 1949.

52. Sunderland, S., and Bradley, K. C.: The cross-sectional area of peripheral nerve trunks devoted to nerve fibres. Brain, *72*:428–449, 1949.

53. Sunderland, S.: The distribution of sympathetic fibres in the brachial plexus in man. Brain, *71*:88–102, 1948.

54. Sunderland, S.: The intraneural topography of the radial, median, and ulnar nerves. Brain, *68*:243–298, 1945.

55. Sylla, S., Papasian, P., Balde, I., Dintimille, H., and Argenson, C.: Les troncs du plexus brachial d'apres 122 dissections chez l'africain de l'ouest. Bull. Soc. Med. Afr. Noire Lang. Franc., *20*:387–392, 1975.

56. Talos Company. Dave Burley and others. Phone conversation. 12 March 1984.

57. Tamura, K.: The funicular pattern of Japanese peripheral nerves. Arch. Jap. Chir., *38*:35–58, 1969.

58. Tarlov, I. M.: Plasma Clot Suture of Peripheral Nerves and Nerve Roots—Rationale and Technique. Springfield, Del., Charles C Thomas, Publisher, 1950, pp. 82–83.

59. Terzis, J. K., Felker, B. L., and Sismour, E. M.: A computerized study of the intraneural organization of the median nerve. (In press.)

60. Turner, W.: Further examples of variations in the arrangement of the nerves of the human body. J. Anat. Physiol., *8*:297–299, 1873.

61. Turner, W.: Some additional variations in the distribution of the nerves of the human body. J. Anat. Physiol., *6*:101–106, 1872.

62. U.S. Mint, Philadelphia, Pennsylvania, Department of Exhibits and Public Services. Phone conversation, 15 March 1984.

63. Vallois, H. V.: Recherches sur la trajet et les anastamoses du nerf musculocutané au niveau du bras. Arch. Anat. Histol. d'Embryol., *1*:183–204, 1922.

64. Vasickova, Z.: Neural anastamoses in the human forearm. Folia Morphol., *25*:396–399, 1977.

65. Walsh, J. R.: The anatomy of the brachial plexus. Am. J. Med. Sci., *74*(N.S.):387–399, 1877.

66. Wickstrom, J., Haslam, E. T., and Hutchinson, R. H.: The surgical management of residual deformities of the shoulder following birth injuries of the brachial plexus. J. Bone Joint Surg., *37A*:27–36, and correction, p. 656, 1955.

67. Woollard, H.: The sympathetic and the brachial plexus. Proc. Anat. Soc. of Great Britain and Ireland. *In* J. Anat., *66*:147–148, 1931.

23

Traumatic Paralysis of the Brachial Plexus: Preoperative Problems and Therapeutic Indications

■

J. Y. Alnot, M.D.

Translated by W. Theodore Liberson, M.D., Ph.D. *

Numerous surgeons have become interested in traumatic lesions of the brachial plexus, and many studies have analyzed the spontaneous course of the disabilities that these lesions engender. The indications and the timing of the tendon transfers that might compensate for the resulting paralysis have also been suggested.

This chapter will deal only with traumatic lesions of the brachial plexus in adults and will not cover obstetrical or post-radiation plexus lesions, lesions due to tumors, or the thoracic outlet syndrome.

For over 15 years there has been a progressive evolution in brachial plexus surgery toward *surgical repair of traumatized nerve structures.* This surgery has become possible because of increased knowledge of the anatomy of the brachial plexus and of the more precise description and classification of lesions involving the plexus.

Millesi and Narakas pioneered this type of surgery in Europe. In 1981 we (Alnot and colleagues) published the results of our first 100 operated cases. Currently our statistics deal with 420 patients operated on from 1974 to 1985. This wide experience has provided a better knowledge of the diagnosis and various clinical pictures of these pathologic lesions as well as their spontaneous course. Approximately 60 to 65% of traumatic lesions

recover spontaneously in the first months following the accident, and secondary palliative surgery by tendon transfers may be considered in certain cases in which only partial recovery has occurred. Thirty to thirty-five per cent of patients do not recover, and their suitability for surgery must be decided upon quickly (by the second or third month), based on the clinical findings and the results of other tests or examinations.

Whatever the clinical picture, all patients with a traumatic paralysis of the brachial plexus that has not shown signs of recovery by the 30th day should have an additional work-up, including myelography and electromyography, so as to come quickly to a decision regarding surgery. A precise knowledge of the anatomy and pathology of the brachial plexus is indispensable in order to evaluate the clinical and other data necessary for diagnosis and therapy.

ANATOMY

It is important to remember two points:

1. The brachial plexus has two components, anterior and posterior, containing mo-

*Special thanks are expressed to Asa Ruskin, M.D., for his contribution to this translation. *W.T.L.*

tor, sensory, and sympathetic fibers that are totally independent from each other (Fig. 23–1).

2. It is possible to establish a topographic brachial plexus "map" consisting of its cords, trunks, or even roots.

Anatomy and Anatomic Variations of the Brachial Plexus

Anatomy

The brachial plexus is formed by the anterior branches of the last four cervical spinal nerves (C5–C8) and of the first thoracic spinal nerve (T1). These nerves unite to form the upper (C5–C6), middle (C7), and lower trunks (C8–T1).

Each trunk is divided into anterior and posterior branches. The anterior branches form the lateral and medial (anterior) cords with their terminal ramifications. The posterior branches form the posterior cord with its terminal ramifications. The anterior groups are primarily involved with the flexors of the upper extremity, whereas the posterior groups are mainly involved with the extensors of the upper extremity. Alnot and Huten described this anatomic picture at the meeting of the French Society of Orthopedic and Trauma Surgery in 1977.

Other anatomic findings are also of clinical interest:

Suprascapular Nerve. This nerve occupies a special place on the topographic map. Despite its posterior origin, it soon modifies its course and becomes located in an anteroinferior and external position in relation to the upper trunk. Clinically, the sparing of this nerve in the presence of upper root paralysis is proof of a more distal lesion of the upper trunk.

Posterior Branch of the Spinal Nerve. The clinical, and especially the electrical, involvement found during pre- or intraoperative study of the paravertebral muscles may have prognostic and localizing significance contributing to the differentiation between pre- and post-ganglionic lesions, even though multi-segmental innervation exists for these muscles.

Long Thoracic Nerve. The origin of this nerve is near the roots. However, the presence of a constant C5, C6 contribution, with very frequent and variable contributions of C7, C8, and T1 (especially C7) implies that

its involvement in brachial plexus paralysis imparts a poor prognosis indicating a very proximal pararadicular lesion spreading over several spinal nerves.

Autonomic Nervous System Fibers. Although the sympathetic pathways and centers are not discussed in this chapter, it should be mentioned that Horner's syndrome results from lesions of the communicating rami of T1 to the stellate ganglion, often indicating a proximal lesion.

Phrenic Nerve. All total brachial plexus injuries require an evaluation of the mobility of the corresponding hemidiaphragm. Diaphragmatic weakness or paralysis is a sign of a C4 lesion. In addition, C4 not only gives rise to the phrenic nerve but is a part of the brachial plexus because of its anastomosis with C5.

Brachial Plexus Collaterals. Certain collaterals of the brachial plexus especially the nerve to the angle of the scapula and of the rhomboids (C4, in addition to C5) may be injured. The superficial cervical plexus and the spinal accessory nerve (innervating the trapezius) can also be injured and therefore must be evaluated.

Anatomic Variations

Variations in Origins of Roots. The neighboring roots contribute to the formation of the plexus by their anastomoses. An anastomosis originating from C4 is found in 63% of cases.

The classic anatomic variations were defined by Seddon as "pre-fixed" when the plexus is formed by C4, C5, C6, C7, and C8 or "post-fixed" when it is formed by C6, C7, C8, T1, and T2. These anatomic variations explain certain clinical findings in relation to pathology.

Variations in the Composition of the Trunks. Variations in the length of the roots and trunks imply that each plexus is different and that surgical difficulties may occur at times, especially at the level of the lower roots, which are very short.

Anterior and Posterior Planes
(Fig. 23–1)

As stated earlier, an understanding of the arrangement of the plexus in an anterior and a posterior group or plane of nerve fibers, independent of each other and having no connecting fibers between them, is very im-

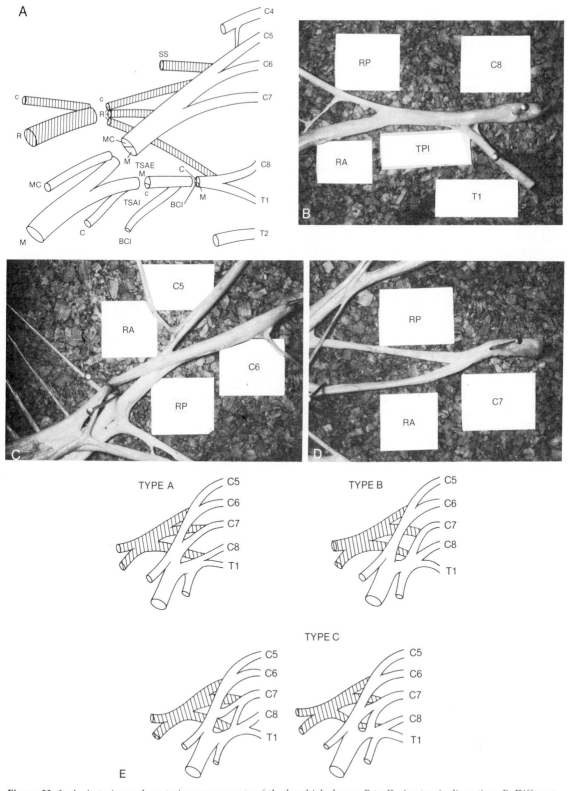

Figure 23–1. *A*, Anterior and posterior components of the brachial plexus. *B* to *D*, Anatomic dissection. *E*, Different anatomic variations based on the contribution of C7 to anterior structures. BCI = medial brachiocutaneous, c = axillary, C = ulnar, M = median, MC = musculocutaneous, RA = anterior structures, RP = posterior structures, SS = suprascapular, TSAE = lateral cord, TSAI = medial cord.

portant. It is possible to study the organization of each group separately by operative microscope dissection in order to follow and track each terminal or collateral branch inside the cords, trunks, and even the roots. This is why we use the term "topographic map."

The topographic map of the posterior group is simple and constant, whereas that of the anterior part is complex because of the divisions of the C7 root. The anterior division of C7 contributes in various ways to the anterior (lateral and medial) cords.

Based on the variations in this distribution one can distinguish three types of plexus—A, B, and C (Fig. 23–1*E*). The variable distribution of the anterior plane of C7, which may or may not give fibers to the ulnar nerve, may help explain the presence of certain confusing clinical pictures.

The Anatomic Study

Two fundamental anatomic points must be considered in dealing with traumatic paralysis of the brachial plexus.

1. As discussed earlier, the brachial plexus is made of two independent planes, anterior and posterior, beginning at its roots and ending at its terminal and collateral branches.

2. Dissection permits one to follow the radicular origin, to track, and to quantitatively evaluate the fibers of each plane inside the cords, trunks, and roots of the brachial plexus and thus to develop a "topographic map." Knowledge of this systematization is of both therapeutic and clinical interest. The innervation of the muscles of the upper extremity is bi- or multi-segmental, thus allowing anatomico-clinical correlation and the creation of clinical schematic diagrams or examination forms. However, the numerous anatomic variations result in different clinical pictures in the presence of the same lesion.

Repair of a lesion by a nerve graft should therefore minimize any disturbance of the cortical representation of the upper extremity by maintaining the arrangement of fibers in the anterior and posterior planes. However, the fascicular systematization is extremely difficult to establish, as one must distinguish between histologic and surgical fascicles, the latter of which may contain several histologic fascicles.

Histologic studies conducted by Bonnel and Margot have as yet been unable to precisely define the organization of these fascicles. However, their findings did indicate that the average number of surgical fascicles found at the root levels is as follows: one to two for C5, four to five for C6, six to seven for C7, two to four for C8, and two to four for T1.

In addition to this fascicular differentiation, the number of nerve fibers composing different roots must also be taken into account. For example, C5 contains 21,000 fibers (14,000 dorsal sensory root fibers and 7000 ventral motor root fibers). Finally, C7 contains on average more fibers than any other root.

PATHOLOGY OF BRACHIAL PLEXUS LESIONS (Fig. 23–2)

Lesions may occur at any level from the spinal cord to the branching of the nerves in the axilla. Such lesions are generally due to stretch injuries and fractures and can be differentiated according to Sunderland's classification (grades 1 to 5), which distinguishes between neurapraxia, axonotmesis, and neurotmesis.

Avulsion of the roots should be added to this classification, as this constitutes a lesion very specific for brachial plexus pathology. The lesions must be defined not only according to their severity but also according to their localization (as has been indicated by Seddon). Proximal supraclavicular lesions can be pre- or post-ganglionic, according to their localization in relation to the posterior root ganglion. More distal lesions are retro- and infraclavicular.

With the exception of direct transection injuries, brachial plexus lesions are secondary to mechanisms that have a common cause, i.e., traction or stretch injuries.

Both peripheral and central mechanisms can be distinguished. There are three possible peripheral mechanisms:

1. The first involves a downward pull of the shoulder away from the cervical column. Ninety-five per cent of these lesions are secondary to motorcycle accidents associated with a fall on the shoulder. The position of arm and the degree of abduction play a definite role. If abduction is 90° with retropulsion of the shoulder, the tension on all the roots is maximum, which explains why this injury may cause total paralysis.

2. The second and less frequent possibility is stretching of the upper extremity in maxi-

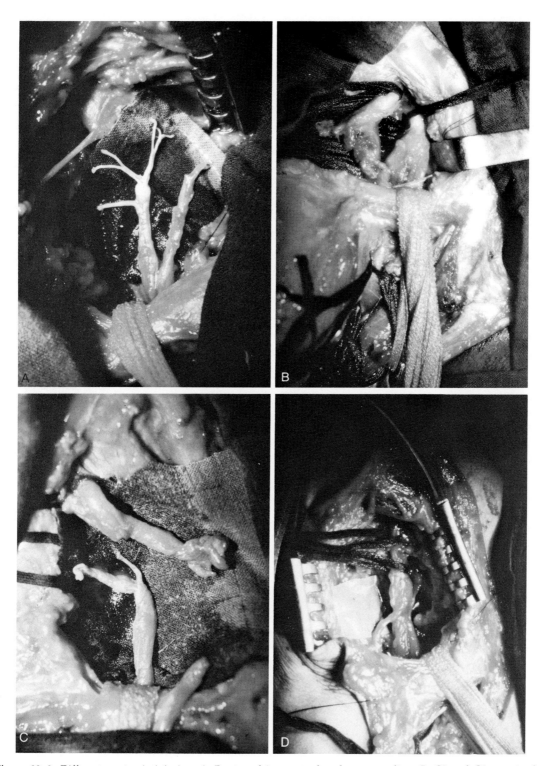

Figure 23–2. Different anatomic injuries. *A*, Root avulsion; note dorsal root ganglion. *B*, C5 and C6 torn in the scalene region with stumps that can be used for grafting. *C*, Rupture of C5 and C6; avulsion of C7. *D*, Stretch injury in continuity in the upper trunk.

mal abduction, which may cause paralysis of C8 and T1.

3. Finally, anteroposterior trauma or dislocation of the shoulder may cause lesions of the cords, especially the posterior cord or the terminal branches of the brachial plexus (axillary, suprascapular, and musculocutaneous nerves). This may be accompanied by lesions due to stretching of all the roots.

The central mechanism, secondary to extreme movements of the cervical column caused by violent trauma to the head, can induce intrinsic stretching of the rootlets at the level of the cord without associated lesions of the dura.

Pathologic lesions due to traction or stretching are not localized but spread over a significant length of roots or trunks (Fig. 23–3).

Lesions of this type can occur at any level from the emergence from the spinal cord down to the infraclavicular region. The presence of a nerve gap requires repair by nerve grafts in the majority of cases.

Several points should be noted. Rupture of the roots can occur at different levels, with some fascicles broken in the vertebral canal and others in the scalene region, associated with a true longitudinal laceration. Repair, if possible, should be directed to nerve structures that have lost some or most of their potential for axonal regeneration.

Very proximal lesions can cause retrograde degeneration associated with lesions of the anterior horn cells or with damage to the sensory cells of the posterior root ganglia equivalent to an avulsion injury. This could explain the failure of some repairs of atrophic roots.

The rupture can occur more or less distally, involve a larger or smaller segment of the root or trunk, and therefore be more or less suitable for the surgical repair. Rupture can be incomplete with persistence of one or several fascicles. This explains to a certain extent the partial recuperation that sometimes occurs over time.

These fascicles must be treated carefully during surgical exploration, as they cause difficult problems of identification.

The lesions can be found at different levels on the plexus, which can be explained by the existence of several points of relative fixation at the transverse processes, the level of the coracoid process, or the pectoralis minor or costocoracoid ligament.

The clavicle, the costoclavicular space, and the presence of a dislocated humeral head may also play some role in certain mechanisms of brachial plexus lesions. Thus, both supraclavicular (the most frequent) and some infraclavicular lesions must be considered.

In our series of 420 patients operated on between 1974 and 1985, 315 cases (75%) involved supraclavicular lesions and 105 cases (25%) were retro- or infraclavicular lesions. Double-level lesions (supra- and infraclavicular) must also be considered.

During forced abduction of the arm, the middle part of the plexus is temporarily fixated in the region of the coracoid process. The terminal branches can then be torn, and there will be some concomitant supraclavicular lesions caused by sudden turning of the head to the uninjured side.

Thus, supraclavicular lesions can be associated with infraclavicular lesions either at or below the level of the cords. Lesions below cord level can involve the musculocutaneous nerve, which has a relative fixation when entering the coracobrachialis muscle; the axillary nerve in the quadrangular space of Velpeau; or the suprascapular nerve at the level of the coracoid notch. The frequency of double-level lesions (15% of all supraclavicular lesions) justifies exploration of the entire plexus during surgical intervention.

Finally, avulsion of the roots is a special type of lesion. The tearing of the roots at their origin from the spinal cord causes irreversible lesions that cannot be repaired surgically.

At the spinal cord level, avulsion can be confirmed by posterior laminectomy, and in some of our rare cases in which surgery was done by this approach, there was complete disappearance of the root without a scar visible at the cord.

One cannot stress enough the importance of such radicular avulsions. A root immobilized in the cervical region may be pulled by violent traction that tears off the dural membranes first and then the root itself. Surgical intervention through the cervical approach permits one to recognize this lesion. However, it is possible to have the roots remain in the vertebral canal or within the dural fold, resulting in an appearance of continuity in the cervical region that creates difficult diagnostic problems.

When the injury is peripheral, the fact that the dura is torn (evidenced by pseudomeningocele at myelography) means that trauma may directly involve the ventral and dorsal rootlets. In the majority of cases, these

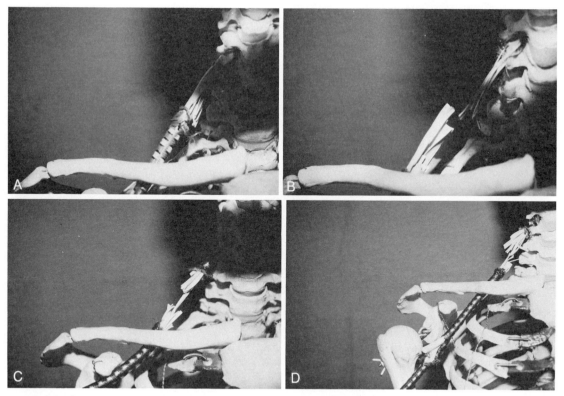

Figure 23–3. Schematic examples of various injuries. *A* and *B*, Longitudinal multilevel ruptures. *C*, Partial injuries. *D*, Double level injuries.

are torn at the spinal cord level, particularly root C7 and especially roots C8 and T1, which become horizontal as a result of arm abduction. Because of their oblique course, roots C5 and C6 will often be torn more distally in the scalene space. When the injury is central, the tearing of rootlets without injury to the dura explains the diagnostic difficulties, which can be resolved only by a posterior laminectomy.

Knowledge of pathology of brachial plexus trauma allows classification of the lesions as a basis for interpreting clinical and other findings. Several classifications are used, notably the one of Millesi. However, they are all complex and involve a large number of variables. The classification that we propose defines the lesions according to the involved root level and whether paralysis is partial or total (Table 23–1). During spontaneous improvement, differentiation must be made between resolution in the entire region of a theoretical root distribution or simply improvement in one or two muscles of this segmental territory. The classifications are indispensable for study of results following surgical repair. In addition, the use of diagrams showing different lesions and their repair facilitates follow-up examinations (Fig. 23–4).

DIAGNOSIS

Knowledge of all the anatomic and pathologic factors involved in brachial plexus lesions, together with the clinical examination and other diagnostic studies, permits one to diagnose the lesion, to determine which

Table 23–1. CLINICAL AND PATHOLOGIC FINDINGS IN BRACHIAL PLEXUS INJURIES

Clinical Findings	
C5, C6 C5, C6, C7, C8, T1 C7, C8, T1	*Total* (complete motor and sensory paralysis) or *partial* (incomplete motor or sensory paralysis)

Pathologic Findings	
Supraspinal ganglion plexus	Roots
Infraspinal ganglion plexus	Roots
Supra- and retroclavicular plexus	Trunks
Infraclavicular plexus	Cords and nerves

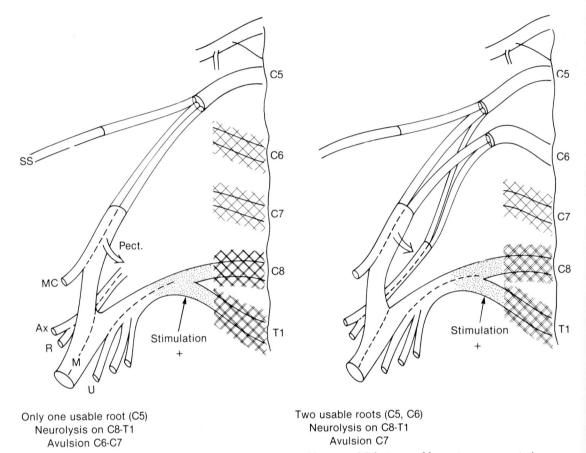

Only one usable root (C5)
  Neurolysis on C8-T1
  Avulsion C6-C7

Two usable roots (C5, C6)
  Neurolysis on C8-T1
  Avulsion C7

Figure 23–4. Examples of nerve repair with one or two usable roots. With two usable roots, some posterior areas may be grafted. Grafts connect the anterior level of the root to the anterior level of the distal plexus and the posterior level of the root to the posterior level of the distal plexus.

roots, trunks, and cords are involved, and to detect any associated lesions.

Clinical Examination

The initial clinical examination is an essential step toward establishing a topographic diagnosis and sometimes determining the exact type of lesion, which aids in prognosis.

Muscle Examination

This examination must be completed muscle by muscle, recognizing that it can be difficult because of possible simultaneous contractions of muscle groups having similar functions.

The results should be recorded on a special form that is useful for follow-up examinations. The involved roots should be recorded and differentiation between radicular trauma

and paralysis at the level of trunks or cords should be noted, taking into consideration the possible individual anatomic variations and the presence of bi- or multi-segmental innervation. Finally, these forms should record the degree of muscle atrophy and the presence of contractures or joint stiffness, which are helpful in determining the degree of improvement at periodic follow-up examinations.

At longer intervals, it is possible to compare these data with sensory examination findings by constructing special charts that include all the clinical findings as well as certain test results.

The severity of the trauma is evaluated by means of the manual muscle test, using the international scale of 1 to 5. This scale has the drawback of recording muscles as different as the biceps and those of the hypothenar region at the same level, but it must be retained because it is needed for future comparisons. However, we will have to add to this description an indication of the fatigability of the reinnervated muscles and some idea of the overall function of the shoulder, elbow, and hand.

Sensory Examination

This examination should evaluate both subjective and objective sensory disturbances. Objective sensory deficit (hypesthesia, anesthesia, or sometimes hyperesthesia) must be recorded on a special form indicating sensory root distribution. The results of sensory testing are sometimes difficult to evaluate and must be confirmed by several examinations. In cases of extensive paralysis, disturbances in deep sensation must also be checked.

Disturbances of subjective sensitivity, expressed by pain, must be thoroughly evaluated. This pain may be one of two main types:

1. Pain associated with "pins and needles" sensations or an "electric current" sensation, induced by percussion or palpation of the cervical and supraclavicular as well as the axillary region. This aspect of the cervical examination is of extreme significance because the spontaneous pain, exacerbated by local percussion, indicates a neuroma of a root, trunk, or cord. Recognizing changes in this symptom is extremely important because this painful "electrical current" sensation can remain localized and fixed, indicating a total local rupture, or can change location and be found during successive examinations first in the cervical, then in the supraclavicular, and finally in the axillary regions (Tinel's sign). This sign may be mobile, permitting one to follow the degree of axonal regeneration, which plays a role in determining prognosis and surgical indications.

2. At times, pain has no precise distribution. This type of extremely painful causalgia results in difficult pathogenic and therapeutic problems perhaps related to sympathetic nervous system participation. It appears that these causalgias, which occur only rarely immediately after an accident, are seen especially in total paralysis with damaged lower roots, the roots richest in sympathetic fibers. The pathogenesis of these causalgias is, however, difficult to determine. This type of pain, which is often intolerable, is seen more often in the long-standing nonoperated cases.

Sympathetic Nervous System Disturbances

This evaluation is a part of the initial clinical examination. One should look for rapidly appearing vasomotor disturbances (e.g., anhidrosis), cyanosis, edema of the soft tissues, or cutaneous trophic lesions, especially of the hand. Radiologically, there is a very pronounced demineralization of carpal and finger bones, which causes stiffness and secondary trophic disturbances. The presence of Horner's syndrome (myosis, ptosis, and enophthalmos) should also be determined. Although this syndrome may regress, it is always in an incomplete fashion during the 6 months following the accident.

Complete Neurologic Examination

This includes a systematic search for the signs of spinal cord involvement (pyramidal signs in the lower extremities, temporary bladder problems, blood in the cerebrospinal fluid). Even discrete findings are proof of avulsion of the roots.

Search for Associated Lesions

Associated lesions indicate the extent and seriousness of the initial trauma. However, they make formulation of the overall prognosis more difficult, particularly when dealing with multiple trauma and fractures. Vascular lesions must be searched for, and restoration of the continuity of a ruptured subclavian or axillary artery is desirable in all cases.

Evaluation of Results

At the completion of the preliminary clinical examination, an initial evaluation must be made.

The statistical analysis of a study dealing with our first 100 operated cases showed the frequency of motorcycle or motorbike accidents as the cause of these injuries. This explains the high incidence of this type of injury among young people, especially males, who favor this mode of transportation (Table 23–2).

The clinical examination, together with the other tests, permits identification of the nerve lesions in relation to the involved roots, taking into consideration the anatomic variabil-

Table 23–2. STATISTICAL ANALYSIS OF 100
PATIENTS UNDERGOING BRACHIAL PLEXUS
REPAIR

Etiology
Traffic injuries (94 of 100 cases; 69 of which involved
motorcycle injuries)

Sex
93 males; 7 females

Age (years)
Under 15:	4 cases
15–24:	71 cases
25–40:	19 cases
Over 40:	6 cases

ity and diversity of pathologic lesions. Two types of lesions can be distinguished:

1. Supraclavicular root palsies (75%, of which 15% are double-level lesions). These can be further divided into involvement by upper, middle, and lower and total plexus palsies. Upper plexus paralysis includes C5, C6 plus/minus C7, or involvement of the entire upper trunk. It is a frequent finding, constituting 20 to 25% of the cases worldwide (22% in our series). Lower plexus paralysis involves C8 and T1. It accounts for only 2 to 3% of cases worldwide (3% in our series). Middle plexus paralysis (C7) is never an isolated lesion but is associated with either an upper or a lower paralysis. Total paralysis (C5, C6, C7, C8, T1) is the most frequent, involving 75 to 80% of the cases worldwide (75% in our series). It is associated with motor involvement of the entire upper limb but sometimes spares the serratus anterior muscle (7 of 100 lesions). There are sensory disturbances of varying degrees and often significant sympathetic involvement. The lesion may be total or predominate in the lower or upper roots. From a pathologic viewpoint, the majority of cases have a typical picture, with avulsion or irreversible damage to T1, C8, and C7 associated with stretching. In addition, there is rupture of C5 and C6 in the scalene region or more distally, where the lesions are accessible to repair by grafting.

2. Infraclavicular plexus palsy with lesions of the cords or terminal branches of the plexus (25%). Several clinical forms can be distinguished, including posterior cord syndrome, isolated involvement of the terminal branches, and lesions associated with fractures of the humerus. Posterior cord syndrome is accompanied by paralysis of the deltoid at the shoulder level, but some func-

tion of the supra- and infraspinatus muscles is retained. The axillary and radial nerves are paralyzed, sometimes with involvement of the nerve branches innervating the teres major and latissimus dorsi muscles. A second clinical form is isolated involvement of the terminal branches, namely the suprascapular and axillary nerves, as well as the musculocutaneous nerve. Finally, some cases are associated with a fracture of the humerus, the paralysis of the radial nerve complicating the diagnostic problem.

In cases of traumatic brachial plexus palsies, the most important questions are those related to the prognosis and the patient's future. It is difficult to answer these questions at an early stage, but certain factors permit us to formulate a prognosis. These include the clinical examination, other tests and evaluations, and the clinical course.

Clinically, certain findings can be considered favorable or unfavorable. Favorable clinical findings include paralysis of the brachial plexus appearing after a shoulder dislocation. This has a 90% chance of complete recovery, which is important to know in order to reassure the patient. Also considered favorable is incomplete paralysis, e.g., of a muscle, graded 1 or 2 in each myotome, associated with absence of or only slight objective sensory disturbances. Unfavorable findings include severe initial trauma, as the extent of the brachial plexus lesion is directly proportional to the violence of the initial trauma.

In our 100 first cases, we noted 58 fractures and 22 arterial ruptures of the upper limb (Figs. 23–5 and 23–6). Because of its multisegmented innervation and the origin of branches from the exit of the vertebral canal, involvement of the serratus anterior indicates very extensive proximal lesions (7 of 100 cases). Horner's syndrome indicates severe proximal lesions of the lower roots C8 and T1 (31 of 100 cases). The presence of pain or of spinal cord involvement also indicates an unfavorable prognosis.

The prognosis also depends on the early clinical course, which is determined on the basis of repeated examinations and whether or not Tinel's sign shifts from the supraclavicular region to the axillary region and finally to the upper extremity nerves. In the case of multiple lesions or of a complete and a partial lesion, the interpretation is often difficult and a precise localization cannot be made. On the other hand, persistence of a syndrome of nerve irritation that remains in

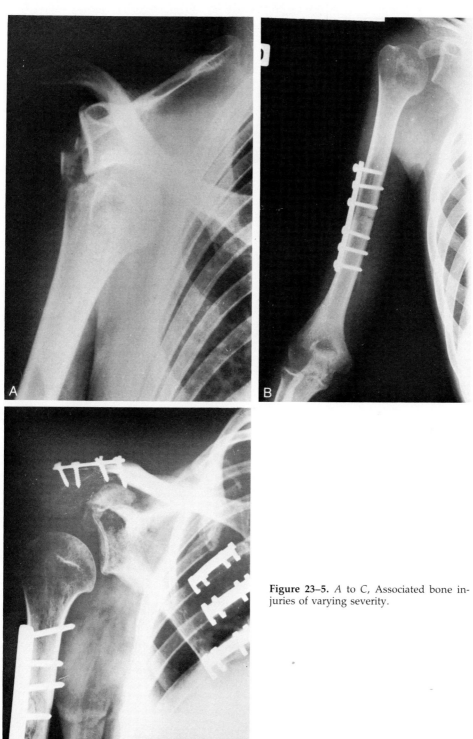

Figure 23–5. *A* to *C*, Associated bone injuries of varying severity.

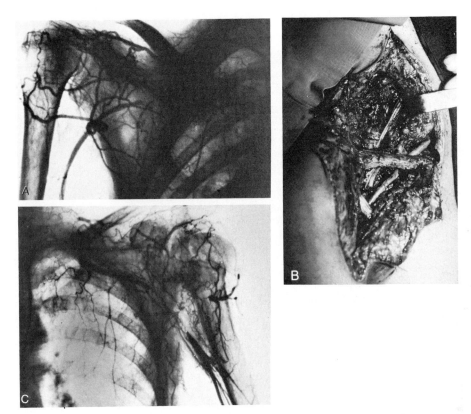

Figure 23–6. *A to C,* Arterial ruptures repaired by venous graft at the same time as the plexus reconstruction.

the supraclavicular region (Tinel's sign) indicates a neuroma and root rupture.

Other Tests and Examinations

Myelography and electromyography permit one to make as precise a diagnosis as possible of the pathologic lesions.

Together with Frot, we have described diverse radiologic abnormalities. We have also performed 400 myelograms of the cervical region and have compared these with the findings at surgery in our first 100 operated cases. A normal myelogram clearly shows a fine edge, which corresponds to the juxtaposition of the two ventral and dorsal roots and which divides the root space into two areas (Fig. 23–7).

Radiologically, lesions are classified as injuries of either the dura or the roots.

1. Lesions of the dura (Fig. 23–8). The presence of a pseudomeningocele, either large or small, indicated either a root avulsion or a very proximal lesion at the entrance of the vertebral canal in the majority of cases

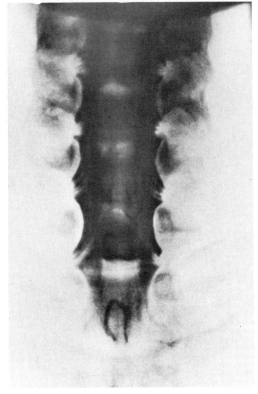

Figure 23–7. Myelography: normal view.

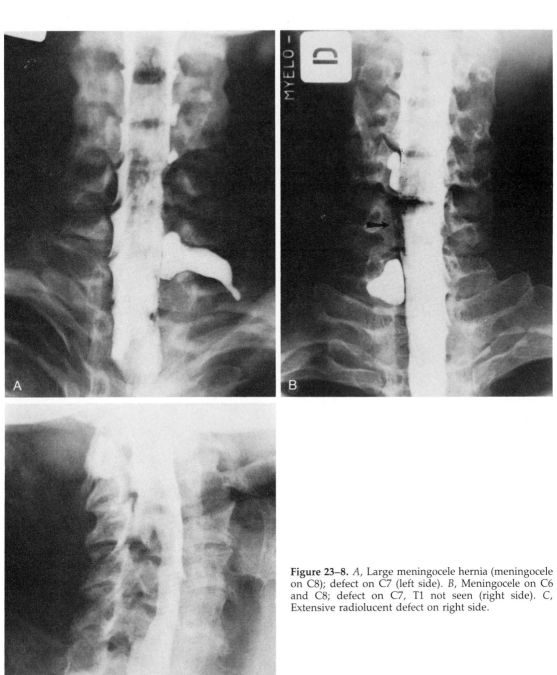

Figure 23–8. *A*, Large meningocele hernia (meningocele on C8); defect on C7 (left side). *B*, Meningocele on C6 and C8; defect on C7, T1 not seen (right side). *C*, Extensive radiolucent defect on right side.

(i.e., a lesion that cannot be repaired surgically). Continuity of the nerve after injury to the dura seems to be very rare, and recovery after severe traction lesions does not occur in most cases. If the clinical picture justifies it, a precise diagnosis can be made by posterior laminectomy.

In our first 100 operated cases, surgical exploration showed the following pathologic findings. There were 88 cases of total avulsion of the roots and 11 cases of apparent roots in continuity that did not respond to electrical stimulation. In these cases we observed no subsequent clinical recovery, and the avulsion or stretch lesions were apparently located at the rootlet level.

In one case a very large pseudomeningocele of C7 had a diverticulum that extended to C8 and T1, which led us to make an incorrect diagnosis of pseudomeningocele of these lower roots. This is one of those rare cases in which the findings at surgery did not coincide with the preoperative studies, and the possibility of this type of diagnostic error must be kept in mind.

The appearance of extensive lacunae and defects have the same significance and often coincide with a pseudomeningocele on an adjacent root. In two cases of extensive lacunae, laminectomy confirmed the presence of root avulsion and the existence of adhesions between the medulla and the dura.

2. Root lesions (Fig. 23–9). These lesions are seen only if there is no meningeal lesion, such as just discussed. Following an injury, however, the two meningeal membranes surrounding the root are modified; their parallel appearance is lost and they have a tendency to merge. The root itself may show diverse abnormalities, including a simple Lipiodol ball lesion, stretching of a root with disappearance of the central edge, and an opaque or even an absent root. These abnormalities raise the suspicion of a root lesion but do not allow evaluation of its severity. As a rule, these are partial stretch lesions that could be subjected to neurolysis if the root were in continuity. However, in a certain number of cases there is a complete rupture caused by longitudinal laceration. This results in a fibrous root that has only 25 to 50% of its nerve fibers available for possible regeneration, and the potential for subsequent regrowth is difficult to determine.

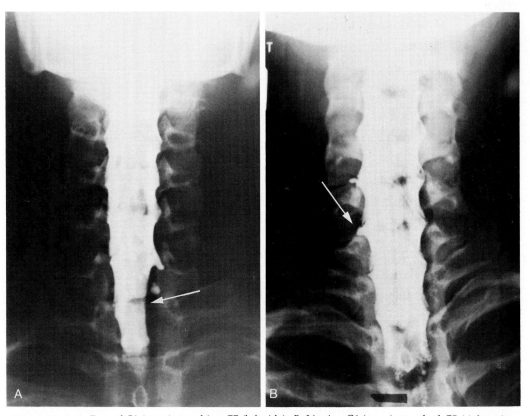

Figure 23–9. *A,* Tear of C8 (*arrow*) stretching C7 (left side). *B,* Lipping C6 (*arrow*) stretched C5 (right side).

We consider careful myelography with a CT scan an extremely reliable examination and a part of the preoperative assessment. However, the radiographs of the meninges and the roots must not be interpreted without taking other factors into consideration. Associated lesions are frequent and can be indicative of a more extensive injury. For example, an opaque root located between two pseudomeningoceles confirms the presence of a lesion of some severity.

Finally, the radiologic study may indicate a specific root lesion but does not always correspond with the clinical picture because of anatomic variability. Myelography will aid in identifying two distinct clinical pictures: (a) An abnormal myelogram indicates a root lesion, the severity of which must be determined in relation to the factors just discussed. In most cases pseudomeningoceles indicate a root avulsion and are most often localized on C7–C8–T1. (b) A normal radiologic study of the meninges and roots in a patient with total paralysis raises hope either for a spontaneous recovery or for the discovery of more distal lesions accessible to direct repair. In most of our patients with normal myelograms we have found either root continuity (second or third degree lesion) with progressive recovery or a rupture in the scalene region or more distally. Repair by graft is then done if the nerve is likely to regenerate.

However, a normal radiologic study can be associated with an irreversible total lesion. This may occur in some rare cases when the root has disappeared following an avulsion in the vertebral canal. In three of our own cases the T1 root was apparently in continuity without a lesion, but no subsequent clinical regeneration was observed. These findings favor an avulsion by a central mechanism, but they can be confirmed only by laminectomy or by scanning using contrast medium.

An operative plan can be formulated based on the clinical findings and the diagnostic studies.

Finally, electromyography is part of the evaluation. Two successive studies should be done to indicate the presence or absence of reinnervation not detected by clinical examination. Such reinnervation indicates the existence of first-degree lesions, i.e., of the upper roots (proximal muscles), in the third or fourth month after the accident.

Psychological Evaluation

We must also discuss the psychological problems presented by these patients and attempt to respond to their legitimate anxiety. Patients frequently ask: Is healing possible? When will this occur? When can surgery be done if this is necessary? What kind of results can I hope for and what kind of work will I be able to do?

SURGERY

Timing of Surgery

The first months after the accident are a period of possible regeneration, and based on our experience, surgery is not indicated at this time except for repair of any associated vascular lesions, which must be treated as soon as possible. In the case of severe ischemia, emergency surgery is necessary to repair the vascular damage; assessment of the nerve lesions can also be done during this procedure.

Nerve repair should be done as a secondary procedure because it seems impossible to determine the site at which the grafts must be done during emergency operations.

In addition, initial treatment of the associated bone and joint injuries must begin. Traction of the upper extremity upon the roots must be avoided. The limb should be immobilized in a simple splint (the arm in abduction, internal rotation, and forward flexion). Active mobilization should be started as soon as possible, as well as passive mobilization to prevent joint stiffness. The clinical course should be followed by repeated clinical examinations to determine motor and sensory function. By the 30th day, assessment should be completed by electromyography and, if regeneration is not present, by myelography.

Surgical Indications

The need for surgery will depend on the degree of preliminary regeneration. A certain number of patients (approximately two thirds of the cases worldwide) recover spontaneously in the first months; in other patients the decision to intervene surgically must be made after considering all the factors just discussed. Based on our series of 420 patients operated on between 1974 and 1985, surgical exploration by the cervico-axillary approach should be considered after 2 to 4 months if no clinical or electromyographic regeneration has occurred in one or more root segments. This delay in performing surgery is calculated from the date at which the patient was first seen. In our series, surgical exploration for the first 100 operated cases took place between the sixth and eighth months (extremes being 30 days and 18 months). We currently undertake exploration at around the third month.

The prognosis depends on the extent and type of the pathologic lesions, but in all cases is predominantly determined by the presence or absence of hand involvement.

As the therapeutic indications depend on the type of pathologic lesions, it is essential to evaluate these lesions preoperatively by the clinical and other diagnostic examinations.

Total Sensory and Motor Paralysis

In this type of injury a decision regarding surgery must be made during the second or third month following the accident (Fig. 23–10). Some patients recover spontaneously in a shorter time. However, if this does not occur, it is useless to wait for the 7 or 8 months that are normally required for proximal reinnervation.

Several clinical pictures may be described:

1. *Total paralysis without any regeneration during the second or third month.* In this type of injury the myelogram shows some meningoceles on root C8 and T1 and often on root C7. C6 may appear abnormal and C5 is generally normal radiologically. This standard radiographic picture corresponds in most cases to total paralysis, and we can predict preoperatively that a nerve graft will be possible from C5 and sometimes from C6.

In cases of total paralysis with avulsion of lower roots C7, C8, and T1, when only one

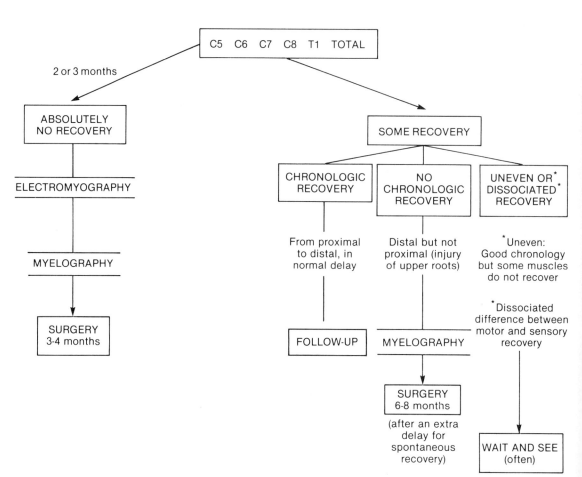

Figure 23–10. Preoperative planning (direct nerve repair) in total brachial plexus palsies.

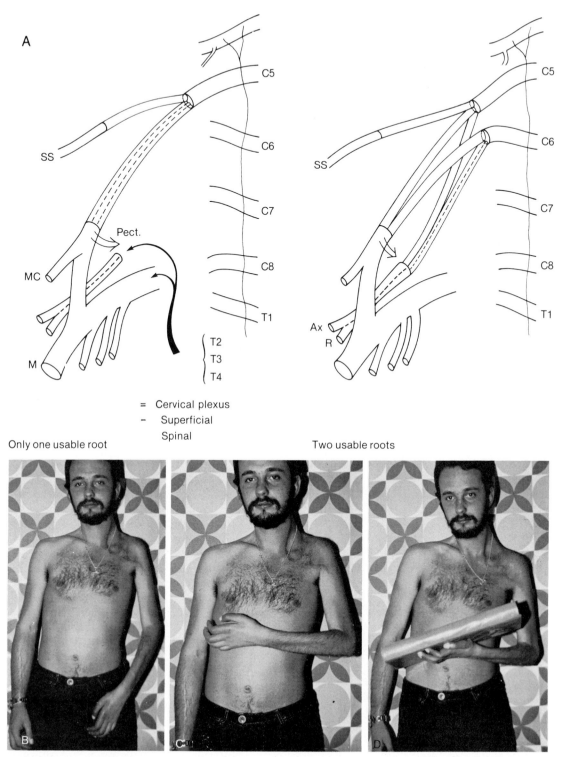

Only one usable root   Two usable roots

= Cervical plexus
– Superficial
   Spinal

Figure 23–11. *A*, Priorities in repair with one or two usable roots, preventing axonal waste. *B* to *D*, Clinical result of one usable root grafted onto suprascapular nerve and lateral cord.

or two roots are available for grafting (usually C5 and C6), *it is important to make a choice because the entire plexus cannot be bridged* (Fig. 23–11). Our procedure is now well established, and our goal *is to obtain reinnervation of the proximal regions*.

When only one root is available for grafting, our choice of the structure to repair is either the suprascapular nerve or the lateral cord above the pectoral loop. The objective is to obtain stabilization of the paralytic shoulder, to repair the pectoralis major in order to hold objects against the thorax, and to restore elbow flexion and certain palmar protective sensitivity (Fig. 23–11*B* to *D*). It is important to inform these patients that their hand will be permanently paralyzed.

With two roots to graft, in addition to the above structures, we can also bridge some parts of the posterior cord (radial or axillary nerves). Every effort is made to bridge the anterior plane of the root grafts with the anterior plane of the plexus and the posterior plane of the root with the posterior plane of the plexus.

2. *Total paralysis without any regeneration by the second or third month*. Myelography shows the presence of meningoceles on all the roots, and at surgery a spinal cord avulsion from C5 to T1 is found. It is necessary to perform neurotization of the intercostal nerves, the spinal accessory nerves, or the nerves of the superficial cervical plexus to provide a better trophic state of the upper limb and to restore some degree of flexion to the elbow by giving priority to neurotization of the musculocutaneous nerve. Amputation is warranted only in exceptional cases and should never be used to treat severe pain.

3. *Initial total paralysis with spontaneous regeneration in the first months*. Healing may occur from proximal to distal or distal to proximal segments. In proximal to distal regeneration, in some cases more or less complete healing can occur starting at the shoulder, then the elbow, and finally the hand. In total paralysis after dislocation of the shoulder, this favorable course is frequent in 80 to 90% of cases, but sometimes takes 6 to 12 months. In other cases, the course is still favorable from proximal to distal but some additional findings must be noted. Tinel's sign that does not progress indicates a distal rupture or, more rarely, fibrosis causing a block of nerve conduction. Certain muscles in the same root area may not regenerate. As a rule, this is caused by partial traction le-

sions that may improve following secondary neurolysis. Surgery may be decided upon around the fifth or sixth month, when either neurolysis or repair of a partial proximal rupture or a total distal lesion is performed.

In some cases of distal to proximal healing, paralysis is reversed quickly and totally in C8 and T1 segments, to a lesser degree in C7, and not at all in C5 and C6. Surgical exploration must be done early because a large number of patients have repairable extrascalenic lesions of upper roots or upper trunk.

Upper Root Paralysis (C5, C6, C7) (Fig. 23–12)

The prognosis is determined by the fact that the hand is either normal or only partially involved and therefore has some useful functions. A decision regarding surgery must be made early, as the lesion, which is often distal, involves the roots in the scalene region or at the level of the upper trunk. Nerve repair with satisfactory functional results is therefore possible owing to the proximity of the lesion to the effector muscles. The possibility of palliative interventions must not delay the initial nerve repair, as the results of direct reinnervation of muscles are always superior to those achieved with the best of transplants.

Lower Root Paralysis (C7, C8, T1)

In these cases a decision regarding surgery will be based upon results of the clinical examination and other diagnostic studies. Here again, the prognosis is determined by the degree of hand function and the severity of the nerve lesions. Myelography will reveal the presence or absence of pseudomeningoceles, and based on the degree of diagnostic certainty of the existence of avulsion of different roots, the clinical status should be reevaluated and a decision regarding surgical exploration made.

If pseudomeningoceles involve the lower roots, surgery is not justified. However, if the myelograms are normal but spontaneous regeneration has not occurred, surgery is appropriate for assessment and eventual nerve repair.

It is important to remember that although some C8 and T1 roots in the scalene region or even some more distal lesions of the trunk and cords can be repaired by nerve grafts,

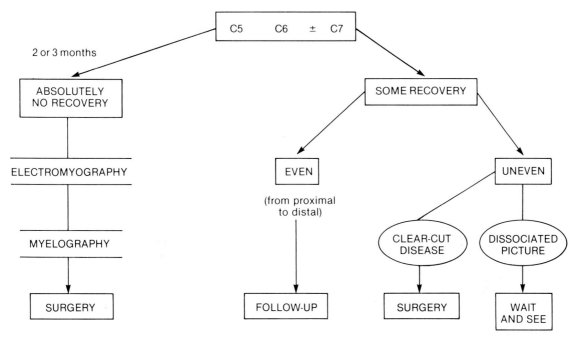

Figure 23–12. Preoperative planning (direct nerve repair) in upper brachial plexus palsies.

the distance between the nerve lesions and the hand precludes reinnervation of the intrinsic muscles.

Paralysis Due to Subclavicular Lesions

The prognosis is based on the results of the clinical examinations and the experience of the surgeon. Bone or joint lesions at the scapular or scapulothoracic level are frequent and suggest a retro- or subclavicular localization of the plexus lesions. Myelography is normal, and electromyography often shows diffuse signs that are difficult to evaluate. Our present tendency is to operate quickly on these patients, who can be divided into two groups:

1. Those with distal lesions at the level of the terminal branches of the plexus (suprascapular, axillary, musculocutaneous nerves) together with frequent associated injuries, e.g., injury to the suprascapular nerve accompanied by axillary nerve lesions. Clinically, the sensory and motor paralysis indicates a complete rupture. This is important because of the good results obtained by nerve repair if surgery is done early (before the sixth month).

2. Those with lesions at the cord level, behind and under the clavicle. This type of injury is often associated with vascular lesions, creating difficult diagnostic problems. It is in these cases that the correct diagnosis takes the longest time.

Long-standing Paralysis

In paralysis that has been present for several years after the accident, only pain constitutes an indication for neurolysis. Based on the present experience in microsurgery following early exploration of brachial plexus lesions, intractable pain is exceptional; we have never had to use a stimulator to control pain in such cases.

CONCLUSION

From 1974 to 1985, we have performed surgical exploration on 420 patients with traumatic paralysis of the brachial plexus. Problems of preoperative diagnosis are fundamental, and the clinical evaluation and other studies (myelography, electromyography) must be used to formulate coherent therapeutic indications.

If surgery is indicated, the preoperative assessment must anticipate any pathologic lesions that may be encountered in order to allow the surgery to develop an operative

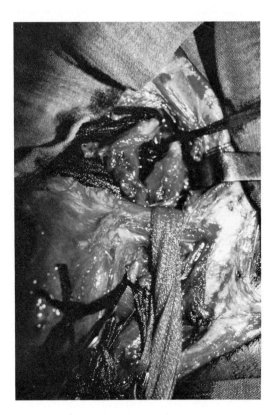

Figure 23–13. Total brachial plexus traumatic lesion (right side). Grafts are to be placed in an appropriate proximal stump.

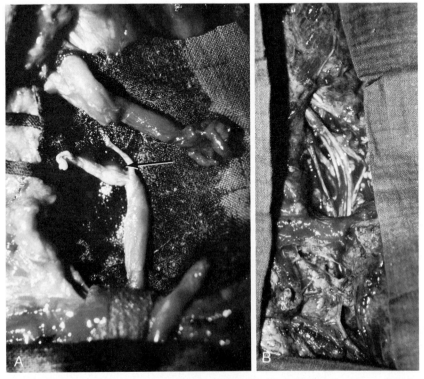

Figure 23–14. *A* and *B*, Stretched C5 and C6 roots. C7 is avulsed (*A*). Note C7 dorsal root ganglion (*arrow*). Repair is by grafting (*B*), but the prognosis is poor because of the questionable ability of the proximal stumps to regenerate.

plan. Surgical exploration will permit one to evaluate these lesions without exacerbating the patient's condition and to determine the possibilities for repair by nerve grafting. Three factors must be considered prior to repair.

1. Evaluation of the proximal structures. We must emphasize the essential difference between avulsions with neuroma and those having an atrophic appearance with reduced density. In the first case (Fig. 23–13), the grafts will be performed on a proximal stump rich in axons with a good chance of reinnervation. In the second case (Fig. 23–14), the potential for nerve regrowth is limited (a) by longitudinal laceration, with some of the fibers being ruptured distally and the others proximally in the vertebral canal close to their exit from the spinal cord; (b) by retrograde degeneration; and (c) by reactive fibrosis. The nerve graft will be then done on a root that has lost 40 to 60% of its fibers, and some of our poor results may be explained by the pathology of the additional proximal lesions.

2. Evaluation of the length of the graft and the graft bed.

3. The choice of structures to be repaired, as discussed earlier (see Fig. 23–11).

The results must be analyzed critically, and we must credit any regeneration as being due to the nerve repair only if there is no other possible explanation for healing. In any event, the results can be evaluated only after sufficient time has elapsed because reinnervation after nerve grafting is always delayed. This requires 2 to 3 years, depending on the type of lesion and its location (roots, trunks, cords, and terminal branches) and *must be evaluated according to the function of the structures to be repaired and therefore the therapeutic objectives to be achieved.*

When evaluating motor function, the classic 8 months' delay for healing of the shoulder must be increased to 12 to 15 months in order to determine return of useful function. Some patients experience a return of function that is difficult to assess. These patients do not have any active movement of the shoulder secondary to inferior dislocation of the humeral head. In addition to determining function based on the international scale of 0 to 5, it is advisable to take into account the fatigability of the reinnervated muscles and the total function of the shoulder, elbow, and arm.

Return of sensory function is difficult to evaluate. However, recovery of function of bridged structures confers considerable protective sensitivity and definite improvement in the trophic state of the extremity.

Finally, the pain syndrome must be treated. The majority of our patients who underwent surgery do not have pain or have only some intermittent pain localized in the hand in the form of cramps or "electrical currents" that does not necessitate any medical treatment.

It is important to stress that surgical interventions with nerve repair for any given region considerably modify the afferents originating in the upper limb and that almost no patients have pain after surgery. This last observation is a very important point that indicates the value of the surgical treatment.

Increased knowledge of pathologic lesions and progress in microsurgery also indicate the importance of the path that treatment of brachial plexus lesions has taken.

Precise indications taking into consideration the spontaneous course of this condition as well as the long-term results (over 2 years) confirm that direct repair of nerve lesions provides increasingly frequent functional results that justify this type of surgery. The best results evidently occur in the upper root partial palsies involving C5–C6 supraclavicular lesions and also in infraclavicular palsies. However, in total root paralysis, the increasing percentage of useful return of function, depending upon the roots grafted and the actual structures repaired, suggests that this type of surgery must be carried out after precise indications.

24

Brachial Plexus Injuries: Management and Results
■

Hanno Millesi, M.D.

Surgical repair of brachial plexus injuries for individual cases was initially reported in the last century. However, serious attempts to solve the problem of brachial plexus injuries were first undertaken during the 1940s and 1950s by Seddon, Bateman, Merle d'Aubigné, and others. The main problem was distinguishing between *supraganglionic lesions*, which had no chance for spontaneous recovery, and *infraganglionic lesions*, in which there was hope for direct repair (if continuity was lost) and for spontaneous recovery (if continuity was preserved). Different clinical tests were developed to permit this differentiation.

Seddon restored continuity by nerve grafts in five patients with upper brachial plexus lesions and achieved useful recovery in two of these patients.[19a, 20] He achieved useful flexion of the elbow joint in one patient with root avulsion by transfer of intercostal nerves via a nerve graft (ulnar nerve) from intercostal nerves 3 and 4 to the musculocutaneous nerve.[18]

Thus, the basic procedures for surgical repair were already outlined: (1) nerve grafting for loss of continuity by interruption, and (2) neurotization by nerve transfer in cases of avulsion. In spite of these successes, a feeling of dissatisfaction concerning the chances for surgical repair spread among the involved surgeons. At the 10th SICOT Meeting (Société Internationale de Chirurgie Orthopédique et Traumatologique) in Paris in 1966, there was a roundtable discussion on brachial plexus injuries under the chairmanship of Seddon and Merle d'Aubigné, with

participation of all authorities in this field. The conclusions were pessimistic.

The treatment at that time could be summarized as follows: All efforts were made to establish the diagnosis of a supraganglionic lesion and to prove that a loss of continuity had indeed occurred, if necessary by utilizing surgical exposure. If this diagnosis, with its associated poor prognosis, had been proved, early upper arm amputation was recommended, an arthrodesis of the shoulder joint was performed, and the patient was fitted with an upper arm prosthesis. If the loss of continuity could not be proved, conservative treatment was continued for at least 2 years while awaiting spontaneous recovery.

Seddon stated in 1972 that surgery has nothing to offer a patient with a root lesion, except to clarify the diagnosis and to shorten the period of waiting prior to amputation if continuity was lost. Intraneural neurolysis was not accepted as a procedure because of the danger of damaging parts of the brachial plexus having some chance of spontaneous recovery.

Seddon did not continue with his early successful attempts to treat upper brachial plexus lesions by restoring the continuity with nerve grafts because of the development of Clark's operation,[6] which employed transfer of part of the pectoralis major muscle and offered a good chance of achieving active elbow flexion in partial brachial plexus lesions. Merle d'Aubigné[11] (1976) reported on a retrospective study of patients treated during the 1950s and early 1960s. Two observations were made: (1) The patients treated by amputation and fitted with a prosthesis did not use the prosthesis for daily activities. (2) Some patients had a partial return of important functions, even after 5 or 6 years. It is evident that continuity was preserved in these patients but that spontaneous recovery was retarded by external constriction or by a very severe lesion, producing grade III to IV damage based on Sunderland's classification.[22]

Surgical developments since the 1960s have followed two pathways.

Nerve Transfer. Following Seddon's experience, Tsuyama et al.[23] utilized the transfer of intercostal nerves to the musculocutaneous nerve. Kotani et al.[7, 8] utilized the transfer of intercostal nerves and the accessory nerve in different ways. The transfer is performed by an end-to-end coaptation, exposing the entire length of the intercostal nerve to a far distal level. The brachial plexus itself is not explored. The indication for surgery is based on clinical investigation with proof of root avulsion. The weak point of this treatment is that in only 11% of all complete brachial plexus lesions are all five roots avulsed. In 86% of all root lesions with complete brachial plexus palsy, one to four roots are not avulsed but are only interrupted or have developed a lesion in continuity. In these cases a neurotization does not allow the chance of restoring the continuity of interrupted roots or of accelerating spontaneous recovery in lesions in continuity of some roots by neurolysis.

Management of Brachial Plexus Injuries by Microsurgery. The development of microsurgical techniques for repair of brachial plexus injuries has two advantages. By careful microsurgical dissection, it is possible to perform intraneural neurolysis of lesions in continuity with safe preservation of parts having only a first, second, or third degree lesion, according to Sunderland's classification.[22] Microsurgical nerve grafting offers the chance of achieving useful recovery of function by restoring continuity, even in cases involving long defects. Also, it is not necessary to make a desperate attempt to achieve an end-to-end neurorrhaphy by placing the patient in an uncomfortable position and reducing the distance between the two stumps by bone resection of the shaft of the humerus.

Early experiences with microsurgical nerve grafting of peripheral nerves and brachial plexus lesions were first reported in 1967 and

1968. In 1969 I presented my results of brachial plexus management by microsurgical techniques at a local meeting in Lausanne, Switzerland, at the invitation of Claude Verdan. Narakas discussed my paper, but he could not yet present results of his own. My paper from this conference, given in 1969, was finally published in 1973.[13] Some years later, Narakas also published a series of successful cases. This was very important because in the early years of treatment of brachial plexus lesions (between 1967 and 1970), the majority of surgeons did not believe that recovery could be achieved by brachial plexus surgery.

Since the new approach treats interruptions, avulsions, and lesions in continuity by surgery, the indications for this type of surgery have broadened. The exact preoperative estimation of the amount of damage is, of course, still important, but it is no longer decisive prior to performing surgery. The only situations in which surgery is not indicated are first and second degree lesions that have a good chance for spontaneous recovery.[22]

If spontaneous recovery is retarded in first and second degree lesions, it can be accelerated by external or internal neurolysis. The same is true for third degree lesions, which may possibly have some spontaneous recovery after many years, according to Merle d'Aubigné.[11] In third degree lesions with severe fibrosis and in all fourth degree lesions, resection and restoration of continuity by nerve grafting are indicated. If there is an interruption, continuity is restored by nerve grafting, and if there is an avulsion of more than two roots, neurotization by nerve transfer is indicated.

Direct surgery of the brachial plexus can be performed along with wide exposure and routine osteotomy of the clavicle or by limited exposure with maximal preservation of anatomic structures.

New techniques have been developed during the past 10 years. Celli and Bonola[4, 5] reported on intercostal nerve transfer, mobilizing the intercostal nerves up to the dorsal end of the intercostal space and bringing them into contact with the brachial plexus by rerouting. The motor components of the cervical plexus were utilized as donors for neurotization.[3] The accessory nerve was once again used as a donor, based on the experience that it could be utilized after giving its first branch to the trapezius muscle without completely denervating this muscle and that the trapezius muscle in some cases is innervated by an additional motor branch forming the cervical plexus.[1, 17]

In recent years vascularized nerve grafts have also been used to treat brachial plexus lesions.

Surgery to manage brachial plexus lesions is currently performed in a number of centers throughout the world. Different centers may have different experiences because the clinical material differs. Thus, there are some variations between my first group of patients, operated upon between 1962 and 1974, and my second group of 152 patients, operated upon since 1974. In the following pages I will describe my personal experience, based on these studies.

INDICATIONS FOR SURGERY

Primary Repair

In the case of an open wound, the brachial plexus may be transected. If there is a clean cut, primary nerve repair is indicated, and an end-to-end neurorrhaphy may be possible. In the case of a blunt injury, the subclavian artery and/or the subclavian veins are usually involved. The vascular repair is the primary objective, and the brachial plexus repair should be performed as an early secondary procedure. If there is a closed injury with a fracture of the clavicle, the fragments may compress the brachial plexus, and an osteosynthesis of the clavicle is therefore indicated. A large hematoma raises the suspicion of a rupture of the subclavian artery. Surgical exposure, possible evacuation of the hematoma, and vascular repair are necessary. In all other types of closed injury, there is no indication for immediate surgery.

Secondary Repair

The main objective of the early phase of treatment after a closed injury is to establish the diagnosis. The presence of a first degree lesion can be excluded by electrophysiologic investigations. In this case the conductivity of motor fibers remains intact despite the presence of paralysis because Wallerian degeneration does not occur (the axons being uninterrupted). The exclusion of a second degree lesion is more difficult. In this case conductivity of the motor fibers is lost owing to Wallerian degeneration, and early signs of recovery may appear only several months after the injury.

All other cases are subject to surgical exploration. If an avulsion or an interruption can be proved, the surgical exploration should be performed as early as possible. In all other cases, surgical exploration is indicated if there are no signs of incipient recovery within 5 or 6 months. If spontaneous recovery is evident in certain parts of the brachial plexus but is not apparent in other parts, exploration has to be reconsidered. The same is true for cases in which recovery had started but has come to a standstill.

A contraindication to surgery is a poor general state of the patient. In the case of concomitant severe craniocerebral trauma, careful neurologic examinations have to be performed, as there is danger of deterioration of the cerebral situation because of the long operation over several hours, the general anesthesia, and the extreme position of the head and neck.

TECHNIQUE OF EXPLORATION

The baseline of our exploratory technique is to achieve sufficient access with minimal damage to the anatomic structures. We believe that as much soft tissue as possible, including the subclavian muscle, should be preserved to achieve adequate soft tissue cover of the brachial plexus. If it is not possible to do a sufficient survey, the exposure has to be enlarged, and in this case we do not hesitate to perform an osteotomy of the clavicle with immediate repair by plate and screws. If there is a pseudarthrosis of the clavicle or a clavicular fracture that has healed in a poor position, a correction of the bony lesion is imperative.

Even if a clear diagnosis has been established by preoperative studies, in a proximal lesion each root should be explored individually, and a diagnosis of avulsion must be confirmed separately for each root. Experience has shown that in a series of cases in which the diagnosis of "root avulsion" seemed to be well established, one or two roots were not avulsed. These roots had preservation of continuity and had shown spontaneous recovery, which would have been lost if the surgeon had decided to perform a nerve transfer immediately. This is especially important in cases in which the ulnar nerve has been selected as a donor for nerve grafting. If an intervertebral canal is empty and the root with its spinal ganglion is outside the canal, a root avulsion is clearly proved. There are cases, however, in which the rootlets are avulsed but the root is still in the intervertebral canal, and therefore the avulsion is not evident. These situations offer a diagnostic problem that might be solved by electrophysiologic studies to record evoked potentials in the electroencephalogram.

Incision. The incision follows the dorsal border of the sternocleidomastoid muscle, turns at the level where the lateral fibers of this muscle insert at the clavicle, follows the clavicle, turns again, and crosses the pectoralis major muscle. After another turn it follows the free border of the pectoralis major muscle and reaches the upper arm with a zig-zag course. If necessary, it can be extended along the medial aspect of the upper arm or along the free border of the pectoralis major muscle to the lateral aspect of the thorax in case of an intercostal nerve transfer.

Supraclavicular Dissection. A triangular skin flap is lifted in the supraclavicular fossa. The external jugular vein is ligated and resected. Dissection enters the supraclavicular fossa and meets the scalenus anterior muscle. The phrenic nerve is defined on top of this muscle and is followed in a proximal direction. It usually originates from root C4, which belongs to the cervical plexus, and is usually intact. The phrenic nerve may also have a contribution from C5. After C4 is explored, the level of the roots is defined and the dissection is continued in caudal direction to reach C5, C6, and eventually C7. The transverse cervical artery is defined and saved. The omohyoid muscle is also defined and saved.

Infraclavicular Dissection. A triangular skin flap is raised in the infraclavicular area. The cephalic vein is defined in the deltopectoral sulcus. Entering this space, the pectoralis minor muscle is defined and isolated in order to place a rubber sling around its belly.

The dissection then enters the space medial to the pectoralis minor muscle. Here the lateral cord is encountered first. The dorsal cord is defined dorsally and the subclavian artery medially. Dissection between the subclavian artery and the lateral cord exposes the medial cord. This dissection is difficult because all the branches from the lateral cord

to the pectoralis major muscle must be preserved.

If this area is full of scar tissue, the same dissection is performed lateral to the pectoralis minor muscle. If scar tissue also extends to this area, the major nerves and vessels are exposed at the lateral aspect of the upper arm, and the dissection is performed from this level into the axillary groove and the infraclavicular fossa. To achieve this, the pectoralis major muscle has to be isolated, but it is not transected. The dissection always follows the rule that the anatomic structures must be defined in normal regions, and the damaged parts are explored from normal areas.

Establishing a Connection Between the Supra- and Infraclavicular Zones of Dissection Underneath the Clavicle. To gain better access to the area underneath the clavicle, the clavicular origin of the pectoralis major muscle is disinserted. The deltopectoral fascia is transected. The subclavian muscle is then isolated and separated from the clavicle, and the suprascapular vessels are defined. The soft tissue above the clavicle is separated from the clavicle and isolated. The clavicle is now isolated as well and can be pulled in a cranial, anterior, and caudal direction to provide sufficient space for the further dissection.

By these maneuvers the wound in the infraclavicular area is connected underneath the clavicle with the wound cavity in the supraclavicular area. The common wound cavity is crossed by the following structures: transverse cervical vessels, omohyoid muscle, supraclavicular soft tissue, clavicle, subclavian muscle, and pectoralis minor muscle. Above, between, and below these structures are different levels of access:

1. The supraclavicular fossa is easily accessible.

2. The area underneath the clavicle can be accessed (a) between the supraclavicular soft tissue, the transverse cervical artery, and the omohyoid muscle on one side and the clavicle on the other side; (b) between the clavicle and the subclavian muscle; or (c) by lifting the clavicle and the subclavian muscle.

3. The infraclavicular fossa is approached between the subclavian muscle and the pectoralis minor muscle.

4. The depth of the axillary groove is approached either laterally from the pectoralis minor muscle from above or from the upper arm from below.

ANATOMY OF BRACHIAL PLEXUS LESIONS

Between 1975 and 1981, 185 patients with brachial plexus lesions were operated on. In 152 patients the anatomic findings after exploration were sufficiently well documented to be able to include these patients in a study classifying the exact type of injury. Forty-nine patients had suffered a partial brachial plexus palsy; 103 patients had complete brachial plexus palsy.

Complete Brachial Plexus Lesions. Of 103 patients with a complete brachial plexus lesion, 21 had a peripheral lesion and 82 a root lesion. Of the 82 patients with a root lesion, 76 showed a normal configuration of the brachial plexus (C5, C6, C7, C8, T1). In two patients a prefixation was present (C4, C5, C6, C7, C8). In four patients the brachial plexus had a strong contribution from C4 (C4, C5, C6, C7, C8, T1).

Altogether 414 roots were involved. Of these, 226 roots were avulsed, 127 roots were interrupted, and 61 roots had preservation of continuity. Avulsions, interruptions, and lesions in continuity were distributed to the different roots as shown in Table 24–1.

In 12 patients (14.6% of all root lesions), all five roots were avulsed. One patient had five roots avulsed, but there was a strong stump available after interruption of the contribution from C4. In ten patients (12%) four roots were avulsed and one root was interrupted. In 26 patients (31.7%) three roots were avulsed, and the remaining roots were interrupted or in continuity. Twelve patients (14.6%) had two root avulsions with interruption or a lesion in continuity of the remaining roots. Seventeen patients (20.7%) had an avulsion of one root, and four patients (4.9%) had only a root interruption without avulsion.

In summary, of 82 patients with *root lesions*, 12 patients (14.6%) had a pure root avulsion and 4 (4.9%) had a pure interruption. More than 80% had a combined lesion. Of the 21 patients with *peripheral lesions*, 11 had a diffuse lesion of the entire plexus, making neurolysis and nerve grafting of particular parts necessary. In two patients the damage was restricted to the peripheral portion and involved mainly cords. In eight patients the amount of damage was so severe that continuity had to be restored by nerve grafts between trunks or cords and peripheral nerves.

Partial Brachial Plexus Lesions. Forty-nine patients had a partial brachial plexus lesion. In two patients the entire brachial plexus was involved, and the only remaining function was some ineffective muscle contraction. In two patients the lesion was restricted to the lower roots (C8 and T1). In one patient the lesion involved mainly the middle part of the brachial plexus (C7). Forty-four patients had a paralysis corresponding to an upper brachial plexus lesion. Four of these patients also had a lesion at the cord level. In three patients the complete lesion of the upper brachial plexus was combined with a partial denervation of the lower roots. Thirty-seven patients had a pure lesion of the upper part of the brachial plexus. Two patients in the latter group had an avulsion of roots C5, C6, and C7, three patients had an interruption of the same roots, and seven patients had a lesion in continuity of C5, C6, and C7. In eight patients the roots C5 and C6 were avulsed, in twelve patients these roots were interrupted, and in five there was a combined lesion of C4, C5, C6, or C7 in different combinations. Fifteen of 44 patients had one or more roots avulsed, and 24 of 45 patients had one or more roots interrupted. In 4 of 44 patients a neurolysis of the roots was performed, and in 4 of 44 patients a lesion was localized at cord level. In four patients C4 contributed to the brachial plexus.

This anatomic study again confirms the fact that pure lesions are exceptions and that the rule is a combined lesion with some roots avulsed, some roots interrupted, and others in continuity.

SELECTION OF TECHNIQUE FOR REPAIR

Available Techniques

Neurolysis. The individual structures of the brachial plexus are exposed in normal areas. The dissection continues toward the lesion, and, because of adhesions of the structures to the surrounding tissue, an external neurolysis always has to be performed to achieve a complete survey on the brachial plexus. Where and to what extent continuity was lost are established during this procedure.

If the individual structures of the brachial plexus seem to be uninjured, the operation can be completed as an external neurolysis.

Table 24–1. DISTRIBUTION OF AVULSIONS, INTERRUPTIONS, AND LESIONS IN CONTINUITY

	C4	C5	C6	C7	C8	T1	Total
Avulsion	1	22	39	68	53	43	226
Interruption	5	57	40	10	6	9	127
Lesion in continuity	—	3	3	4	23	28	61

This is especially true for first and second degree lesions (based on Sunderland's classification[22]) with external compression. If there is a third degree lesion with fibrosis of the epi- and interfascicular epineurium that is compressing the fascicles but with intact fascicular structures, an internal neurolysis is indicated. If the dissection within the nerve reveals that the fascicles are completely fibrotic and hard or that the fascicular structure has been lost, the involved segments are excised and continuity is restored by nerve grafting. Between these extremes are many variations. In patients with partial loss of fascicular pattern but only "soft" fibrosis, the decision as to whether to perform resection is very difficult and has to be made individually.

Neurorrhaphy. End-to-end coaptation without interposing nerve grafts is possible in only rare cases, especially those involving clean transection.

Nerve Grafting. In cases of root lesions with available proximal stumps, continuity is restored by nerve grafting between these stumps and the trunks or the cords at the level where these structures seem to be normal again. If the entire plexus is fibrotic, nerve grafting should be performed between roots and stumps of peripheral nerves.

In peripheral lesions, continuity may be restored between trunks and peripheral nerves or between cords and peripheral nerves. Free grafting of peripheral nerve trunks has proved to be unsuccessful owing to the large diameter of these nerves in relation to the surface. In the vast majority of cases we used free cutaneous nerve grafts derived from the sural nerves, the cutaneous antebrachii medialis nerves, the cutaneous femoris lateralis nerves, and the superficial branch of the radial nerve. In some instances we used the ulnar nerve as a free graft with good success after the nerve had been split longitudinally into minor subunits.

Nerve trunks and cutaneous nerves can be used as vascularized nerve grafts. Improved results have been expected from this procedure but so far have not been reported.

If the ulnar nerve is used as a donor, the existence of a root avulsion of C8 and T1 has to be proved by direct vision. In 8 of 82 patients in whom an avulsion of the root T1 was expected based on clinical investigations, this root was not avulsed, and four of these patients had useful recovery of the non-avulsed T1. Utilization of the ulnar nerve as a graft, based on clinical studies, would have made this recovery impossible and would have actually harmed the patients.

Neurotization by Nerve Transfer

Intercostal Nerves. In contrast to Tsuyama et al.[23] and Celli and Bonola,[4] we prefer to explore the intercostal nerves in the midaxillary line, leaving the innervation of the intercostal muscles behind this line intact. The intercostal nerves are transected at this level and a nerve graft is applied to the proximal stump, which connects the intercostal nerve with a selected peripheral nerve. We believe that the intercostal nerve has more motor fibers in its cross section at this level than at a more distal level. Loss of motor fibers along the small branches to the intercostal muscles and ventrally to the midaxillary line is thus avoided. In earlier procedures we tried to neurotize many different muscles by intercostal nerve transfer (see later discussion). These attempts failed. Although there was some regeneration in different muscles, patients did not learn to perform useful motions. We learned that it is much better to restrict intercostal nerve transfer to a limited number of peripheral nerves, mainly to the musculocutaneous nerve.

Accessory Nerve. We initially did not use the accessory nerve, as suggested by Kotani et al.,[7] because we believed that the complete denervation of the trapezius muscle was an unacceptable functional loss. We subsequently learned from Alnot[1] and Narakas[17] that the accessory nerve can be utilized without complete denervation of the trapezius muscle if it is transected peripheral to its first branches to the trapezius muscle even in cases in which the trapezius muscle does not receive independent innervation from the cervical plexus. Therefore, in recent years we have used the accessory nerve on many occasions.

Cervical Plexus. Brunelli[3] has drawn attention to the possibility of utilizing the motor parts of the cervical plexus for neurotization. As a result of this development there are now three easily accessible structures available to achieve neurotization in three different functional areas of the arm. The utilization of these different donors (intercostal nerves, accessory nerve, cervical plexus) for neurotization is not an alternative; they should be combined.

Techniques in Peripheral Brachial Plexus Lesions with Complete Palsy

These lesions (found in 21 of 103 patients) are characterized by the finding that the function of the long thoracic nerve (innervating the serratus anterior muscle) and in many cases the function of the suprascapular nerve remained intact following injury. In 19 patients the lesion was localized at the level of the trunks and cords and in 2 patients at the level of the cords. In some patients neurolysis alone was sufficient, and in others neurolysis was performed together with a few individual nerve grafts to more severely damaged portions. In 13 patients nerve grafts were the main treatment, the grafts being applied between trunks and peripheral nerves in 12 patients and between cords and peripheral nerves in 11 patients. Useful recovery occurred in 10 of 13 patients.

Techniques in Complete Brachial Plexus Palsy with Root Avulsion

An avulsion of *all five roots* was observed in 12 of 82 patients with complete palsies with root lesions. In five of seven patients with sufficiently long follow-up, reinnervation occurred with useful motion after increasing the force of exercise or after palliative surgery. We have utilized the accessory nerve to neurotize the suprascapular nerve. Motor parts of the cervical plexus are connected with the axillary nerve, and the intercostal nerves are used to reinnervate the long thoracic nerve and the musculocutaneous nerve. In addition, two intercostal nerves, usually intercostal nerves II and III, are connected with the median nerve in order to bring sensibility into the median nerve area.

One patient had an avulsion of five roots, but there was an interrupted root C4 contributing to the brachial plexus, which could be used. The patient had useful recovery in the shoulder joint.

If four roots were avulsed (10 of 82 patients), root C4 or C5 was always interrupted and could be utilized as a proximal stump. This root was connected by cutaneous nerve grafts with the peripheral stump of the upper trunk. In addition, intercostal nerve transfer was performed to neurotize the median nerve for sensibility (intercostal nerves II and III or III and IV) and the musculocutaneous nerve (intercostal nerves V, VI, and VII). Seven patients can now be evaluated; three had useful recovery. The failures are probably due to the fact that the available root stump was also partially avulsed and did not prove to be a good donor for axon sprouts. One of these patients had spontaneous recovery in the ulnar wrist flexor and in the ulnar finger flexors, indicating that the diagnosis of avulsion of T1 was incorrect.

In cases of *three root avulsions* (26 of 82 patients) we have to distinguish two typical situations: In 16 patients roots C7, C8, and T1 were avulsed and root C5 and C6 interrupted. In some patients root C5 was connected by nerve grafts with the lateral cord and root C6 with the dorsal cord, both without additional neurotizations. In other patients roots C5 and C6 were connected with the suprascapular nerve and the dorsal cord, the median nerve was neurotized by intercostal nerves II and III, and the musculocutaneous nerve was neurotized by intercostal nerves IV, V, and VI (Fig. 24–1).

The second group consisted of three patients with interruption of C5, avulsion of C6, C7, and C8, and preserved continuity of T1. In these patients T1 was treated by neurolysis, C5 was connected by nerve grafts with the upper trunk, a nerve transfer of three intercostal nerves (III, IV, and V or V, VI, and VII) was performed to neurotize the musculocutaneous nerve, and two intercostal nerves were connected with the median nerve.

The remaining seven patients with avulsion of three roots showed individual variations in damage. Of the 26 patients, 20 could be followed sufficiently long. Fourteen had useful recovery, five had recovery without sufficient strength, and one failed to recover at all.

In patients with *two root avulsions* (12 of 82

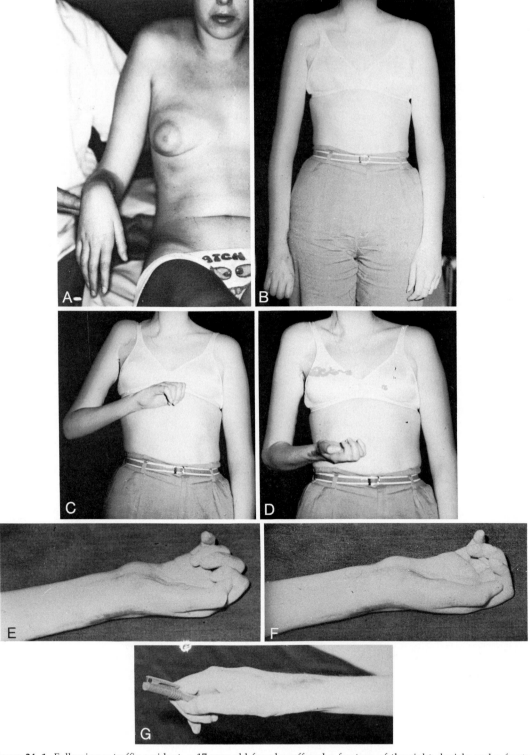

Figure 24–1. Following a traffic accident, a 17-year-old female suffered a fracture of the right clavicle and a fracture of the right transverse process of several cervical vertebrae. Complete palsy of the right brachial plexus resulted (*A*), and avulsion of C6, C7, and C8 was proved by computed tomography. The Tinel-Hoffmann sign was positive at the lateral cervical triangle. Although some surgeons might have immediately performed a nerve transfer without exploration, it should be a rule to first ascertain that actual damage to the roots has occurred. Exploration demonstrated a viable root stump with neuroma formation at C5. The avulsion of C6, C7, and C8 was confirmed.

Legend continued on opposite page

patients), the lower roots were usually involved and the upper roots were available as proximal stumps for repair. Continuity was restored between the upper roots and the dorsal and lateral cord, and in some instances also with the medial root of the median nerve. Nine of the 12 patients could be followed, with five showing useful recovery of function.

In patients with *one root avulsion* (17 of 82 patients), root C7 was avulsed in 13 instances, root C6 in two cases, and root T1 in two instances. Continuity was restored between the available root stumps and the suprascapular nerve, the dorsal cord and the lateral cord, respectively, and the superior and intermediate trunk. Eleven patients have had a sufficiently long follow-up for evaluation. Eight of them achieved useful functional recovery.

There were four patients in whom three, four, or five roots were interrupted without an avulsion. Continuity was restored between the proximal stumps and the distal stumps at the trunk or cord level. Three patients could be followed. All three had useful recovery of function.

Techniques in Partial Brachial Plexus Lesions

The five patients with lower brachial plexus lesions, C7 lesions, and irregular partial lesions were treated by neurolysis and individual nerve grafts to areas with major damage. Four of them could be followed, and all four had useful recovery of function. Four patients with upper brachial plexus lesions had a lesion at the fascicular level. They were treated by neurolysis and nerve grafts to individual nerves (axillary, radial, or musculocutaneous). All four patients had useful recovery of function. In one patient radial nerve function did not return with sufficient strength, and, therefore, a tendon transfer

had to be performed. In three patients roots C5 and C6 had to be repaired by nerve grafts, and there was, in addition, partial damage to the lower roots, which was treated by neurolysis. Thirty-seven patients had a pure upper brachial plexus lesion with roots C8 and T1 intact. In three patients the roots C5, C6, and C7 were interrupted and repaired by nerve grafts. Two of these patients had useful recovery of function.

In two patients roots C5, C6, and C7 were avulsed. In one patient intercostal nerve IV was connected with the axillary nerve, intercostal nerve V with the musculocutaneous nerve, and intercostal nerves VI and VII with the radial nerve. There was good recovery in the deltoid and in the biceps muscles; however, radial nerve function had to be strengthened by tendon transfer. In the other patient the accessory nerve was connected with the axillary nerve and the suprascapular nerve by two nerve grafts, resulting in satisfactory recovery of shoulder motion. Motor parts of the cervical plexus were connected with the radial nerve and useful recovery was achieved. Intercostal nerves II, III, and IV were connected with the musculocutaneous nerve, obtaining useful recovery of the biceps muscle.

In seven patients the continuity of roots C5, C6, and C7 was preserved. Neurolysis was performed, and useful recovery occurred in all six patients who could be followed.

Eight patients had an avulsion of roots C5 and C6. Nerve transfer was performed, using the accessory nerve for the suprascapular or the axillary nerves, intercostal nerves for the musculocutaneous nerve, and in one case the cervical plexus for the musculocutaneous nerve. Six patients could be evaluated, with three showing useful recovery of function. In 12 patients roots C5 and C6 were interrupted and continuity was restored by nerve grafts. Nine patients could be evaluated, with five having useful recovery of function. Five patients had a different combination of inter-

---

Figure 24–1 *Continued.* It was decided to restore continuity between the stump of C5 and the superior trunk by free cutaneous nerve grafts (sural nerve) and to neurotize the musculocutaneous nerve by connecting its distal stump with the proximal stumps of the intercostal nerves V, VI, and VII, using nerve grafts. Two intercostal nerves (III and IV) were linked with the median nerve. The root T1 appeared badly damaged and without possibility of regeneration. It was tempting to harvest the ulnar nerve either as a free graft after longitudinal splitting or as a vascularized graft. Since there was some hope, the root T1 was neurolized.

One and a half years later, the state of the patient was as follows: There was functional return of the deltoid muscle and no subluxation of the humerus. Atrophy had improved (*B*). There was strong elbow flexion (*C*) with supination (*D*). Return of finger flexion of median innervated muscles (*E*) and return of function of the flexor carpi ulnaris (ulnar nerve innervated) were also noted. After arthrodesis of the wrist joint and transfer of the flexor carpi ulnaris to the finger extensors, some extending function could be achieved (*F*) and a primitive grip was restored (*G*).

ruption and avulsion of roots C4, C5, C6, and C7. Useful recovery occurred in four of the five patients.

POSTOPERATIVE CARE

The operation is completed with careful hemostasis and reattachment of the clavicular origin of the pectoralis major muscle. If nerve grafts were applied, the patient is immobilized by a head-arm-trunk plaster cast. The immobilization is maintained for 8 days. After that time, careful passive motion is resumed and treatment with exponential current is commenced. The postoperative care is extremely important. The patient needs psychological and social support and is regularly seen and supervised by the surgeon. It is important to avoid depression and to provide the patient with a meaningful occupation during the long period of treatment. Average patients require 6 to 10 months until signs of reinnervation in the muscles of the arm and forearm occur. Patients with neurotization especially need sophisticated guidance. They have to become aware that, for example, the biceps muscle is innervated when they breathe or cough and they must therefore learn to perform voluntary motions without breathing and coughing. This is a very long process that requires much patience on the part of the patient and the therapist.

Often simultaneous innervation of antagonists occurs, which results in neutralization of each antagonist as far as the functional effect is concerned. Sometimes this situation is overcome by the more important muscles becoming the stronger ones; however, in many cases surgical intervention is necessary.

PALLIATIVE SURGERY

Two completely different situations have to be distinguished: (1) palliative surgery in cases of partial brachial plexus lesions and (2) palliative surgery in cases of complete brachial plexus lesions with partial recovery.

Palliative Surgery in Partial Brachial Plexus Lesions

In this situation there is a well-defined loss of function, but the remaining muscles are more or less normal. For this reason the muscles, which may be considered for use as a transfer, can be regarded as normally functioning.

Upper Brachial Plexus Lesions
Shoulder. Arthrodesis of the shoulder joint has been recommended by different authors. However, prolonged immobilization of the shoulder joint in abduction and elevation leads to stiffness of the shoulder joint and an effect similar to arthrodesis. In all these cases it is extremely important that the serratus anterior muscle works well. Normal function of the trapezius muscle is also a requirement. Control of the shoulder joint and some abduction can be achieved by transfer of the trapezius muscle to the collum humeri. The pectoralis major or minor muscle can be considered for external rotation. The position of the arm can be improved by a rotatory osteotomy of the humerus shaft, as far as external rotation is concerned. However, we believe that an additional active force for external rotation is important.

Elbow Flexion. According to Steindler,[21] strong elbow flexion can be achieved in cases of upper brachial plexus lesions by transfer of the common head of the forearm and finger flexors from the epicondylus medialis humeri to the humerus shaft about 5 cm above. Another possibility is the transfer of the lateral part of the pectoralis major muscle, according to Clark[6] or the transfer of the latissimus dorsi muscle, according to Zancolli and Mitre.[25]

Radial Nerve Palsy. When C7 is involved, the patient also has a palsy similar to a radial nerve palsy. In this situation a tendon transfer (as for radial nerve palsy) can be performed.

Lower Brachial Plexus Lesions and Irregular Partial Brachial Plexus Lesions. In the case of a lower brachial plexus lesion, palliative surgery can be performed as for a combined high median and ulnar nerve lesion.

Palliative Surgery in Complete Brachial Plexus Lesions with Partial Recovery

Full recovery after brachial plexus lesions can be expected only in patients who have limited damage to the fascicular structures and in whom the permanent palsy was due to external compression or compression by fibrosis of the epifascicular epineurium. In more severe lesions in continuity and in all patients with loss of continuity, full recovery does not occur. Treatment must be regarded as successful if at least some muscles regain voluntary innervation with sufficient force to perform useful movements. Because of the long period of denervation, muscles are often overextended, and in this case tendon shortening improves functional efficiency. In other cases a less important muscle may resume active motion and an important muscle may not. In this situation palliative surgery is required.

Shoulder Joint. If recovery after direct repair is associated with subluxation of the shoulder, transfer of the horizontal fibers of the trapezius muscle to the collum humeri improves the situation. External rotation can be achieved by transfer of the pectoralis major or minor muscle, if these muscles have regained function. Rotatory osteotomy may be an additional measure.

Elbow Joint. In some patients only the triceps resumes forceful contractions and the biceps remains paralyzed. Transfer of the triceps tendon to the biceps tendon results in sufficiently strong elbow flexion to improve this situation.

In other patients the biceps and the triceps muscles are innervated simultaneously, neutralizing each other when contracting. If this situation does not resolve spontaneously and if the patient does not learn to innervate the two muscles independently, a transfer of the triceps tendon to the biceps results in strong elbow flexion, with both muscles now acting as elbow flexors. Extension is accomplished by gravity.

Hand. If the patient has control of the shoulder joint and active elbow flexion, he can also control supination. An arthrodesis of the wrist joint in adults and a tenodesis of the wrist joint in children provide stability of the hand in this situation. Arthrodesis can be the basis for reconstruction of a primitive grip. This can be achieved by the following procedures:

1. Arthrodesis of the thumb in opposition, using a bone graft between metacarpals I and II, arthrodesis of the interphalangeal joint of the thumb, and tenodesis of the flexor pollicis longus tendon.

2. Arthrodesis of metacarpal II to metacarpal V in the flexed position.

3. Tenodesis of the flexor digitorum profundus in order to fix the interphalangeal joint in flexion and in opposition to the thumb. This opposition is strengthened if the patient supinates the forearm.

If at least one muscle, e.g., the brachioradialis, is available at the forearm, this muscle is used to activate the flexor digitorum profundus tendons. If two muscles are available, one is used for flexion and one for extension of the finger joints. If three muscles are available, the third muscle is used to activate the flexor pollicis longus tendon.

Another important function is pronation. This may be achieved by transfer of the flexor carpi ulnaris muscle if several muscles are available in the forearm.

Additional Operations

The occurrence of a pain syndrome is characteristic for brachial plexus lesions. Based on our experience before brachial plexus surgery was developed, it seems that the frequency of a pain syndrome is much lower after direct surgery compared with that of untreated lesions. After direct operation on the brachial plexus the pain syndrome very often disappears slowly. The pain and discomfort experienced by the patient first move toward the periphery and then gradually disappear.

We had to perform surgery in four patients because of the pain syndrome. All four patients had a cervical chordotomy performed by neurosurgeons. In three patients surgery was successful; in the fourth additional stereotactic operations had to be done in order to achieve control of the pain.

In two patients forearm amputation was performed because it was considered more useful to have a forearm stump with good control fitted with a prosthesis and to remove the uncontrolled and unesthetic hand.

One patient had useful partial functional recovery. The patient was able to grip but there was no sensibility in the thumb and index finger. In this case we performed a microsurgical dissection of the fascicle groups forming the digital nerves to the thumb and index finger and followed them as long as possible in a central direction within the median nerve. This was possible until about the middle of the forearm. Intercostal brachial nerves, coming from T2 and T3, were explored and used as proximal stumps. The intercostal brachial nerves and the distal stumps of the fascicle groups, going to thumb and index finger, were united with sural

Table 24–2. RESULTS IN 134 PATIENTS WITH COMPLETE BRACHIAL PLEXUS LESIONS*

Type of Surgery	Total Number of Patients	Treatment Completed— Follow-up Sufficiently Long	Useful Recovery	Percentage
Neurolysis	20	16	11	68.7
Neurorrhaphy	2	2	2	—
Nerve grafts	82	65	47	72.3
Nerve transfer	30	20	10	50.0
Total	134	103	70	67.9

*From Millesi, H.: Clin. Plast Surg., *11*:115, 1984.

nerve grafts 31 cm in length. The result was return of protective sensibility in the thumb and the index finger.

RESULTS

For each group of patients included in the anatomic study results have been defined as "useful" and "not useful." This raises the question of how results after brachial plexus surgery can be evaluated.

The basic questions that had to be answered in the early years of brachial plexus surgery were: Is it worthwhile to perform brachial plexus surgery? Are all the efforts justified by the actual results? We know that we rarely can achieve normal function, except in the few patients with limited damage to the fascicular structures. On the other hand, the severity of the functional loss has to be considered. With severe loss of function, the arm is not only useless but is an obstacle. This is the reason why amputation was recommended in the past. However, return of even minimal function means a great deal to the patient, as the arm is no longer an obstacle and can be used as a supportive limb. If this can be achieved, the result can be regarded as a useful one. How-

ever, the following conditions must be fulfilled:

1. There must be no subluxation of the shoulder joint. Some active control of the shoulder must be present. Elevation of the shoulder is not really necessary, but the patient needs some amount of external rotation.
2. There should be strong flexion of the elbow joint. This is the most important function.
3. There should be control of the wrist joint. If this is not possible in any other way, an arthrodesis will allow active supination. If forearm muscles resume function, the result must be regarded as good. We then can consider a procedure to reconstruct pronation and even obtain some type of gripping function, as outlined above.

The following figures are based on all of the 206 patients operated upon between 1962 and 1980. The 152 patients referred to earlier are included. In 165 patients the treatment is already completed and the follow-up is sufficiently long to permit an evaluation. The vast majority of these patients were treated by one surgeon. In recent years two more surgeons have contributed to the material.

Surgery was performed on 134 patients with *complete lesions*. The results can be evaluated in 103 patients, and 70 of them have

Table 24–3. RESULTS IN PARTIAL BRACHIAL PLEXUS LESIONS

Type of Lesion	Total Number of Patients	Treatment Completed— Follow-up Sufficiently Long	Useful Recovery	Percentage
Upper brachial plexus lesion	63	54	42	77.7
Lower brachial plexus lesion	6	6	6	—
Irregular lesion	3	2	2	—
Total	72	62	50	80.6

Table 24–4. RESULTS IN UPPER BRACHIAL PLEXUS LESIONS
ACCORDING TO THE TYPE OF SURGERY

Type of Surgery	Total Number of Patients	Treatment Completed— Follow-up Sufficiently Long	Useful Recovery	Percentage
Neurolysis	25	23	22	95.6
Nerve grafts	34	28	21	75.0
Nerve transfer	13	11	7	63.6
Total	72	62	50	80.6

achieved useful recovery (68%). For details see Table 24–2.

Of the 72 patients with partial brachial plexus lesions, 62 have completed treatment and have had a sufficiently long follow-up to evaluate results; 50 (80.6%) achieved useful recovery of function (Table 24–3).

SUMMARY

At the time of the accident the brachial plexus can be repaired primarily if there is a clean transection. In the case of a clavicular fracture and/or severe bleeding caused by rupture of the subclavian artery, the hematoma has to be evacuated to avoid compression of the brachial plexus. For the same reason the fracture should be stabilized as soon as possible and the artery repaired. The reconstruction of the brachial plexus is performed as a secondary procedure.

In case of a closed injury all efforts should be directed toward clarifying the diagnosis and excluding patients with good chances of spontaneous recovery. The remaining patients should undergo direct repair. According to the amount of damage, external or internal neurolysis, neurorrhaphy, nerve grafting, or neurotization by nerve transfer is performed (Table 24–4).

Direct surgery is followed by a period of intensive physiotherapy. Social and psychological care is extremely important. Patients should resume work as soon as possible. If they are not able to resume their former profession, they have to be prepared for another job that can be performed wtih one arm and one hand. The entire treatment is planned and supervised by the surgeon. After a sufficiently long period, usually 1½ years following direct repair, the amount of functional return is analyzed. At that time decisions are made whether to perform ade-quate palliative surgery in order to make maximum use of the restored function.

References

1. Alnot, Y.: Personal communication at the 1st Congress of the International Confederation of the Societies for Surgery of the Hand. Rotterdam, May 15–18, 1980.
2. Bateman, J.E.: Trauma to Nerves in Limbs. Philadelphia, W.B. Saunders Company, 1962.
3. Brunelli, G.: Neurotization of avulsed roots of the brachial plexus by means of anterior nerves of the cervical plexus. Int. J. Microsurg., 2:55–58, 1980.
4. Celli, L., and Bonola, A.: Intercostal nerve transplant in brachial plexus lesion with tearing of the nerve root. Surgical technique. Proceedings of the 13th Congress of the Société Internationale de Chirurgie Orthopédique et Traumatologique. Copenhagen, July 6–11, 1975.
5. Celli, L.: Conference at the Giornate Internazionale di Chirurgia. Taranto, Italy, June 8–10, 1978.
6. Clark, J.P.M.: Reconstruction of biceps brachii by pectoral muscle transplantation. Br. J. Surg., 34:180, 1946.
7. Kotani, P.T., Toyoshima, Y., Matsuda, H., Suzuki, T., Ishikazi, Y., Iwani, H., Yamano, K., Inoue, H., Moriguchi, T., Ri, S., and Asada, K.: The postoperative results of nerve transfer of the brachial plexus injury with root avulsion. Proceedings of the 14th Annual Meeting of the Japanese Society for Surgery of the Hand, Osaka, 1971.
8. Kotani, P.T., Matsuda, H., and Suzuki, T.: Trial surgical procedures of nerve transfer-to-avulsion injuries of plexus brachialis. Abstracts of the 12th Congress of the Société Internationale de Chirurgie Orthopédique et Traumatologique. Israel, October 9–13, 1972.
9. Merle d'Aubigné, R.M.: Personal communication at the 10th Congress of the Société Internationale de Chirurgie Orthopédique et Traumatologique. Paris, September 4–9, 1966.
10. Merle d'Aubigné, R.M., and Deburge, A.: Etiologie, évolution et pronostic des paralysies traumatiques du plexus brachial. Rev. Chir. Orthop., 53:23, 1967.
11. Merle d'Aubigné, R.M.: Personal communication at the Symposium über ausgewählte Probleme d. Plastischen u. Rekonstruktiven Chirurgie. Vienna, November 16–17, 1976.
12. Millesi, H.: Zum Problem der Überbrückung von Defekten peripherer Nerven. Wr. Med. Wschr., 118:182, 1968.

13. Millesi, H.: Résultats tardifs de la greffe nerveuse interfasciculaire. Chirurgie réparatrice des lésions du plexus brachial. Rev. Médi. Suisse Romande, *93:7*, 511, 1973.

14. Millesi, H., Ganglberger, J., and Berger, A.: Erfahrungen mit der Mikrochirurgie peripherer Nerven. Chir. Plast. Reconstr., *3:47*, 1967.

15. Millesi, H., Meissl, G., and Katzer, H.: Zur Behandlung der Verletzungen des Plexus Brachialis. Vorschlag einer integrierten Therapie. Bruns' Beitr. Klin. Chir., *220:4*, 429, 1973.

16. Narakas, A.: Plexo braquial, terapéutica quirúrgica directa, técnica, indicación operatoria y resultados. *In* Palazzi Coll, S. (ed): Cirurgia de los Nervios Periféricos. Madrid, Tipografía Artística Alameda, 1972, pp. 339–404.

17. Narakas, V.: Personal communication at the 1st Congress of the International Confederation of the Societies for Surgery of the Hand. Rotterdam, May 15–18, 1980.

18. Seddon, H.J.: Nerve grafting. J. Bone Joint Surg., *45B:447*, 1963.

19. Seddon, H.J.: Personal communication at the 10th Congress of the Société Internationale de Chirurgie Orthopédique et Traumatologique. Paris, September 4–9, 1966.

19a. Seddon, H.J.: Surgical Disorders of the Peripheral Nerves, 1st Ed. Edinburgh, Churchill Livingstone, 1972.

20. Seddon, H.J.: Surgical Disorders of the Peripheral Nerves, 2nd Ed. Edinburgh, Churchill Livingstone, 1975, p. 194.

21. Steindler, A.: Traumatic Deformities and Disabilities of the Upper Extremity. Springfield, Ill., Charles C Thomas, Publisher, 1946.

22. Sunderland, S.: A classification of peripheral nerve injuries producing loss of function. Brain, *74:491*, 1951.

23. Tsuyama, N., Sakaguchi, R.T., Hara, T., Kondo, S., Kaminuma, M., Ijichi, M., and Ryn, D.: Reconstructive surgery in brachial plexus injuries (39–40). Proceedings of the 11th Annual Meeting of the Japanese Society for Surgery of the Hand, Hiroshima, 1968.

24. Yeoman, P.M., and Seddon, H.J.: Brachial plexus injuries: treatment of the flail arm. J. Bone Joint Surg., *43B:493*, 1961.

25. Zancolli, E., and Mitre, E.: Latissimus dorsi transfer to restore elbow flexion. J. Bone Joint Surg., *55A:1265*, 1973.

25

Motorcycle Brachial Plexopathy

■

Julia K. Terzis, M.D., Ph.D.
W. Theodore Liberson, M.D., Ph.D.
Hallene A. Maragh, M.D.

Motorcycle accidents are quite frequently the cause of brachial plexus palsy (BPP) in adult patients. Such patients contribute to about 30% of adults with BPP treated by microsurgery by one of us (JKT). It is well known that these patients incur the most devastating injuries to the brachial plexus. With this in mind, we analyzed our data for these patients, and our findings are discussed in this chapter.

MECHANISM OF INJURY

Although obviously there is no documented description of the types of accidents leading to BPP in these patients, one may safely assume that the following factors were involved:

1. *High velocity injury.* This was true for 17 of 19 of our patients; the two other patients were traveling at a low speed at the time of the accident.

2. *Traction* upon the plexus in any of the three classic directions: downward, upward, and sideward.

3. Additional *fractures and dislocations*, particularly those of the humerus and clavicle, as well as *vascular lesions*, some of which resulted in hematomas.

Despite these various factors, it seems that these patients have a more uniform background of traumatic mechanisms than that of other adult patients with BPP in whom factors such as direct compression lesions by trauma or tumors, gunshot wounds, neuropathy, etc., complicate the analysis of the mechanisms of BPP.

POPULATION

The population for this study consists of 19 patients—18 males and 1 female. Most of our patients are young (Fig. 25–1); the average time from injury to surgery is relatively

AGE DISTRIBUTION

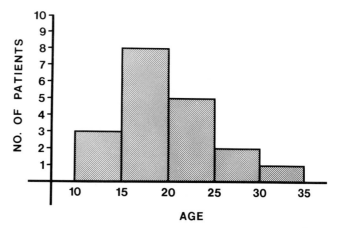

Figure 25–1. Age distribution of injured motorcyclists. Note preponderance of subjects under age 20.

Table 25–1. INTERVAL BETWEEN INJURY AND
RECONSTRUCTIVE SURGERY

Months	0–6	6–12	12–18	>18
Number of patients	10	2	3	4

short (Table 25–1); and left-sided injuries
slightly predominate (Table 25–2). Table 25–3
shows the incidence of vascular lesions, and
Table 25–4 shows the incidence of fractures
and dislocations.

PRESURGERY AND POSTSURGERY FOLLOW-UP TESTING

In addition to a complete clinical examination, the following tests were carried out:

1. *Videotapes*. These were recorded in each
case prior and following surgery as part of
routine follow-up. The videotapes show the
initial deficit and the improvement of active
range of motion over time. Photographs were
taken the same day as the taping.

2. *Manual Muscle Test*. All muscles innervated by the brachial plexus were scored
according to the classic scale of 0 to 5 (5 being
normal strength).

3. *Sensibility Testing*. This was performed
using static two-point discrimination, moving two-point discrimination, constant touch,
Ninhydrin testing, and thermography which
have been used as objective methods to evaluate peripheral nerve injuries.

4. *Electromyography (EMG)*. EMG and conduction velocity testing were done routinely.
These tests included a search for fibrillations
and positive sharp waves in the cervical erector spinae and extremity muscles; determination of the amount of voluntary activity
(single motor unit potentials indicating a
number of motor units present); poor, incomplete, or full interference pattern; and evaluation of sequential conduction velocities.

5. *Cervical Myelography*. All patients undergoing surgical exploration had a cervical myelogram.

Table 25–2. INCIDENCE OF EXTREMITIES
AFFECTED (LEFT VS. RIGHT)

	No. of Patients	Per Cent
Total	19	100%
Left	11	58%
Right	8	42%

Table 25–3. INCIDENCE OF VASCULAR
INJURIES

	No. of Patients	Per Cent
Total	19	
Vascular injuries:	7	36%
Axillary	4	21%
Brachial	2	10%
Subclavicular	1	5%

6. *Computed Tomography (CT)*. In order to
increase the resolution of the myelogram and
improve the accuracy of the myelographic
prediction, CT of the cervical spine can be
done following a metrizamide cervical myelogram.

7. *Angiography*. An angiogram was performed on patients who had a previous vascular injury or who were found to have a
vascular abnormality.

8. *Additional Radiologic Examinations*: These
included views of the cervical spine, shoulder, clavicle, humerus, and forearm to determine multiple levels of injury that may have
occurred from associated fractures. Radiographs of the chest during inspiration and
expiration were done to detect the presence
of diaphragmatic paralysis.

Pathologic Findings

Figure 25–2 shows all the drawings made
during surgical exploration classified according to: (1) relative sparing of the hand (eight
patients), (2) sparing of the shoulder (four
patients), and (3) global plexus involvement
(seven patients).

Table 25–5 shows the distribution of roots
involved and whether the roots were severed
or avulsed. As in the case of obstetrical BPP
(see Chapter 38), C7 is involved more often
than any other root. Moreover, just as in
obstetrical palsies, when C8 was involved,

Table 25–4. INCIDENCE OF FRACTURES AND
DISLOCATIONS*

Type of Injury	No. of Patients
Without fracture	3
Fracture of humerus	2
Fracture of clavicle	6
Fracture of forearm and arm	9
Shoulder dislocation	4

*Some of our patients had fractures of several bones
and/or shoulder dislocations.

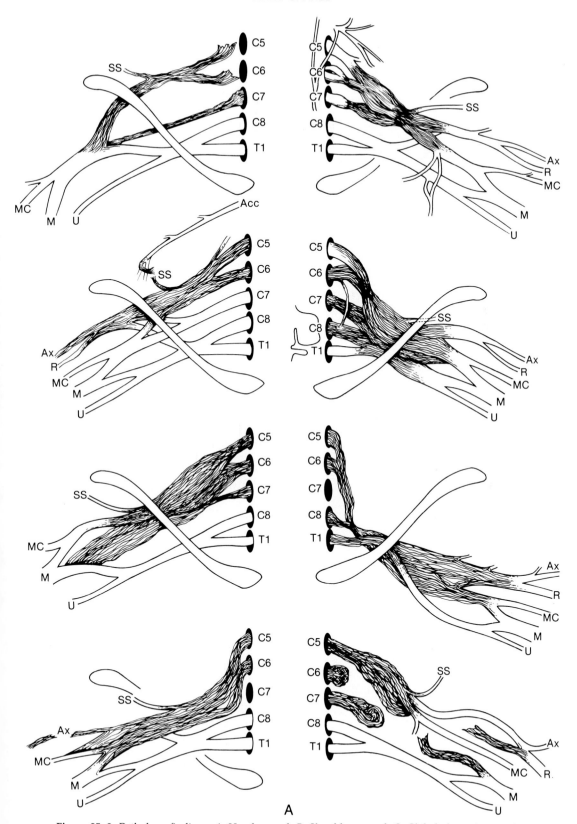

A

Figure 25–2. Pathology findings: *A*, Hand spared; *B*, Shoulder spared; *C*, Global plexus (see text).

Illustration continued on following page

SHOULDER SPARED

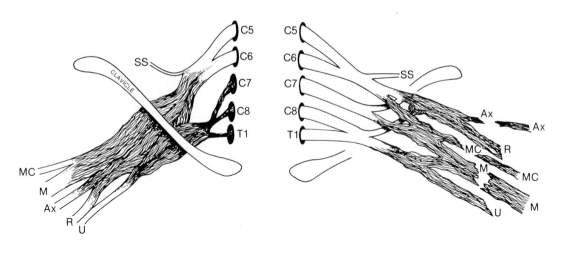

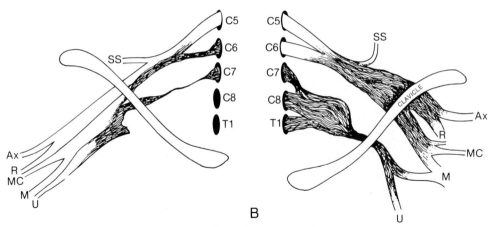

B

Figure 25–2 *Continued*

Illustration continued on opposite page

Table 25–5. DISTRIBUTION OF INVOLVED
ROOTS

	C5	C6	C7	C8	T1
Damaged	15	16	16	12	12
Intact	3	2	1	6	6
Avulsed	3	4	12	10	8
Ruptured	1	1	1	0	0
% Avulsed	20%	25%	75%	83%	67%

this root was avulsed in the great majority of cases (83%).

In order to pinpoint possible differences between patients who either had no fractures or vascular lesions or sustained fractures and/or dislocations, with or without vascular lesions, we analyzed the data related to these groups of patients. We were particularly interested in the distribution of patients with (1) "shoulder spared," (2) "hand spared," and (3) "global plexus" involvement (Table 25–6). There was a predominant trend (without statistical significance) showing an increased number of "hand spared" patients in the presence of shoulder dislocations, with or without fractures. This suggests that a fall on the shoulder or other mechanisms causing such dislocations affected the long upper cervical nerves more often than the short lower nerves. This is in agreement with the study of Alnot (see Chapter 23).

GLOBAL PLEXUS

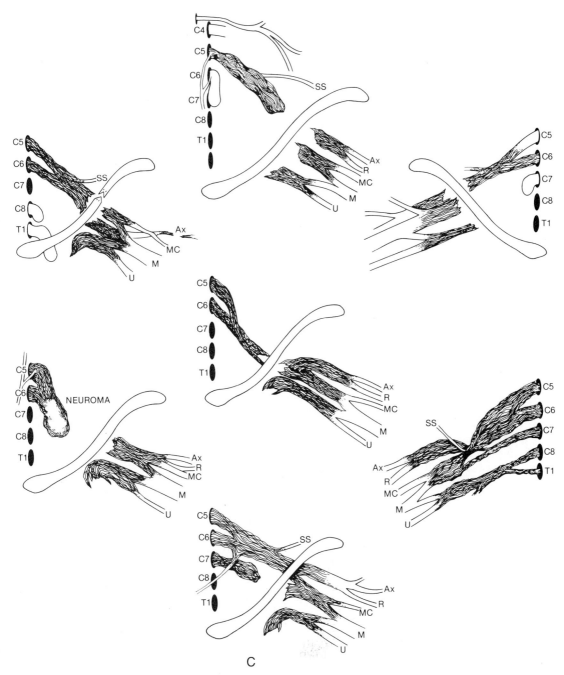

Figure 25–2 *Continued*

When we addressed the major finding of our study, namely the predominant involvement of the C7 spinal nerve and root, we found this to be equally true for patients with fracture-dislocation and for patients without fractures. All these patients (with one exception) had involvement of the C7 nerve (Table 25–7).

Traction Exerted on Different Components of the Brachial Plexus According to Arm Position. In an investigation carried out on a cadaver by one of us (HAM), traction on the spinal nerves in the downward (anatomic) position of the arm (no abduction) was the greatest on the upper spinal nerves, including C7 (Fig. 25–3). When the arm was

Table 25–6. DISTRIBUTION OF PATIENTS WITH "HAND SPARED," "SHOULDER SPARED," OR "GLOBAL PLEXUS" IN DIFFERENT SUBGROUPS

Subgroup	Number of Patients			
	Total	Hand Spared	Shoulder Spared	Global Plexus
No fractures around the shoulder	8	3	2	3
Fractures around the shoulder and vascular lesions	11	5	2	4
Fracture of clavicle	6	2	1	2
Fracture of clavicle and vascular injuries	5	1	2	2
Fracture of clavicle and shoulder dislocation	10	5	1	4
Shoulder dislocation	4	3	0	1
Fracture of humerus	2	1	0	1
Fracture of humerus and dislocation	6	4	0	2
Fracture of forearm and hand	9	4	1	4

abducted to 90°, the traction on nerve C8 increased. When the arm was abducted and elevated to 160°, traction was at its maximum on nerve C8, then T1, and then C7. When the arm was elevated 180° but placed in forward flexion, the clavicle compressed the trunks. These findings were exaggerated by pulling the head to the opposite side. It was noteworthy that whatever the position of the arm when submitted to traction, the C7 spinal nerve was always stretched.

It is unwise to consider the direction of the pull upon the arm without considering other factors. The partial attachment of these nerves or roots to the bones, muscles, joints, capsules, or the dura may segmentally distort the effect of traction in certain directions. Indeed, we observed such partial attachments to the anterior and medial scalene muscles in the cadaver.

Results of Presurgery Testing

Myelograms suggesting the presence or the absence of root avulsion were confirmatory in 21 of 35 patients (60%).

Table 25–7. DISTRIBUTION OF C7 ROOT INVOLVEMENT

	Avulsed	Damaged	Total
Patients without fractures	5	3	8
Patients with fractures and vascular lesions	8	2	10

As stated earlier, *electromyography* was used prior to surgery to predict the localization and the extent of the lesion and following surgery to document the healing process. Five electromyographers were involved in this series of patients. Two methods were used, just as in patients with obstetrical brachial palsy (see Chapter 38).

1. Results of stimulation of distal structures of the plexus at surgery were compared with presurgical EMG findings. In all cases in which the surgeon (JKT) found that an electrically stimulated distal structure of the plexus activated a certain muscle, the electromyographer noted the absence of motor unit potentials preoperatively in only 27% of instances (for the same muscle). However, in all the instances in which the surgeon found "no response" to electrical stimulation, the corresponding percentage of pathologic EMG findings increased to 92%. The correlation was therefore evident.

2. The conclusions of the electromyographer concerning the probable involvement of a particular plexus structure were divided in a number of statements, e.g., "the posterior cord is least involved" or "there is probably avulsion of C7 root." The statistical analysis of these statements showed that they were correct in 80% of instances.

Reconstructive Considerations

Once a brachial plexus injury is diagnosed, the indications for surgery are as follows:

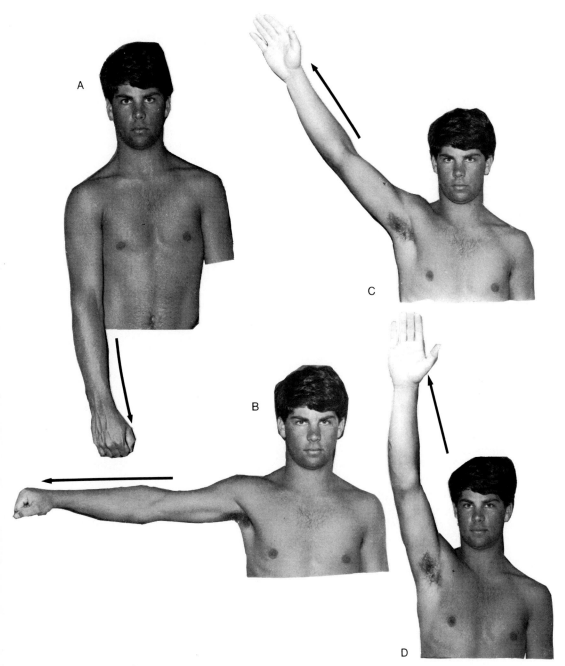

Figure 25–3. Investigated positions of the arm: A, B, and C are positions in the frontal plane of the body. In D, the arm is in forward flexion. The direction of the pull is indicated by the arrows (see text).

1. *Primary Repair*: This is performed in patients with an open wound without major vessel injury, as may occur with penetrating wounds.

2. *Secondary Repair*: This is performed in patients with (a) major vessel injuries, (b) closed plexus injuries, or (c) in whom primary repair was contraindicated.

Secondary repair is usually done between 8 and 12 weeks after the initial surgery, when the diagnosis of first-degree injury (neurapraxia) has been excluded and all appropriate investigations to localize the sites of injury have been completed. The importance of timely repair in peripheral nerve injuries has been emphasized by the findings in our clinic.[14]

Techniques of surgical intervention include:

1. *Neurorrhaphy*. In very exceptional cases, an end-to-end coaptation may be accomplished in patients with sharp, clean, penetrating lacerations of the brachial plexus structures.

2. *Neurolysis*. External neurolysis is used for the first- and second-degree lesions with evidence of external compression.[12] If there is evidence of interfascicular fibrosis, internal neurolysis is performed.

3. *Nerve Grafting*. This technique may be used for both nonvascularized and vascularized grafts.[9]

   a. Nonvascularized grafts. These consist of devascularized cutaneous nerves and are used when there is a good vascular bed or when an epineurectomized trunk graft is used in selective circumstances. Recently, nonvascularized grafts have been replaced by the vascularized nerve grafts.

   b. Vascularized nerve grafts.[3, 4, 13] The benefits of vascularized grafts are that the grafts

      (1) May be used in a scarred bed.

      (2) May be used as a carrier for devascularized grafts, ensuring their revascularization.

      (3) Provide the best milieu for axonal growth.

      (4) Allow trunk grafts such as the ulnar nerve to be transferred in cases of documented C8 and T1 avulsion. Because its normal vascular anatomy is maintained, a vascularized trunk graft is free of ischemia, which prevents structural damage in the endoneurial tube and provides the best environment for growth of the axon.[8]

      (5) Bridge large nerve gaps. Because of the delay of the axon in reaching the distal coaptation, a neuroma may develop at this site, which prevents the axon from bridging the distal coaptation. The delay may be reduced by vascularized nerve grafts, and recent experimental and clinical observations suggest that nerve regeneration by means of vascularized nerve grafts is faster than by conventional grafting techniques.[7, 14] In fact, Terzis has documented axonal growth rates of up to 7 cm/month for vascularized nerve grafts.

4. *Neurotization*. The transfer of a peripheral nerve to neurotize a recipient nerve is well documented by the transfer of the spinal accessory nerve to the denervated suprascapular nerve. This principle is employed for motor and sensory neurotization of the brachial plexus. To achieve a functional reinnervation, it is believed that a number of viable axons comparable to that provided by the parent nerve must be provided. The source of motor and sensory nerves and their axonal counts have been reported[5, 10] (see also Chapters 29 to 32). In this series, the transferred nerves are limited to the spinal accessory nerve and intercostal nerves T3 to T9. The spinal accessory nerve has been used only for transfer to the suprascapular nerve to achieve shoulder stability and abduction of 30°. The intercostal nerve has been used for transfer to the musculocutaneous nerve and the lateral head of the median nerve.

5. *Direct Muscular Neurotization*. This involves the direct placement of a nerve into a muscle to achieve nerve-muscle coaptation and is used primarily in cases of irrevocable injury to the parent nerve.

In this series, the length of the interposition nerve grafts ranged from 5 to 32 cm. Devascularized nerve grafts were used up to a length of 20 cm and vascularized nerve grafts were used up to a length of 32 cm. Vascularized nerve grafts were used in seven patients. In all patients, vascularized nerve grafts were utilized in association with devascularized nerve grafts.

At surgical exploration, evaluation of the plexus is carried out by clinical, electrical, and histologic techniques. Clinically, the structures of a plexus are examined to determine their size, vascular patterns, extent of scarring, and texture. In addition, the intervertebral foramina are palpated to determine if they were occupied or are empty of their contents. The roots and nerves are electrically stimulated with a disposable nerve stimulator with DC current of the magnitude of 0.5, 1 and 2 mA, and respective muscle groups are observed for contraction. This is carried out proximal and distal to the areas of injury of the plexus structures. Electrophysiologic recordings of compound action potentials may be carried out with microsurgical isolation of individual nerve fascicles or groups of nerve fascicles with questionable functional integrity.[15] Histologic assessment by frozen section is used to quantify the axons that are viable and to identify ganglion cells, which confirms a preganglionic avulsion of the mixed spinal root.

These evaluations allow the surgeon to identify structures that are completely or partially avulsed, ruptured, or present as a neuroma in continuity. Nerves that are ruptured will not respond to stimulation distal to the site of injury, whereas lesions in continuity may or may not respond to stimulation. If there is no response, the damaged areas are resected proximally to identify the presence of any viable axons. In the case of lesions in continuity responding to stimulation, resection may be complete if the response to stimulation is poor. Similarly, the proximal stump is studied histologically to identify viable axons. Neurolysis of this portion of the plexus may be indicated when the responses are decreased but still adequate.

In this series, 18 of 19 patients were injured at a supraclavicular level, and the reconstruction involved the donor nerves near the level of the cord. The frequency of use of donor nerves is depicted in Table 25–8. A neurolysis procedure was performed in six patients.

Functional restoration of a plexus injury demands an order of priority. The order followed in this series was as follows: restoration of (1) shoulder stability, (2) elbow flexion, (3) shoulder abduction, (4) hand sensibility, (5) long flexors, (6) long extensors, and (7) external shoulder rotation.

Donor roots and nerves are used to restore derivatives of C5, C6, and C7, the upper and

Table 25–8. FREQUENCY OF USE OF DONOR NERVES

Donor Nerves	Frequency of Use
C5	10 patients
C6	11 patients
C7	2 patients
C8	2 patients
T1	2 patients
Spinal accessory nerve	3 patients
Intercostals	5 patients

middle trunks, and the lateral and posterior cords. Functional recovery of the intrinsic muscles has been universally poor.[1, 6, 12] and at present is not a priority. The desirable minimal goal is to provide an extremity that has a stable shoulder, active elbow flexion, and sensibility of median nerve distribution. This guarantees that the extremity serves as a useful helper to the other extremity. Furthermore, secondary surgery or orthotic devices may be required to restore a hand grip. With this priority in mind, donor nerves that are graded as excellent or good are distributed to muscles with the highest priority. Donor nerves of poorer quality are used for muscles that have low priority or that have poor recovery rates, based on experience, in spite of being reconstructed with adequate donor nerves. These less viable muscles have been the long extensors of the wrist and fingers.

Postsurgical Results

Only 11 of our 19 patients have been followed for more than 18 months. These patients will be discussed here. In no case was the recovery of any patient downgraded and many patients showed improvement. In most patients this improvement was only partial, with the exception of two or three outstanding individual cases. Figures 25–4 to 25–12 show the scatter of individual manual muscle test scores for different muscles (indicated in some figures by their initials) in different subjects, as a function of the time elapsed from surgery.

In all these patients the initial presurgery score was equal to 0. For example Figure 25–4 shows the improvement of the strength of the brachioradialis and extensor carpi ra-

Text continued on page 373

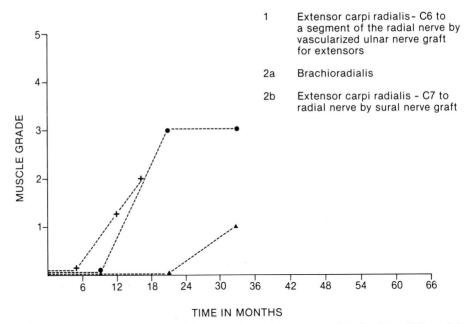

1   Extensor carpi radialis - C6 to
     a segment of the radial nerve by
     vascularized ulnar nerve graft
     for extensors

2a   Brachioradialis

2b   Extensor carpi radialis – C7 to
     radial nerve by sural nerve graft

Figure 25–4. Increase with time after surgery of the manual muscle test score of the brachioradialis and the extensor carpi radialis. Graph 1 represents the recovery in the extensor carpi radialis in a patient in whom C6 was the donor nerve to the segment of the radial nerve for the long extensor. Graphs 2a and 2b represent the recovery of the brachioradialis (2a) and ECR (2b) of patient in whom C7 was the donor nerve to the radial segment of the posterior cord.

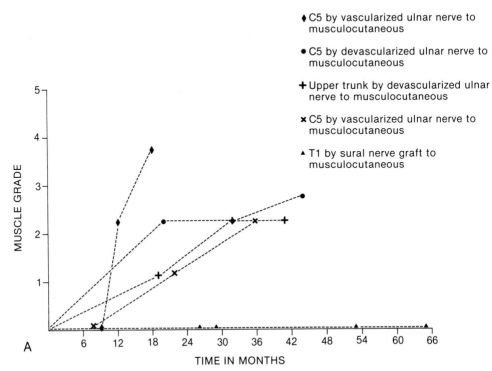

♦ C5 by vascularized ulnar nerve to
  musculocutaneous

● C5 by devascularized ulnar nerve to
  musculocutaneous

✛ Upper trunk by devascularized ulnar
  nerve to musculocutaneous

✗ C5 by vascularized ulnar nerve to
  musculocutaneous

▲ T1 by sural nerve graft to
  musculocutaneous

Figure 25–5. *A,* Increase with time after surgery of the manual muscle test scores of the biceps after grafting of the musculocutaneous nerve to different roots in five patients.

Illustration continued on opposite page

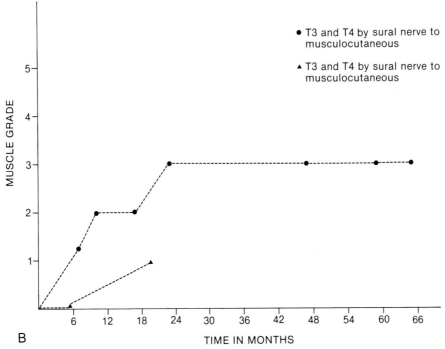

B

Figure 25–5 *Continued. B,* Results with grafting of the intercostal nerves to the musculocutaneous nerve via sural nerves (in two patients).

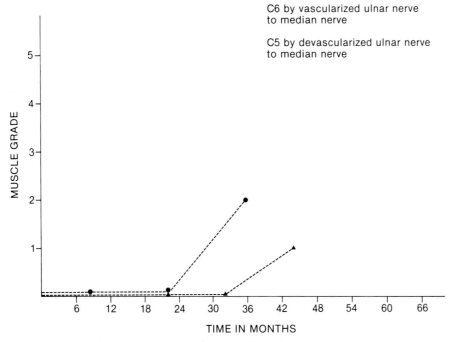

Figure 25–6. Increase with time after surgery of the manual muscle test scores in the flexor of the forearm after grafting to the median nerve of different brachial plexus structures.

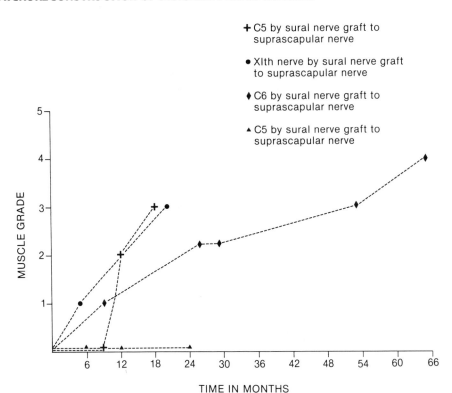

Figure 25–7. Increase with time after surgery of the manual muscle test scores of the supraspinatus after grafting to the suprascapular nerve by spinal accessory nerve, and C5 and C6 roots with interposition sural nerves. Recovery in four patients is shown.

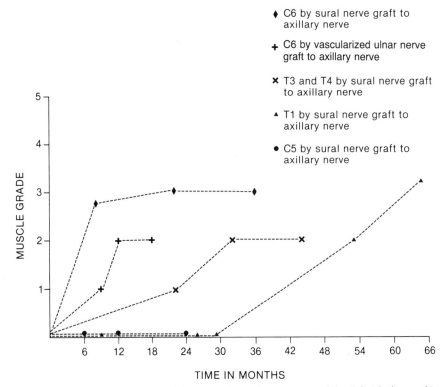

Figure 25–8. Increase with time after surgery of the manual muscle test scores of the deltoid after grafting the axillary nerve by several donor nerves including intercostals.

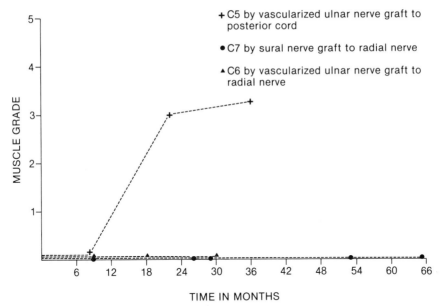

Figure 25–9. Increase with time after surgery of the manual muscle test grades of the triceps after grafting the posterior cord and radial nerve in three patients.

dialis muscles following bridging by the vascularized sural nerve of the stump of the C7 spinal nerve and the posterior cord or the radial nerve. This figure shows the longer delay in improvement of the extensor carpi radialis after grafting the C7 spinal nerve. Figure 25–5A shows the analogous findings for the biceps (grafting the musculocutaneous nerve to either the C5 spinal nerve or

upper trunk or to the T1 spinal nerve). The same nerve was grafted in two instances to the intercostal nerves (Fig. 25–5B). Figure 25–6 shows analogous data related to the long flexors of the hand (note the prolonged "silent period"). Data from grafting of the suprascapular nerve to the spinal accessory, C5 and C6 roots in four patients are provided in Figure 25–7. Figure 25–8 refers to the

Figure 25–10. Improvement of the muscle strength as a function of time elapsed from surgery. In this figure, instances of neurolysis are represented as well as those very few cases in which despite the absence of voluntary action of the muscle the corresponding nerve was not considered in need of any surgical repair. The letters represented on the figure are the initials of the muscles examined in five patients.

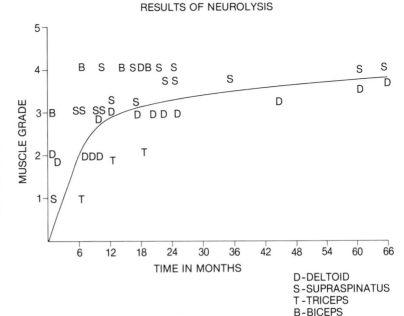

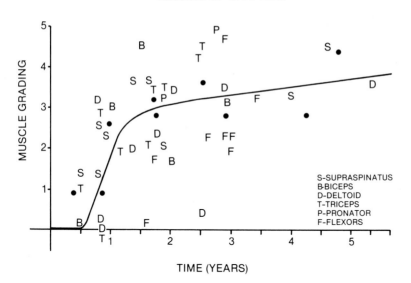

Figure 25–11. The same relationship as in Figure 25–10. However, this figure is related to the results with interposition grafts in seven patients.

grafting of the axillary nerve to C5, C6, T1, and the intercostal nerves (rarely successful). Figure 25–9 shows the effect on the strength of the triceps after grafting the posterior cord or the radial nerve to C5, C6, and C7.

Figures 25–10 and 25–11 represent the combined experience with many patients. These graphs were drawn from (1) cases in which the corresponding nerve structures were neurolysed or considered to be sufficiently uninvolved to be left intact (Fig. 25–10) and (2) cases in which interposition grafts were performed (Fig. 25–11).

In patients with an interposition graft, there was a "silent period" for almost a year when no progress was recorded. Following this silent period, improvement was gradual,

taking place over several years but never reaching the normal score of 5. Patients with neurolysis or no repair experienced practically the same improvement over several years or more. However, the improvement started shortly after surgery without any significant silent period. Figure 25–12 shows the average tracings corresponding to those of Figures 25–10 and 25–11, so that the two types of improvement may be compared.

DISCUSSION

Our approach to management of adult traumatic plexopathies is depicted in the following examples of two patients with supra-

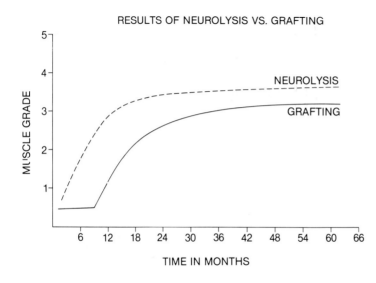

Figure 25–12. The average tracings related to the results with grafting are compared with the tracings related to the instances in which only neurolysis was done. One can see that if the "silent period" is disregarded, both grafts are almost superimposable.

clavicular and one with infraclavicular motorcycle plexopathy.

Case 1

J.A., a 17-year-old white male, had a left-sided motorcycle plexopathy associated with a neuroma in continuity of C5 and C6 at the trunk level proximal to the suprascapular nerve. C7, C8, and T1 were avulsed.

The reconstruction, accomplished 4 months after injury, involved grafting C5 to the suprascapular and lateral pectoral nerves by sural nerves. In addition, the C5 nerve was grafted by a vascularized ulnar nerve to the musculocutaneous nerve, and C6 was grafted by a vascularized ulnar nerve to the axillary and radial nerves and also by a vascularized ulnar nerve to the median nerve. The examination at 18 months revealed the following recovery: deltoid, grade 2; supraspinatus, grade 3; biceps, grade 4 and supinator, grade 3. All other muscles had no recovery at 18 months (Fig. 25–13).

Case 2

S.B., a 23-year-old white male, presented 22 months after injury with a total left-sided plexopathy associated with avulsion of the C5 spinal nerve and extensive injury of other brachial plexus structures.

The reconstruction was as follows: C6 was grafted to the suprascapular nerve, C7 and T1 to the radial nerve, C8 to the median nerve, and T1 to the musculocutaneous and the axillary nerves. Devascularized ulnar and sural nerve grafts were employed. The recovery at 5 years revealed return of motor power in only the supraspinatus, grade 4; and deltoid, grade 3+; there was no recovery distally. There was no return of sensibility (Fig. 25–14).

Case 3

R.F., a 14-year-old white male, presented with an infraclavicular motorcycle plexopathy. The injury was at the level of the lateral, posterior, and medial cords (see Fig. 25–15).

Reconstruction was carried out by interposition sural nerve grafts to the median, musculocutaneous, and axillary nerves. External neurolysis was performed to the posterior cord, radial nerve, and suprascapular nerve. At 8 months after surgery, the neurolyzed nerves had achieved return of motor power in the supraspinatus, deltoid, and triceps to a grade of 4 and by 32 months to a grade 5–. The extensors of the wrist and the fingers had no recovery. In addition the grafted nerves had achieved a return as follows: biceps grade 5– at 32 months. The flexor muscles

achieved a grade of 3 at 32 months. Intrinsic muscle recovery at 32 months was achieved in median and ulnar nerves by a grade of 3.

In order to emphasize that good recovery may result if the donor nerves are of good quality and provide an adequate axon population, the following two cases of plexopathies are presented.

Case 4

A.C., a 28-year-old-black male, suffered a gunshot plexopathy to the left plexus. The injury involved predominantly the upper trunk. Reconstruction was done at 2 weeks by interposition sural nerve grafts, C5 to the suprascapular nerve and posterior cord, and C6 to the musculocutaneous constituents of the lateral cord. The remaining portion of the lateral cord was neurolyzed. Recovery at 28 months revealed the supraspinatus, deltoid, biceps, and pectoralis major muscles achieving a grade of 5– (Fig. 25–16).

Case 5

R.H., a 25-year-old white male, presented with severe blunt trauma caused by a fallen tree associated with a compound fracture of the left clavicle and complete transection of the musculocutaneous and ulnar nerves and a neuroma in continuity of the posterior cord. Reconstruction was by interposition graft of the musculocutaneous and ulnar nerves and neurolysis of the posterior cord. Recovery at 2 years revealed: biceps, grade 5–; flexor digitorum profundus to the ring and little fingers, grade 5–. There was no recovery of the flexor carpi ulnaris or of the ulnar intrinsics. Sensibility to the ulnar nerve distribution recovered to a level of protective sensibility. Posterior cord recovery was limited to only the triceps, grade 5–, and the extensor carpi ulnaris, grade 5– (Fig. 25–17).

Several major findings are emerging from the analysis of this study.

Relative Incidence of the Involvement of Different Roots. The classic subdivision of BPP into Erb's palsy (5th and 6th roots) and Klumpke's palsy (8th and T1 roots) might suggest that C7 is relatively spared. In fact, just as with the obstetrical BPP, the 7th root is the most vulnerable to injury, whereas proportionally the 8th root is the most frequently avulsed. It may well be that some of the extrinsic factors (direction of traction) are common in both situations, although this is difficult to visualize exactly. Our study on the cadaver does show that C7 is involved

Text continued on page 379

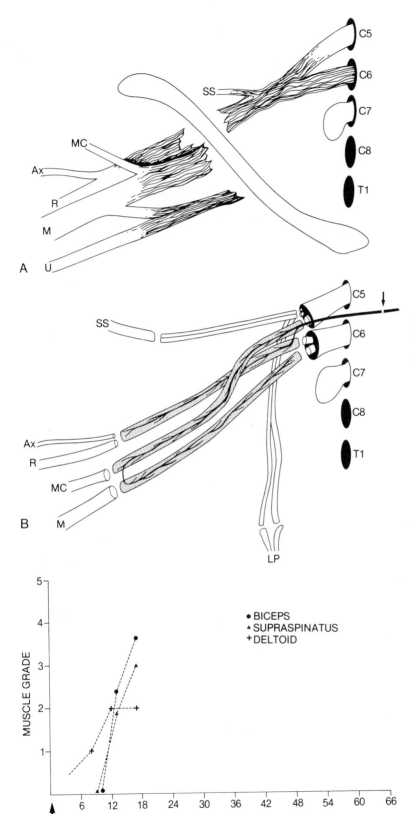

Figure 25–13. *A*, Schematic drawing of rupture of the upper trunk and avulsion of C7, C8, and T1. The sac at C7 depicts the presence of a meningomyelocele. *B*, The repair of the brachial plexus is shown. The suprascapular and lateral pectoral with interposition sural nerve graft. The axillary, radial, musculocutaneous, and median by a vascularized ulnar nerve. Arrow points to microvascular anastomoses. *C*, Recovery over 18 months is graphically shown (by manual muscle test score as a function of time after surgery) for the biceps, supraspinatus, and deltoid.

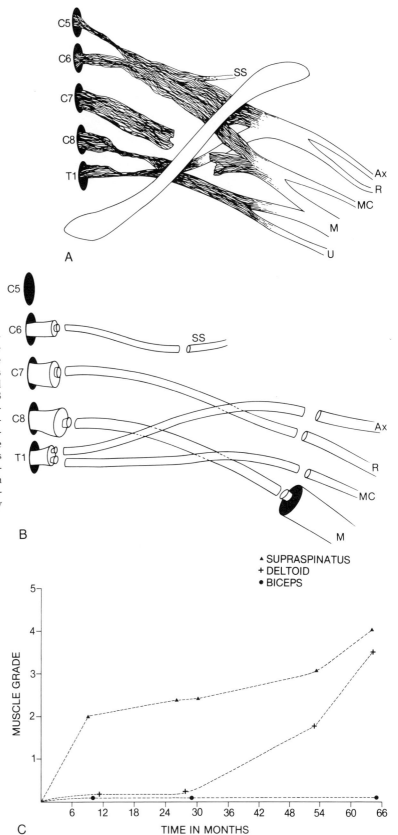

Figure 25–14. *A*, Schematic drawing of avulsion of C5 and rupture of C6, C7, C8, and T1. *B*, The repair of the brachial plexus is shown. C6 by devascularized sural to suprascapular, C7 to radial, C8 to median, and T1 to musculocutaneous. These were all accomplished by interposition devascularized ulnar nerve grafts (see text). *C*, Recovery over 65 months is graphically shown (by the manual muscle test grade as a function of time after surgery) for the supraspinatus and deltoid. No recovery was obtained for the biceps.

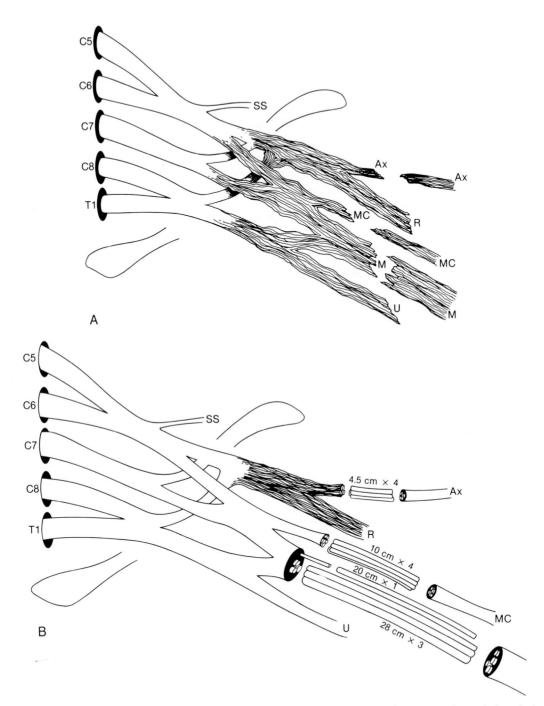

Figure 25–15. *A,* Schematic drawing of an infraclavicular plexus injury. Ruptures of suprascapular, radial, and ulnar nerves. Ruptures of axillary, musculocutaneous, and median nerves. *B,* The repair of the brachial plexus is shown. Neurolysis of suprascapular, posterior cord, and radial nerves was carried out. Sural interposition grafts of axillary, musculocutaneous, and median nerves were done.

Illustration continued on opposite page

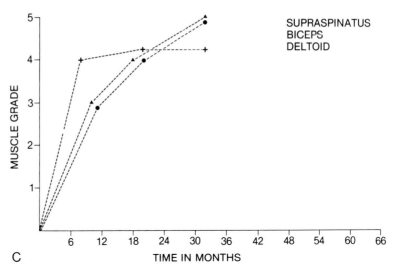

Figure 25–15 *Continued. C,* Recovery over 32 months is graphically shown (by the manual muscle test grade as a function of time after surgery) for the biceps, supraspinatus, and deltoid.

no matter what direction of traction is present. However, the analysis of the common intrinsic factors in both groups is mandatory in order to reach a complete understanding of the findings in both populations of patients.

Obviously, the anatomic relationship of the 5th spinal nerve (high above the clavicle) and the 7th and 8th spinal nerves (nearer the clavicle) may play a critical role in our findings. Also, the adhesions of the roots and of different segments of spinal nerves to the bones, muscles, or dura may be responsible for certain aspects of pathology. We were impressed, however, by the almost complete superimposition of the graph depicting the average number of fascicles found in each spinal root according to Bonnel[2] (Fig. 25–18) and tracings representing the number of severed roots (avulsions and ruptures) of the same spinal nerves or roots in our patient population. Figure 25–18 shows an almost complete correspondence of both tracings. The tracing relating to the number of "good" (intact) roots shows almost a mirror image of the other two.

It is futile to try to explain this relationship. However, it is hardly scientific to consider these findings a coincidence. Quite possibly this represents the "attempt" of nature to prevent injury to the individual roots by compensating those roots that are more exposed to injury by increasing the number of fascicles.

Finally, because of the almost constant involvement of C7, preservation of wrist mobility may be considered to be futile. Therefore, wrists could be fused in most cases, which would liberate a number of axons for other reconstructive aims.

Additional Diagnostic Tests. Because of the importance of the proximal donors and of their physiologic status, additional tests must be developed for evaluation of their condition preoperatively and intraoperatively. One test (described in Chapter 40) seems to be important. This involves the subjective preoperative evaluation by the patient of the digital projections of sensation elicited by the stimulating electrode introduced percutaneously down to the vertebral lamina. Intraoperatively, evoked potential techniques seem to be destined to be of even greater importance than they are now.

Additional Sources for Donors. One must look to the future for other proximal donor sources for interposition grafts, such as those from the noninvolved side. Furthermore, T2 sensory nerves may be grafted to the first and second digital nerves supplying the thumb and index finger for grasp sensitivity.

Electromyography. EMG appears to be helpful not only for prediction of the level and the extent of the lesion, for the follow-up after microsurgical reconstruction, and for evaluation of the muscle prior to secondary surgery but also as a possible source of electrical potentials for myoelectrical orthoses (i.e., electric motors moving a segment of the extremity). The electrogenesis may be insufficient to mobilize the muscle physiologically but adequate to close a switch controlling a

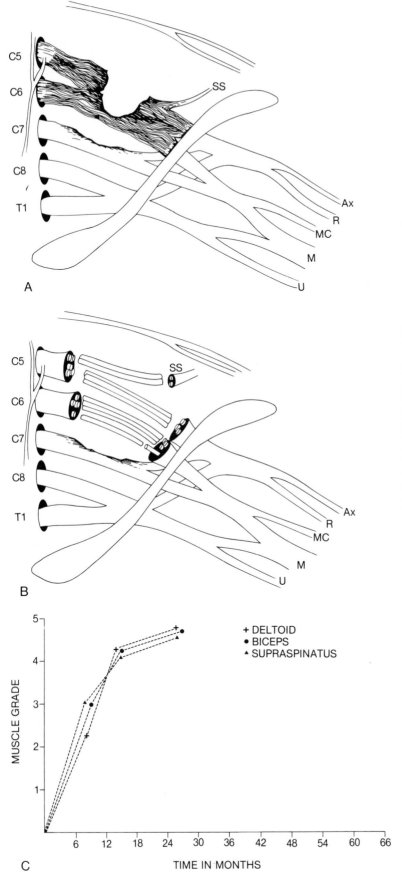

Figure 25–16. *A,* Schematic drawing of a neurotmetic lesion in continuity of the upper plexus proximal to the suprascapular nerve. *B,* Repair of the brachial plexus is shown. The suprascapular nerve and axillary component of posterior cord by interposition sural graft to C5. The upper trunk by segmental repair to area of lateral cord for biceps. The remaining portion of upper trunk was neurolysed. *C,* Recovery over 28 months is graphically shown (by the manual muscle test grade as a function of time after surgery) for the biceps, supraspinatus, and deltoid.

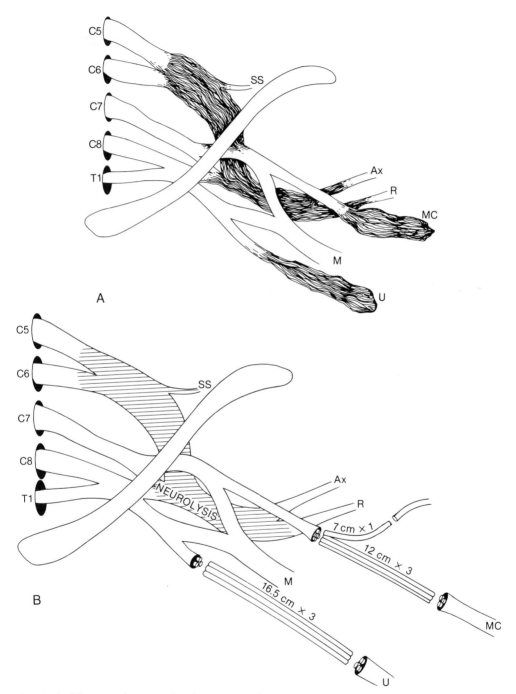

Figure 25–17. *A,* Schematic drawing of end neuromas of musculocutaneous and ulnar nerves. The posterior cord exhibits a severe stretch lesion in continuity. *B,* The repairs of the brachial plexus is shown. The musculocutaneous and ulnar nerves are repaired by interposition sural nerves. Neurolysis of the posterior cord was carried out.

Illustration continued on following page

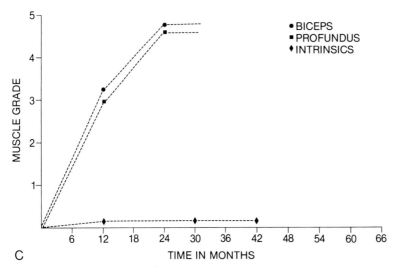

Figure 25–17 *Continued. C,* Recovery over 31 months is graphically shown (by the manual muscle test grade as a function of time after surgery) for the biceps, ulnar profundus, and intrinsics.

motor. Recent attempts at using muscle sounds rather than the muscle potentials should be explored further.

Rehabilitation. Because of the only partial success of microsurgery in most patients, the role of rehabilitation medicine is paramount (see Chapter 38). This is particularly true for the young patients who predominate in our series.

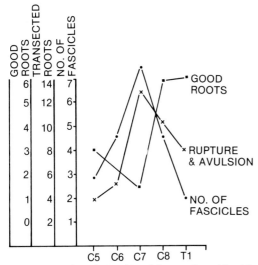

Figure 25–18. The relationship of the number of fascicles found in different roots and the incidence of severed roots observed in this study as a function of the level of emergence of the roots from the cervical cord. Note that the tracing expressing the number of fascicles calculated (on the basis of the Bonnel's study[21]) is almost superimposable on the tracing expressing the number of severed roots found in our study for different cervical levels. The tracing of "good" roots as a function of the level of their emergence from the cervical spine is a mirror image of the two other tracings.

Effects of Fractures and Vascular Lesions. It may be significant that when our population was divided in two groups—(1) 8 patients without additional fractures or vascular lesions and (2) 11 patients with fractures (shoulder, clavicle, etc.) and vascular lesions—the distribution of instances of "hand spared," "shoulder spared," and "global palsy" were different for each group (see Table 25–7). Inasmuch as patients with "hand spared" lesions have the most favorable outcome, the fact that the presence of dislocations and fractures increases the proportion of "hand spared" cases is noteworthy.

Relationship of the Restoration of Muscle Strength to that of the EMG. Despite the fact that needle electromyography expresses the activity of only limited segments of muscle fibers, Fig. 25–19 shows that there is a close relationship between the results of the EMG and the manual muscle scores. For this purpose the EMG was quantified as follows:

0: No voluntarily induced potentials.

1: Some motor units under voluntary control.

2: Incomplete interference pattern.

3: Full interference pattern (the maximal score).

As seen from Figure 25–19, the manual muscle score increases with the increase of the EMG score. However, although the latter score reaches its maximum, the manual muscle test score does not. Figure 25–20 shows the analogous relationship between these two physiologic measurements when only the final score is considered. Again, although the EMG shows the maximal score in certain patients, the maximal muscle test score is

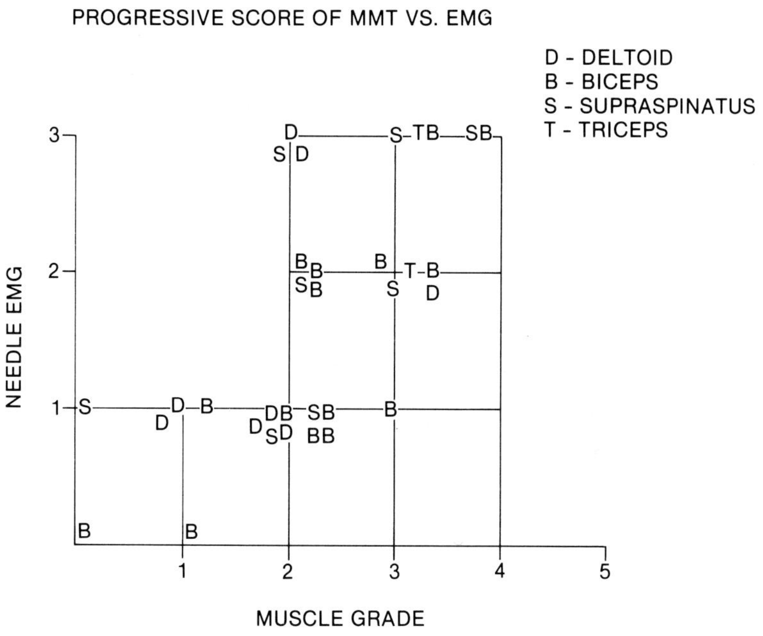

PROGRESSIVE SCORE OF MMT VS. EMG
D - DELTOID
B - BICEPS
S - SUPRASPINATUS
T - TRICEPS
NEEDLE EMG
MUSCLE GRADE

Figure 25–19. Relationship between the EMG score and those of the manual muscle test (MMT) score. The latter are those of the classic manual muscle test (0–5, five being the normal score). The EMG scores are as follows: 0: no voluntary potentials; 1: only few motor unit potentials under voluntary control; 2: incomplete interference pattern; 3: complete interference pattern. Note the relationship between these two measurements (composed on the basis of seven patients' follow-up).

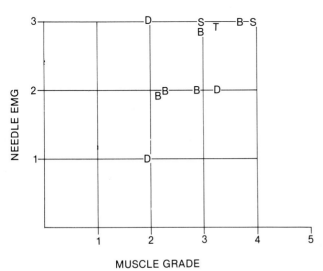

FINAL SCORE FOR EMG AND MMT
D - DELTOID
B - BICEPS
S - SUPRASPINATUS
T - TRICEPS
NEEDLE EMG
MUSCLE GRADE

Figure 25–20. Same relations as in Figure 25–19 and the same number of patients. However, only final scores are represented on the graph. Note that while EMG scores reach the maximum, the MMT scores lag behind them.

achieved rarely. The EMG reflects neural restoration, whereas the manual muscle test score also depicts deficits such as the deterioration of the tendon gliding mechanism, joint stiffness, etc. (for further discussion, see Chapter 40).

Intractable Pain. Intractable pain is experienced by some patients prior to surgery but is no longer a dominant problem after surgery.

CONCLUSIONS

1. *No patient's condition was downgraded* by microsurgery, and some improvement was found in the majority of patients.

2. *EMG and even myelography* have only a partial predictive value for the presence of root avulsions. Complementary tests are therefore desirable, e.g., vertebral "electrical Tinel" sign prior to surgery and evoked potentials during surgery (see Chapter 40).

3. *C7 is the most frequently involved root* and C8 the most frequently avulsed. The relationship of these findings to extrinsic factors (direction of pull) as well as to intrinsic factors (projecting the clavicle over the plexus, different number of fascicles in different roots) and to adherence to bones, muscles, joints, and dura was discussed earlier. Involvement of the C7 root and spinal nerve (see Table 25–8) may influence the attitude of the surgeon in relation to the fusion of the wrist.

4. *The increased proportion of "hand spared" cases* in patients with shoulder fractures, and particularly with dislocations, is noteworthy.

5. *Follow-up of muscle strength testing* reveals the presence of a prolonged "silent period" for patients with grafted nerve structures. Following this silent period, the improvement is comparable to that found in patients with neurolysis. Figure 25–12 shows that if one shifts the tracing of averages in the case of grafting to the left (so that the "silent period" remains at the left from the origin of coordinates), both tracings are almost superimposable initially. Later on, those tracings corresponding to nerve grafts do not show final scores as high as those in the case of neurolysis. Obviously, the initial damage in the latter case was not as devastating as in the former. Three years and occasionally more are required in order to reach the final score.

The delayed and less complete recovery of patients with grafts underscores the importance of rehabilitation procedures in these cases (see Chapter 10). Moreover, it is noteworthy to mention that a persistent intractable pain syndrome was extremely rarely seen in our patients after surgery.

References

1. Alnot, J. Y.: Infraclavicular lesions. Clin. Plast. Surg., *11*:121, 1984.
2. Bonnel, F.: Microscopic anatomy of the adult human brachial plexus: an anatomical and histological basis for microsurgery. Microsurgery, *5*:107, 1984.
3. Bonney, G., Birch, R., Jamieson, A. M., and Eames, R. A.: Experience with vascularized nerve grafts. Clin. Plast. Surg., *11*:137, 1984.
4. Breidenbach, W., and Terzis, J. K.: The anatomy of free vascularized nerve grafts. Clin. Plast. Surg., *11*:65, 1984.
5. Brunelli, G., and Monini, L.: Neurotization of avulsed roots of brachial plexus by means of anterior nerves of cervical plexus. Clin. Plast. Surg., *11*:149, 1984.
6. Kline, D. S., and Judice, D. J.: Operative management of selected brachial plexus lesions. J. Neurosurg., *58*:631, 1983.
7. Koshima, I., and Harii, K.: Experimental study on vascularized nerve grafts: morphometric and biochemical analysis of axonal regeneration of nerves transplanted into scar. Paper presented at the 7th Symposium on Microsurgery, New York, June 19–23, 1983.
8. Lundborg, G.: Structure and function of the intraneural microvessels as related to trauma neuroma formation and nerve function. J. Bone Joint Surg., *57A*:938, 1975.
9. Millesi, H.: Nerve grafting. Clin. Plast. Surg., *11*:105, 1984.
10. Narakas, A. O.: Thoughts on neurotization or nerve transfer in irreparable nerve lesion. Clin. Plast. Surg., *11*:153, 1984.
11. Sedel, L.: The management of supraclavicular lesions. Clin. Plast. Surg., *11*:121, 1984.
12. Sunderland, S.: A classification of peripheral nerve injuries producing loss of function. Brain, *74*:491, 1951.
13. Taylor, I. E., and Ham, F. J.: The free vascularized nerve graft. Plast. and Reconstr. Surg., *57*:413, 1976.
14. Terzis, J. K.: Personal communication.
15. Terzis, J. K., Dykes, R. W., and Hakstian, R. W.: Electrophysiological recordings in peripheral nerve surgery. A Review. J. Hand Surg., *1*:52, 1976.

26

The Management of Supraclavicular Lesions: Clinical Examination, Surgical Procedures, Results

■

Laurent Sedel, M.D.

In many circumstances, brachial plexus palsy occurs as a limited lesion of the upper roots or trunks when the hand has almost returned to normal. Duchenne described this condition many years ago, which is now known as Duchenne's palsy. Sometimes the clinical features are somewhat different, as the hand is more severely paralyzed. These cases are very interesting because corrective surgery occasionally gives a very good result, with complete recovery of the upper limb. These results are far better than those obtained after classic palliative procedures.

We shall present our experience in 44 patients with upper trunk lesions from a group of 170 patients who had brachial plexus operations. These 44 patients had a normal hand or at least some muscle activity at this level. These types of palsy present three major questions: Which palsies will recover spontaneously? How does the surgeon determine the type of lesion, its site, and its severity before surgery? How does the surgeon decide between neurolysis and grafting? We will try to answer these questions.

Of the 44 patients with partial palsies in whom surgical exploration showed a supraclavicular lesion, only 28 were followed for more than 2 years. Therefore, results can be evaluated in only those 28 patients, and these cases will be presented in detail.

Four patients were female and 24 were male. Their ages ranged from 15 to 59 years with a mean of 23 years. Table 26–1 shows the etiology of the injuries and Table 26–2 lists the associated lesions.

It is interesting to note that none of the patients had a vascular lesion, a condition that is very frequent in patients with infraclavicular lesions. Therefore, a partial brachial plexus palsy with an arterial main trunk lesion usually indicates an infraclavicular rather than a supraclavicular lesion.

PREOPERATIVE FINDINGS

Neurologic Status. Some of the post-traumatic lesions were partial at the time of injury; others were complete initially but later recovered at the forearm and hand level. Eleven patients initially presented with complete paralysis but showed some signs of recovery at the hand level within a few days or at less than 3 weeks. Twelve patients presented with an initial partial palsy. With time, their muscle strength increased, but they showed no recovery in the areas initially affected. Four patients had lesions due to direct trauma or tumor; the initial status is unknown for one patient.

Table 26–3 shows the neurologic status at time of operation.

Table 26–1. ETIOLOGY OF
SUPRACLAVICULAR INJURIES

Injury	No. of Patients
Motorcycle accident	20
Automobile accident	2
Direct trauma	3
Wound	2
Tumor	1

Pain. Nine patients had mild pain (graded 1), two had severe pain (graded 2), one had very severe pain (graded 3), and sixteen had no pain.

Type and Site of Lesion. Predicting the exact type and site of the lesion is the most difficult aspect of managing these palsies. The surgical procedure will usually solve this problem, but to perform a good repair it is important to know as much as possible about the exact extent of the lesion.

The clinical examination must be carried out very precisely. The motor and sensory findings are recorded diagrammatically. If the supraspinatus is spared, this is of great value in predicting a nonavulsed C5. Knowledge of the exact trauma incurred can also be of great importance in predicting the site of the lesion.

The site and intensity of Tinel's sign must be very carefully noted. If it is found easily, this usually implies a proximal neuroma and therefore a good operative prognosis. Sometimes it may be possible to palpate these neuromas.

The electrodiagnostic examination may include conduction velocity studies; electromyography to record spontaneous potentials with and without stimulation (the cervical paravertebral and the supraspinatus muscles are particularly important); and evoked potentials,[2, 8, 15] the presence of which is a sign of the absence of a preganglionic avulsion, as is the F wave recording.[3]

Table 26–3. NEUROLOGIC STATUS AT TIME
OF OPERATION FOR SUPRACLAVICULAR
LESIONS

Type of Involvement	No. of Patients
Erb's palsy	8
C5, C6, C7 (three of these patients had a weak hand)	12
C5, C6, C7, C8	2
C7, C8	2
Other	2

Cervical myelography is required for every patient in whom surgery is contemplated. However, it is not required for those with a tumor or a penetrating lesion. At the beginning of our experience, we did not request a myelogram for all patients with partial palsies. In retrospect, we think that not obtaining a myelogram was a mistake that can possibly explain some paradoxical poor results.

The usual techniques are employed, i.e., lumbar puncture and tilting of the patient. The contrast dye used has been Lipiodol emulsion or, more recently, Amipaque. Plain films and tomograms are taken and the abnormal side is compared with the normal side. The irregularities of the roots at their origin or the meningeal pouches must be well defined. Myelography facilitates accurate prognosis. It also helps the surgeon because the presence of a meningeal pouch means that the corresponding root need not be explored. Of our 28 patients, 13 underwent cervical myelography and 15 did not. Of the 15 patients who did not undergo myelography, in retrospect, 12 should have had this study performed and only 3 did not require it.

One myelogram showed no abnormality, three were difficult to interpret because of poor quality, and nine showed abnormalities, i.e., meningeal pouches or root irregularities (Table 26–4). We must emphasize that some

Table 26–2. LESIONS ASSOCIATED WITH
SUPRACLAVICULAR LESIONS

Lesion	No. of Patients
Isolated palsy without fracture or luxation	17
Fracture of the clavicle	6
Fracture of the humerus	2
Fractures of the scapula and forearm	1
Fracture of the cervical spine	1
Fractures of the clavicle, scapula, and forearm	1

Table 26–4. MENINGEAL POUCHES OR ROOT
IRREGULARITIES FOUND ON CERVICAL
MYELOGRAPHY

Level	No. of Patients
C7	1
C7, C8	2
C5, C6, C7, C8	1
C6, C7, C8, T1	1
C6, C7	2
C8, T1	1
C8	1

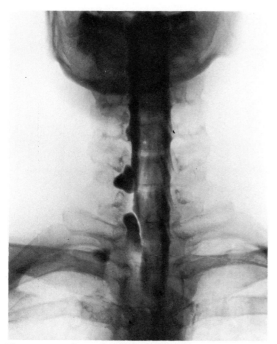

Figure 26–1. Case 15 (see text and Table 26–5). Myelogram of a patient who had many muscles active at hand level (flexor digitorum profundus, flexor carpi, extensor digiti communis). (From Sedel, L.: Clin. Plast. Surg., *11*:124, 1984.)

of these pouches at the C8–T1 level were seen in patients with normal hand function. Therefore, we must conclude that inferior pouches are not always evidence of avulsion (Fig. 26–1).

SURGICAL PROCEDURES

All operations were performed between 3 weeks and 16 months after injury. The indications for surgery in patients with traumatic closed lesions were that the palsy remained complete in one region or unchanged for many months. We now realized that delay for many months is undesirable and currently propose earlier exploration if no clinical or electrical recovery has occurred in one region after 2 months.

The operation was performed under general anesthesia. Neuromuscular blocking agents such as curare, which would prevent a stimulated muscle from contracting, were avoided.

The incision, which is made above the clavicle, is L-shaped, with one limb parallel to the sternocleidomastoid muscle and one parallel to the clavicle. The skin flap is carefully raised and the lateral jugular vein is ligated. The sternocleidomastoid is retracted, and dissection is continued into the prescalenic area, where lymph nodes and fat are removed. The phrenic nerve is identified on the surface of the scalenus anterior muscle and followed upward until it crosses the lateral aspect of that muscle. Precisely behind this point is the C5 root. C6 is lower and more medial and its direction is less vertical. C7 is more horizontal, more posterior, and more medial. It is not necessary to look for C8 and T1, as they are usually intact in these cases.

Sometimes the incision must be continued at the infraclavicular region to find the distal part of the musculocutaneous or the radial nerve. In some instances, it is necessary to divide the clavicle for better exposure.

Lesion Appraisal and Classification. Determining the type of lesion is sometimes very difficult and is based on palpation of the plexus, electrical stimulation, and careful dissection of the nerves after opening the epineurium under microscopic visualization. The clinical history, neurologic status, and operative findings must be taken into account to classify the lesion.

Three different situations are encountered: (1) Clear evidence of traction injury, leaving a gap and either large neuromas or no root proximal to the gap. This is a type 3 lesion according to our classification.[16] (2) A lesion in continuity, in which electrical stimulation is positive and only one muscle contracts. This is a type 4 lesion. (3) A lesion in which the nerves appear to be severely damaged but seem to be in continuity. Electrical stimulation is negative, and the roots seem intact but proximally become thinner and thinner. For the second situation, neurolysis gives generally poor results, and resection and grafting are preferable. The third situation corresponds to root avulsion, which could have been seen on the myelogram but this was not always done. These types of lesion explain the sometimes poor results of isolated neurolysis.

Reparative Procedures. Details of the techniques are described elsewhere. We used neurolysis in 10 cases, suture in 1, nerve grafting in 14, and nerve transfer in 2. Microsurgical techniques were used for major repair (nerve grafting, suture, and nerve transfer) and sometimes for neurolysis.

Assessment after operation was based upon the clinical examination, the usefulness

Table 26–5. RESULTS OF MAJOR REPAIRS IN PATIENTS WITH SUPRACLAVICULAR OR UPPER TRUNK LESIONS*

Case No.	Age	Initial Lesion	Lesion Type	Delay (months)	Lesion Site	Grafted Nerve	Donor Nerve	Graft	Graft Length (cm)	Results		Follow-up (years)	Grade	Comments
1	23	Partial	Stretching	6	C5, C6	Upper trunk	C5, C6	++ / +++	5 / 5	Biceps / Deltoid / Br. rad.	4+ / 4 / 1	3½	2 (rotator cuff palsy)	Humerus derotation refused
2	43	Complete	Stretching	5	C5, C6	Upper trunk	C5, C6	++ / ++	5 / 5	Deltoid / Biceps / Br. rad.	5 / 3+ / 0	4	2 (rotator cuff palsy)	Humerus derotation proposed
3	24	Partial	Crush and wound	16	C5–C6 partial C7 partial	TSAE TSP	C6, C5	++ / +++	7 / 8	No recovery		4	3	Latissimus dorsi transfer
4	49	Partial	Tumor excision	2	Post. division of upper trunk	Suture				No recovery		4	3	Shoulder arthrodesis refused
5	41	Partial	Section	2	C7, C8	C7, C8	C7, C8	+++++ / +++++	2 / 2	Nearly complete recovery		4	1	
6	25	Partial	Stretching, vascular lesion	12	C5, C6, C7	Post. cord neurolysis C5, C6	C7	+++++	6	Biceps / Triceps	4+ / 4+	5	2	Shoulder arthrodesis palliative transfer for radial palsy
7	29	Partial	Stretching	8	Upper trunk, C7 avulsed	Upper trunk	C5, C6	++ / +	6 / 6	Biceps / Deltoid	4+ / 3	4	2	Shoulder arthrodesis refused
8	23	Complete	Stretching	6	C5, C6 avulsed	Upper trunk	C5	+++	5	Biceps / Deltoid	4+ / 3	2	2	
9	23	Partial	Stretching	3	C5 neuroma, C6, C7 avulsed	MC	C5	++++	10	Biceps	4+	4	2	Shoulder arthrodesis refused

No.	Age	Type	Cause	Lesion		Level	Roots			Muscles				Result
10	20	Complete	Stretching	C5 avulsed, C7 avulsed, C6 neuroma	8	Upper trunk	C6	++++	6	Biceps / Deltoid / Ext. carp.	4+ / 4 / 4	3	2	Shoulder arthrodesis
11	23	Complete	Stretching	C5 post. cord	3	Post. cord	C5	+++	8	Triceps / Br. rad. / Ext. carp. / Biceps	4 / 1 / 1 / 4	3	2	Transfer for radial palsy
12	20	Complete	Stretching	Upper trunk rupt. C7 fibrotic (neurolysis)	3	Upper trunk	C4, C5, C6	++ / ++ / +++	6 / 6 / 6 / 5	Biceps / Deltoid / Ext. carp. / Br. rad.	4+ / 4 / 4 / 3	4	2	
13	15	Complete	Stretching	C5–C6 strongly damaged	3	C5	C4	+++++++ / ++	5	Biceps / Triceps / Deltoid	3 / 3 / 0	4	3	
14	16	Partial (flexor digiti intact)	Stretching	C5, C6 rupture, C7 avulsed	5	MC	C5, C6	+++ / +++	10 / 13	Biceps / Triceps / Ext. carp.	2 / 4+ / 0	6	2	Shoulder arthrodesis triceps transfer on biceps tendon transfer for radial palsy
15	20	Complete	Stretching	C5 rupture, C6 fibrotic, C7 avulsed	13	TSAE neurolysis	C5	+++	11	Deltoid / Biceps	4 / 4+	3	3 (the hand is very weak)	
16	46	Complete	Stretching	C5, C6, C7 avulsed	9	MC	T2, T3, T4	+++	6	Biceps	1	4	3	Wrist arthrodesis
17	36	Partial	Crush injury	C5, C6, C7 avulsed	10	MC	T3, T4, T5	+ / ++	8	Triceps / Biceps	4 / 0	5	3	Weak hand

TSAE = lateral cord, TSP = posterior cord, Br. rad. = brachioradialis, Ext. carp. = extensor carpi.
*From Sedel, L.: Clin. Plast. Surg., 11:122, 1984.

of the arm, and the patient's occupation. We distinguished three grades:

1. Manual work can be performed with normal strength.

2. Manual work can be performed with limited strength.

3. Manual work cannot be performed. The limb can be used for daily activities such as cutting meat or tying shoe laces.

The results of nerve graft, suture, and neurolysis or transfer will be analyzed separately.

Analysis of the 17 Major Repairs (Table 26–5; Figs. 26–2 and 26–3). Eight patients initially had complete palsy but recovered some hand function spontaneously before operation. Usually, function of the hand is good; if it is weak, the results are less beneficial. The overall function is graded 1 for the patient who had a section of C7 and C8. She regained almost complete use of her hand after grafting.

Ten patients had very good recovery, graded 2. They had a nearly normal hand and good elbow function following the repair. Three of them also attained good shoul-

der function. Four had shoulder arthrodesis or transfer for radial palsy; they sometimes regained good elbow function after tendon transfer (Case 14).

Six patients had a poor result, graded 3. Two of them (Cases 16 and 17) had an intercostal nerve transfer, which was successful in one patient but the muscle strength was insufficient. One patient had a graft 16 months after injury (Case 3). One patient had only a damaged stump of C5 to be used as the proximal donor site (Case 13). Another patient (Case 14) had a suture after tumor excision, which may be the wrong procedure. The latest patient (Case 15) regained a very weak hand function. He is therefore also graded 3 despite the fact that he regained good deltoid and biceps function.

Analysis of the 11 Neurolysis or Exploration Procedures (Fig. 26–4). The overall results were two patients, grade 1; 7 patients, grade 2; and two patients, grade 3.

The grade 1 results correspond to special lesions: one tumor excision of C7 (Case 28) and one limited neurolysis of C5 (Case 25). The grade 2 results correspond to limited

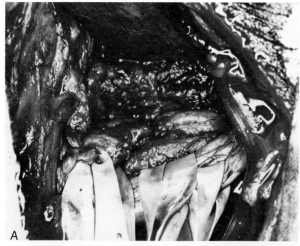
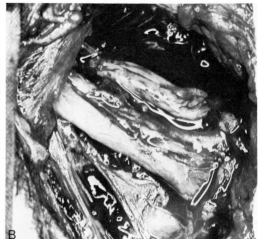
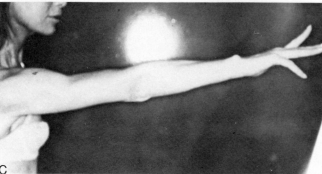

Figure 26–2. Case 5 (see text and Table 26–5). *A*, Section of C7 and C8. Intraoperative view at 2 months after injury. *B*, Repair with eight grafts. *C*, Nearly complete recovery at 4 years.

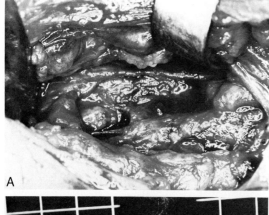

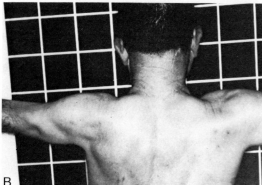

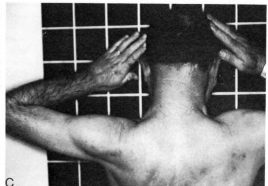

Figure 26–3. Case 2 (see text and Table 26–5). *A*, Operative view of C5 and C6 after dissection of the extremities. *B* and *C*, Very good recovery after 4 years.

recovery with persisting palsy either in the deltoid muscle (Cases 21, 24, 26), the rotator cuff (Cases 18, 19), the triceps (Case 20), or the biceps (Case 22). In fact, two of these patients (Cases 11 and 22) had no recovery compared with the preoperative state. The two patients with grade 3 results had no recovery at all. Therefore, 4 of 11 patients had no recovery. We think that their lesions could correspond to avulsion lesions that were not diagnosed during the surgical pro-

cedure. A myelogram would have detected this but was not done.

In conclusion, we think that the best results after neurolysis alone are those obtained when a limited lesion is found. If another type of lesion is present, the results are less satisfactory. We also conclude that a myelogram is beneficial even in patients with limited palsy.

CONCLUSION

This review of 28 patients with upper trunk lesions and some preservation of hand function led to the following conclusions:

1. The importance of performing a myelogram even when some clinical features indicate a limited lesion.

2. The good prognosis following upper trunk grafting done within 12 months of injury and when two roots are available. When only one root is available, the results are still good but recovery is limited and a palliative procedure is usually needed.

3. The absence of any aggravation of injury postoperatively.

4. The overall conclusion that operative

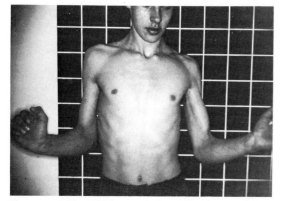

Figure 26–4. Case 25 (see text). Recovery after neurolysis of C5. Recovery of the rotator cuff, the deltoid, and the median radials, which were totally paralyzed.

exploration and repair in patients with upper trunk lesions are strongly recommended.

References

1. Alnot, J. Y., Jolly, A., and Frot, B.: Traitement direct des lésions nerveuses dans les paralysies traumatiques du plexus brachial chez l'adulte. A propos d'une série de 100 cas opérés. Int. Orthop. SICOT, 5:151–168, 1981.
2. Bonney, G.: Prognosis in traction lesions of the brachial plexus. J. Bone Joint Surg., *41B*:4–35, 1959.
3. Deboichet-Perez de Lasota, A.: Etude électromyographique des paralysies traumatiques du plexus brachial humain. Thèse, Paris, 1980.
4. Frot, B.: La myélographie cervicale opaque dans les paralysies traumatiques du plexus brachial. Rev. Chir. Orthop., *63*:67–72, 1977.
5. Harris, W. R., Rathbun, J. B., Wortzman, G., and Humphrey, J. G.: Avulsion of lumbar roots complicating fracture of the pelvis. J. Bone Joint Surg., *55A*:1436–1442, 1973.
6. Jolly, A.: Traitement chirurgical direct des lésions par élongation du plexus brachial chez l'adulte (100 cas opérés). Thèse, Paris, 1980.
7. Kotani, T., Matsuda, H., and Suzuki, T.: Trial surgical procedures of nerve transfer to avulsion injuries of brachial plexus. *In* Proceedings of the 12th Congress of the International Society of Orthopaedic Surgery and Traumatology, Tel Aviv, 1972, p. 348.
8. Landi, A., Copeland, S. A., Wynn-Parry, C. B., and Jones, S. J.: The role of somatosensory evoked potentials and nerve conduction studies in the surgical management of brachial plexus injuries. J. Bone Joint Surg., *62B*:492–496, 1980.
9. Leffert, R. D., and Seddon, H. J.: Infraclavicular brachial plexus injuries. J. Bone Joint Surg., *47B*:9–22, 1965.
10. Lejars, F.: Lésions traumatiques des nerfs. *In* Traité de Chirurgie d'Urgence, 4th Ed. Paris, Masson et Cie, 1904.
11. Lusskin, R., Campbell, J. B., and Thompson, W. A. L.: Post-traumatic lesions of the brachial plexus: treatment by transclavicular exploration and neurolysis or autograft reconstruction. J. Bone Joint Surg., *55A*:1159–1176, 1973.
12. Merle d'Aubigné, R., and Deburge, A.: Etiologie, évolution et pronostic des paralysies traumatiques du plexus brachial. Rev. Chir. Orthop., *53*:23–42, 1967.
13. Millesi, H.: Indications et résultats des interventions directes. Rev. Chir. Orthop., *63*:82–87, 1977.
14. Narakas, A.: Surgical treatment of traction injuries of the brachial plexus. Clin. Orthop., *133*:71–90, 1978.
15. Seddon, H. J.: Surgical Disorders of the Peripheral Nerves, 2nd Ed. Edinburgh, Churchill Livingstone, 1975.
16. Sedel, L.: Traitement palliatif d'une série de 103 paralysies par élongation du plexus brachial. Rev. Chir. Orthop., *63*:651–666, 1977.
17. Sedel, L.: The results of surgical repair of brachial plexus injuries. J. Bone Joint Surg., *64B*:54–66, 1982.
18. Tavernier, B.: Discussion: paralysie radiculaire totale du plexus brachial. Lyon Chir., *29*:90–92, 1932.

27

Infraclavicular Lesions
■
J. Y. Alnot, M.D.

Based on anatomicopathologic findings, traumatic brachial plexus lesions can be classified as either infraclavicular or supraclavicular.

In our study of 420 patients undergoing surgery, 105 (25%) had infraclavicular lesions, with lesions of the cords or terminal branches of the plexus (Figs. 27–1 to 27–3), whereas 315 (75%) had supraclavicular lesions, of which 15% were double level.

ETIOLOGY

The causes of infraclavicular lesions are diverse and include:

1. Anteromedial shoulder dislocation, which caused most of the isolated lesions of the axillary nerve and of the posterior cord.

2. Violent downward and backward movement of the shoulder, which caused stretching of the plexus.

3. Complex trauma with multiple fractures of the clavicle, the scapula, or the upper humerus, which caused more diffuse lesions of the cords and terminal branches, often accompanied by vascular damage.

4. Knife or gunshot wounds.

As previously mentioned, 15% of the supraclavicular lesions in our study were double level. These lesions occur when the arm is forced violently into abduction and the middle part of the plexus is blocked temporarily in the coracoid region. Terminal branches are thus torn away, and supraclavicular lesions occur when the head is concomitantly jerked violently to the opposite side.

Supraclavicular lesions may therefore be associated with infraclavicular lesions affecting the cords or more distal sites, e.g., the musculocutaneous nerve, which is tightly attached at its entry into the coracobrachialis; the axillary nerve in the quadrangular space; or the suprascapular nerve in the coracoid notch.

The relative frequency of these double level lesions justifies a thorough exploration of the plexus at the time of surgery. However, in this chapter we are principally concerned with *post-traumatic infraclavicular lesions*, as these hold the greatest possibility for repair.

CLINICAL DESCRIPTION AND DIAGNOSIS

Several clinical pictures can be observed.

Posterior Cord Injury

Motor deficit findings are typical. Active abduction and external rotation of the shoulder are still possible in a limited way in cases of posterior cord lesions because the supra- and infraspinatus muscles, which are innervated by the suprascapular nerve, are unaffected, whereas the deltoid and teres minor muscles, which are innervated by the axillary nerve, are paralyzed. Active internal rotation may also be limited if the lesion is proximal, preceding the origin of nerves that innervate the teres major and latissimus dorsi muscles.

Findings are less characteristic for the sensory deficit. There may be anesthesia or

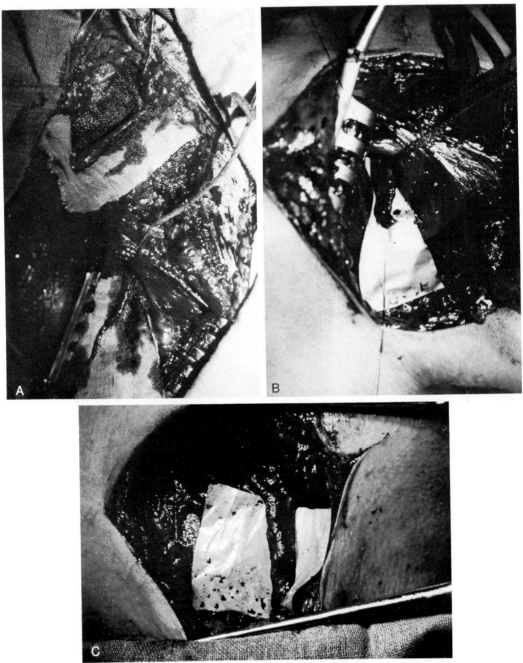

Figure 27–1. *A*, Two associated injuries: suprascapular nerve and axillary nerve. *B* and *C*, Isolated injuries of the axillary nerve: *B*, Nerve rupture in the axillary area just under the pectoralis minor muscle. *C*, A posterior approach must be used to find the distal end of the nerve, which is transected in the quadrangular space.

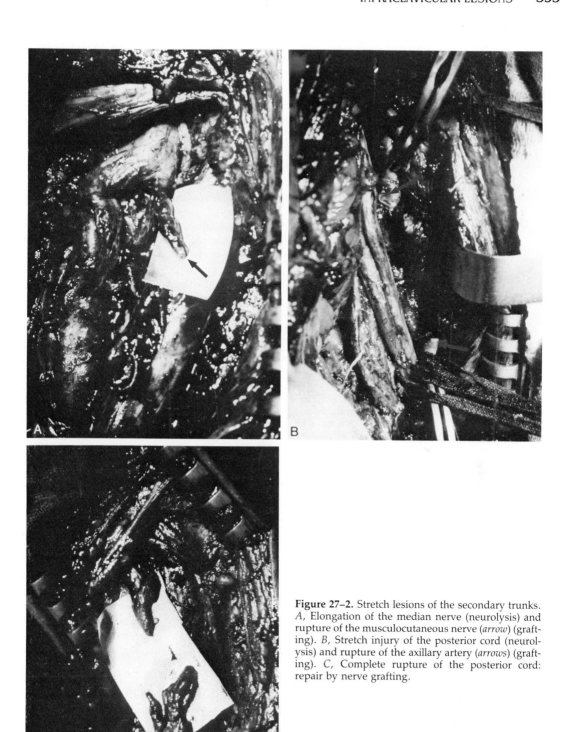

Figure 27–2. Stretch lesions of the secondary trunks. *A*, Elongation of the median nerve (neurolysis) and rupture of the musculocutaneous nerve (*arrow*) (grafting). *B*, Stretch injury of the posterior cord (neurolysis) and rupture of the axillary artery (*arrows*) (grafting). *C*, Complete rupture of the posterior cord: repair by nerve grafting.

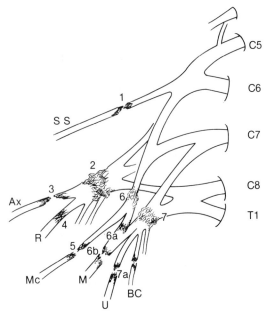

Figure 27–3. The different anatomic-pathologic infraclavicular plexus injuries. 1 = rupture of the suprascapular nerve; 2 = rupture of the posterior cord above and below the origin of the nerve to the latissimus dorsi and teres major muscles; 3 = rupture of the axillary nerve; 4 = rupture of the radial nerve; 5 = rupture of the musculocutaneous nerve; 6 = rupture of the lateral cord; 6a = rupture of the lateral head of the median nerve; 6b = rupture of the median nerve; 7 = rupture of the medial cord; 7a = rupture of the ulnar nerve and brachial cutaneous nerve. (From Alnot, J. Y.: Clin. Plast. Surg., *11*:128, 1984.)

hypesthesia of the lateral aspect of the shoulder and of the dorsal aspect of the first intermetacarpal space ("snuffbox" region). However, absence of sensory deficits should be considered a favorable sign.

Isolated or Associated Injuries of a Terminal Branch of the Plexus

Lesions may involve the *musculocutaneous or radial nerves*. The typical clinical picture in these cases does not pose a diagnostic problem. However, lesions of the *axillary nerve* must be given special consideration (Fig. 27–4A and B). Axillary nerve lesions may occur alone or associated with other distal nerve lesions of the suprascapular, musculocutaneous, or radial nerves. All of these nerves contribute to shoulder function, especially abduction. The axillary and suprascapular nerves contribute directly and the musculocutaneous and radial nerves indirectly (by the biarticulation function of the biceps and triceps).

Although the general clinical picture is that of a paralytic shoulder, certain etiologic and clinical factors should point to the diagnosis of the involvement of one or another of these nerves. The most frequent cause of isolated axillary nerve lesions is anterointernal shoulder dislocation. In 80% of cases, this results in a neurapraxia with total recuperation in 4 to 6 months time.

Trauma caused by violent downward and backward movement of the shoulder leads to more widespread lesions involving the cords or terminal branches (see Fig. 27–3). These are often multiple, e.g., axillary nerve plus suprascapular nerve or musculocutaneous nerve. Because of stretching, the terminal branches are torn from their points of relative fixation (i.e., the quadrangular space for the axillary nerve, the coracoid notch for the suprascapular nerve, and the point of entry into the coracobrachialis for the musculocutaneous nerve).

Clinically, total paralysis of abduction and of external rotation is observed when injury to the axillary nerve is associated with injury to the suprascapular nerve (Fig. 27–4C and D). Shoulder flexion is possible because the shoulder is stabilized by the long part of the biceps.

When lesions are confined to the axillary nerve alone, the deficit can be variable, but there is always some active abduction of the shoulder, even if it is limited (Fig. 27–4A and B). This abduction, which is accompanied by some external rotation, is possible because the supra- and infraspinatus muscles, innervated by the suprascapular nerve, are unaffected. The stabilization of the humeral head by the supraspinatus muscle and the action of the long part of the biceps explain why shoulder flexion and abduction can sometimes be normal. Ignorance of this fact often leads to errors or delays in diagnosis.

Lesions of the Lateral Cord and Medial Cord

Injury to the lateral cord is rare. As the musculocutaneous nerve and the lateral head of the median nerve are affected, the motor deficit consists of paralysis of elbow flexion, associated with a deficit of the pronator muscles of the forearm and wrist and finger flexors. When the lesion is proximal, the lateral pectoral nerve is injured, resulting in partial or total paralysis of the upper part of

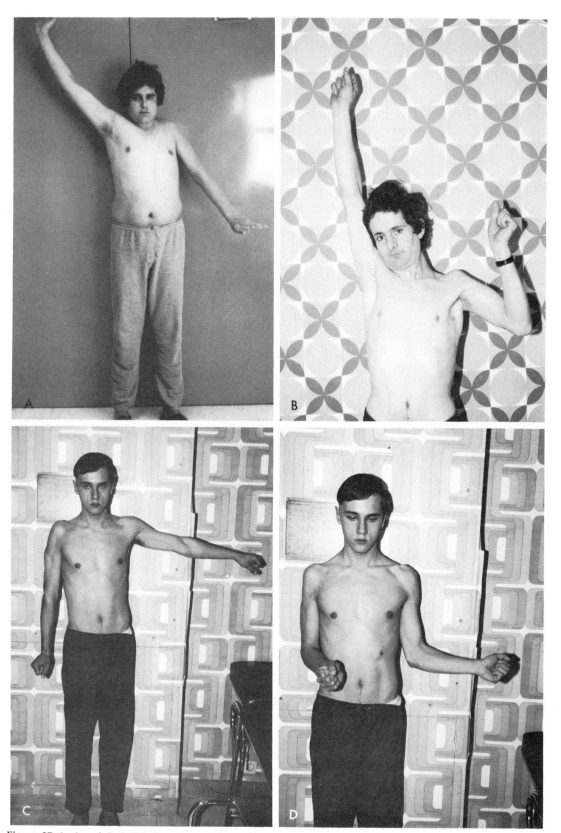

Figure 27–4. *A* and *B*, Isolated rupture of the axillary nerve. *C* and *D*, Associated ruptures: axillary nerve and suprascapular nerve. (From Alnot, J. Y.: Clin. Plast. Surg., *11*:129, 1984.)

partial or total paralysis of the upper part of the pectoralis major muscle. A sensory deficit is manifested in the forearm and particularly in the thumb.

Injury to the medial cord is even more rare. Clinically, there is upper medioulnar paralysis, which is total in the area of the ulnar nerve and only partial in the area of the median nerve, in particular the flexor pollicis longus and flexor digitorum profundus muscles of the index fingers. This should alert one to the possibility of a medial cord injury, especially if there is concomitant anesthesia in the area of the medial cutaneous nerve or partial paralysis of the inferior part of the pectoralis major muscle caused by a lesion of the medial pectoral nerve.

Lateral and medial cord lesions are caused locally by bone fractures or open wounds (glass and knife wounds). X-rays permit a precise evaluation of associated lesions of the shoulder area, including fractures of the clavicle, the scapula, the upper part of the humerus, or the first rib.

The presence of concomitant distal lesions may account for a more complex clinical picture. Lateral and medial cord lesions may occur together, and the resulting clinical picture is hard to differentiate from that due to injuries to roots or supraclavicular trunk lesions. Either lateral or medial cord lesions may be associated with radial nerve lesions due to fracture of the humeral diaphysis, which leave the triceps muscle unaffected. Vascular lesions may also be present and must be repaired if there is interruption of the subclavian and axillary arteries. The development of a severe ischemic syndrome has sometimes necessitated emergency vein graft.

Nerve repair is rarely undertaken at the same time as arterial repair, either because the surgeon is not experienced in the procedure involving peripheral nerve repair or because widespread longitudinal stretch lesions make it impossible to determine the exact extent of damage. Therefore, a nerve graft must be performed later under better conditions. However, reoperation in these cases of combined nerve and vascular lesions is difficult, as it entails a long and dangerous dissection to identify the injured plexus components. Thus, if possible, nerve repair should be undertaken during the emergency operation, nerve and vein grafts being done separately.

If vascular repair has not been done, it is important to establish arterial continuity as a secondary procedure, even though vascularization of the upper limb may seem satisfactory because of collateral substitution. Improved vascularization is a very important factor favoring nerve regeneration.

Lesions During Surgical Procedures

Surgical treatment of recurrent shoulder dislocation by the Latarget technique, involving lateral displacement of the coracoid process with the coracobrachialis, modifies the pathway of the musculocutaneous nerve and sometimes that of the posterior cord. These nerves may be injured during the surgical approach or strangulated during muscle repair.

The presence of abnormal postoperative pain should arouse one's suspicion. Paralysis of active elbow flexion or abduction is an indication for immediate revision. Although paralysis can be due to contusion caused by retraction, we found that of five patients reoperated in the sixth month following the primary procedure, four had nerve lesions necessitating repair by graft and one required secondary suture. In three of these patients, early reoperation could have freed the nerves trapped in sutures and permitted clinical recuperation by simple neurolysis.

THERAPEUTIC INDICATIONS

Therapeutic indications for managing infraclavicular lesions are derived from clinical examinations and tests.

Electromyograms are useful in detecting subclinical reinnervation, and cervical myelography is most often necessary.

Classic syndromes are easily diagnosed by the informed clinician or surgeon, but atypical syndromes indicating multiple associated lesions can make diagnosis difficult. In these cases the possibility of supraclavicular lesions should be eliminated; supraclavicular lesions are not likely to be present when there is no sign of irritation in the cervical area and myelography is normal.

Surgical exploration should be considered in the absence of clinical or electromyographic recuperation. Surgery should be done after the third or fourth month, except, of course, in the case of lesions caused by knife or gunshot wounds, which should be operated upon earlier (Fig. 27–5).

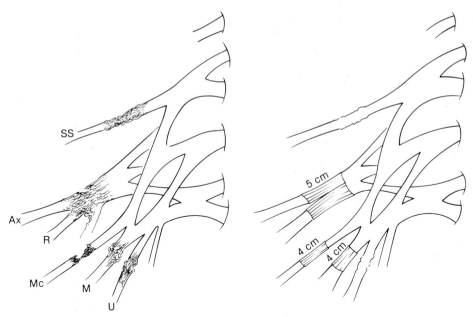

Figure 27–5. Classic injuries: Stretch of suprascapular nerve (neurolysis). Rupture of the posterior cord (grafting). Rupture of the musculocutaneous and median nerves (grafting). Stretch of the ulnar nerve (neurolysis).

In 60% of infraclavicular lesions, recuperation is spontaneous, and an early favorable prognosis can be made when the electromyogram shows signs of subclinical reinnervation. The rate of functional return is related to the distance between the level of the nerve lesion and the corresponding muscles. In the absence of recuperation, these relatively distal lesions should be repaired surgically, as they can be treated by neurolysis or a graft with much better results than those obtained for supraclavicular lesions. Statistics show satisfactory results for reinnervation of proximal shoulder and elbow muscles (with an 80% success rate), less satisfactory results for reinnervation of forearm and hand muscles (with a 60 to 70% rate for flexors and extensors of the wrist and hand), and total failure for the reinnervation of the intrinsic hand muscles.

CLINICAL DATA

Of our 420 patients with traumatic brachial plexus palsy, who had neurolysis or grafting procedures between 1974 and 1985, 75 had infraclavicular lesions. The patients were classified as follows:

1. *Seven patients with isolated musculocutaneous lesions (six grafts and one secondary suture):* Results were good in all seven patients, with function of elbow flexors graded at 3 +, and 4.

2. *Seventy-three patients with cord lesions:* Fifty-nine of these patients had posterior cord lesions treated by neurolysis or graft. Associated lesions of median and musculocutaneous nerves occurred in 30% of these patients. There were also twelve patients with lateral cord lesions and seven with medial cord lesions. Results are, in any case, difficult to analyze because of associated lesions and combined procedures (neurolysis and grafts) in the same patient.

3. *Twenty-five patients with axillary nerve lesions:* Nine of these were associated with other injuries, four with lesions of the suprascapular nerve and five with lesions of the musculocutaneous nerve. Sixteen were isolated lesions. In all cases of axillary nerve lesions the patients were young men between 10 and 30 years of age, and the average delay between injury and operation was 9 months.

Lesions were located at points of relative fixation: the quadrangular space for the axillary nerve, the coracoid notch for the suprascapular nerve, and the entry into the coracobrachialis for the musculocutaneous nerve. Except for one case of gunshot wounds, lesions were caused by stretching and because of their extent were repaired by a graft. In four patients terminal branches were torn from muscle sites, which resulted in the equivalent of an avulsion and offered no real possibility of repair. Brunelli has attempted to treat these lesions by directly implanting the nerve graft into the muscle, but the results have been equivocal.

Associated Axillary Nerve Lesions

Results are good in patients after neurolysis of the suprascapular nerve and graft of the axillary nerve. On the contrary, results have been disappointing in the three patients with associated axillary and suprascapular nerve ruptures (Figs. 27–6 and 27–7). The

suprascapular nerve could not be repaired in these three patients.

Despite adequate deltoid muscle contraction and good electromyogram results for the three muscle segments, the clinical picture has shown little improvement because of complex problems of rotator cuff lesions, especially of the supraspinatus muscle, complicating restoration of shoulder function.

Results have been satisfactory in the five patients with associated axillary and musculocutaneous nerve lesions. The reinnervation of the deltoid muscle and of elbow flexors

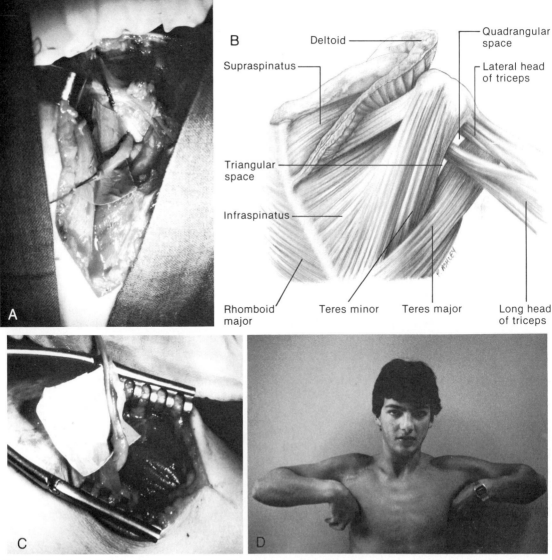

Figure 27–6. *A* and *B*, Isolated rupture of the axillary nerve in the quadrangular space. Posterior approach to expose the distal end of the axillary nerve. The grafting is started from the back (*C*) and the grafts are tunneled through the quadrangular space anteriorly to coapt with the proximal nerve end. *D*, Results 2 years postoperatively.

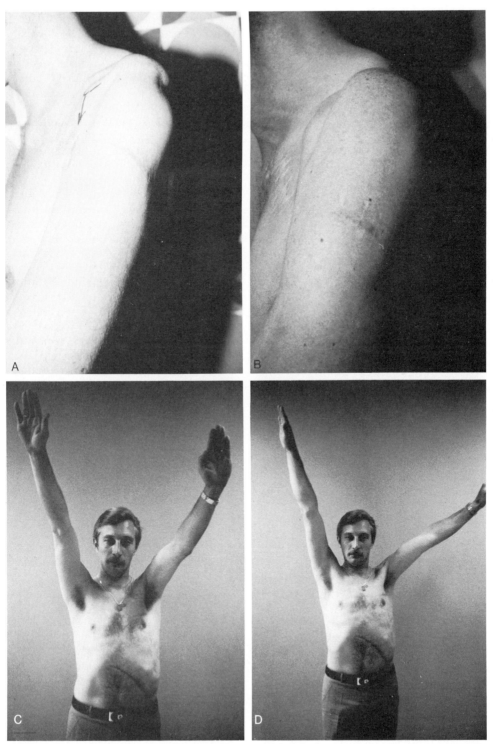

Figure 27–7. Isolated rupture of the axillary nerve. *A*, Preoperative state. *B* to *D*, Postoperative results.

has permitted recovery of useful elbow function and reinforced shoulder abduction.

Isolated Axillary Nerve Lesions

Of the fifteen patients with isolated axillary nerve lesions, the axillary nerve could not be repaired in three and the nerve graft was directly implanted in the muscle without clinical effect in one. Secondary suture with good clinical results was possible in one patient, and recuperation of the three muscle divisions of the deltoid was graded at 3+ after 1 year of follow-up.

Twelve patients had nerve graft, and eleven of them had good results after 1 year of follow-up. Clinical recuperation has apparently taken so long because the deltoid muscle has few "motor units." Recuperation takes place in the following order: beginning with the posterior part, then the middle part, and finally the anterior part. In the one remaining patient, follow-up is still insufficient, but at 6 months the electromyogram showed signs of reinnervation.

The clinical picture in isolated axillary nerve lesions is quite variable. Certain patients have normal active motion of the shoulder, although there is total paralysis of the deltoid muscle. Although debatable, surgical repair in these often very young patients would seem justified by the frequency of rotator cuff lesions after a certain age. In other patients there is lack of function of the shoulder, and surgery is generally indicated 4 to 6 months after trauma, if there is no sign of clinical or electromyographic recuperation.

CONCLUSIONS

Treatment of brachial plexus injuries requires thorough knowledge of these anatomicopathologic lesions. The indications for repair by nerve graft or neurolysis should also be known. Clinical diagnosis, although sometimes difficult, should permit early surgical exploration (4 to 6 months after trauma).

The most important fact is that prognosis for infraclavicular lesions is better than that for supraclavicular lesions. However, several points should be stressed.

First, the majority of lesions are caused by stretching and often result in widespread longitudinal nerve injury. In certain cases, only sections can be repaired by secondary suture. In all other cases, the length of the nerve graft and the quality of surrounding tissues must be considered in the evaluation of results.

Second, in the case of distal lesions a clear distinction should be made between lesions that are relatively near to the corresponding muscles and those that are farther away. Suprascapular, axillary, musculocutaneous, and radial nerve lesions occur near motor end organs. Nerve repair by graft is followed by satisfactory recuperation in 70 to 80% of cases. However, certain difficulties in nerve repair should be pointed out. For example, the distal end of the suprascapular nerve is hard to locate, and repair of the axillary nerve is difficult when it is torn from the muscle. Lateral and medial cord, median nerve, and ulnar nerve lesions are farther from motor end-organs. In these cases, even though repair may be of good quality, the results are equivocal. Reinnervation of wrist and hand flexors occurs in 60% of patients, but there is a complete absence of recuperation of intrinsic hand muscles. Nevertheless, reinnervation provides protective sensibility, in particular in the area of the median nerve.

Third, the frequency of concomitant lesions should be noted, especially the association of posterior cord lesions with those of the musculocutaneous nerve, the median nerve, or the ulnar nerve. Also, bone and vascular lesions affect the overall prognosis.

References

1. Alnot, J. Y., Allieu, Y., Bonnel, F., Cadre, N., Frot, B., Huten, B., Mansat, M., Millesi, H., Narakas, A., and Sedel, L.: Paralysie traumatique du plexus brachial chez l'adulte. Symposium Société Française Chirurgie Orthopédique et Traumatologique. Rev. Chir. Orthop., 63:17–125, 1977.
2. Alnot, J. Y., and Huten, D.: Systématisation du plexus brachial. Rev. Chir. Orthop., 63:27–34, 1977.
3. Alnot, J. Y., Jolly, A., and Frot, B.: Traitement direct des lésions nerveuses dans les paralysies traumatiques du plexus brachial chez l'adulte. (100 cas opérés). Int. Orthop., 5:151–168, 1981.
4. Jolly, A.: Traitement chirurgical direct des lésions par élongation du plexus brachial chez l'adulte. Thèse Paris. Hopital Bichat, 1980.
5. Millesi, H.: Surgical management of brachial plexus injuries. J. Hand Surg., 2:367–379, 1977.
6. Narakas, A.: Surgical treatment of traction injuries of the brachial plexus. Clin. Orthop., 133:71–90, 1978.
7. Privat, J. M., Mailhe, D., Allieu, Y., and Bonnel, F.: Hémilaminectomie cervicale exploratrice et neurotisation précoce du plexus brachial. In: Plexus Brachial et Médecine de Rééducation. Paris, Masson, 1982, pp. 66–73.
8. Sedel, L.: The results of surgical repair of brachial plexus injuries. J. Bone Joint Surg., 64:54–66, 1982.
9. Sunderland, S.: Nerves and Nerve Injuries, 2nd Ed. Edinburgh, E. S. Livingstone, 1978.

28

Experience with Vascularized Nerve Grafts

■

George Bonney, M.S., F.R.C.S.
Rolfe Birch, F.R.C.S.
Angus M. Jamieson, F.R.C.S.
Rosemary A. Eames, M.R.C.P., M.R.C.(Path.)

EXPERIMENTAL STUDIES

Twelve ex-breeder beagles were divided into three groups. The dogs were induced with pentothal and anesthesia was maintained with nitrous oxide, oxygen, and halothane. The sixth cervical nerve was exposed in the neck and the supraclavicular nerve was excised.

Technique

Group I: Vascularized Ulnar Nerve Graft—C6 to Supraclavicular Nerve. In Group I (four animals) the ulnar nerve was exposed in the foreleg and the ulnar artery was identified. The nerve was removed with the vessel after its branches were electrocoagulated. An artery of similar caliber was identified in the suprascapular region and microvascular anastomoses were carried out using 11–10 nylon (Fig. 28–1A).

One of the venae comitantes was also anastomosed. The distal vessels of the graft were coagulated. When the clamps were released, there was a satisfactory circulation through the graft in all four dogs. The ulnar nerve was then anastomosed to the proximal stump of C6 and to the distal stump of the supraclavicular nerve using 10–0 nylon. The wounds were closed, and all the animals recovered.

Group II: Pedicle Graft—Ulnar Nerve to C6: Avulsion C8/T1. In Group II (Fig. 28–1B), a laminectomy was carried out and roots C8 and T1 were avulsed from the spinal cord. The ulnar nerve was exposed in the forearm and mobilized after division distally. The nerve was passed subcutaneously in the upper leg to the neck and anastomosed to the proximal stump of C6 as a pedicle graft. The pedicle was not cut to produce predegeneration.

Group III: Avascular Ulnar Graft—C6 to Suprascapular Nerve. In Group III (Fig. 28–1C) the ulnar nerve was taken as an avascular graft and anastomosed between root C6 and the suprascapular nerve. All the animals recovered without complication.

The animals were re-explored under general anesthesia 6 weeks following the primary operation and specimens of the nerve grafts were taken. The dogs were then killed with veterinary Pentothal Forte. The specimens were fixed in 4% glutaraldehyde buffered in phosphate, post-fixed in 1% osmium tetroxide, and after dehydration embedded in Araldite. Sections measuring 1 μm were cut on a L.K.B. ultra-microtome and stained with 1% toluidine blue.

Results

The macroscopic appearance of the nerve grafts in Group I and Group III was different.

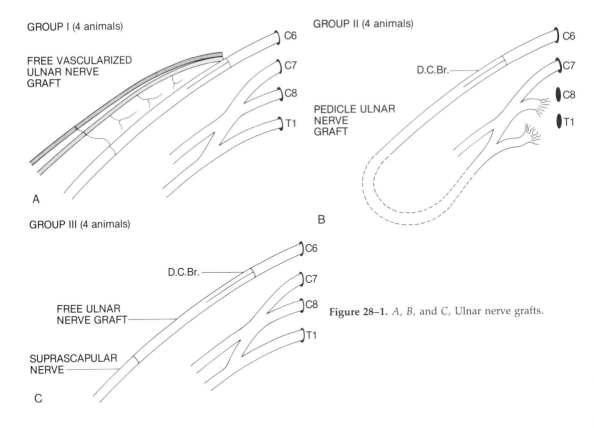

Figure 28–1. *A, B,* and *C,* Ulnar nerve grafts.

The avascular nerve grafts were fibrotic and shrunken and difficult to dissect (Fig. 28–2*A*). The vascularized grafts had the appearance of a normal nerve and retained their length. Fibrosis was apparent only at the anastomosis sites (Fig. 28–2*B*). The Group II pedicle grafts had an intermediate appearance, with more fibrosis than Group I but less than Group III.

Group I. Sections taken from C6 proximal to the level of the proximal anastomosis were normal. In one animal there was very mild damage in the periphery of one fascicle, with three or four regenerating clusters.

At the level of the proximal coaptation, the epineurium was greatly thickened by a cuff of well-vascularized fibrous tissue. The numerous small blood vessels present appeared normal and there was no thromboses. The perineurium was closely applied to this cuff and appeared slightly thickened.

No normal myelinated nerve fibers re-

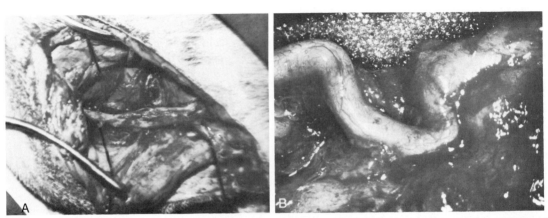

Figure 28–2. *A,* Re-exploration avascular graft. Note fibrosis and shrinkage. *B,* Re-exploration vascular graft. Good longitudinal circulation in the graft.

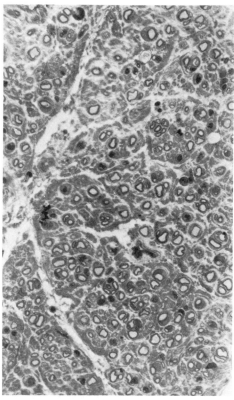

Figure 28–3. Transverse section at the level of the proximal suture showing numerous regenerated myelinated fibers (Group I, D 11 × 840).

mained in the endoneurium. A mild increase in endoneurial collagen was present. Myelin debris was scanty, and an increase in the number of Schwann cells was apparent. Regenerated myelinated nerve fibers were abundant, many of the fibers having attained an overall diameter of 5 μm (Fig. 28–3). Some regenerative clusters were present. No inflammatory cells were seen in the endoneurium, and there was no evidence of neuroma formation.

At a level of 1 cm below the proximal anastomosis, excellent regeneration was still apparent, although myelin debris was more obvious. At levels 2 cm (Fig. 28–4) and 4 cm (Fig. 28–5) below the proximal anastomosis, regeneration was present, but at the 4-cm level the nerve fibers were of a smaller diameter and had correspondingly thinner myelin sheaths; they were also present in fewer numbers. More myelin debris was present than at the level of the proximal anastomosis.

Small blood vessels were quite numerous in both the epineurium and the endoneurium and appeared normal. At the level of the

distal anastomosis the epineurium was again thickened and highly vascular; the perineurium appeared normal. In all four animals, early regenerating myelinated fibers were present, although these were not numerous (Fig. 28–6). There was a marked Schwann cell proliferation, and axonal sprouting was evident.

Group II. The results in this group, in which material was taken at the level of the anastomosis between C6 and the ulnar nerve and at 1-cm intervals distally up to 4 cm, were essentially similar to those in Group I. However, the appearance of the sections was different because of the presence in the grafted nerve of variable numbers of surviving normal myelinated fibers from C6, thus giving a dual population (Figs. 28–7A and B). At 4 cm below the anastomosis, regeneration was similar to that at the same level in Group I. Vascularization also appeared similar, and at the level of the anastomosis there was again a thick fibrous cuff of epineurium containing numerous blood vessels. Here, also, no neuroma formation was seen.

Group III. At the level of the proximal

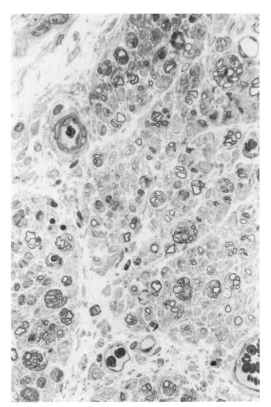

Figure 28–4. Section 2 cm distal to the proximal repair showing numerous thinly myelinated regenerated fibers (Group I, D 11 × 840).

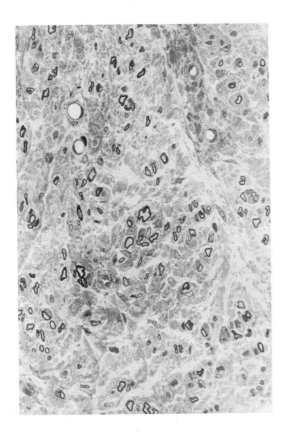

Figure 28–5. Section 4 cm below proximal repair showing scattered regenerated myelinated fibers, less abundant than in Figure 28–2 (Group I, D 12 × 840).

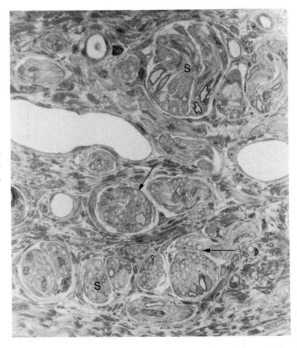

Figure 28–6. Transverse section at level of distal repair showing Schwann cell bundles (S) containing a few thinly myelinated regenerated fibers and numerous sprouts (*arrows*) (Group I, D 12 × 840).

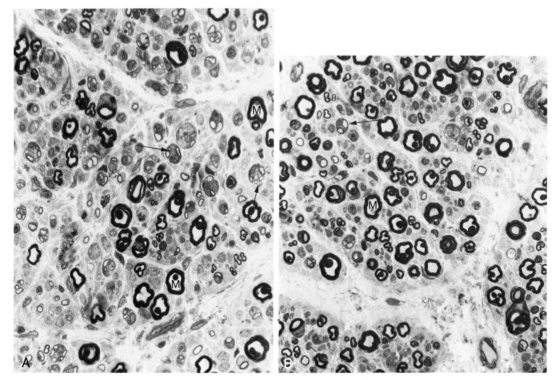

Figure 28–7. *A* and *B*, Transverse sections 2 cm and 4 cm below proximal repair showing normal surviving myelinated fibers (M) together with small regenerated fibers (*arrows*) (Group II, D 9 × 840).

anastomosis, the nerve fascicles surrounded by perineurium were embedded in a thick pad of fibrous tissue that contained few blood vessels. In all four animals, the pad was at least twice the size of the cuff present at this level in Groups I and II, and vascularization was obviously much less rich. The perineurial sheaths were not unduly thick. *Marked endoneurial fibrosis was present in all animals.* Regenerated myelinated fibers were present, but were generally of much smaller diameter (maximum 3 μm) than corresponding fibers in Groups I and II, and in all animals there was evidence of neuroma formation, with groups of small fibers ramifying in several directions (Fig. 28–8) accompanied by much fibrous tissue. There were increased numbers of both Schwann cell nuclei and fibroblasts. No inflammatory cells were seen. At 1 cm below the anastomosis, regeneration was even less evident, only relatively few small myelinated fibers being present (Fig. 28–9). Endoneurial fibrosis was still quite marked at this level, and myelin debris was present.

At 2 cm below the anastomosis, a few tiny myelinated fibers were present in only one animal. In the other three animals no myelinated fibers could be found by light micros-

copy. At 3 and 4 cm below the anastomosis, no regenerated fibers were seen in any animal; myelin debris was fairly prominent, and some endoneurial fibrosis was apparent. Fibrous epineurial thickening was also present and was much greater than in either of the other two groups of animals. Although small blood vessels (mainly of capillary size) were present, they were not as numerous as at corresponding levels in Groups I and II.

Discussion

The results demonstrated that there was much more potential for regeneration in the vascularized grafts and that this occurred earlier than in the avascular grafts. The pedicle graft demonstrated satisfactory vascularization. However, without predegeneration,[5] *many of the Schwann tubes were blocked by surviving sensory axons.*

CLINICAL FINDINGS

The ulnar nerve is used as a graft in repair of injuries of the brachial plexus only when

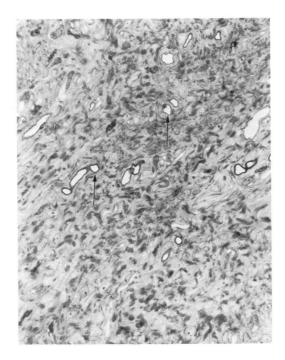

Figure 28–8. Level of proximal repair showing neuroma formation with only a few ramifying regenerated fibers (*arrows*) and large amounts of collagen (Group III, D 17 × 840).

there is definite evidence of preganglionic avulsion of C8 and T1. Operative diagnosis is much easier in patients explored within 4 or 5 days of injury. In the majority of our patients, however, the severity of associated injuries dictates delay. In these patients, demonstration of conduction in sensory fibers of the ulnar nerve either by the histamine test[1] or by sensory potential studies[2] is important evidence of preganglionic injury to C8 and T1. The myelograph is less reliable; we have seen several cases of recovery to the level of the first thoracic root even when a pouch was shown on myelography.

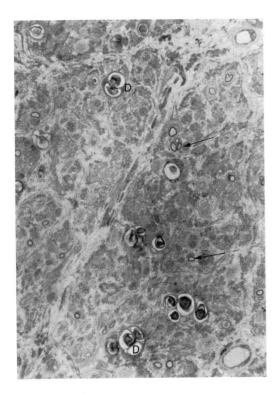

Figure 28–9. Section 1 cm below repair site; very few small regenerated fibers (*arrows*) and clumps of myelin debris (D) (Group III, D 17 × 840).

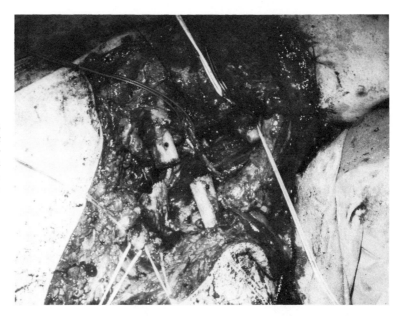

Figure 28–10. The brachial plexus exposed: C5, C6 postganglionic rupture (*right*). C7, C8, T1 preganglionic avulsion (*left*) pulled down below the clavicle. (From Bonney, G., et al.: Clin. Plast. Surg., *11*:138, 1984.)

Of the clinical findings, pain, felt in the anesthetic hand, is a strong indicator of avulsion of the lower roots of the plexus. A Claude Bernard–Horner syndrome is less certain.

TECHNIQUE

The supraclavicular plexus is exposed through a transverse incision in the neck. The transverse cervical and other blood vessels are preserved. If a postganglionic rupture at, for example, C5 and/or C6, with preganglionic avulsion at C7, C8, and T1, is found, the incision is extended to expose the axillary plexus (Figs. 28–10 to 28–12).

The ulnar nerve, with the accompanying artery and vena comitans, is exposed in the forearm and removed. Collateral vessels passing with the nerve in the cubital tunnel occasionally allow extension of the vascularized segment of the nerve into the arm.

The graft is laid in place between the roots and the distal nerve stumps, deep to the clavicle. If only C5 is available, one strand of graft is used to the lateral cord/musculocutaneous nerve. C6 and C7 are usually large enough to take at least two strands of ulnar nerve.

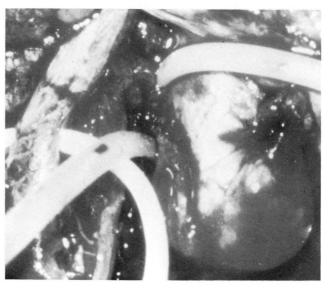

Figure 28–11. Close-up of C5 showing good bundles. The phrenic nerve is seen to the left (× 10).

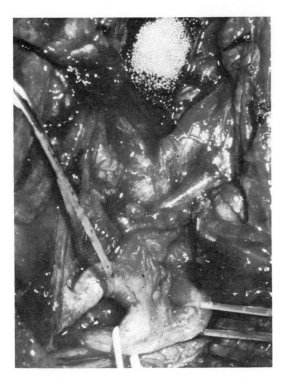

Figure 28–12. The middle and lower trunks, with posterior root ganglia of C7, C8, and T1 coiled up in the axilla (× 6).

The vascular anastomosis precedes the neural repair. The ulnar artery is interposed as a loop into an arterial circulation, most commonly by end-to-end suture to the transverse cervical artery both distal and proximal. In other cases, in which the suprascapular or subclavian arteries are used to supply the graft, end-to-side anastomosis is performed. Good circulation through the graft is usually evident within minutes of releasing the clamps. Venous return picks up after 5 min-

utes (Fig. 28–13), and a vena comitans is then chosen for anastomosis to an adjacent vein.

The neural repair is now performed. The nerve can be sectioned to allow a double vascularized strand (Figs. 28–14 to 28–16) nourished by a U loop; rarely, three strands can be developed, supplied by the vascular pedicle. Accessory grafts, using sural nerve, avascular ulnar nerve, or medial cutaneous nerve of the arm, may be necessary.

The wound is then closed. The arm is

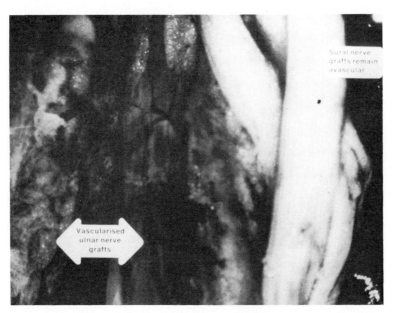

Sural nerve grafts remain avascular

Vascularised ulnar nerve grafts

Figure 28–13. Close-up of two vascularized strands of ulnar nerve; avascular sural nerves to the right (× 10). (From Bonney, G., et al.: Clin. Plast. Surg., *11*:138, 1984.)

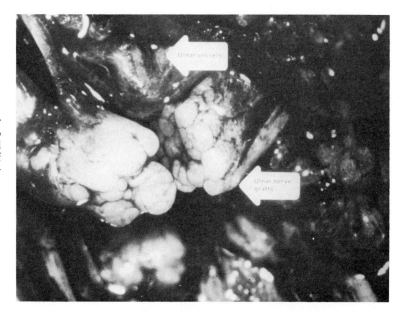

Figure 28–14. A "U" loop of ulnar nerve, here prepared in two strands for suture to the lateral cord distally. Note the pedicle of the ulnar vessels (× 6). (From Bonney, G., et al.: Clin. Plast. Surg., 11:139, 1984.)

supported in a body sling for 2 weeks, and the neck is supported by a soft cervical collar. Anticoagulants are not used.

DISCUSSION

Since 1977, over 100 repairs of brachial plexus injuries have been performed at St. Mary's, the Royal National Orthopaedic, and the Robert Jones and Agnes Hunt Orthopaedic Hospitals. The vascularized ulnar nerve graft has been used in over 30 cases; results of the first 12 cases are summarized in Table 28–1. It is our impression that recovery in these patients is better than when sural nerve or avascular ulnar nerve has been used in similar lesions. However, functional return is limited. In all cases, shoulder control is imperfect, and in no case has significant hand function returned by means of grafts. More recently, we have extended the technique to reinnervate the median nerve. Time will tell whether this is worthwhile.

The reasons for failure are obscure. However in both Case 2 and Case 6, it is possible that at least one of the proximal roots had a higher preganglionic injury within the spinal canal. It is now our practice to stimulate nerve roots at exploration and record cortical

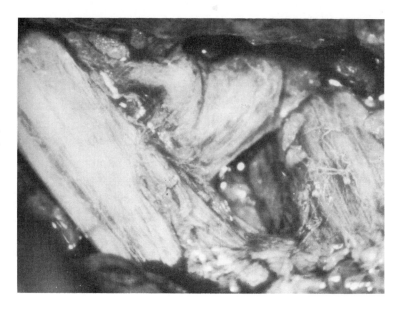

Figure 28–15. The neural repair completed; two strands of ulnar nerve sutured to lateral cord (× 6).

Table 28–1. RESULTS OF VASCULARIZED ULNAR NERVE GRAFTS

Case	Age	Sex	Time Interval—Accident to Operation	Findings at Operation	Mode of Repair	Results	Function
1	17	M	4 months	5/1978 Postganglionic C5, C6 Preganglionic C7, C8, T1	Gap 15 cm 1 vascularized strand, C6—lateral cord 1 avascular strand C6—lateral cord 1 avascular strand C5—posterior cord	No worthwhile recovery	—
2	19	M	4 months	7/1978 Postganglionic C5 Preganglionic C6–T1	Gap 16 cm 1 vascularized strand, C5—lateral cord	Biceps 3+ at 6 months Biceps 4 at 1 year	Elbow flexion useful
3	18	M	4 months	11/1978 Postganglionic C5 Preganglionic C6–T1	Gap 12 cm 1 vascularized strand, C5—lateral cord	No recovery	—
4	17	M	5 days	11/1978 Postganglionic C5, C6, C7 Preganglionic C8, T1	Gap 12 cm 1 vascularized strand upper trunk—lateral cord 1 avascular strand upper trunk—lateral cord 1 avascularized strand, C7-posterior cord (gap 15 cm)	Biceps 3+ at 6 months Biceps 4 at 2 years Lat. dorsi 4 Triceps 3+	Full time at work Limb useful as paper weight; elbow flexion useful in carrying
5	18	M	5 days	9/1979 Postganglionic C6 Preganglionic C6–T1	Gap 18 cm 1 vascularized strand, C5—lateral cord	Biceps 4 at 1 year Biceps 4+ at 2 years FCR FDS3 Protective sensation in index, thumb, and palm	Elbow flexion useful at work and hobby (carpenter)
6	22	M	6 months	3/1980 Postganglionic C5, C6 Preganglionic C7, C8, T1	Gap 15 cm 2 vascularized strands, C5—lateral cord 6 strands sural nerve, C6—medial head, median nerve	None	Using flail arm splint At work full time
7	22	M	13 months	4/1980 Postganglionic C5 Preganglionic C6–T1	Gap 18 cm 1 vascularized strand, C5—lateral cord 1 vascular sural strand used to supplement	No recovery for 2 years At 28 months Biceps 3+ Awaiting derotation osteotomy humerus	Using flail arm splint Not at work
8	18	M	3 months	8/1980 Postganglionic C5, C6 Preganglionic C7–T1	Gap 18 cm 1 vascularized ulnar, C5—lateral cord 1 avascular ulnar C6—lateral cord 2 surals, C6—medial head, median nerve	At 7 months biceps recovery Biceps 4+ at 2 years FCR FDS 2 Protective sensation in thumb and palm	Full time at work Elbow flexion useful

Table continued on opposite page

Table 28–1. RESULTS OF VASCULARIZED ULNAR NERVE GRAFTS *Continued*

Case	Age	Sex	Time Interval— Accident to Operation	Findings at Operation	Mode of Repair	Results	Function
9	19	M	6 months	9/1980 Postganglionic C5, C6 Preganglionic C7– T1	Gap 12 cm 1 vascularized strand, C5—lateral cord 1 vascularized strand, C6—lateral cord	Recovery commenced at 1 year At 2 years, biceps 4+ FCR FDS 3 Protective sensation in hand	Derotation osteotomy improved function from the elbow flexion Not at work
10	17	M	2 months	10/1980 Postganglionic C5, C6 Preganglionic C7, C8, T1	Gap 9 cm 1 vascularized strand across the upper trunk	Recovery commenced at 1 year At 1 year, biceps 4, triceps 4, lat. dorsi 4, supraspinatus 3, infraspinatus 3	Uses flail arm splint flexion and extension independent Limb useful as a paper weight Full-time student
11	23	M	5 months	11/1980 Postganglionic C5, C6 Preganglionic C7, C8, T1	Gap 10 cm 2 vascularized strands, C5 C6 to lateral cord Sural to suprascapular nerve	Recovery commenced at 1 year At 2 years, biceps 4+, lat. dorsi 3+, FCR FDS 2 No hand sensation	Full time at work Uses splint Elbow and wrist flexion useful
12	19	M	7 months	11/1980 Postganglionic C5, C6 Preganglionic C7, C8, T1	Gap 10 cm 1 vascularized strand, C5—lateral cord 1 avascular strand C6—lateral cord	Biceps 4 at 2 years	Full time at work Elbow flexion useful

Note: All these young men were injured in motorcycle accidents. Follow-up in all cases minimum 2 years. From Bonney, G. et al. Clin. Plast. Surg., *11*:140–141, 1984.

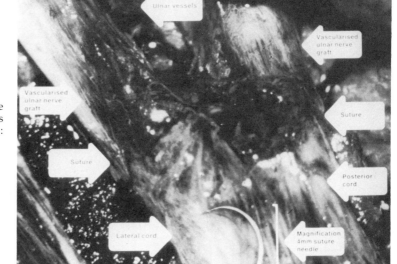

Figure 28–16. After release of the clamps; good perfusion of grafts (× 6). (From Bonney, G., et al.: Clin. Plast. Surg., *11*:139, 1984.)

evoked potentials through scalp electrodes.[4] This technique may prove of value in diagnosing such "double" lesions. We have been encouraged by recent experience with computed tomographic scans, using dilute radiopaque medium to outline the spinal roots of C5, C6, and C7 within the spinal canal. In one recent case, an intradural tear was clearly shown at C6; at operation this root appeared healthy.

Taking the ulnar artery has given rise to justifiable anxiety about circulation in the hand. The operation is performed only when there is a detectable radial pulse. Allen's test is useful in confirming adequate blood flow through that vessel. The majority of our patients with preganglionic avulsion injuries experience pain in the anesthetized hand. This pain is often extremely severe. In some of the patients described earlier, pain returned with neural regeneration. However the majority find the pain tolerable or absent by 2 years, and the transcutaneous nerve stimulator is more effective in a limb with partial sensory recovery than in a completely insensitive upper limb.[3]

We should emphasize that neural repair is only one part of a rehabilitation program for these severely injured young people. Many find the flail arm splint, or modifications of it, useful. Retraining for work and treatment for pain are essential parts of the rehabilitation program.[7]

Acknowledgments: We wish to thank Dr. C. Green, Veterinary Surgeon, and the staff of the Department of Comparative Anatomy, Medical Research Centre, Northwick Park Hospital, London; Mrs. M. Naylor, Mr. R. Bowden, and the pathology technicians, The National Hospital for Nervous Diseases, London; and the Photographic Departments at the National Hospital for Nervous Diseases and St. Mary's Hospital, London. The animal study was made possible with a research grant from the North West Thames Regional Health Authority.

References

1. Bonney, G.: The value of axon responses in determining the site of lesion in traction injuries of the brachial plexus. Brain, *77*:588–609, 1954.
2. Bonney, G., and Gilliatt, R. W.: Sensory nerve conduction after traction lesions of the brachial plexus. Proc. R. Soc. Med., *51*:365–367, 1958.
3. Frampton, V. M.: Pain control with the aid of transcutaneous nerve stimulation. Physiotherapy, *68*: 77–81, 1982.
4. Jones, S. J., Wynn Parry, C. B., and Landi, A.: Diagnosis of brachial plexus traction lesions by sensory nerve action potentials and somatosensory evoked potentials. Injury, *12*:376–382, 1981.
5. Strange, F. G. St. C.: Case report on pedicled nerve graft. Br. J. Surg., *37*:331, 1950.
6. Taylor, G. I., and Ham, F. J.: The free vascularized nerve graft. Plast. Reconstr. Surg., *57*:413, 1976.
7. Wynn Parry, C. B.: Rehabilitation of the Hand, 4th Ed. London. Butterworths, 1981, pp. 157–180.

29

Paralysis in Root Avulsion of the Brachial Plexus: Neurotization by the Spinal Accessory Nerve

■

Y. Allieu, M.D.
J. M. Privat, M.D.
F. Bonnel, M.D.

In root avulsion of the brachial plexus due to traumatic stretching of the plexus, the only possible reinnervation of the distal part is by anastomosis with the neighboring nerves. The first anastomosis or "neurotization" was done in 1963 by Seddon,[16] who reinnervated the biceps and the brachialis muscles by anastomosing the distal part of the musculocutaneous nerve with the second, third, and fourth intercostal nerves.

The recent resurgence of interest in surgery specifically on the brachial plexus has given a new momentum to neurotization techniques. Narakas,[13–15] Allende and Mana,[1] and Tsuyama and Hara[18] have introduced neurotization of the musculocutaneous nerve by the intercostal nerves. It is also possible to reinnervate the avulsed plexus by the other neighboring nerves. Kotani et al.[11] carried out neurotization of the musculocutaneous nerve, superior trunk, and radial nerve by the spinal accessory nerve. We have followed the same techniques and have come to similar conclusions. In this chapter we will discuss 21 of our cases of neurotization by the spinal accessory nerve in root avulsion of the brachial plexus. First, however, the anatomico-surgical basis of neurotization will be outlined.

ANATOMICO-SURGICAL BASIS OF NEUROTIZATION BY THE SPINAL ACCESSORY NERVE

The spinal accessory nerve has a close relationship with the superior part of the brachial plexus in the supraclavicular fossa. This nerve can be anastomosed directly, without an intermediary graft, with the fourth and fifth cervical roots or the upper trunk. There is also a close relationship between the spinal accessory nerve and the suprascapular nerve, which allows direct anastomosis (Fig. 29–1).

Use of the spinal accessory nerve may vary. All the fibers of this nerve, before crossing the sternocleidomastoid muscle, may be utilized for neurotization of the brachial plexus, but, theoretically, at the price of complete paralysis of the sternocleidomastoid and trapezius muscles. The latter muscle, however, may receive fibers posteriorly from the deep cervical plexus, which is why in certain patients there is incomplete paralysis of the trapezius muscle after section of the spinal accessory nerve. In that case, the surgical approach will be difficult, and it is necessary to use a long intermediary graft

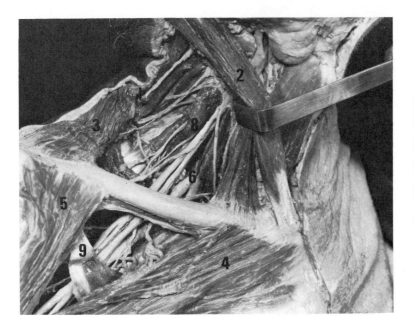

Figure 29–1. (1) Anterior view of the brachial plexus elements and the spinal accessory nerve, (2) sternocleidomastoid muscle, (3) trapezius muscle, (4) pectoralis major muscle, (5) deltoid muscle, (6) subclavian artery, (7) scalenus anterior muscles, (8) scalenus medius muscle, and (9) pectoralis minor muscle. (From Allieu, Y., et al.: Clin. Plast. Surg., 11:134, 1984.)

between the spinal accessory nerve and the plexus.

Taking the spinal accessory nerve in the supraclavicular fossa spares the sternocleidomastoid muscle. It is possible to carry out a direct anastomosis with the two primary cervical root nerves and the upper trunk. However, if we want to neurotize the musculocutaneous nerve itself, an intermediary graft is needed. Taking the spinal accessory nerve more distally in the deep surface of the trapezius muscle allows use of some fibers to that muscle.

The technique described by Kotani[11] involves direct anastomosis between the terminal part of the spinal accessory nerve within the trapezius muscle and the musculocutaneous nerve, along with interposition of short intermediary grafts between the muscular branches of the spinal accessory nerve destined for the trapezius muscle and the remainder of the musculocutaneous nerve. This approximation of the terminal segments during the anastomosis is possible only after an extensive endoneurolysis of the musculocutaneous nerve within the lateral cord of the plexus and after section of the clavicle. In addition, postoperative immobilization in a fixed position is obligatory. We have attempted this technique in one patient without success, in spite of very favorable conditions. However, the patient developed clavicular pseudarthrosis, which caused elevation of the shoulder. Direct anastomosis was therefore impossible.

We have had the same results in our cadaver dissections. Thus, we have gone back to our initial technique, i.e., interposed grafts between the spinal accessory nerve in the supraclavicular fossa and the part of plexus to be neurotized (Fig. 29–2), and we have used this technique in all our cases.

Anastomoses between the spinal accessory nerve and branches of the divisions of the deep cervical plexus are constant. These branches are very numerous and are much larger than is classically taught.[6–8] The presence of numerous anastomotic branches poses a problem because of the presence of sensory and motor sensory fibers. In addition, experience shows that the size of the spinal accessory nerve varies according to the individual subject. This suggests that there is a balance between the spinal accessory nerve and the deep cervical plexus (Fig. 29–3). This may be important because it could explain the poor results in certain cases of neurotization and incomplete paralysis of the trapezius muscle after section of the spinal accessory nerve.

This anatomico-surgical study suggests that in certain cases it is necessary to join the spinal accessory nerve to branches derived from the deep cervical plexus that may carry a certain number of motor fibers. Systematically, the fascicular surface of the spinal accessory nerve is significantly less than that of the musculocutaneous nerve and of the upper trunk of the brachial plexus (Fig. 29–4). The fascicular surface of the spinal acces-

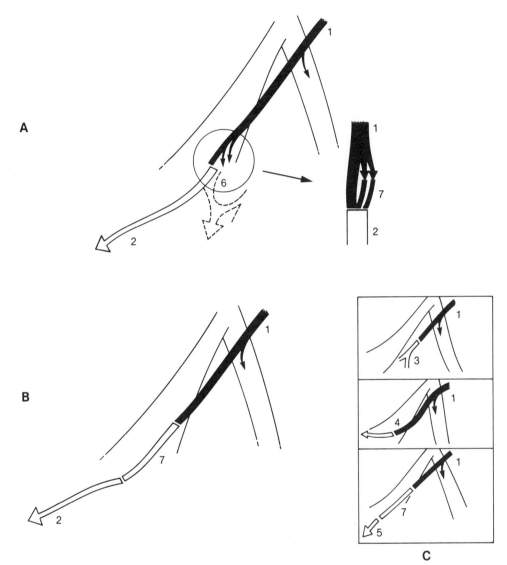

Figure 29–2. (1) Spinal accessory nerve, (2) musculocutaneous nerve, (3) superior trunk (or fifth and sixth cervical root nerves), (4) suprascapular nerve, (5) radial nerve, (6) middle trunk, and (7) intermediary grafts. *A,* Kotani and Mastuda techniques. Anastomosis of the direct part of the spinal nerve on the musculocutaneous nerve. It is necessary to carry out retrograde endoneurolysis for this anastomosis. In order to approximate the extremities, the authors utilize shortening of the clavicle. *B,* Anastomosis of the spinal nerve with the musculocutaneous nerve in the supraclavicular fossa (using the interposed grafts). This is the technique that we use at the moment. *C,* Techniques no longer used: *Top,* Direct anastomosis of the spinal nerve with the superior trunk or fifth or sixth cervical root nerve. *Middle,* Direct anastomosis of the spinal nerve with the suprascapular nerve. *Bottom,* Anastomosis of the spinal nerve to the radial nerve with intermediary grafts.

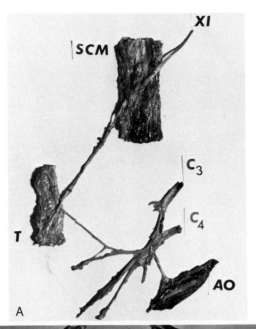

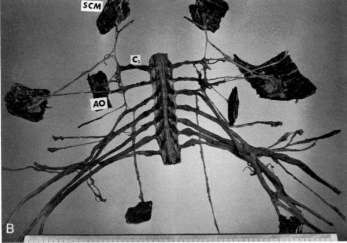

Figure 29–3. Dissection and branches of spinal nerve XI with its course in the sternocleidomastoid muscle (SCM). Branches of the deep cervical plexus giving origin to C3 and C4 toward the trapezius muscle (T). *A,* View of the two plexuses over the same subject. *B,* Detail.

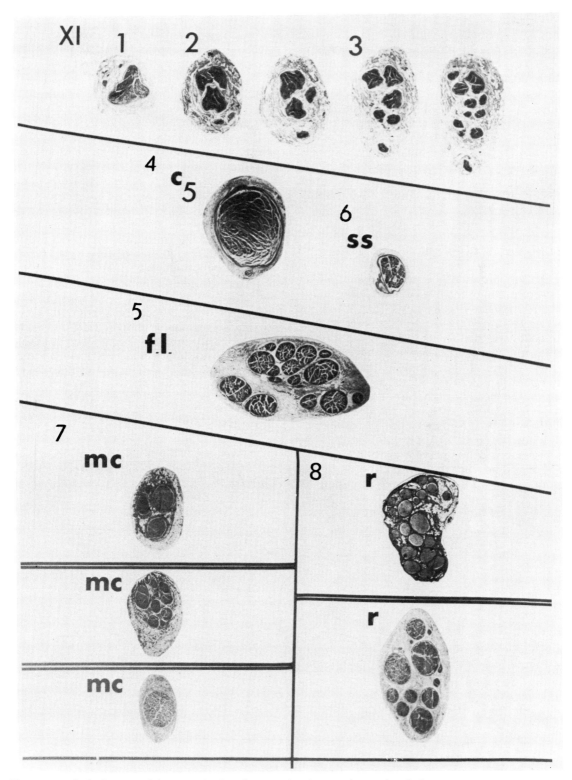

Figure 29–4. Scale diagram of the neurotization elements showing, on the one hand, the incongruence between the spinal accessory nerve and other elements and, on the other hand, the importance of the surrounding connective tissue environment. (1) Spinal nerve in the sternocleidomastoid muscle, (2) spinal accessory nerve in the supraclavicular fossa, (3) spinal nerve as it enters the trapezius, (4) root C5, (5) upper trunk of brachial plexus, (6) suprascapular nerve (SS), (7) musculocutaneous nerve (mc), and (8) radial nerve (r). For the musculocutaneous nerve there are three variations and for the radial nerve two variations. Note the individual variations in arrangement and number of the fascicles.

sory nerve is also a bit smaller or equal to that of the suprascapular nerve. The number of fibers is equally reduced: 1700 in the spinal accessory nerve compared with 6000 in the musculocutaneous nerve and 3500 in the suprascapular nerve.[8] If we compare these 1700 fibers with the 5000 utilizable fibers in the four intercostal nerves, neurotization by the spinal accessory nerve seems to be less logical than by the intercostal nerves. Whether it is preferable to use the spinal accessory nerve (which innervates more muscle) or the intercostal nerves (which have more fibers) is still undecided.

SURGICAL TECHNIQUE

At the present time we use only direct neurotization of the musculocutaneous nerve by the spinal accessory nerve (Fig. 29–5). To date, 15 procedures have been carried out. Initially, we tried to place the suture directly over the spinal accessory nerve without an intermediary graft. In two cases we attempted to anastomose the spinal accessory nerve directly with the suprascapular nerve and in two other cases with the upper trunk. However, because of disappointing results, we now connect all utilizable fibers to the musculocutaneous nerve.

For the neurotization of this nerve by the spinal accessory nerve, two intermediary grafts varying from 70 to 200 mm (average 150 mm) are needed. They are taken from the external saphenous or intercostobrachial nerve under microscopic control after the epiperineural sutures are done. This surgery should follow the general principles of reconstructive surgery of the brachial plexus. It is necessary to provide the best site for the graft, which means that as much of the subcutaneous (adipose) tissue as possible and the blood vessels in the supraclavicular fossa should be used. If results of preoperative studies or exploratory laminectomy are available at the time of neurotization, extensive dissection in the supraclavicular fossa can be avoided. Therefore, the grafts are in better condition. It is obligatory to verify the integrity of the musculocutaneous nerve up to its entrance into the coracobrachialis muscle. The distal part of the nerve must also be dissected. In fact, the lesions frequently occur in two stages, particularly when the nerve penetrates the muscle. An undiagnosed associated distal lesion makes neurotization of the proximal musculocutaneous nerve useless.[4, 5, 14]

RESULTS

The results of 21 cases of neurotization of the spinal accessory nerve are now available after more than 2 years of follow-up. In all

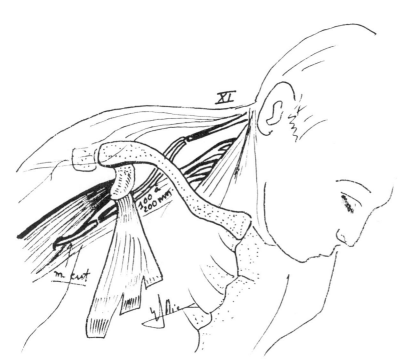

Figure 29–5. Anastomosis of the spinal accessory nerve with the interposed grafts. (From Allieu, Y., et al.: Clin. Plast. Surg., 11:134, 1984.)

cases, the root avulsion of the brachial plexus had been diagnosed and confirmed before operation (by exploratory semilaminectomy). In all cases, the fifth and sixth cervical roots were avulsed. In nine cases, the brachial plexus was completely avulsed (from C5 to T1). The interval between the time of the accident and the operation varied from 1 month to 15 months. All the patients were young (under 40 years of age; average age, 20 to 30 years). In most cases the paralysis was due to a motorcycle accident. The results are summarized in Table 29–1. The analysis of these results shows several significant points:

Neurotization of the suprascapular nerve has not been successful despite use of numerous fibers and direct anastomosis between the spinal accessory nerve and the suprascapular nerve. Results of anastomosis of the spinal accessory nerve with the upper trunk of the brachial plexus, either directly (two cases) or by short grafts (one case), are discouraging. This can be explained by dispersion of fibers. In fact, a significant number of fibers within the spinal accessory nerve from the upper trunk run in many directions, and this nonfocalization explains the poor result.

One of our patients had the following results on muscle testing: biceps, 3; brachialis, 2; pectoralis major, 4; and teres major, 1. In this patient, if all the fibers had been concentrated within the biceps muscle, the results would have been better. Two other patients have shown scattered recovery on electromyography but no clinical improvement.

We have anastomosed the spinal accessory nerve to the radial nerve in one patient with moderate results. Anastomosis between the spinal accessory nerve and the musculocutaneous nerve in 15 patients showed inconsistent results (see Table 29–1). However, the poor results are essentially from the initial group of patients, and technical problems should therefore be considered. Generally, however, the results were moderate.

Movement against weight allows only a certain orientation of the hand. It is therefore necessary to distinguish two types of patients regarding the extension of paralysis:

1. With complete paralysis of the brachial plexus, the patient has only slight flexion of the elbow and a nonfunctional and insensible hand. Surgery can be justified in these patients. All the patients who were asked preferred to keep their arm rather than undergo amputation (provided intolerable pain was not present). Nevertheless, in certain patients the results in relation to amputation should be discussed, not only for the relief of pain but from a functional point of view. It is important to warn the patient of the moderate result of neurotization procedures in case he prefers the more radical surgery.

2. If there is incomplete brachial plexus paralysis (paralysis of C5–C6 or C6–C7), it is possible to grade the biceps muscle at 2, which provides flexion of the elbow with the help of Steindler's effect. It is also possible to increase the flexion of elbow by a tendon transfer. In two cases, we have transferred the pectoralis minor muscle after neurotization (Lecoeur's technique). However, this isolated transfer with insufficient neurotization was not enough to provide flexion of the elbow.

In two cases the result was good: one muscle was graded as 4 and the other as 5. Elbow flexion is absolutely normal in these patients (Fig. 29–6). These good results were confirmed by stimulation of the spinal accessory nerve, which flexed the elbow. The first patient had localized avulsion of C5–C6 and the second had complete avulsion of the brachial plexus. The latter benefited from the neurotization of the radial nerve by intercostal nerves as well and had motor recovery of the triceps muscle graded as 4. In spite of their rarity, the two good results encourage us to keep using this technique because we

Table 29–1. NEUROTIZATION BY THE SPINAL ACCESSORY NERVE IN 21 PATIENTS FOLLOWED FOR 2 OR MORE YEARS

Nerve Neurotized	Results		
	Poor or Absent*	Moderate†	Good‡
Suprascapular (n = 2)	2		
Upper trunk (n = 3)	2	1	
Musculocutaneous (n = 15)	5	7	3
Radial (n = 1)		1	

*No recovery or muscle recovery less than 3 during muscle testing.
†One muscle can be marked at 3 during muscle testing.
‡One muscle can be marked at 4 or 5 during muscle testing.

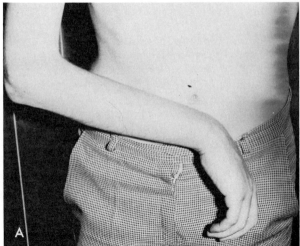

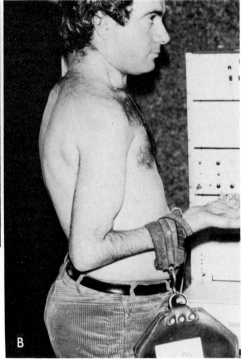

Figure 29–6. Result of the neurotization of the musculocutaneous nerve by the spinal accessory nerve. *A*, Biceps, 3 years after the neurotization of the musculocutaneous nerve in complete avulsion of the brachial plexus. *B*, Biceps, 5 years after the neurotization of the musculocutaneous nerve in complete avulsion of the brachial plexus. The associated neurotization of the radial nerve by the intercostal nerve makes contraction of the triceps muscle possible after 4 years. This is our best result following neurotization.

have never had such innervation after neurotization by the intercostal nerves alone.

It should be emphasized that apart from one exceptional patient who recovered despite a 15-month interval between the time of injury and the operation, the best results have been obtained following surgery before the third month. In addition, in all cases the primary results were obtained at least 1 or 2 years after surgery and final recovery took up to 4 years postoperatively. The patient should be warned about the long recovery period.

The trapezius muscle can be sacrificed in taking the spinal accessory nerve for neurotization. There are two consequences:

1. One of the patients showed incomplete paralysis of the trapezius muscle and another has completely recovered from trapezius muscle paralysis after 3 years. These two cases correspond to two poor results of neurotization of the musculocutaneous nerve. With positive results (moderate or good), postoperative paralysis of the trapezius muscle in most cases is complete.

2. Paralysis of the trapezius muscle alters the mobility of the shoulder girdle and finally, as a result of scapulohumeral arthrodesis, prevents shoulder movement.

Thus, we must note in cases of root avulsion whether there is preoperative paralysis of the serratus anterior muscle or of other muscles that stabilize the scapula. Additional paralysis of the trapezius muscle does not alter the total functional deficit of the shoulder. Of course, conservation of the stabilizing muscles of the shoulder, particularly the serratus anterior muscle, prevents sacrifice of the spinal accessory nerve. In the contrary case, this nerve can be used to flex the elbow.

On comparison, the results that are obtained in cases of nerve grafting (when the proximal stump of the nerve is present) even at level of C5, are better than those obtained with neurotization. It is important, therefore, to be certain of avulsion before carrying out the neurotization.

If there is no sign of preganglionic involvement before operation and if laminectomy shows total or partial integrity of anterior small roots, exploration of the cervical region to find the cervical root stumps (ventral branches of the spinal accessory nerve) should be mandatory. Dissection should be extended high into the intervertebral foramen and, if necessary, the vertebral artery should be freed for use of the prevertebral segment. This may be done by the Verbiest technique. Preoperative electromyography registers the cerebral potential produced by stimulation of the stump of the nerve and can precisely resolve all technical problems. Neurotization should be considered only as the last solution.

CONCLUSIONS

The results of neurotization by the spinal accessory nerve for root avulsion of the brachial plexus are generally moderate. In partial paralysis of the brachial plexus, elbow flexion can be ameliorated by tendon transfer. In complete paralysis, keeping an insensible and nonfunctional extremity only for flexion of the elbow is a matter for discussion. This flexion allows certain useful activities of daily living and movement of a nonfunctional hand, which is always preferable to a prosthesis. However, a prosthesis is practically always required in the long term.

It seems possible that our results may improve in the future. Increased knowledge of the anatomy of the spinal accessory nerve and cervical plexus and improvements in surgical technique may be helpful. Paralysis of the trapezius muscle after taking the spinal accessory nerve can be considered a poor risk because the shoulder will be nonfunctioning. Finally, among the techniques of neurotization,[9, 10, 15, 18] transfer of the spinal accessory nerve seems the best to us in spite of inconsistent results.

References

1. Allende, B. T., and Mana, Y. E.: Transferencia de nervios intercostales a plexo braquial. Rev. Ortoped. Traumatol. Latino-Am., 16:79–82, 1977.
2. Allieu, Y., Privat, J. M., and Bonnel, F.: Paralysis in root avulsion of the brachial plexus. Neurotization by the spinal accessory nerve. Clin. Plast. Surg., 11:133–137, 1984.
3. Allieu, Y.: Exploration et traitement des lésions nerveuses dans les paralysies traumatiques par élongation du plexus brachial chez l'adulte. Rev. Chir. Orthop., 63:89–107, 1977.
4. Allieu, Y., Connes, H., and de Godebout, J.: L'exploration et le traitement direct des lésions nerveuses dans les paralysies traumatiques par élongation du plexus brachial chez l'adulte. Les lésions traumatiques des nerfs périphériques. Monographie du Groupe d'Etude de la Main. Expansion Scientifique, Française Ed., 1979, pp. 165–180.
5. Allieu, Y., Privat, J. M., and Bonnel, F.: Les neurotisations par le nerf spinal (nerf accessorius) dans les avulsions radiculaires du plexus brachial. Neurochirurgie, 28:115–120, 1982.
6. Bonnel, F., and Rabischong, P.: Anatomy and systematization of the brachial plexus in the adult. Anat. Clin., 2:289–298, 1981.
7. Bonnel, F., Allieu, Y., Bruner, P., Gilbert, A., and Rabischong, P.: Anatomical and surgical principles of the brachial plexus in newborn children. Int. J. Microsurg., 2:12–15, 1980.
8. Bonnel, R., Allieu, Y., Sugata, Y., and Rabischong, P.: Anatomico-surgical basis of neurotizations for root avulsions. Anat. Clin., 1:291–296, 1979.
9. Brunelli, G.: Neurotization of avulsed roots of brachial plexus with nerves of cervical plexus. Oberval Ed. New Techniques in Microsurgery. 1979, pp. 145–148.
10. Celli, L., Mingione, A., and Landi, A.: Nuove acquisizioni di tecnica chirurgica nelle lesioni del plesso brachiale: indicazioni alla neurolisi autonest. E Trapianti Nervosi Clinica Orthopedica dell Universita di Modena, 1979, pp. 1–7.
11. Kotani, P. T., Matsuda, H., and Suzuki, T.: Trial surgical procedures of nerve transfer to avulsion injuries of the plexus brachialis. Orthopaedic Surgery and Traumatology. Proceedings of the 12th Congress of the International Society of Orthopaedic Surgery and Traumatology, Tel Aviv. 1972, pp. 348–350.
12. Mansat, M., LeBarbier, P., and Mansat, A.: Mécanismes lésionnels dans les traumatismes fermes du plexus brachial. Les lésions traumatiques des nerfs périphériques. Mongraphie du Groupe d'Etude de la Main. Expansion Scientifique, Française Ed., 1979, pp. 157–164.
13. Narakas, A.: Plexo braquial, terapeutica quirugica directa tecnica. Indicacion operatoria, resultados cirurgia de las nervios perifericos, 1972, 339–404.
14. Narakas, A.: Surgical treatment of traction injuries of the brachial plexus. Clin. Orthop., 133:71–90, 1978.
15. Narakas, A. Third symposium on lesions of the brachial plexus. Int. J. Microsurg., 2:103–106, 1972 (Abstract).
16. Seddon, H. J.: Nerve grafting. J. Bone Joint Surg., 45–B:447–461, 1963.
17. Seddon, H. J.: Surgical Disorders of the Peripheral Nerves. Edinburgh, Churchill Livingstone, 1972.
18. Tsuyama, N., and Hara, T.: Intercostal nerve transfer in the treatment of brachial plexus injury of the root avulsion type. Orthopaedic Surgery and Traumatology. Proceedings of the 12th Congress of the International Society of Orthopaedic Surgery and Traumatology, Tel Aviv, 1972, pp. 351–353.

30

Intercostal Neurotization of the Peripheral Nerves in Avulsion Plexus Injuries

■

Vinko V. Dolenc, M.D., Ph.D.

Surgical treatment of brachial plexus lesions, especially those involving avulsion of the roots, constitutes a newly introduced microsurgical field, which has been given increasing attention in the last decade.

The level of the morphologic interruption of the nerve structures is the most important factor influencing the functional results of constructive or reconstructive surgery. The lesion may lie anywhere along the brachial plexus structures, from the spinal cord down to the formed peripheral nerves in the axilla supplying the upper extremity. Traction lesions, implying division of the rootlets at the point of connection with the spinal cord at the ventral rootlet entry zone (VREZ) and at the dorsal rootlet entry zone (DREZ), pose the most demanding problems for surgical reconstruction.

The level of the lesion dictates the type of surgery to be employed: either reconstructive, in cases in which the upper stump is preserved and the lesion lies distal to the spinal ganglia, or constructive, in cases of avulsion injury, in which the lesion is located central to the spinal ganglia at the rootlet entry zone (REZ). In the latter we have to look for new sources of neurotization, e.g., the intercostal nerves.

The clinical picture of paralysis affecting the upper extremity may be the same even though the injury occurs at various levels of the brachial plexus. Usually, the injury to the brachial plexus involves various segments at various levels. There is a direct and logical relation between the distribution and extent of the injury and the direction and amount of the injury-producing force exerted upon the individual structures. Sudden violent downward or upward pulling of the arm causes avulsion of the upper roots, which may be associated with laceration of the lower roots and vice versa. Avulsion of all roots of the brachial plexus occurs, although rarely, as a result of very violent and sudden pulling of the arm with the head/or neck turned to the opposite side.

The diagnostic procedures for determining the exact location and degree of the brachial plexus lesion comprise thorough clinical neurologic examinations: electromyography (EMG), electroneurography, and cervical myelography. The presence of clinical signs suggesting accompanying bone and/or vascular lesions calls for further appropriate diagnostic evaluation. The diagnostic procedures should be carried out within the third to fifth week following injury to the brachial plexus. Surgery, if required, should be performed very soon after injury, so that valuable time is not lost. Thanks to accurate and timely diagnosis followed by appropriate surgical therapy, the patient can begin physiotherapy at the end of the second month after injury. Intensive physiotherapy should occupy most of the patient's time over the ensuing 2 to 3 years.

DIAGNOSTIC PROCEDURES

By determining the distribution and the severity of the neurologic deficits, we can at

425

least approximately evaluate the degree and level of the brachial plexus injury. Differentiation of laceration of the brachial plexus from avulsion of the roots is not possible on clinical grounds alone. When the EMG findings accord with those of electroneurography, the lesion is very likely situated peripheral to the spinal ganglia. EMG findings evidencing complete denervation in one or several segments, in the presence of normal electroneurographic findings in the same distribution, suggest avulsion of the root(s). In such cases, further diagnostic proof is supplied by positive cervical myelography. At the point of root avulsion where the dura and the arachnoidea have been torn, contrast medium is seen to escape from the spinal channel along the root sleeves into the paravertebral space (Fig. 30–1).

With cervical myelography, pseudocysts are visualized paravertebrally. Normal myelographic findings do not exclude the presence of the suspected avulsion of the root(s).

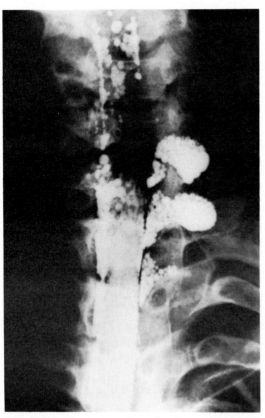

Figure 30–1. Cervical myelography shows pseudocysts paravertebrally on the left side at the level of C7, C8, and T1. A filling defect is seen at the level of C6 and C7 more to the left side of the spinal canal.

More reliable, although not absolute, confirmation of the avulsion of the root(s) is provided by positive myelographic findings, i.e., visualization of the escape of contrast medium from the subarachnoid space of the cervical segment of the spinal channel through the lateral foramina. A filling defect (Fig. 30–1), either observed at the same level as the paravertebral cysts accompanying avulsion of the roots or visualized slightly more proximally or distally in the cervical portion of the spinal channel, is not suggestive of a hematoma situated in the spinal channel (epidurally), as was often believed in the past, but indicates that the passage of the contrast medium is possibly obstructed by the torn or adherent arachnoidea.

CLASSIFICATION OF PATIENTS

During the period from 1972 to 1980, 158 patients with lesions of the brachial plexus were operated on by the author. Patients with avulsion of the roots were divided into three groups (A, B, and C), whereas patients with more peripheral lesions were placed in a separate group (D). The groups were further classified as follows: Group A comprised 31 patients with avulsion of all the C5–T1 nerve roots of the brachial plexus. Group B consisted of 25 patients with avulsion of either one, two, three, or four roots and complete laceration (interruption) of the nonavulsed roots of the brachial plexus. Complete paralysis of the affected upper extremity was the finding shared by Groups A and B. Group C comprised ten patients: seven patients with avulsion and/or laceration situated very close to the spinal cord of the proximal roots C5 and C6, and three patients with the same lesion of the two distal roots C8 and T1 but with the other three roots and other structures of the brachial plexus being morphologically and functionally almost completely intact. Group D consisted of 92 patients who sustained local injuries to the brachial plexus, such as stab wounds, gunshot wounds, fracture of the clavicle, dislocation of the humerus at the shoulder, etc. Their neurologic deficits varied widely, ranging from the loss of function of a single component (e.g., axillary nerve) to complete paralysis of the arm corresponding to the underlying morphologic lesion of the brachial plexus.

SURGERY

As indicated in Figure 30–2, the line of skin incision for the entire brachial plexus exposure begins at the mid-third of the sternocleidomastoid muscle and runs along its lateral aspect down the clavicle, crosses the clavicle, and in the pectoral region turns laterally in the direction of the axilla. It proceeds from the axillary crease down the inner aspect of the arm, thus permitting exposure of all the peripheral nerves of the upper extremity at the level where normal anatomic conditions of the nerves, veins, and arteries are preserved. The thoracic extension of the skin incision along the dorsal axillary line of the chest wall is not made unless one is certain that the intercostal nerves will be needed for surgical repair. In that case the incision is carried down as far as necessary but not beyond the level of T10. The pectoralis major muscle is divided in the tendinous part near its insertion in the humerus. After being separated from the deltoid muscle and the cephalic vein, the medial part of the muscle is rotated medially. When both the pectoralis major and the pectoralis minor muscles are divided, enough tissue should be left laterally for a firm repair at the time of closure. There is no need to divide the clavicle and the subclavius muscle. At oper-

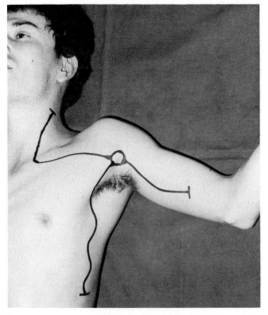

Figure 30–2. The line of skin incision for exploration of the entire brachial plexus, intercostal nerves, and peripheral nerves of the upper arm.

ation, the shoulder is moved up and down to permit visualization of the plexus situated below and behind the clavicle. We expose the trunks and the roots of the brachial plexus by supraclavicular division of the platysma as well as of the anterior scalene muscle, taking care not to compromise the phrenic nerve, which is usually situated on the medial half of the anterior aspect of the muscle. There is no need to sever the omohyoid muscle, as it can be pushed upwards and backwards. Usually, division and ligation of the cephalic vein and the external jugular vein are required.

Dissection of the brachial plexus begins at the upper third of the upper arm, with exposure of the main nerve and vascular structures. We proceed upwards to the pectoral, supraclavicular, and paravertebral regions. After ascertaining that the avulsed root(s) will have to be reconstructed by means of the intercostal nerves, we proceed to dissect these nerves, using horizontal incisions made between the bundles of the serratus muscle and extended to the intercostal space(s). After pushing apart the ribs, blunt dissection through the external and internal intercostal muscles is used to reach the lower intercostal margin. The intercostal nerve is exposed and divided. The distal end of the proximal stump is pulled out above the muscles. This is made possible by additional dissection of the nerve backwards along the rib. Utmost care must be taken not to damage the intercostal artery adjacent to the nerve and/or pleura. Every attempt should be made to leave the lymph nodes and the veins in the axilla intact. Therefore, the brachial plexus is dissected as laterally as possible, and the dissection of the intercostal nerves begins in the third intercostal space.

Twenty-two of 31 Group A patients with avulsion of all the C5–T1 nerve roots underwent repair of axillary, musculocutaneous, radial, and median or ulnar nerves. For grafts, both sural nerves from the lower extremity and the ulnar or median nerve from the affected upper extremity were employed. One graft only was used for connecting the axillary nerve to the third intercostal nerve and the musculocutaneous nerve to the fourth intercostal nerve. The radial nerve and the ulnar and median nerves were repaired with three grafts and three intercostal nerves each (Fig. 30–3). In all cases the so-called proximal coaptation between the intercostal nerves and grafts was done as far posteriorly

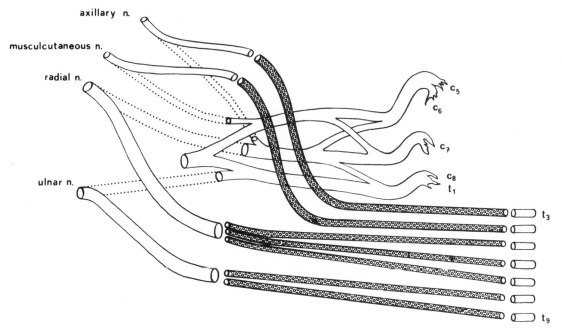

Figure 30–3. Reconstruction of individual peripheral nerves with intercostal nerves in avulsion of all the five roots of the brachial plexus. (From Dolenc, V. V.: Clin. Plast. Surg., *11*:144, 1984.)

as possible, but at least as far as the dorsal axillary line (in order to obtain more motor nerve fibers) and the distal coaptation (between the grafts and the peripheral nerves) in the axilla or on the brachium (to obtain the peripheral nerves).

Exploration of the entire brachial plexus not followed by repair was carried out in nine patients of the group. The exploration was undertaken in the hope of finding that

some of the roots were at least partially spared. However, because of severe muscular atrophy coupled with scarring of all the muscles and the lapse of more than a year from trauma to time of surgery, any functional reinnervation of the fibrosed muscles was hopeless, and surgical repair of the brachial plexus using intercostal nerves was not undertaken.

In Group B patients, avulsion of either one,

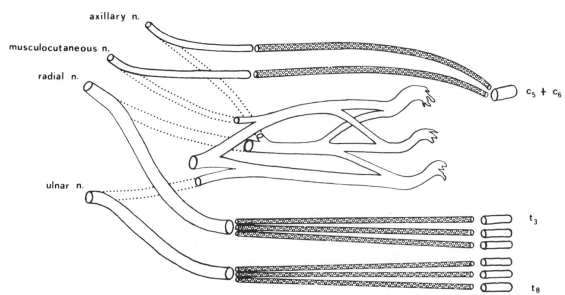

Figure 30–4. Reconstruction of individual peripheral nerves in combined injuries with avulsion of some roots and rupture of the remaining ones. (From Dolenc, V. V.: Clin. Plast. Surg., *11*:145, 1984.)

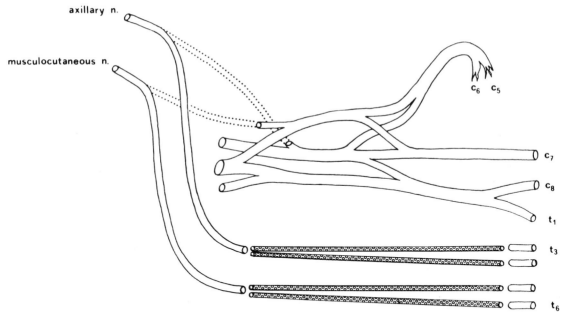

Figure 30–5. Reconstruction of the axillary nerve and musculocutaneous nerve in avulsion of the roots C5 and C6. (From Doulenc, V. V.: Clin. Plast. Surg., *11*:145, 1984.)

two, three, or four roots with the concomitant interruption of the remaining root(s) was managed by grafting the peripheral nerves and the upper stumps of the interrupted roots and the intercostal nerves when the number of the roots available was insufficient (Fig. 30–4). The latter also applied when the avulsed roots outnumbered the ruptured ones.

In Group C patients with avulsion of the upper two roots (C5, C6) but without injury to the other roots or structures of the brachial plexus, the peripheral nerves were grafted with the intercostal nerves (Fig. 30–5). The axillary nerve of the patients sustaining avul-

sion of C5 and C6 was grafted to intercostal nerves T3 and T4, whereas the musculocutanous nerve was grafted to intercostal nerves T5 and T6. In avulsion of C8 and T1, four grafts were used to repair the ulnar nerve and part of the median nerve or the medial fascicle of the brachial plexus and intercostal nerves T3–T6 (Fig. 30–6).

RESULTS

The patients operated on for avulsion of the brachial plexus were followed for 2 to 6 years. Regeneration of the peripheral nerves

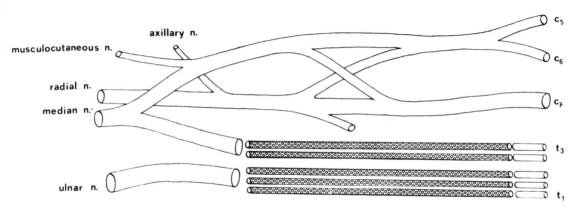

Figure 30–6. Reconstruction of individual peripheral nerves in avulsion of the roots C8 and T1. (From Doulenc, V. V.: Clin. Plast. Surg., *11*:146, 1984.)

took 4 years; however, some functional improvement was to be expected in even the fifth and sixth years postoperatively. Motor reinnervation was evaluated according to the proposed clinical criteria and rated on the 6-point scale, as follows: M0 = complete paralysis; M1 = muscular contraction without effect; M2 = muscular contraction with visible effect, excluding gravity; M3 = active movement against gravity; M4 = active movement against gravity and resistance; and M5 = active movement against strong resistance.

Return of sensory function was designated as either protective sensation or good sensory function. Pain in the affected arm was recorded separately.

All the patients with avulsion of all C5–T1 roots who underwent reconstruction of individual peripheral nerves with grafts and central stumps of intercostal nerves used the new sources of neurotization and attained good active motility in the shoulder and elbow joints but showed poorer motor function in the wrist and finger joints. Two years postoperatively none of the patients had dislocation of the shoulder (Fig. 30–7).

Active abduction of the shoulder joint was rated from M3 to M4 in all but two patients. The rates for active flexion of the elbow ranged from M3 to M4 in all but three patients. Rating of active extension in the elbow

was as follows: M4 in six patients, M3 in three patients, and M2 in four patients. Active movements in the wrist (flexion and/or extension) were rated M2 in five patients and M1 in four patients. The remaining patients could not perform any active movement of the wrist joint. Six patients were able to perform very weak, but evident, flexion movements in the interphalangeal joints, which were scored from M3 to M1. Reinnervation of the intrinsic musculature was nil.

Sensory function was restored to the level of good protective sensation in 16 patients, who no longer ran the risk of sustaining burns or other injuries because of skin anesthesia. Preoperative phantom pain was present in two patients subjected to surgical reconstruction with grafts and intercostal nerves for avulsion of all the roots of the brachial plexus. The pain gradually ceased within 4 years after surgery. The only problem experienced later was discomfort in the affected arm related to weather changes and emotional stress.

Of 25 Group B patients who underwent nerve repair by grafting peripheral nerves to intercostal nerves for complete paralysis of the upper extremity following avulsion of one to four roots with concomitant injury to the remaining root(s) or trunks, 21 patients regained function, which was rated from M4 to M1.

Similar findings were observed in restoration of sensory function. The skin of the fingers was no longer dry and rough and regained its previous moisture and elasticity. Three patients complained of occasional pain in the affected extremity, predominantly in the areas innervated by the interrupted roots of the brachial plexus; however, no adjunctive treatment was required.

Very good postoperative functional return was observed in the eight Group C patients with complete loss of function of the axillary and musculocutaneous nerves following avulsion of roots C5 and C6. All the patients performed abduction in the shoulder and flexion in the elbow joint, with the rates ranging from M2 to M4. Dislocation of the shoulder joint was no longer present and almost normal configuration of the shoulder was restored (Fig. 30–8). The two Group C patients with complete loss of function in the ulnar nerve due to avulsion of roots C8 and T1 showed good postoperative recovery. Abduction and adduction of the fingers were rated M3 (Fig. 30–9).

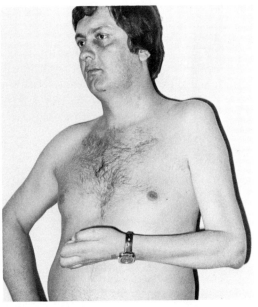

Figure 30–7. Final results 5 years after reconstruction of peripheral nerves with intercostal nerves for avulsion of all the five roots (see Fig. 30–3).

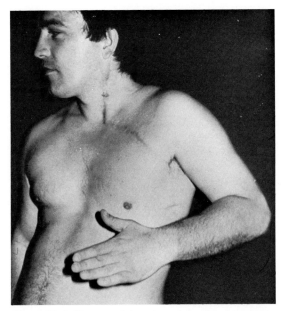

Figure 30–8. Very good function of the deltoid and the biceps muscles following intercostal neurotization (see Fig. 30–5).

All Group C patients regained good protective sensation. None of them had any pain in the areas supplied by the nerves that had sustained root avulsion.

No patient in Groups A, B, or C experienced problems in either the areas innervated by the sural nerves used in grafting or the areas supplied by the intercostal nerves, the central stumps of which had been used for the neurotization of the denervated skin and muscles of the paralyzed arm.

DISCUSSION

Injuries to the brachial plexus are the third most frequent cause of lesions of the peripheral nervous system, following closely injuries to the median and ulnar nerves. About 75% of brachial plexus injuries require no surgical repair, since appropriate physiotherapy can restore either complete or satisfactory function of the affected upper extremity. Only 25% of the patients sustaining trauma to the brachial plexus require surgical therapy. Of all the patients with morphologic interruption of the brachial plexus structures, at least 60% show lesions of the structures distal to the roots. The other 40% have injuries associated with avulsion of the root(s). The great majority of patients with avulsion of the root(s) need surgical repair of individual peripheral nerves by means of grafts and new sources of neurotization. So far, the

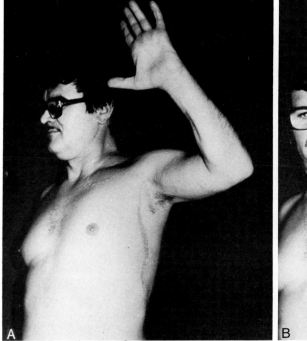
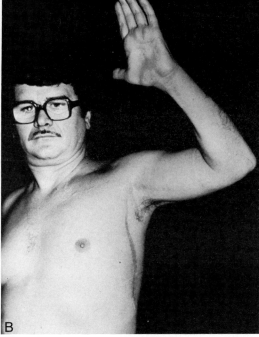

Figure 30–9. Functional return following reconstruction with intercostal nerves for avulsion of the roots C8 and T1 (see Fig. 30–6). Note the satisfactory extension in the metacarpophalangeal joints of the fourth and fifth fingers as well as abduction (*A*) and adduction (*B*) of the fifth finger.

intercostal nerves have proved to be the most suitable source for neurotization of the degenerated peripheral nerves arising from groups of axons of the avulsed roots. The most frequent problem connected with this technique of peripheral nerve reconstruction, however, is the low number of available motor axons.

In avulsion of all the roots, the number of axons of the intercostal nerves ipsilateral to the injured brachial plexus is too small to match the number of axons of the peripheral nerves. In patients requiring neurotization of the nerves of only one or two avulsed proximal roots (C5 and C6), a single nerve, e.g., the axillary and/or the musculocutaneous nerve, is repaired with two or three intercostal nerves. Similarly, in patients with injury to the ulnar nerve and partial damage of the median nerve with avulsion of the lower roots (C8 and T1), several intercostal nerves can be employed for one peripheral nerve of the arm. The procedure, however, is complicated by the disproportion between the number of axons of the intercostal and peripheral nerves and the distance of the effector muscles. In avulsion of three or more roots, neurotization with intercostal nerves proves inadequate because of the insufficient number of axons and the length of the individual nerves (e.g., the radial, median, and ulnar nerves) and therefore fails to create conditions conducive to good, or at least satisfactory, reinnervation of denervated muscles of the upper arm and, to a still lesser degree, of the hand.

The most severe cases of avulsion of all the roots and those cases involving two, three, or four roots and interruption of the other roots have both proved refractory to successful reconstruction that would restore useful active motion of the fingers of the affected arm. This does not imply that no reinnervation at all occurs in the musculature of the forearm and hand, but rather that it is of no use to the patient. In patients sustaining avulsion of the two proximal roots of the brachial plexus, as well as those with more serious injuries involving avulsion of several or all the roots, good and useful reinnervation of the denervated muscles situated on the upper arm was observed after repair with intercostal nerves. The function of the deltoid muscle improves so as to enable a certain range of active abduction and prevent subluxation in the shoulder joint. Still better movement can be produced in combination

with anteflexion. Active flexion in the elbow and visible clinical contraction of the biceps muscle are further evidence of good intercostal neurotization of the muscles of the arm.

Reinnervation of the muscles of the forearm and hand more peripherally attains a certain degree of useful contraction in patients with avulsions of either one or two roots, whereas reinnervation fails to occur in patients with avulsions of all the roots of the brachial plexus. The problem of poor reinnervation of the distal musculature of the forearm and hand is due not only in the scarcity of axons, which take a very long time to reach the denervated and scarred muscles, but also to the patient's inability to employ the reinnervated muscles and his failure to perform active movements by making use of the intercostal axons. The post-trauma muscular wasting, which was observed in all patients, was reduced in many cases later, so that some muscular contraction was inducible by electrical stimulation of the corresponding nerve. On the other hand, the patients were unable to produce voluntary contractions. The earlier mentioned muscular contractions were carried out only in combination with forced inhalation. Patients with the muscles of the upper arm reinnervated exclusively by means of intercostal neurotization were able to produce abduction in the shoulder to a greater or lesser degree and perform flexion in the elbow when breathing normally. With forced inhalation the range of the two movements was considerably increased. Movement of the arm more distal to the elbow was not performed unless assisted by forced inhalation. The problem lies not only in the inadequate reinnervation of the distal musculature following intercostal neurotization of the injured peripheral nerves of the arm, but also in the patient's incomplete re-education and lack of adjustment to altered body image. Further difficulties arise when the more distal intercostal nerves are employed to reinnervate the more distal muscles of the upper extremity. The final outcome of rehabilitation is compromised by the cumulative effect of the deficient number of axons and the distance of the effectors, as well as by the negative influence of the intricate function of the muscles or groups of muscles producing movements of the fingers, which are much more sophisticated than the relatively simple abduction in the shoulder joint and flexion in the elbow.

Inability to carry out voluntary contraction

despite good reinnervation of the previously denervated muscles was observed in some patients who had direct reconstruction or repair by grafting of the same groups of axons of the proximal and distal ends for interruption of the more distal structures of the brachial plexus. The fact that regeneration of the previously degenerated axons of the distal end is affected by the corresponding groups of axons of the upper stump suggests that the patient forgets particular movements as a result of the long interruption of "the center-periphery line" and is unable to reproduce them even after anatomic continuity has been restored and function of the peripheral neuron regained. In some patients hypnosis has proved successful for the recall of the forgotten movements. This seems to apply also to patients in whom the intercostal nerves were used as the new source of neurotization of injured nerves.

In addition to various forms of physiotherapy used to restore the function of the paralyzed extremity, ranging from passive exercises to electrical stimulation, breathing exercises were included in the program to make the patients realize that the activation of the intercostal nerves on the side of the reconstructed brachial plexus and peripheral nerves brings into action the muscles of the affected arm. After achieving good voluntary movement with forced inhalation, the patients were subjected to hypnotherapy designed to enable them to produce particular movement(s) by means of normal breathing. Hypnosis was only partially effective. None of the patients was able to achieve "full command" of the primary function of the intercostal nerves employed in neurotization of the arm and make full use of it in order to perform voluntary contraction of the arm muscles.

Clinical as well as electromyographic improvement in voluntary contraction was found when forced inhalation was used, although fairly good movements were also obtained with normal breathing. The effect seems to be better if structures pertaining to the two related functions are in close proximity. Therefore, in rupture of two roots with concomitant avulsion of the remaining three roots, the former are reconstructed by connecting the proximal root ends to the distal ones or to the corresponding nerves via grafts. Central stumps of the divided roots are employed for neurotization of at least one of the avulsed roots. Thus, better reinervation can be expected as a result of the lesser difference in function between the two cervical roots as compared with that between the cervical root and the intercostal nerves. Another advantage of this procedure is that more intercostal nerves are available for reconstruction of fewer remaining avulsed roots.

CONCLUSIONS

The major problem of functional restoration of the brachial plexus nerves in cases of avulsion of the roots is the inadequate neurotization of the affected nerves because the number of axons of the peripheral nerves greatly exceeds that of the axons of the intercostal nerves. As a result of this disproportion, when treating avulsion of all the roots of the brachial plexus, it is advisable to reconstruct only some of the nerves (e.g., the axillary, musculocutaneous, median, and, possibly, the radial nerve) and sacrifice the ulnar nerve for grafts. Ideally, better use should be made of the scarce axons of the intercostal nerves. This aim is attainable only by the most meticulous microsurgical grafting of the intercostal nerves with the individual bundles of the major peripheral nerves. Such reconstruction should be carried out together with stimulation of individual bundles of the peripheral nerves with the aim of determining which of the groups of fibers are responsible for individual movements. The procedure should be carried out not later than 1 to 2 weeks after injury, when at least some axons have not yet undergone Wallerian degeneration. In the first week after injury, one cannot determine with certainty, either by clinical examination or by electromyography, whether the patient with complete paralysis and sensory loss over the arm has sustained an avulsion of the roots or an injury to the brachial plexus more distally. The diagnostic tools currently employed for early recognition of the nerve injury are somatosensory evoked potentials, cervical myelography, and operative exploration. The latter is diagnostically the most reliable procedure and should be planned so that in cases of avulsion of the roots or serious damage to other structures of the brachial plexus, surgery can be modified from a diagnostic to a therapeutic procedure.

A universally adopted code of management of brachial plexus lesions is still lacking. Yet all of us who daily encounter the severe disability secondary brachial plexus trauma that arises despite meticulous microsurgical technique and prolonged and persistent physiotherapy and who realize that a wide range of unknown underlying biologic factors interfere with the final outcome of therapy are aware that the problem cannot be solved by current operative and/or physiotherapy measures only. We need to optimize our knowledge and facilities and exploit every new achievement in the field. The road traveled so far has been short but broad, and no person can see its end.

31

Neurotization of Avulsed Roots of the Brachial Plexus by Means of Anterior Nerves of the Cervical Plexus

■

Giorgio Brunelli, M.D., F.I.C.S., F.A.S.S.H.

At times, the surgeon repairing brachial plexus lesions cannot use sutures or grafts because one, some, or all of the roots have been avulsed and the proximal stump is not visible. Until some years ago, these lesions could not be treated. However, as the palsy is irreparable without surgery, attempts are now being made to use intercostal nerves to neurotize avulsed roots.[1-4, 6-8]

Different techniques have been suggested in order to take many (four or five) intercostal nerves posteriorly before fibers are lost, but results have not been good.[5, 7, 9, 10] Even when taking five intercostal nerves posteriorly and passing them anteriorly by means of sural nerve grafts (which is a difficult, long, and bloody operation), one can count on obtaining only a small number of fibers (3000 or 4000). These fibers are mixed and motor and sensory fibers cannot be distinguished. Therefore, half the fibers will be lost.

In my experience, the first four intercostal nerves at the axillary line can supply less than 3000 fibers. As the function of many of these fibers is lost because of misconnections, one can roughly anticipate only a maximum of 1500 fibers for a brachial plexus that generally has 120,000 to 160,000 fibers. Furthermore, the motor fibers that can reach motor fibers in denervated roots (or motor branches) are semiautomatic fibers that require a very long process of cortical reorgan-

ization. Therefore, effectiveness of neurotization remains more theoretical than practical, and clinical results are very poor.

This very poor supply of fibers can provide only very weak movement—and only if all these fibers are distributed on only one nerve (e.g., the musculocutaneous nerve for biceps movement). If the fibers are distributed on more than one nerve, no useful movement is obtained because of extreme weakness and co-contractions with antagonist muscles.

For these reasons and in order to be able to perform a quicker and less traumatic operation, I wanted to utilize other donor nerves. I therefore studied the possibility of using some nerves of the cervical plexus in order to neurotize the brachial plexus.[3] Only anterior nerves of cervical plexus can be found and used. The cervical plexus most often has eight anterior superficial nerves, four motor (Fig. 31–1) and four sensory. These are the motor nerves for the sternocleidomastoid, trapezius, levator scapulae, and rhomboid muscles and the auricular, transverse cervical, supraclavicular, and supra-acromial sensory nerves. To determine if and to what extent classic anatomy of these small nerves could be validated, 12 cervical plexuses in cadavers were dissected to confirm the existence of these nerves and their possible variations. Myelinated fibers of each nerve were counted to determine how many

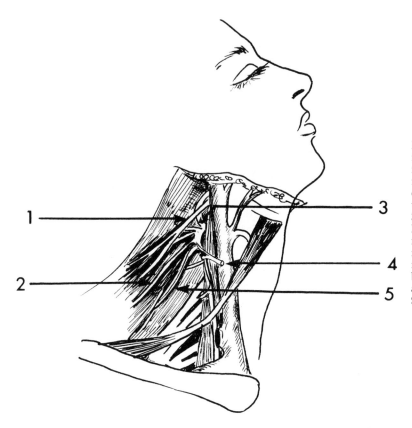

Figure 31–1. The five motor nerves that can be used to neurotize avulsed brachial plexus roots: 1 = cranial nerve XI (accessory) nerve, 2 = nerve of cervical plexus to trapezius muscle, 3 = nerve of cervical plexus to levator scapulae muscle, 4 = nerve of cervical plexus to sternocleidomastoid muscle, 5 = nerve of cervical plexus to rhomboid muscle. (From Brunelli, G., and Monini, L.: Clin. Plast. Surg., *11*:150, 1984.)

fibers would be available if these nerves were used as donor nerves. Results were as follows:

Sensory Nerves:

One, two, or more supra-acromial nerves, for an average of 560 fibers.

One, two, or more supraclavicular nerves, for an average of 620 fibers.

One auricular nerve, for an average of 740 fibers.

One transverse cervical nerve, for an average of 730 fibers.

Possibly other small sensory nerves, for an average of 600 fibers.

Motor Nerves:

One nerve to the sternocleidomastoid muscle, for an average of 800 fibers.

One or more (often two to five) small nerves to the rhomboid muscle, for an average of 880 fibers.

One nerve to the levator scapulae muscle, for an average of 920 fibers.

One nerve to the trapezius muscle, for an average of 740 fibers.

Possibly other motor nerves arising from the anterior aspect of the third cervical ansa, for an average of 750 fibers.

Totals: 3250 sensory fibers and 4090 motor fibers.

Clinical observations, together with the anatomic dissection, showed that in some cases all the nerves of the cervical plexus were very large, whereas in other cases they were very small. The superior nerve for the sternocleidomastoid muscle sometimes was absent. The nerve for the rhomboid muscle was absent in one case, was very large in three cases, and was made up of many small nerves in several cases. The levator scapulae muscle was often absent. In many cases it was possible to find and to electrically stimulate other motor nerves for posterior muscles that were large enough to be used as donor nerves for neurotization. Thus, the motor nerves for the sternocleidomastoid, trapezius, levator scapulae, and rhomboid muscles and the sensory auricular, transverse cervical, supraclavicular, and supra-acromial nerves can be easily recognized by their anatomic position and their response to electrical stimulation.

Anatomic research and clinical experience have shown that severance of these four sensory nerves results in a narrow, irregular area of anesthesia that extends from the ear to the acromion. The borders of this area are partly replaced distally by T1 and medially by contralateral C3. Severance of the four motor nerves causes a partial palsy of the trapezius and sternocleidomastoid muscles (which are also innervated by the spinal accessory nerve) and of the rhomboid and levator scapulae muscles, which are innervated by the brachial plexus.

SURGICAL TECHNIQUE

A large incision is necessary, extending from the subclavicular region to the cranial part of the sternocleidomastoid muscle, in order to expose both the third cervical ansa (from which the nerves to be taken originate) and the distal terminal nerves of the brachial plexus (which are to be neurotized). As mentioned previously, many anatomic variations are possible. Superficial sensory nerves can be found easily and cut as distally as possible. However, motor nerves have to be searched for by careful dissection and with the help of electrical stimulation to ascertain that they are indeed motor nerves. Then the terminal nerves to be neurotized must be found and cut as proximally as possible. For motor nerves, a connection between the donor and recipient nerves has to be made by means of sural nerve grafts. Because of their greater length, sensory nerves generally can be directly sutured on the median nerve. The combination of neurotizations of different donor nerves on different recipient terminal nerves and the search for and use of the eleventh cranial nerve (to be discussed) will be adapted to the severity of each individual case.

Using these eight nerves provides many advantages:

1. A great number of fibers are available.
2. Anastomosis of well-defined pure motor and sensory nerves is possible.
3. The motor nerves are voluntary motor nerves with autonomous function (see Fig. 31–4).
4. In some cases direct anastomoses (without grafts) are possible, especially for sensory nerves.

In brief, approximately 4100 motor fibers and 3250 sensory fibers are available that we can easily recognize and correctly distribute on nerves to be neurotized without making errors during connection or causing loss of function.

Initially, I tried to neurotize C5 and C6 roots by suturing the sensory nerves on the posterior part of the avulsed roots distal to ganglions and by suturing the motor nerves on the anterior part. This was a mistake because the roots are made up of a very large number of mixed fibers that were impossible to differentiate. As a result, neurotization was not worthwhile because the function of many of the fibers was destroyed. I now distribute the motor nerves on well-chosen distal branches of the plexus whose fibers are easily identified (e.g., the nerves of the trapezius and rhomboid muscles on the suprascapular nerve in order to stabilize the shoulder and the nerves of the sternocleidomastoid and levator scapulae muscles on the musculocutaneous nerve in order to obtain flexion of the elbow while all the sensory fibers are sutured to the median nerve in order to restore some sensibility to the hand).

Another technique is that of neurotizing the axillary nerve in order to obtain abduction of the arm by means of the eleventh cranial nerve (Figs. 31–2 to 31–8). In other cases the spinal accessory nerve can be transferred on the musculocutaneous nerve while the axillary nerve is neurotized by means of nerves of the sternocleidomastoid and levator scapulae muscles. The eleventh cranial nerve must also be taken when one of the nerves of the cervical plexus is too short or is absent. All sensory nerves are brought onto the median nerve.

Twenty-nine patients have been operated on since 1977. As at least 3 years of follow-up are required to obtain complete results in brachial plexus injuries and as the initial technique was incorrect (distributing the donor nerves on several roots and losing most of the fibers), the results are only now becoming significant.

The donors used for the neurotization of the brachial plexus by means of superficial nerves of the cervical plexus are much richer than those used for neurotization by means of intercostal nerves.

By converging the motor fibers on two or three motor nerves and the sensory fibers on the median nerve, the best results are obtained, even if they are limited results because of the severity of the lesions (Fig. 31–9). Limited avulsions of one or two roots can give better results, as the same number of donor axons are available to neurotize a smaller number of distal avulsed axons. If only one root is avulsed, this root can be neurotized, rather than peripheral nerves, and a good result is anticipated (Fig. 31–10). On the other hand, in total avulsions (or

Text continued on page 444

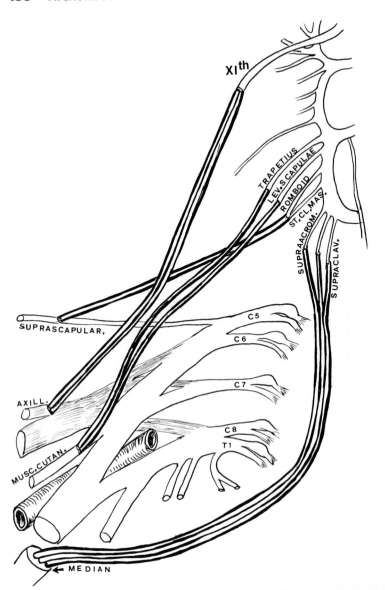

Figure 31–2. Scheme of typical neurotization for total avulsion of the brachial plexus. In other cases, cranial nerve XI can lead to the musculocutaneous nerve. (From Brunelli, G., and Monini, L.: Clin. Plast. Surg., *11*:151, 1984.)

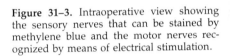

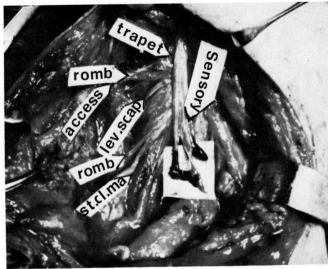

Figure 31–3. Intraoperative view showing the sensory nerves that can be stained by methylene blue and the motor nerves recognized by means of electrical stimulation.

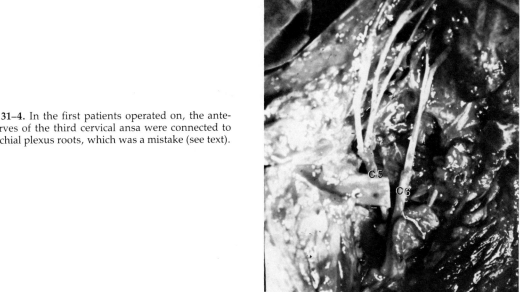

Figure 31–4. In the first patients operated on, the anterior nerves of the third cervical ansa were connected to the brachial plexus roots, which was a mistake (see text).

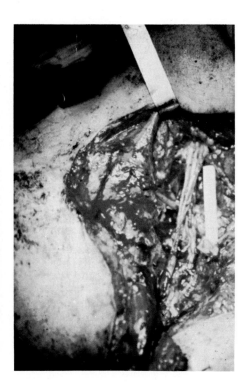

Figure 31–5. Example of connection with the distal branches of the brachial plexus.

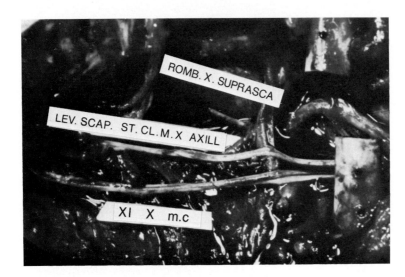

Figure 31–6. Another example of connection of the anterior nerves of the third cervical ansa to distal branches of the brachial plexus by means of sural nerve grafts.

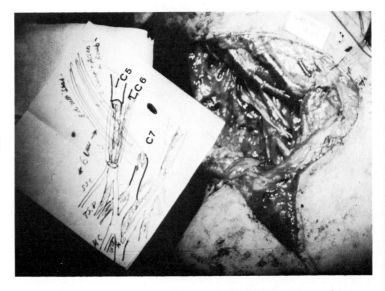

Figure 31–7. Another example in which roots C5 and C6 were found (C7 was missing) and were neurotized by means of the third cervical ansa.

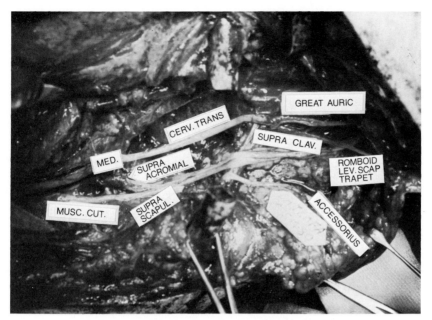

Figure 31–8. Surgical view showing the repair done.

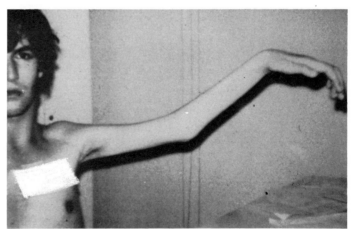

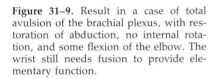

Figure 31–9. Result in a case of total avulsion of the brachial plexus, with restoration of abduction, no internal rotation, and some flexion of the elbow. The wrist still needs fusion to provide elementary function.

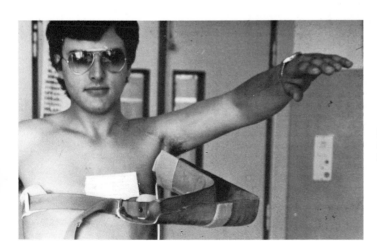

Figure 31–10. Result at 6 months in a case of isolated avulsion of C5 neurotized by means of cervical nerves.

Table 31–1. NEUROTIZATION OF AVULSED BRACHIAL PLEXUS BY ANTERIOR CERVICAL NERVES: MOTOR RECOVERY*

No. of Cases	Neurotized Nerve	Donor Nerves	Result	Other Neurotized Nerve	Donor Nerves	Result
Total palsy (5)†	1 Suprasc.	Rhomboid, lev. scap.	Active abduction 45°; no intrarot.	MC	SCM, trapezius	Elbow Act. Flex. to 90°
	1 Suprasc.	Rhomboid, lev. scap.	Act. abd. 35°; no intrarot.	MC	SCM, trapezius	Elbow Act. Flex. to 80°
Upper palsy (21)‡	1 Suprasc.	Rhomboid (3), lev. scap.	Act. abd. 50°, slight; no intrarot.	MC	11th cranial (no SCM)	Elbow Act. Flex. to 80°
	1 Suprasc.	Rhomboid (4), lev. scap.	Act. abd. 50°; no intrarot.	MC	SCM, trapezius	Elbow Act. Flex. to 100°
	1 Suprasc.	Rhomboid (1), SCM	Act. abd. 45°; no intrarot.	MC	Lev. scap., trapezius	Elbow Act. Flex. to 80°
	1 Suprasc.	Rhomboid (1), SCM	Act. abd. 30°; no intrarot.	MC	Lev. scap., trapezius	Elbow Act. Flex. to 70°
	1 Suprasc.	Rhomboid (3), lev. scap.	Act. abd. 80°, impossible; intrarot.	MC	SCM, trapezius	Elbow Act. Flex. to 80°
	1 Suprasc.	Rhomboid (1), SCM	Act. abd. 50°; no intrarot.	MC	Lev. scap., trapezius	Elbow Act. Flex. to 90°

1 Suprasc.	Rhomboid (4), trapezius	Act. abd. 50°; no intrarot.	MC	Lev. scap., SCM	Elbow Act. Flex. to 80°
1 Suprasc.	Rhomboid (1), trapezius	Act. abd. 50°; no intrarot.	MC	Lev. scap., SCM	Elbow Act. Flex. to 100°
1 Suprasc.	Rhomboid (4), trapezius	Act. abd. 60°; no intrarot.	MC	Lev. scap., SCM	Elbow Act. Flex. to 90°
1 Suprasc.	Rhomboid (2), trapezius	Act. abd. 45°; no intrarot.	MC	Lev. scap., SCM	Elbow Act. Flex. to 30°
1 Suprasc.	Rhomboid (4)	Act. abd. 45°; no intrarot.	MC	Lev. scap., SCM	Elbow Act. Flex. to 90°
Radialis	11th cranial	Elbow ext. 3–4			
Lower palsy (3)§ 1 Median nerve	Rhomboid, trapezius	Unchanged	Ulnar	Lev. scap., SCM	Unchanged
1 Median nerve	Rhomboid, trapezius, Lev. scap., SCM	Extrinsic flexor 2–3			

*Total of 29 cases: 18 assessed; 11 too recent to be assessed.
†Three operated on by earlier technique; poor results not taken into consideration.
‡Ten too recent to be assessed.
§One too recent to be assessed.
MC = musculocutaneous; SCM = sternocleidomastoid; lev. scap. = levator scapulae.
Suprasc. = suprascapular; intrarot. = internal rotation.
Axillary recovery due to cranial nerve XI has not been evaluated in this table.

Table 31–2. NEUROTIZATION OF AVULSED BRACHIAL PLEXUS BY ANTERIOR CERVICAL NERVES: SENSORY RECOVERY*

No. of Cases	Neurotized Nerve	Protective Sensibility	Two-Point Discrimination	Area of Reinnervation	Paresthesia
Total palsy (5)†	1 Median	Yes	No	Palm of hand	Paresthesia in donor area
	1 Median	Yes	No	Proximal hand	No
Upper palsy (21)‡	1 Median	No	No		No
	1 Median	No	No		No
	1 Median	Yes	30 mm. (?)	Hand and fingers	No
	1 Median	Yes	No	Proximal part of palm	Paresthesia of hand
	1 Median	Yes	No	Palm of hand	No
	1 Median	Yes	30 mm. (?)	Hand and fingers	Paresthesia in donor area
	1 Median	Yes	No	Palm and index finger (?)	No
	1 Median	Yes	No	Palm and fingers	No
	1 Median	Yes	No	Palm	Pain in palm
	1 Median	No	No		Paresthesia in hand
	1 Median	No	No		No
Lower palsy (3)§	1 Median	No	No		Paresthesia in hand
	1 Median	Yes	No	Palm of hand	No

*Total of 29 cases: 18 assessed; 11 too recent to be assessed.
†Three operated on by earlier technique; poor results not taken into consideration.
‡Ten too recent to be assessed.
§One too recent to be assessed.

large avulsions), the number of donor fibers available must be carefully assessed and the neurotization limited to a few well-chosen muscles, or the results will be unsatisfactory. Of course the results assessed as good are satisfactory only as related to the single muscles, whereas function of the limb is very poor. Nevertheless, this is still a useful result compared with the previous situation of total palsy. As results are not yet standardized, one can only compare the present state with the previous palsy or with the results one could expect by the neurotization by means of intercostal nerves. This comparison seems to show that much better results can be anticipated when cervical nerve transfer is used.

Results are outlined in Tables 31–1 and 31–2.

SUMMARY

Using nerves of the cervical plexus to neurotize the brachial plexus provides a certain number of well-differentiated sensory and voluntary motor fibers. The number of fibers is certainly less than that of a normal plexus but is much more and of much better quality than that obtainable using intercostal nerves. If we distribute these fibers on well-chosen branches of the brachial plexus, limiting the neurotization to a few selected structures, useful recovery of essential movements of the shoulder and elbow is possible. Sensation of the hand will also recur to a certain extent. Subsequent palliative operations (e.g., different types of arthrodeses) can provide a limb that can be useful even if still paralyzed and severely impaired.

References

1. Alnot, J. Y., et al.: Étude clinique et paraclinique plus evolution spontanée des paralysies du plexus brachial. 50th Reun. Ann. S.O.F.C.O.T., Paris, November, 1975, p. 4.
2. Alnot, J. Y., Mansat, M., Huten, B., Bonnel, F., Narakas, A., Cadre, N., Sedel, L., Millesi, H., and

Allieu, Y.: Simposium sur la paralisie traumatique du plexus brachial chez l'adulte. Rev. Chir. Orthop., *63*:19–126, 1977.

3. Brunelli, G.: Neurotization of avulsed roots of the brachial plexus by means of anterior nerves of the cervical plexus. Int. J. Microsurg., *2*:55–58, 1980.
4. Gilbert, A., Khouri, N., and Carlioz, H.: Exploration chirurgicale du plexus brachial dans la paralisie obstétricale. Rev. Chir. Orthop., *66*:33–43, 1980.
5. Jaeger, R., and Whiteley, W. H.: Avulsion of the brachial plexus. J.A.M.A., *153*:633, 1953.
6. Mendelsohn, R. A., Weiner, J. H., and Keegan, J. M.: Myelographic demonstration of brachial plexus root avulsion. Arch. Surg., *75*:102, 1957.
7. Millesi, H.: Surgical management of brachial plexus injuries. J. Hand. Surg., *2*:367, 1977.
8. Narakas, A.: Plexo brachial. Terapéutica quirùrgica directa. Técnica. Indication operatoria. Resultados. Rev. Orthop. Traumat., *16*:855–921, 1972.
9. Sedel, L.: Traitement palliatif d'une serie de 103 paralysies par élongation du plexus brachial. Rev. Chir. Orthop., *63*:651–677, 1977.
10. Sunderland, S.: Nerves and Nerve Lesions. Edinburgh, Churchill Livingstone, 1972.

32

Thoughts on Neurotization or Nerve Transfers in Irreparable Nerve Lesions

■

Algimantas O. Narakas, M.D.

When a nerve is destroyed beyond repair, instead of using a musculotendinous transfer (which is not always available) to restore lost function, a nerve transfer can be performed. A normal donor nerve can be separated from muscle(s) of lesser functional value and connected to the distal stump of the nerve to be revived. A typical example of this type of transfer is the use of the hypoglossal or the spinal accessory nerve in facial nerve palsy. A sensory territory can be neurotized in the same manner with suitable donor nerves. Direct implantation of terminal rami of a motor nerve or of nerve grafts connected to the main trunk into muscle is also termed neurotization, but in this chapter we will discuss only the former method as applied to brachial plexus injuries.

The transfer of the proximal stump of an intentionally transected healthy nerve into the distal stump of an irreparably damaged one, below the site of the lesion, was first carried out in brachial plexus injuries by two British specialists, the neurologist Harris and the surgeon Low, at the turn of the century.[6] After some neurophysiologic considerations, they inserted half of the distal fascicles of the spinal nerve C5, damaged at the foramen, into the healthy spinal nerves C6 or C7 in three patients with Erb's palsy. Their results were not reported. However, the partial section of the donor nerves seemed not to have any consequences.

The American surgeon Tuttle,[17] describing one case of plexus injury in 1913, mentioned neurotization with the spinal accessory nerve as a current technique, but no other cases of nerve transfer were found by the author in a search of the literature of that period. Spontaneous neurotizations by rami of the phrenic nerve (probably the ramus leading from C5 to the phrenic nerve) were reported more than 50 years ago in obstetrical palsies. This has been observed more recently in both children and adults.

Vulpius and Stoffel,[18] in the 1920s, rerouted some of the five to seven available rami of the nerves to the pectoral muscles onto musculocutaneous or axillary nerves when they were unable to repair the nerves by direct suture. Foerster[5] used the same technique, employing in addition the nerves to latissimus dorsi or the subscapularis muscles when repairing isolated lesions of the axillary nerve.

Neither neurotization nor brachial plexus surgery seems to have been popular between World War I and World War II. The Russian surgeon Lurje[8] applied these techniques more widely in patients with Erb's palsy in the 1940s. Yeomann,[19] working with Seddon,[13] first had the idea of performing neurotization when radicular avulsions were present and used intercostal nerves for that purpose. Fantiš and Slezák[4] (and other Eastern European surgeons), followed by Kotani et al.[7] and Tsuyama and Hara,[16] also employed this technique, sometimes using the

Table 32–1. FIBER COUNTS
(APPROXIMATION) IN SOME DONOR
NERVES FOR NEUROTIZATION*

Spinal accessory terminal rami	1500–1700
One intercostal nerve	1200–1300
Long thoracic nerve (only half can be used in upper root avulsion)	1600–1800
Rami to the pectoral muscles	400–600 per ramus

*From Narakas, A. O.: Clin. Plast. Surg., *11*:154, 1984.

spinal accessory nerve for neurotization. Allieu,[1] Brunelli,[2] Celli et al.,[3] Merle,[9] Millesi,[10] Narakas,[11, 12] and Sedel,[14] as well as many other modern pioneers in brachial plexus microsurgery, currently use nerve transfers. Conclusive experimental work has been done in the dog by Tomita et al.[15]

This present chapter is an attempt to provide some guidelines based upon my experience gained after personally performing 83 nerve transfers (between 1969 and 1982) and seeing many patients with brachial plexus injuries treated by other surgeons.

NEUROANATOMIC CONSIDERATIONS

In order to obtain an acceptable reinnervation of the receptor nerve, the donor nerves(s) must supply a comparable number of motor or sensory fibers, or both. Table 32–1 gives the approximate number of myelinated fibers in the donors available for repairing brachial plexus injuries and Table 32–2 shows the number needed. At a glance, it can be seen that adequate reinnervation is beyond the capacity of the majority of the donor nerves. For example, to neurotize C5 with the eleventh cranial nerve will result in insufficient reinnervation of each muscle depending on that root. Therefore, the choice between the deficit created by depriving a

muscle of its innervation and the benefit gained by giving its innervation to another muscle or muscle group must be carefully considered.

NEUROPHYSIOLOGIC CONSIDERATIONS

If two different nerves reinnervate the same muscle, only one will ultimately function. Therefore, we cannot use the accessory nerve in conjunction with some other donor nerve(s) to reinnervate one given receptor. Nerves supplying basic needs must be selected because of the limited availability of donors. Moreover, central and peripheral contingencies must be taken into account.

Peripheral contingencies will be considered first. Some nerves, for example the radial, are made of fibers that command antagonistic muscles; primarily, the radial nerve is an elbow, wrist, and metacarpophalangeal extensor. However, it also innervates the brachioradialis and, in one third of individuals, the lateral part of brachialis muscles, which are elbow flexors. Thus, massive neurotization of the radial nerve with four or five intercostal nerves will not necessarily result in good elbow extension. The same applies to the posterior cord, which contains fibers for shoulder abduction and adduction. In addition, any given spinal nerve at the foramen contains fibers widely distributed in its neurotome. Therefore, neurotization of an avulsed root will not only interfere with the growing axons in a majority of the muscles of that root but will innervate antagonistic groups or create undesired synkinesis.

It seems that centrally, movements as such are represented and are not the function of individual muscles or muscle groups. Any movement of the upper extremity requires

Table 32–2. MYELINATED FIBER COUNTS OF ROOTS OF THE BRACHIAL PLEXUS (EXTREME VALUES) AND PERIPHERAL NERVES (APPROXIMATE VALUES)

Roots	Root Fiber Counts*	Peripheral Nerves	Peripheral Nerve Fiber Counts
C5	7000 to 33000	Suprascapular	3500
C6	12000 to 39000	Axillary	6500
C7	16000 to 40000	Musculocutaneous	6000
C8	14000 to 41000	Median	18000
T1	10000 to 35000	Ulnar	16000
		Radial	19000

*Total fiber counts in a given plexus (all five roots added) vary from 70,000 to 150,000 approximately. (From Narakas, A. O.: Clin. Plast. Surg., *11*:154, 1984.)

the modulated function of several muscle groups, integration and coordination being naturally enhanced by training. This fact is fundamental to musculotendinous transfers, particularly when an antagonist is used. Problems may arise in nerve transfer because donor nerves may not have medullary or cerebral centers that are integrated into the function of the upper extremity. My experience has shown that incorrect sutures between some nerves of the upper extremity, such as the proximal stump of the radial nerve to the distal stump of the median nerve (an error made while reimplanting a limb amputated at the shoulder), may yield a good and coordinated function, whereas neurotization with intercostal nerves, which can result in fair flexion or extension of a joint, will not allow the newly gained function to be harmoniously integrated into the other functions of the limb. It is easy for the patient to demonstrate the function gained by the use of intercostal nerves alone, but not in conjunction with the other available functions present in the extremity, with functions restored by direct repair of plexus trunks, or with functions that were never lost, as in lesions limited to some parts of the plexus.

In addition, nerves such as the intercostals have a very crude, almost binary function. It is not possible, for example, to use three intercostal nerves for elbow flexion and three others for elbow extension. When using intercostal nerves to restore sensation, it must be realized that they have a distribution of modalities different from that of the median or ulnar nerves and that the intercostal nerves are more akin to the radial nerve. The sensory zones supplied by the latter are very sensitive to the slightest touch, as is the skin supplied by the intercostals, but radial nerve dermatomes have a poor two-point discrimination and stereognosis. This applies to a much greater extent to intercostal nerves. The author has found that adult patients with musculocutaneous nerves neurotized with intercostal nerves may develop great cutaneous sensitivity to light touch (e.g., by cotton wool) but have no localization, whereas children with ulnar or median nerves neurotized with intercostal nerves may have a Weber test result of 25 to 30 mm, better than that in the zone on the chest supplied by the contralateral intercostal nerves. This fact implies that the receptor skin area plays a role in the sensory result.

Donor nerves such as the spinal accessory

nerve or the long thoracic nerve of Bell contain very few sensory fibers; nevertheless, some unusual protective type of sensation is gained while using them. This sensation is referred simultaneously to the deep scapular and shoulder area, as well as to the neurotized autonomous zone.

ANATOMICOPATHOLOGIC CONSIDERATIONS

Nerve transfers are particularly indicated in root avulsions. More than 72% of patients with supraclavicular plexus lesions have one, several, or all roots avulsed. In a series of 138 patients undergoing surgery for avulsions, the author has never seen an isolated avulsion of C5. In contrast, seven patients demonstrated an extraforamenally ruptured C5, an avulsed C6, and a stretched or ruptured C7, whereas C8 and T1 were barely injured. Isolated C7 avulsions with extraforamenal lesions to the neighboring spinal nerves were seen in eight instances. Three examples each of C5–C6 avulsions, C5 rupture with C6–C7 avulsions, and C5–C6 and C7 avulsions were seen.

Much more frequent are lower root avulsions such as C8 and T1 (23 instances) and C7, C8, and T1 (26 instances). Avulsions of all five roots or rupture of C5 and avulsion of the other four roots both occurred 13 times.

In avulsions of all five roots, if any reconstructive surgery is considered, neurotization is the only option and the choice of nerves is rather simple. The author favors connecting the spinal accessory or other available motor rami of the cervical plexus with the suprascapular nerve, giving up some scapulothoracic control, and connecting (at least) three intercostal nerves with the lateral part of the lateral cord or directly with the musculocutaneous nerve.

If C5 is not avulsed but is ruptured and the other four roots are avulsed, the reinnervation potential of C5, which can contain more than 10,000 myelinated axons, must not be neglected. C5 is connected by grafts to the suprascapular nerve, the upper division of the posterior cord, and the nerves to the upper part of the pectoralis major muscle, whereas the intercostal nerves are used as described earlier. One or two terminal rami of the spinal accessory nerve can be connected with the rami going from C6 and C7

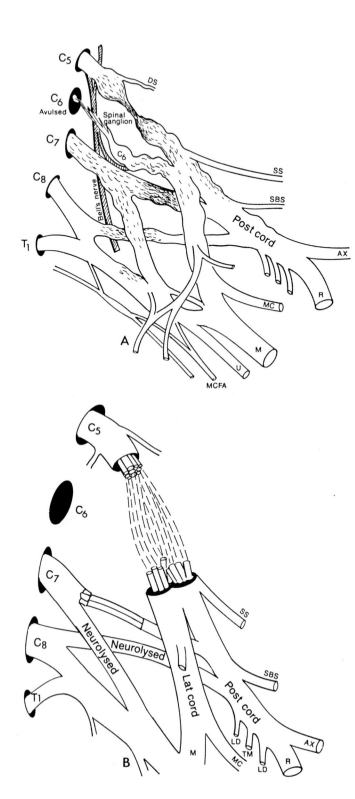

Figure 32–1. *A,* Schematic drawing of a rupture of C5 and avulsion of C6. *B,* The repair of the brachial plexus is shown. AX = axillary nerve, DS = dorsal scapular nerve, LD = latissimus dorsi nerve, MC = musculocutaneous nerve, MCFA = medial cutaneous nerve of forearm, P = pectoral nerve, R = radial nerve, SS = suprascapular nerve, SBS = subscapular nerve, U = ulnar nerve. (From Narakas, A.: Orthop. Clin. North Am., *12*:303, 1981.)

to the long thoracic nerve to improve scapular control.

If C5 and C6 are ruptured extraforamenally and C7, C8, and T1 are avulsed, repair of the suprascapular nerve, the upper division of the posterior cord, and the lateral cord is carried out with grafts from C5 and C6. To neurotize all of the C7 root with any donor nerve has been disappointing. It is better to neurotize only the posterior division of C7 or place C7 directly (or with interposition grafts on some part of C6 that is still uncovered by grafts, while using intercostal nerves to the medial origin of the median nerve (Fig. 32–1).

In the case of avulsion of C8 and T1, neurotization of the medial origin of the median nerve or of the ulnar nerve has been disappointing in adults, but worthwhile for restoring sensation in children. The situation is much more complicated when avulsion injury affects only the upper roots, while the lower ones are not injured and the function of the hand is fair or even good.

According to my personal experience, there is no proper solution for rupture of C5 and avulsion of C6 (Fig. 32–2). To repair C5 by autografts and neurotize C6 has given only fair results for return of C5 function and no return of function for C6. An acceptable solution is to connect all the distal stumps onto C5 only, which then produces abduction in the shoulder with synchronous flexion of the elbow. Another possibility is to connect C5 only to the part of the upper division of the posterior cord that was originally in-

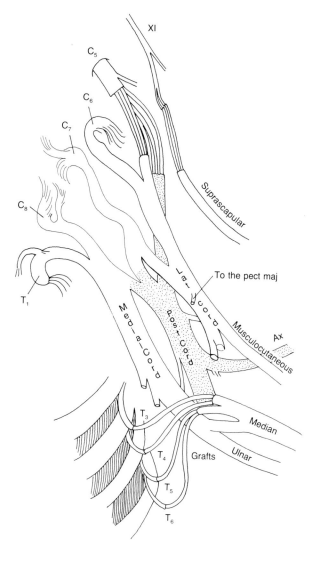

Figure 32–2. Rupture of C5, avulsion of C6 to T1. Some restoration of shoulder function can be attempted by placing the terminal rami of the accessory nerve into the suprascapular nerve and connecting the posterior part of C5 to the upper division of the posterior cord, which contains most of the fascicles for the deltoid, while the anterior part goes to the lateral cord to innervate the pectoralis major and the musculocutaneous nerves. The lateral origin of the median nerve receives four intercostal nerves. The alternative would be to use all C5 into the suprascapular nerve and the posterior cord neurotizing the musculocutaneous nerve with intercostals or the XIth nerve. (From Narakas, A.: Clin. Plast. Surg., *11*:156, 1984.)

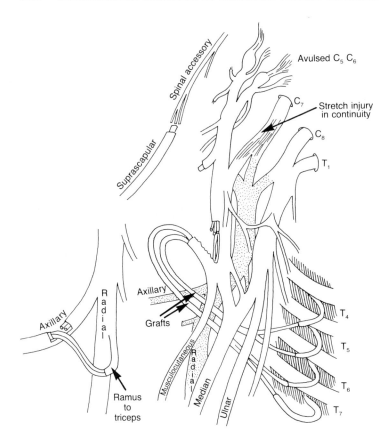

Figure 32–3. An attempt to restore shoulder control and elbow flexion in avulsion of C5 and C6. One ramus of the still functional triceps is diverted into some fascicles of the axillary nerve, while intercostals neurotize the musculocutaneous nerve, the XIth nerve being the suprascapular nerve. (From Narakas, A.: Clin. Plast. Surg., *11*:158, 1984.)

nervated from C5 and C6 and to neurotize the fascicles of the lateral cord. This technique has to be supplemented by musculotendinous transfers (latissimus dorsi, inferior part of the pectoralis major) to restore elbow flexion.

When C5 and C6 are avulsed, scapular control is poor in addition to absence of shoulder function and elbow flexion. A repair can be attempted, as shown in Figure 32–3.

The situation is even more serious when C5–C6 and C7 are avulsed. A fundamental choice has to be made between scapular or shoulder control. Neurotization can then be used to improve the function of the scapulothoracic joint by reinnervating the dorsal scapular and the long thoracic nerves with the eleventh cranial nerve and using intercostals for the musculocutaneous nerve. If good scapular control is restored, the shoulder can be fused and a useful extremity is obtained. Latissimus dorsi transfers cannot be used in the majority of these patients because C7 is damaged or avulsed. There is

Table 32–3. PLEXO-PLEXUAL NERVE TRANSFERS*

Donors	Receptors	Number of Patients	Available Controls	Results	
				Good	*Doubtful, Poor, or Nil*
C5	C5–C6	5	5	5	0
C5	C5–C6–C7	2	2	1	1
C5	C7	1	1	0	1
C6	C7	2	2	2	2
C7	Upper trunk	2	2	1	1
C7	C8	5	5	3	2

*These procedures were carried out when root avulsions were present together with some spinal nerves being ruptured extraforamenally, presenting a usable proximal stump. This stump was the donor, while the distal stump of the same nerve and an avulsed root were the receptors. (From Narakas, A. O.: Clin. Plast. Surg., *11*:158, 1984.)

Table 32–4. NEUROTIZATIONS WITH RAMI OF THE CERVICAL PLEXUS OR WITH INTERCOSTAL NERVES (USUALLY SEVERAL FROM T3 TO T7)*

Donors	Receptors	Number of Patients	Available Controls	Results	
				Good	Doubtful, Poor, or Nil
Long thoracic nerve	C6	1	1	1	0
	Lateral cord	2	2	0	2
	C8	1	1	0	1
Spinal accessory terminal rami to the upper trapezius	Suprascapular nerve	5	2	1	1
Several intercostal nerves	C5 or C6	6	5	1	4
	Lateral cord or musculocutaneous nerve	21	13	9	4
	C7	21	14	7	7
	Posterior cord				
	Axillary nerve	12	8	4	4
	Suprascapular nerve				
	Medial cord C8 or T1				
	Median and/or ulnar nerve	14	9	3 sensory, 1 motor, and sensory result	5

*From Narakas, A. O.: Clin. Plast. Surg., *11*:159, 1984.

no way to compensate for the loss of the triceps. Some elbow extension can be provided by a healthy C8 and partially by gravity, and this can be supplemented by the flexor carpi ulnaris acting in a reverse way.

TECHNICAL CONSIDERATIONS

Donor nerves such as the spinal accessory, the long thoracic, or even the phrenic nerve (as suggested by Chinese surgeons) have to be prepared very distally and their stumps must be cleaned of excess epineurial tissue in order to ensure maximal coaptation between donor and receptor fascicles. Intercostal nerves for motor function are prepared in the mid-axillary line, whereas for sensory neurotization, only their anterior superficial rami need be used at the level of the anterolateral aspect of the thorax. When taking intercostals in women, it is best to avoid denervating the nipple.

CONCLUSIONS

Nerve transfers in reconstructive peripheral nerve microsurgery are still in an experimental phase despite experience accumulated over many years. More knowledge has to be gained with regard to central integration of functions restored in the upper limb

by nerves such as the intercostals, which do not normally participate in the pattern of motion of the upper extremity and which are not usually under voluntary control.

The entire concept of brachial plexus reconstructive surgery is still in its initial stages and suffers from severe lack of fundamental knowledge. Nevertheless, in some situations nerve transfers are rewarding when used to restore one simple function at a time, such as elbow flexion or extension or wrist flexion or extension. However, nerve transfers are particularly disappointing when complex function has to be restored, such as shoulder abduction or finger motion, and the sensation they can provide is at best protective (Tables 32–3 and 32–4).

References

1. Allieu, Y.: Exploration et traitement direct des lésions nerveuses dans les paralysies traumatiques par élongation du plexus brachial chez l'adulte. Rev. Chir. Orthop., *63*:107–122, 1977,
2. Brunelli, G.: Neurotization of avulsed roots of the brachial plexus (preliminary report). Int. J. Microsurg., 2:55–58, 1980.
3. Celli, L., Balli, A., de Luise, G., et al.: La neurotizzazione degli ultimi nervi intercostali mediante trapianto nervoso pedunculato, nelle avulsioni radicolari del plesso brachiale. Chir. Organi di Movimento, *64*:461–464, 1978.
4. Fantiš, A., and Slezák, Z.: On the possibility of reinnervation of total lesions of the brachial plexus

by intercosto-plexual anastomosis (Int. Czech). Cesk. Neurol., *28*:412–418, 1965.

5. Foerster, O.: Die Therapie der Schussverletzungen der peripheren Nerven. *In* Lewandowski: Handbuch der Neurologie. Ergaenzungsband, Berlin, 1929, pp. 1677–1691.

6. Harris, W., and Low, V. W.: On the importance of accurate muscular analysis in lesions of the brachial plexus and the treatment of Erb's palsy and infantile paralysis of the upper extremity by cross-union of nerve roots. Br. Med. J., 2:1035–1038, 1903.

7. Kotani, P. T., Matsuda, H., and Suzuki, T.: Trial surgical procedure of nerve transfers to avulsion injuries of plexus brachialis. Excerpta Med. Int. 12th Congress Series. Series 291 (SICOT Congress, Tel Aviv, 1972), pp. 348–350.

8. Lurje, A.: Concerning surgical treatment of traumatic injury of the upper division of the brachial plexus (Erb's type). Ann. Surg., 127:317–326, 1948.

9. Merle, M.: La chirurgie directe du plexus brachial traumatique. Rev. Readapt. Fonct. Prof. Soc., *6*:45–52, 1980.

10. Millesi, H.: Surgical management of brachial plexus injuries. J. Hand Surg., 2:367–379, 1977.

11. Narakas, A.: Indications et résultats du traitement chirurgical direct dans les lésions par élongation du plexus brachial. Rev. Chir. Orthop., *63*:44–54, 1977.

12. Narakas, A.: Surgical treatment of traction injuries of the brachial plexus. Clin. Orthop., *133*:71–90, 1978.

13. Seddon, H.: Intercostal nerve transfer into the musculocutaneous nerve. *In* Seddon, H. (ed.): Surgical Disorders of the Peripheral Nerves. Edinburgh, Churchill Livingstone, 1972.

14. Sedel, L.: The results of surgical repair of brachial plexus injuries. J. Bone Joint Surg., *64B*:54–66, 1982.

15. Tomita, Y., Tsai, T. M., Burns, J. T., et al.: Intercostal nerve transfer in brachial plexus injuries. An experimental study. Int. J. Microsurg., *4*:95–104, 1983.

16. Tsuyama, N., and Hara, T.: Intercostal nerve transfer in the treatment of brachial plexus injury of root avulsion type. Excerpta Med. Int. 12th Congress Series. Series 291. SICOT Congress, Tel Aviv, 1972, pp. 351–353.

17. Tuttle, H.: Exposure of the brachial plexus with nerve transplantation. J.A.M.A., *61*:15–17, 1913.

18. Vulpius, O., and Stoffel, A.: Orthopädische Operationslehre. 2nd ed. Stuttgart, Enke, 1920.

19. Yeomann, P.: Intercostal nerve transfers in plexus injuries. Personal communication. Symposium on brachial plexus injuries. Lausanne, 1980.

33

Irradiation Plexitis of the Brachial Plexus

■

L. Clodius, M.D.
G. Uhlschmid, M.D.
K. Hess, M.D.

Irradiation plexitis is the most common and the most significant peripheral nerve lesion due to radiation.[45] Spiess,[42] in 1972, ends his monograph on irradiation plexitis of the brachial plexus as follows: "Prognosis of the late irradiation damage syndrome is grave, leading with mostly slow progression in two thirds of our thirty patients with brachial plexus paresis to total functioning disability of the affected limb. A preventive treatment is not known. Neurolysis is difficult and offers at best transient improvement only."

This chapter describes the clinical use of the omentum majus for irradiation-induced plexopathy and outlines the results of this procedure.

EXPERIMENTAL BASIS FOR THE USE OF THE OMENTUM

In the mid-1960s we started an experimental program in dogs to investigate whether the classic concept that lymphedema is confined to the epifascial compartment of an extremity was correct. In one model we achieved a total lymph block of the extremities with the interposition of Etheron, a polyurethane foam, formerly used for breast augmentation.[38] All animals with this total lymph block died as a result of cutaneous fistulas with massive loss of proteins.[10] This model of "malignant" lymphedema was used for

testing the omentum, which bridged the lymph block, in its capacity as a lymphatic "wick."[8, 9] First the pedicled omentum was transferred past the lymph block into the lymphedematous extremity, as had been advocated previously.[14, 33] After McLean and Buncke[30] first published a report of free transplantation of the omentum with microvascular anastomoses for a scalp defect in 1972, we started to use the omentum as a free microvascular graft in our lymphedematous dogs.,[8, 9, 11] Our work showed some success. None of the dogs with "malignant" lymphedema died, and they no longer developed lymphocutaneous fistulas. Instead, following a latent phase, clinical lymphedema became manifest with all its typical histologic changes.[1] Therefore, we concluded that the lymphatic transport capacity of the omentum did not completely match the lymphatic load from the dogs' lymphedematous legs.

In 1973 we were consulted by a patient with secondary lymphedema of the arm following breast amputation, axillary dissection, and postoperative irradiation. The patient had a very annoying lymphocutaneous fistula in the axilla and pain in her arm due to radiation plexitis. We performed a free omental graft, which cured her lymphocutaneous fistula and her pain. However, the lymphedema of the arm did not improve. We then focused our attention on use of an omentum graft for radiation-induced plexopathy.

CAUSES OF IRRADIATION PLEXITIS

Brachial plexus palsy results from the combined effects of surgery: production of scar, leading to compression of the structures within the "thoracic outlet"; removal of x-ray–absorbing fatty areolar tissue with its vascular supply between the skin and the neurovascular bundle; and effects of the direct action of radiation on the neural and perineural structures. This leads to loss of myelin, disappearance of axon cylinders, and obliteration of the peri- and endoneural vasculature. There is a close relationship between the total dose of radiation and the amount of rads administered with a single dose of radiation. The higher the single dose, the greater the danger of neuropathy. Crossfire effects of the anterior and lateral axillary radiation fields have been described in the literature.[2, 28, 34, 37, 39, 42, 44]

The incidence of actinic plexopathy differs according to the statistics of various authors. Stoll and Andrews[44] found neurologic symptoms in 14% of patients after 5775 rads and in 73% after 6300 rads, using 4 MeV megavoltage. Frischbier and Lohbeck,[16] using a 15 MeV betatron, noted signs of plexopathy in 22% of patients given 4000 to 5000 rads; this increased to 47% for doses of 5500 to 6000 rads. If not more than 5000 rads is given to the axillary area within less than 30 to 35 days, the risk of radiation plexitis is minimal.[23]

Radiation, in addition, leads to damage to the vascular system of the nerve, i.e., the epi- and intraneurovascular system. In general, this vascular damage is described as thickening of the vessel walls and proliferation of intimal and subintimal cells, probably due to increased vascular permeability. Later, the circulatory efficiency is compromised by fibrotic and sclerotic changes of the vessels.[2, 21, 39, 43] We have not been able to determine why damage from radiation progresses over decades.

On surgical exploration, we have encountered a tremendous amount of constricting fibrosis in each patient. This also leads to vascular symptoms involving the arm, e.g., diminution or loss of pulsation of the radial artery, with a reduction of blood pressure, was present in one third of the patients seen by Spiess.[42] If the pectoralis minor muscle was not removed when the breast was amputated, we have always found it to be ex-

tensively fibrotic, resulting in considerable narrowing of the outlet between the shoulder joint and the first rib.

SIGNS AND SYMPTOMS OF IRRADIATION PLEXITIS

The diagnosis is not difficult. At their first visit, patients frequently inquire about possible side effects of radiation in relation to their pain and paresthesias. Table 33–1 reports the findings in the 30 patients treated by Spiess. Pain was the leading symptom in all our patients, inducing them to ask for surgical relief. Table 33–2 is a form that we complete based on the questions we ask our patients about pain.

The symptoms are based on the anatomy. The five roots of the brachial plexus (C5–T1) leave the intervertebral foramina to form the upper, middle, and lower trunks. They pass underneath the clavicle and split into anterior and posterior divisions to form the cords. These are named according to their relationship to the subclavian artery. The most proximal cord to be formed, from three posterior divisions, is the posterior cord. Its first branches innervate muscles of the back— subscapular, teres major, and latissimus dorsi (the last of which is innervated by the thoracodorsal nerve). The posterior cord ends in the radial and axillary nerves. The lateral cord is formed from the two anterior divisions of the upper and middle trunks. The pectoralis major muscle is supplied first (by the anterior lateral thoracic nerve). The lateral cord then divides into the musculocutaneous nerve and the lateral head of the median nerve. The musculocutaneous nerve leaves the lateral cord opposite the lower border of the pectoralis minor muscle. The medial cord arises from the anterior division of the lower trunk. Its medial anterior tho-

Table 33–1. SYMPTOMS OF BRACHIAL PLEXOPATHY DUE TO RADIATION ON SURGERY*

Symptom	Frequency
Pain	80% of patients; severe in 50%
Vascular symptoms	One third of patients
Palsy beginning in segments C7 and C8	Two thirds of patients

*Modified from Spiess.[42]

Table 33–2. QUESTIONS FOR PATIENTS WITH BRACHIAL PLEXUS PALSY

Radiated because:		*Histologic findings*:	*When*:
Time interval: x-ray therapy to first symptoms:			*What was the first symptom*:
Pain:	stabbing constant	work dependent	during day
	dull intermittent	when letting arm hang down	during night
Alteration of sensibility:			
where?	when lifting arm		
numb feeling—where?		*Pectoralis minor removed*:	
"fourmillement"—pins + needles			
electricizing—where?			
others—where?			
Palsies: where?	*Arm swelling (lymphedema)*:		
	present since		
Course: progressive loss of sensibility			
decreasing–constant loss of motor power			
The most annoying or disturbing symptom: pain? loss of motor power? loss of sensibility?			
Therapy so far: surgical successful?	has transcutaneous electrical		
medical successful?	stimulation (TENS) been tried?		
physiotherapy successful?			
Respiratory problems:			

racic nerve also supplies the pectoralis major muscle. The medial cord then divides into the medial head of the median nerve and into the ulnar nerve. The ulnar nerve is thus composed chiefly of fibers of C8 and T8, but in over 50% of individuals it also receives a large bundle of C7. The median nerve is formed by the anterior divisions of the lateral and median cords. In 85% of individuals this nerve crosses in front of the axillary artery, close to the insertion of the coracobrachialis muscle. Infraclavicular palsies usually have a cord distribution.

In our patients, all of whom were seen by the neurology service, motor and sensory deficits predominantly involved the ulnar and medial nerves. Of our 12 patients operated on between 1973 and 1980, 9 had moderate to severe secondary arm lymphedema, masking muscle atrophies in the upper arm and forearm.

Various authors have noted different lengths of the latent period between irradiation and the onset of symptoms (Table 33–3). The latent period is extremely variable, ranging between 4 months and 20 years.[3, 31, 32, 42, 44]

Most important for the patient and for therapy is the differential diagnosis between radiation- and metastatic-induced plexopathy. In our opinion there are no specific clinical criteria available to distinguish be-

tween the two causes of plexopathy. Thomas and Colby[47] state "On countless occasions over the years we have been frustrated by the difficulty in distinguishing between metastatic brachial plexopathy and plexus damage resulting from radiation therapy." In addition, the symptom-free interval in tumor patients may last as long as 16 years.[47] The latent period is thus not an index for differential diagnosis. Only multiple biopsies taken at the time of exploration of the plexus will provide the diagnosis in the individual patient. In one of our patients, all biopsies taken from the fibrotic tissues around the brachial plexus were negative for tumor, but a small nodule in the mid-forearm proved to be positive. Therefore, we believe that any clinical diagnosis with therapeutic consequences (based on average incidences of pain, lymphedema, and localization of motor

Table 33–3. BRACHIAL PLEXOPATHY—AVERAGE LATENT PERIOD BETWEEN IRRADIATION AND ONSET OF SYMPTOMS

Time	Reference
20 months	Notter et al.[37]
48 months	Spiess[42]
65 months	Present series
73 months	Thomas and Colby[47]

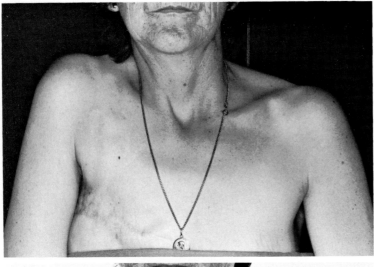

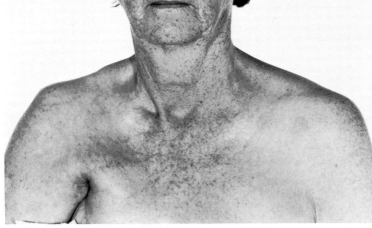

Figure 33–1. Two patients with metastatic brachial plexopathy. (From Clodius, L., et al.: Clin. Plast. Surg., *11*:162, 1984.)

lesions[27]) must be confirmed by biopsies. However, according to Thomas and Colby,[47] it is possible to miss finding tumor tissue even on plexus exploration, especially when the tumor is in the early stages. Local tumor involvement is most probable if there is fullness in the supraclavicular and infraclavicular areas, if the shoulder is retracted toward the neck (Fig. 33–1), if there are venous symptoms such as engorged veins around the shoulder or cyanosis of the arm, and if the symptoms are progressing rapidly.

SURGERY FOR CONSTRICTIVE ACTINIC PLEXOPATHY

Since many surgeons advise against neurolysis for actinic plexopathy,[4, 12, 32, 34–36, 42, 45, 47] what is the goal of our surgery? Resection of the perineurovascular constricting fibrosis will allow for improved or normal axoplasmic flow and will also decompress the epineural and intraneural vascular system. However, we must not only prevent recurrence of constrictive fibrosis with return of pain and palsy, but must also provide revascularization of the nerves by means of the epineural vessels. Both revascularization and prevention of fibrosis are obtained by wrapping the plexus with the omentum (described later in this chapter) (Fig. 33–2 and Table 33–4). In no patient with painful brachial plexus palsy, whether due to radiation and/or tumor, was transcutaneous electrical stimulation (TENS) successful in relieving symptoms.

Surgical Technique

Starting in the mid-upper arm and using a zig-zag incision, the infraclavicular plexus is gradually exposed by resecting all scar tissue and obtaining multiple biopsies. If scar ex-

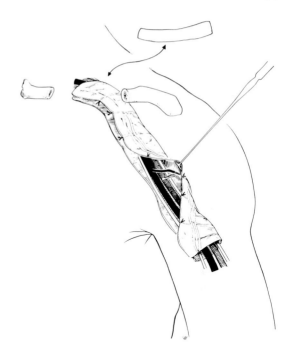

Figure 33–2. Schematic drawing of the positioning of the omentum. For better access to the neurovascular structures at the base of the neck, the clavicle may be temporarily exarticulated or sectioned. (From Clodius, L., et al.: Clin. Plast. Surg., *11*:163, 1984.)

tends above the clavicle, this bone is temporarily cut or disarticulated at its sternal junction. Neurolysis is difficult even under magnification, because the nerve, scar, and tumor are the same color. The surgeon must be prepared for a long, cumbersome, and tedious operation.[13]

What does our "neurolysis" consist of? Following extensive internal neurolysis and the removal of fibrotic tissue between the individual nerve fascicles,[17] we noted a marked loss of motor function in one patient (M. K.) because too much of the microcirculation of the nerves had been destroyed. Therefore, we now do only a very careful external neurolysis, at first preserving the outer investing layer of the epineurium with its essential blood supply for the neural structures. Once all constrictive masses of scar tissue are not only cut but entirely removed from mid-forearm to the base of the neck (and this may take 4 to 6 hours), the thick-

ened superficial epineurium of those nerves that are constricted and flattened is incised longitudinally, again being careful to avoid blood vessels entering the nerves (epineurotomy).[17]

Unfortunately, the scarring that we encounter not only compresses the cross sections of the neural structures but also shortens them. The deleterious effects of stretching on the neural elements have been described by Smith.[41] Typically, patients complain of increased pain when letting the arm hang down (see Table 33–2). Therefore, we make transverse incisions in the epineurium of those cords and nerves that appear particularly tense and tight. For the same reason, we also resorted to shortening the mid-humerus for 5 cm (dorsal approach, plate compression, osteosynthesis) in one patient. The preliminary result in this case was encouraging.

A second team removes the omentum through an upper midline abdominal incision. The part of the omentum incorporating the greater diameter of the gastroepiploic artery (1 to 3 mm) is selected for transplantation. Usually, this is the right gastroepiploic vessel. The abdomen is closed and the omentum is transferred to the axilla. End-to-side anastomoses to the axillary artery and vein are performed using 10–0 sutures. The site of the anastomoses is outside the field of radiation. Once blood flow in the omentum

Table 33–4. BRACHIAL
PLEXOPATHY—OBJECTIVES OF SURGERY

Decompression of:
  Neurovascular bundle
  Proximodistal axoplasmic flow
  Intraneural vascular system
  Endoneurial nutritional blood flow
  Endoneurial edema

Revascularization of neural structures

is established, the omentum is carefully wrapped around the exposed brachial plexus.

It is essential to look for and to avoid any torsion and kinking of the vessels, especially at the site of the venous anastomosis, as the omentum is brought into its final position. Since during neurolysis any remaining lymphatics crossing the axilla are cut, the omentum, proximally in the neck and distally in the mid-upper arm, is carefully appositioned to the path of the subfascial lymphatics.

Postoperatively, the arm is immobilized in 45° abduction in order to avoid any compression of the operative site between the upper arm and the chest wall.

RESULTS

From 1973 until 1980 we have operated on 12 patients with painful plexitis, in whom all biopsy specimens of the constricting fibrotic tissues, examined as frozen sections, proved to be negative. In no patient was there a discrepancy between the frozen section and the definitive histologic findings. No patient showed either improvement or increase of the secondary arm lymphedema that could be attributed to this surgical intervention. The postoperative results and complications are presented in Table 33–5.

One patient (D. I.) consented to having a biopsy of her omentum through a small axillary incision 3 years postoperatively. The omentum was seen to be viable and to have a well-pulsating vasculature. Histologic studies confirmed this finding. We did not perform angiography in any patient to prove the patency of the anastomoses.

The most important result is the relief of severe pain. Four patients (W. L., E. G., M. A., and S. E.) had undergone previous neurolysis. None of them had relief of pain for longer than 9 months following neurolysis.

In one patient (M. A.), when the distal end of the omentum was moved into the nonirradiated tissues of the mid-upper arm toward the end of the operation, a small nodule was found sitting on the deep fascia. The histologic specimen was positive for metastic breast cancer. This patient died of her original tumor (as did patient W. L.). One patient (M. J.) is alive with lung metastases. Another patient (R. P.) died following an accident in 1982, after having had a shoulder girdle amputation for recurrence of tumor in the arm and axilla.

One patient (K. E.) had been completely pain-free for 1 month postoperatively when she was trapped in a snow storm for 11 hours. Her incision, which had healed well even in the heavily irradiated axillary area, broke open within hours (most likely due to prolonged axillary pressure). When we saw her 2 months later, she was again in pain and had a wide, deep, infected fistula where the wound had dehisced. The fistula was excised and the area was covered with a latissimus-musculocutaneous flap. However, this did not improve her pain. We therefore shortened her humerus, as mentioned earlier. This at first abolished her pain completely, but 1½ years after this operation the patient reports that at times she requires analgesics.

One patient (M. K.) developed a small bowel obstruction 1 year postoperatively. This was diagnosed, and the obstructing adhesions were cut.

Table 33–5. RESULTS OF BRACHIAL PLEXOPATHY, NEUROLYSIS, AND OMENTAL GRAFT*

| Patient | Year of Operation | Postoperative Improvement | | Complications |
		Sensory/Motor	*Pain*	
W.L.	1973	Improved/no change	Gone	Died of disease, 1975
R.V.	1974	No change	Gone	—
D.I.	1974	Improved	Almost gone	—
M.A.	1974	No change	Gone	—
E.G.	1974	Improved	Gone	—
M.K.	1975	Worse	Gone	Small bowel obstruction
M.A.	1976	Improved	Gone	Died of disease, 1980
S.E.	1978	No change	Gone	—
M.J.	1978	No change	Gone	Lung metastases, 1982
K.E.	1978	No change	Gone	One month postop. infection
R.P.	1978	No change	Almost gone	Axillary recurrence
B.I.	1980	Improved	Gone	—

*From Clodius, L. et al.: Clin. Plast. Surg., *11*:164, 1984.

DISCUSSION

Resection of constrictive scars and careful neurolysis, combined with a free omental graft, relieved the intense pain of some patients with postactinic brachial plexitis. The positioning of the brachial plexus into well-vascularized, nonirradiated tissue must be the factor that prevents the recurrence of pain, since 4 of our 12 patients had undergone a previous unsuccessful neurolysis. Our results relating to the return of the lost motor and sensory deficits are not good. However, during the reported postoperative control time, there was no progression of loss of sensation and motor power.

The high tolerance of nerves to radiation is related to the absence of mitotic activity of the Schwann cells, vascular endothelial cells, and fibroblasts of the endo- and epineurium under normal conditions.[48] If the mitotic activity of these cells is stimulated by generalized disease or by local trauma, the tolerance phase to the x-ray–inflicted damage ends and clinical symptoms become manifest. In contrast, even high doses of radiation (up to 20,000 rads) did not produce histologic or physiologic changes in peripheral nerves in experimental animals.[7, 22, 24, 40] Experimental compression of the previously irradiated sciatic nerve, however, stimulates the mitotic activity of the Schwann cells and endothelial cells and of the fibroblasts of the endo- and epineurium, and the neural damage is directly related to the dose of radiation.[5] These experimental findings could explain the beneficial long-term effect of the decompression of the radiated nerves, after which the normal reparative processes again become possible.

The main indication for the procedure reported in this chapter is severe pain. If pain is not an indication, we would propose surgery only if repeated neurologic studies demonstrated a rapid progression of motor and sensory losses. We have seen only one patient with this condition but with no pain. She declined surgery, and within 4 years her arm has become totally paralyzed.

So far, we have proposed this intervention only for patients in whom we can exclude metastases. In no patient did we find intra-abdominal tumor spread. One of the advantages of the operation is that it provides the only possibility for establishing the differential diagnosis between delayed radiation-induced plexitis and/or metastatic plexopathy on the basis of multiple biopsies.

We have not employed the pedicled transfer of the omentum, introduced in 1935 by Dick[14] and popularized by Kirikuta[25, 26] and Goldsmith,[19–21] because too many complications have been reported using this method. These include inguinal and spigelian hernias, pulmonary embolism, stress ulcer, upper intestinal obstructions, small bowel gangrene (with death of the patient), gastric torsion, and wound infections. In addition, using the omentum as a free (microsurgical) graft has the following advantages: there is no undermining in the area of the usually tight skin of the chest wall, the size of the omentum is easily adapted to the area it must cover, and the omentum can be placed and wrapped freely around the neural structures.

Goldsmith et al.[19–21] and Yasargil et al.[50] have described the vascularization potential of the omentum for the myocardium, spinal cord, brain, and choroid of the eye. Vascular connections develop between these structures and the omentum. This process may offset the deleterious effects of radiation on the peri- and endoneural vasculature that were described earlier. In our biopsy studies of the tissues around the plexus, we found that even the arterioles were obliterated. Since adequate vascular supply is the most essential factor for functioning of the nerve,[41, 45, 46] revascularization of the neurolysed nerves by the omental graft seems to be the important factor for preventing progression of motor and sensory deficits.

It has been stated that radiation plexopathy will result in an entirely useless extremity in many patients.[47] With careful neurolysis and wrapping of the neural structures with healthy omentum (having significant revascularization potential), the patient can be given the hope of eliminating most or all intractable pain, and the progression of motor and sensory deficits can be stopped.

References

1. Altorfer, J., Hedinger, C., and Clodius, L.: Light and electron microscopic investigation of extremities of dogs with experimental chronic lymphostasis. Folia Angiol., 25:141, 1977.
2. Bakowska, A. J., and Lindop, P. J.: Early and late effects of radiation on the small blood vessels of the mouse ear lobe. *In*: Ditzel, J., and Lewis, D. H. (eds.): 6th European Conference on Microcirculation. Aalborg, 1970. Basel Karger, 1971.
3. Bateman, J. E.: Trauma to Nerves in Limbs. Philadelphia, W. B. Saunders Company, 1962.
4. Burns, R. J.: Delayed radiation-induced damage to the brachial plexus. Clin. Exp. Neurol., 15:221, 1978.

5. Cavanagh, J. B.: Effects of x-irradiation on the proliferation of cells in peripheral nerves during wallerian degeneration in the rat. Br. J. Radiol., *41*:275, 1968.

6. Cavanagh, J. B.: Prior x-irradiation and the cellular response to nerve crush: duration of effect. Exp. Neurol., *22*:253, 1968.

7. Clemedson, C. J., and Nelson, A.: In: Errera, M., and Forssberg, A. (eds.): Mechanisms in Radiobiology, Vol. 2. New York, Academic Press, 1960.

8. Clodius, L., Uhlschmid, G., and Madritsch, W.: Das sekundäre Armlymphödem. Helv. Chir. Acta, *40*:659, 1973.

9. Clodius, L., Uhlschmid, G. and Madritsch, W.: Chirurgische Möglichkeiten der Lymphödembehandlung. Folia Angiol., *11*:304, 1973.

10. Clodius, L., and Wirth, W.: A new experimental model for chronic lymphedema of the extremities. Chir. Plast. (Berl.) *12*:115, 1974.

11. Clodius, L.: The experimental basis for the surgical treatment of lymphedema. In: Clodius, L. (ed.): Lymphedema. Stuttgart, Georg Thieme, 1977.

12. Contamin, F., Mignot, B., Ecoffet, M., Ollat, H., and Jouneau, P.: Les atteintes plexiques post-radiothérapeutiques. Sem. Hôp. Paris, *54*:1225, 1978.

13. Daniel, R. K., and Terzis, J. K.: Reconstructive Microsurgery. Boston, Little, Brown and Company, 1977, Chapter 9.

14. Dick, W.: Ueber die Lymphgefässe des menschlichen Netzes, zugleich ein Beitrag zur Behandlung der Elephantiasis. Bruns Beitr. Klinik Chir., *162*:296, 1935.

15. Flaggman, P. D., and Kelly, J. J.: Brachial plexus neuropathy. Arch. Neurol., *37*:160, 1980.

16. Frischbier, H. J., and Lohbeck, H. U.: Strahlenschäden nach Elektronentherapie beim Mammacarcinom. Strahlentherapie, *139*:684, 1970.

17. Frykman, G. K., Adams, J., and Bowen, W. W.: Neurolysis. Orthop. Clin. North Am., *12*:325, 1981.

18. Goldsmith, H. S.: Pedicled omentum versus free omental graft for myocardial revascularization. Dis. Chest, *54*:37, 1968.

19. Goldsmith, H. S.: Longterm evaluation of omental transposition for chronic lymphedema. Ann. Surg., *180*:847, 1974.

20. Goldsmith, H. S., Duckett, S., and Chen, W.-F.: Spinal cord vascularization by intact omentum. Am. J. Surg., *129*:262, 1975.

21. Goldsmith, H. S., Chen, W.-F., and Palena, P. V.: Intact omentum for ocular revascularization. Invest. Ophthalmol., *14*:163, 1975.

22. Hicks, S. P., and Montgomery, P. O'B.: Effects of acute radiation on the adult mammalian central nervous system. Proc. Soc. Exp. Biol. Med., *80*:15, 1952.

23. Hildebrand, J.: Lesions of the Nervous System in Cancer Patients. New York, Raven Press, 1978.

24. Janzen, A. H., and Warren, S.: Effect of roentgen rays on the peripheral nerve of the rat. Radiology, *38*:333, 1942.

25. Kirikuta, I., and Goldstein, M. B.: L'épiploonplastie vesicale, méthode pour le traitement des fistules vésico-vaginales. Obstet. Ginecol., *2*:163, 1956.

26. Kirikuta, I.: L'emploi du grand epiploon dans la chirurgie du sein cancereux. Presse Méd., *71*:1, 1963.

27. Kori, H. S., Foley, K. M., and Posner, J. B.: Brachial plexus lesions in patients with cancer: 100 cases. Neurology, (New York), *31*:45, 1981.

28. Linder, E.: Ueber das funktionelle und nerphologische Verhalten peripherer Nerven längerer Zeit nach Bestrahlung. Fortschr. Röntgenstr., *90*:618, 1959.

29. Lungborg, G., and Branemark, P. J.: Microvascular structure and function of peripheral nerves. Adv. Microcirc., *1*:66, 1968.

30. McLean, D., and Buncke, H. J.: Autotransplant of omentum to large scalp defect with microsurgical revascularization. Plast. Reconstr. Surg., *49*:268, 1972.

31. Maruyama, Y., Mylrea, M. M., and Lagothetis, J.: Neuropathy following irradiation. An unusual late complication of radiotherapy. Am. J. Roentgenol., *101*:216, 1967.

32. Match, R. M.: Radiation-induced brachial plexus paralysis. Arch. Surg., *110(A)*:384, 1975.

33. Mowlem, R.: Treatment of lymphedema. Br. J. Plast. Surg., *1*:48, 1948.

34. Mumenthaler, M.: Armplexus-paresen im Anschluss an Röntgenbestrahlung. Schweiz. Med. Woschr., *94*:1069, 1964.

35. Mumenthaler, M.: Some clinical aspects of peripheral nerve lesions. Europ. Neurol., *2*:257, 1969.

36. Mumenthaler, M.: Läsionen des Plexus cervico-brachialis. In: Mumenthaler, M., and Schliack, H. (eds.): Läsionen peripherer Nerven. Stuttgart, Georg Thieme, 1982.

37. Notter, G., Hallberg, O., and Vikterlöf, K. J.: Strahlenschäden am Plexus brachialis bei patienten mit Mammacarcinom. Strahlentherapie, *139*:538, 1970.

38. Regnault, P.: One hundred cases of retromammary implantation of Etheron, followed up for 30 months. Transactions, 3rd International Congress of Plastic Surgery, International Congress Series 66. Amsterdam, Excerpta Medica Foundation, 1964.

39. Rubin, P., and Casarett, G. W.: Clinical Radiation Pathology, Vol. I. Philadelphia, W. B. Saunders Company, Chapter 2.

40. Smahel, J., and Clodius, L.: Unpublished experimental data, 1982.

41. Smith, J. W.: Factors influencing nerve repair. II. Collateral circulation of peripheral nerves. Arch. Surg., *93*:433, 1966.

42. Spiess, H.: Schädigungen am peripheren Nervensystem durch ionisierende Strahlen. Berlin, Springer Verlag, 1972.

43. Stearner, S. P., Derine, R. L., and Christian, E. J. B.: Late changes in irradiated microvasculature. Rad. Res., *65*:351, 1976.

44. Stoll, B. A., and Andrews, J. T.: Radiation-induced peripheral neuropathy. Br. Med. J., *1*:834, 1966.

45. Sunderland, S.: Nerves and Nerve Injuries, 2nd ed. Edinburgh, Churchill Livingstone, 1978.

46. Tarlov, I. M., and Epstein, J. H.: Nerve grafts: the importance of an adequate blood supply. J. Neurosurg., *2*:49, 1945.

47. Thomas, J. E., and Colby, M. Y.: Radiation-induced or metastatic brachial plexopathy. J.A.M.A., *222*:1392, 1972.

48. Thomas, P. K., and Cavanagh, J. B.: Neuropathy due to physical agents. In Dyck, P. J., Thomas, P. K., and Lambert, E. H. (eds.): Peripheral Neuropathy, Vol. I. Philadelphia, W. B. Saunders Company, 1975.

49. Vaubel, W. E., Schwarz, G., and Sörensen, R.: Die Omentum-Transposition und ihre röntgenologisch sichtbaren Folgen am Magen. Dtsch. Med. Wschr., *97*:1731, 1972.

50. Yasargil, M. G., Yonekawa, Y., Denton, I., Piroth, D., and Benes, I.: Experimental intracranial transplantation of autogenic omentum majus. J. Neurosurg., *39*:213, 1974.

34

Diagnostic Value of Peripheral and Spinal Somatosensory Evoked Potentials in Traction Lesions of the Brachial Plexus

■

S. J. Jones, M.A., Ph.D.

The prospects for spontaneous recovery following a traction injury of the brachial plexus depend on the level as well as the extent of axonal damage. The prime necessity is for anatomic continuity to be preserved, and this is more likely to be the case in mild lesions with involvement confined to the upper roots (C5 and C6) or trunk. Wynn Parry[8] reported that two thirds of such patients treated conservatively regained elbow flexion, whereas the proportion was less than one third for patients with involvement of the lower roots (C7 to T1) also.

Among patients who do not recover and who undergo surgical exploration, a large number are found to have roots avulsed from the spinal cord, with involvement of sensory axons on the proximal side of their dorsal root ganglia ("preganglionic" lesion). Neither spontaneous recovery nor surgical repair appears to be possible in such cases. However, it was reported by Narakas[7] that up to one third of patients who were surgically explored had postganglionic ruptures of the upper trunk that might have been amenable to grafting. This has led to renewed efforts in developing preoperative investigative techniques, by which it is hoped to select the patients most likely to benefit from surgery.

In addition to certain clinical features re-flecting the level of axonal damage,[8] the preservation or abolition of axon reflexes (histamine flare)[1] and sensory nerve action potentials (SNAPs)[2] in an anesthetic part of the arm may indicate whether the roots concerned are avulsed from the spinal cord or are damaged more distally. There is some interindividual variability in the segmental innervation of the arm, but in patients with complete C5–T1 lesions, it is usually possible to decide for each root whether the lesion is likely to be pre- or postganglionic. When the arm is only partially denervated, however, it may be difficult to arrive at a similar estimate without knowing the proportion of fibers still in continuity with the spinal cord. One means of ascertaining this is to record somatosensory evoked potentials (SEPs) from the cervical spine and/or the sensory cortex in response to stimulation of peripheral nerves and to compare their amplitudes with those of analogous responses obtained from the intact arm. The degree of attenuation can then be compared with the attenuation of the input volley, thereby indicating the degree of involvement on both sides of the dorsal root ganglia. The picture obtained is only partially root-specific (to be discussed), but may be of value when considered in conjunction with clinical features.

BACKGROUND TO THE SEP TECHNIQUE (WITH REFERENCE TO BRACHIAL PLEXUS LESIONS)

When a brief electrical shock is delivered transcutaneously to the median nerve at the wrist with an intensity just above the motor threshold, the ascending volley (composed mostly of orthodromic activity in sensory axons but with a small contribution from antidromic activity in motor fibers) can be recorded by skin-surface electrodes located over the elbow, the axilla, and the brachial plexus. At the last site (Erb's point, or just above the midpoint of the clavicle), the response takes the form of a positive/negative biphasic wave, with the negative peak usually occurring 9 to 10 msec after the stimulus and therefore referred to as "N9" (Fig. 34–1). The peak-peak amplitude of this potential is usually in the range of 3 to 15 μv,[4] which may be comparable with the background "noise" level. It is necessary, therefore, to compute the average of a number of responses, with the effect of attenuating the "noise" (not related in time to the presentation of the stimulus) while leaving consistent stimulus-locked signals unaffected. A normal N9 should require no more than 100 individual responses on the average, but at least 500 stimuli may be required to resolve a pathologic response of less than 0.5 μv.

There are now recording machines available with the capacity of averaging and displaying recordings from two, four, or even eight electrodes simultaneously, such that the peripheral volley can be examined at the same time as spinal and cortical evoked potentials are recorded from the cervical spine and the scalp. The major cervical response (N13) occurs 3 to 4 msec after N9 and can be recorded between the second and seventh dorsal processes. Since the amplitude is normally between 1 and 5 μv, an average of at least 200 responses will be required from a normal arm and more when there is a lesion of the dorsal roots. An additional electrode located over the hand area of the sensorimotor cortex contralateral to the stimulated arm will record an initial negative potential (N20), reflecting the arrival of the sensory volley at the level of the cortex. N20 and succeeding cortically generated potentials are more easily recorded than subcortical components, but their amplitude is less affected by reduction of the peripheral volley, possibly because amplification can take place at synapses in the brain stem and thalamus. For this reason, N13 is preferred as a quantifiable measure of activity arriving at the central nervous system.

The activity present at any location on the body surface can only be recorded relative to some other "reference" site on the body. The location of the second electrode is umimportant for recording N9, but N13 may be difficult to measure unless the reference site is located on the scalp, usually at a mid-frontal position.

With regard to the application of SEP techniques (as well as for more obvious reasons), it is useful to remember that brachial plexus traction injuries are usually unilateral. It is therefore possible to use the intact arm as a

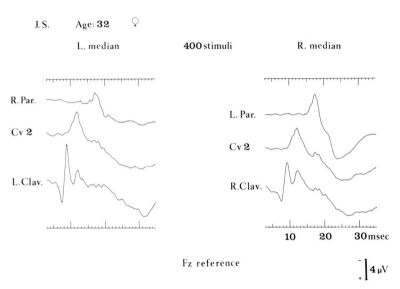

J. S.   Age: **32**   ♀

L. median   **400** stimuli   R. median

R. Par.

Cv 2

L. Clav.

L. Par.

Cv 2

R. Clav.

10   20   30 msec

Fz reference

$^-$| **4** μV
$_+$

Figure 34–1. Major SEP components following stimulation of the left and right median nerves at the wrist in a normal subject. N9 (peripheral volley) is the sharp peak recorded over the ipsilateral clavicle; N13 (reflecting activity in the dorsal horns and possibly the brainstem) is the triangular wave recorded over the second cervical vertebra; and N20 (reflecting the arrival of the sensory volley at the cortex) is the initial negative (upgoing) deflection recorded from the contralateral parietal region. The figure also illustrates left-right amplitude differences in the order of 40 per cent, which are sometimes encountered even in normal individuals. (From Jones, S. J.: Clin. Plast. Surg., *11*:168, 1984).

control and to obtain a more accurate measure of fiber loss than if it were necessary to compare the patient with a group of control subjects. The largest left/right amplitude differences encountered for the three major SEP components (N9, N13, N20) in a group of 12 normal volunteers were between 40 and 60% of the amplitude on the larger side (Fig. 34–1),[4] but when there is clinical evidence of a lesion, a decrement of 30% on the involved side can usually be regarded as significant. Equalization of the effective stimulus strength on the left and right can be difficult when the usual criterion (the presence of a small motor response) is not applicable on one side. In practice, however, it is usually adequate to adopt the same values of intensity (volts or amps) and duration and subsequently to increase the intensity on the involved side in order to be sure that any residual fragment of N9 is not missed.

It was initially supposed, and later borne out by surgical exploration of patients with pathologic lesions, that the great majority of sensory fibers constituting the median nerve at the level of the wrist would derive from the C6 and C7 roots. The C5 root does not appear to be significantly represented, except in rare patients in whom the brachial plexus is "pre-fixed" (deriving from C4 to C8 instead of C5 to T1). However, in some patients with complete ruptures of the C6 and C7 roots a substantial cortical response was still present following median nerve stimulation, presumably mediated by a small number of fibers entering the spinal cord at C8 and/or T1 level. The number of such fibers was apparently insufficient to give rise to any consistent N9 or N13, and the presence of N20 could probably be attributed to amplification through central synapses. For present purposes, therefore, the N9 and N13 components evoked by median nerve stimulation at the wrist could be assumed to derive virtually exclusively from the C6 and C7 roots, and results obtained from patients with localized damage to one or the other of these suggested that they are represented in approximately equal proportions.

In order to provide corresponding evidence concerning the state of the C8 and T1 roots, the stimulus can be delivered to the ulnar nerve. The preferred locus of the stimulating electrode is at the elbow, since here it is more likely to recruit fibers deriving from T1. SEP latencies are shorter by 3 to 4 msec from the proximal site, and the amplitude of the ulnar nerve N13 is smaller than the corresponding median nerve response by approximately 50%. The ulnar nerve N9 is often of comparable amplitude to the median nerve component, but tends to exhibit wider variability between individuals. Surgical exploration confirmed that ulnar nerve responses did reflect the location of the lesion in the C8 and T1 roots fairly accurately (to be discussed), but the results were of lesser prognostic value, since these roots are more often avulsed from the spinal cord. Furthermore, even when the damage is exclusively postganglionic, it is unlikely that there will be any useful recovery of motor function in the hand, since by the time regenerating axons have attained the requisite length, the intrinsic muscles of the hand will usually have atrophied.

REVIEW OF SEP FINDINGS IN 100 LESIONS

Material

Ninety-nine patients, between 6 and 47 years of age, with a mean age of 21 years, were studied. The lesion involved the left arm in 51 patients and the right in 49 (one patient had a bilateral lesion). Ninety-three patients were male and six were female, and approximately 90% had sustained the injury in motorcycle accidents. Clinically there was complete involvement of all roots from C5 to T1 in 63 cases, partial involvement mainly of the upper roots (C5 to C7) in 36, and a partial lower root lesion (C8, T1) in one. The mean time elapsed since the accident was 10 months, but this figure was distorted because one patient was examined 22 years after the injury. In approximately 60% of cases SEPs were recorded less than 6 months after the trauma. Thirty-five patients were surgically explored, two prior to and the remainder after electrophysiologic examination.

Methods

The patients sat semireclined in an armchair and were requested to relax and remain still. Jaw movements (swallowing, talking, etc.) were particularly discouraged, and if muscular artifacts remained a problem the patient was asked to open his mouth slightly. Recording electrodes were located over the midpoint of both clavicles, the spinous processes at T3, C7, and C2, the mastoid processes, and the hand area of the sensorimotor cortex (2 cm posterior to the vertex and 7 cm toward the tragus of the ear on both sides). All sites were referred to an electrode on the midline of the scalp 12 cm above the nasion, except the mastoid processes, which were referred to the sensorimotor hand area contralateral to the stimulus.

The stimulus was delivered via a saddle-type bipolar electrode strapped to the arm over the median nerve at the wrist and the ulnar nerve at the elbow. An earthing electrode (ECG plate) was located proximally on the same limb. The stimulus (initially a capacitor discharge with a time constant of 50 μsec, later a square-wave constant current impulse with a duration of 200 μsec) was delivered at a rate of 2 or 3/second with an intensity sufficient to produce a moderate motor response on the intact side (2 to 5 times the sensory threshold). This was easily tolerated for up to 3 minutes. On the involved side the stimulus was set at the same level for at least one run, but subsequently was often increased in intensity and/or duration. The amplifier high-frequency response was less than 3 dB down at 5kHz and the time constant was 1 second. Up to 1600 responses were averaged in groups of 400 for each stimulation site, with the facility of later computing the "grand average" of repeated runs. The recording epoch was 32 msec, starting 3 msec after the stimulus, and each input channel was sampled 8 times/msec. Although the available apparatus permitted eight channels to be recorded simultaneously, for most purposes it was only necessary to measure the N9 component at the ipsilateral clavicle and N13 over the second cervical vertebra.

Results

Having first divided the cases into 63 complete and 37 partial lesions, SEP findings were interpreted as follows:

1. An attenuation of N9 by more than 30% compared with the intact arm, with N13 attenuated to a similar (or sometimes a lesser) degree, was taken to indicate a postganglionic lesion of one or both involved roots (Fig. 34–2). With complete C5–T1 lesions, N13 was invariably absent, and if N9 was also absent, a postganglionic lesion was presumed for the appropriate roots.

2. N9 attenuated by less than 30%, with N13 either absent or attenuated by more than 30%, was taken to indicate a preganglionic lesion of the involved roots (Fig. 34–3).

3. N9 present but attenuated by more than 30%, with N13 either absent or attenuated to a greater degree than N9, was taken to indicate a combination of pre- and postganglionic involvement in the C6–C7 or the C8–T1 roots, depending on which peripheral nerve was stimulated (Fig. 34–4).

There were three patients (including the patient with the bilateral brachial plexus lesion) in whom injury to the other arm made quantitative assessment difficult. In an additional four patients, the results were of

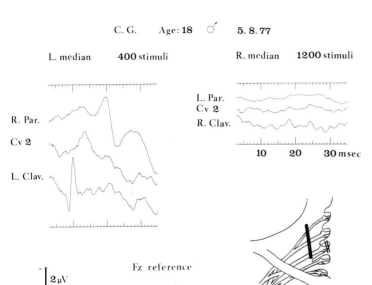

C. G.   Age: 18   ♂   5. 8. 77

L. median   400 stimuli   R. median   1200 stimuli

R. Par.

Cv 2

L. Clav.

L. Par.
Cv 2
R. Clav.

10   20   30 msec

Fz reference

2 μV

Figure 34–2. Partial right brachial plexus lesion affecting the roots from C5 to C7, in which absent SEPs are suggestive of postganglionic involvement. A rupture of all three roots was confirmed at surgery, and there was the possibility of additional, more distal damage to C7. (From Jones, S. J.: Clin. Plast. Surg., 11:169, 1984.)

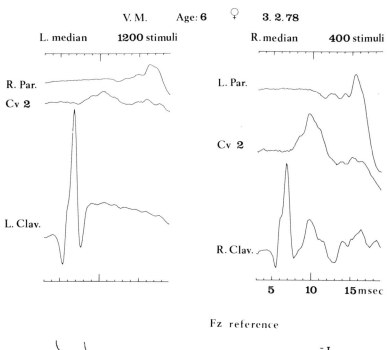

V. M.   Age: **6**   ♀   **3. 2. 78**

L. median   **1200** stimuli   R. median   **400** stimuli

R. Par.
Cv 2

L. Par.

Cv 2

L. Clav.

R. Clav.

5   10   15 msec

Fz reference

$2\mu V$

Figure 34–3. Partial left brachial plexus lesion, affecting the C5 and C6 roots. The complete preservation of N9 on this side, although N13 was attenuated by at least 50 per cent, was suggestive of a preganglionic lesion at C6. At surgery the roots were apparently in continuity, but further electrophysiologic investigations confirmed an intradural preganglionic avulsion of the C5 and C6 roots. (From Jones, S. J.: Clin. Plast. Surg., *11*:170, 1984.)

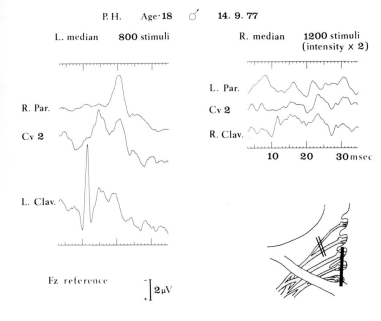

P. H.   Age·**18**   ♂   **14. 9. 77**

L. median   **800** stimuli   R. median   **1200** stimuli
(intensity × 2)

R. Par.
Cv 2

L. Par.
Cv 2
R. Clav.

10   20   30 msec

L. Clav.

Fz reference $2\mu V$

Figure 34–4. Complete right brachial plexus lesion, in which the presence of N9 with amplitude reduced by about 70 per cent was suggestive of a combination of pre- and postganglionic involvement at C6 and C7 (the high noise level makes it difficult to tell whether there is any residual cervical or cortical response; however, none was expected since the stimulus was not perceived by the patient). At surgery the C7, C8, and T1 roots were found to be avulsed from the spinal cord, while a more distal lesion in continuity was discovered for C5 and C6. (From Jones, S. J.: Clin. Plast. Surg., *11*:170, 1984.)

doubtful validity owing to the possibility of additional distal damage to nerves on the involved side. Nevertheless, an estimate of the locus of the brachial plexus lesion was made in each case, using all available information.

A breakdown of the interpretation of SEP findings is given in Table 34–1. For a large proportion of partial lesions involving upper roots only, the ulnar nerve responses were either normal or not recorded. Two patients with partial lesions had normal median nerve responses, one having exclusive lower root involvement (the other arm not being available for comparison owing to multiple fractures) and the other having clinical involvement of the C5 root only.

Considering first the 63 complete lesions, 21 were adjudged to be postganglionic for C6–C7 and C8–T1 on the grounds of complete absence of median and ulnar nerve SEPs. The median response was flat in a total of 28 cases, and the ulnar response was flat in 30. The N9 component was identifiable in 35 median and 32 ulnar nerve recordings, but in only one and five recordings, respectively, was N9 not significantly attenuated compared with the intact arm. In the remaining 34 and 27 recordings, N9 was present but was significantly attenuated, suggestive of a preganglionic lesion of at least one root but with a degree of postganglionic involvement also. Although N9 was identifiable in a slightly larger proportion of median nerve

recordings, the mean amplitude compared with the intact arm was 21% for median and 37% for ulnar nerve responses (scoring individuals up to a maximum of 100%, even in rare cases in which the response was larger on the involved side).

The most striking difference in the overall pattern for the 37 partial lesions was that a much greater proportion appeared to be postganglionic for the C6 and C7 roots. Exclusively preganglionic involvement was suggested in five cases, and in an additional five it was possible that one root might be damaged proximal and the other distal to the dorsal root ganglion (a preganglionic lesion of both with additional postganglionic involvement would also be possible). Ulnar nerve responses, when recorded, were usually suggestive of some postganglionic damage to the lower roots, and the one patient with exclusive lower root involvement appeared to have a preganglionic lesion of C8 and T1, with the upper roots intact.

Correlation with Findings at Surgery

On attempting to relate preoperative SEP indications with the appearance of the roots and brachial plexus at surgery (usually performed several months after the trauma), it became apparent that simple classification into pre- and/or postganglionic lesions for each root was a gross oversimplification. Many patients had identifiable ruptures or avulsed roots (with the dorsal root ganglia still attached), but there were also many instances of "missing" roots (violently avulsed from the spinal cord) and roots that appeared to be in anatomic continuity with no clear indication as to where the locus of conduction failure might be. Nevertheless the agreement between preoperative and surgical findings was adjudged to be "good" (Table 34–2) when the prediction of the locus of the lesion was confirmed by the surgeon without evidence of significant axonal damage elsewhere.

"Fair" agreement was claimed when SEP indications were only partially confirmed. In such cases the reason for the discrepancy was usually clear—often a violently avulsed or missing root giving rise to an attenuated N9, which had been interpreted as indicating postganglionic involvement. In some "fair" cases the SEP findings were considered to have been helpful if the indication of at least

Table 34–1. SEP INDICATIONS IN 100 BRACHIAL PLEXUS LESIONS

Estimated Locus of Lesion	Upper Roots (C6, C7)	Lower Roots (C8, T1)
Complete lesions of C5–T1 (N = 63):		
Postganglionic	28	30
Preganglionic	1	5
Pre- and Postganglionic	34	27
Normal or not assessed	0	1
Partial lesions of C5–C7 (N = 37):		
Postganglionic	25	10
Preganglionic	5	4*
Pre- and Postganglionic	5	0
Normal or not assessed	2*	23

*Includes one patient with clinical involvement of the lower roots (C8, T1) only. (From Jones, S. J.: Clin. Plast. Surg., 11:171, 1984.)

a degree of postganglionic involvement was confirmed without discovery of an additional preganglionic lesion of the same fibers. In patients with complete C5–T1 involvement, if the amplitude of N9 was required to be less than 25% that of the intact arm (instead of less than 70%) before postganglionic involvement was assumed, the classification of the agreement between preoperative and surgical findings could be changed from "fair" to "good" in three cases for median and two for ulnar nerve investigation. These, therefore, were also included in the "helpful" subdivision of the "fair agreement" category.

Finally, the "poor agreement" category includes cases in which the major locus of the lesion was incorrectly estimated by the SEP technique. Sometimes the reason for this became clear, e.g., the discovery of an avulsion of some or all roots in addition to the predicted postganglionic lesion of the same fibers. The discrepancy was also understandable when a postganglionic lesion had been predicted (absent N9) but no roots could be discovered in the supraclavicular fossa. In other cases in which N9 was attenuated or absent but avulsed roots were found, the anticipated postganglionic lesion was not discovered but may have occurred distal to the exposure.

It is clear from Table 34–2 that surgical findings did not fully confirm median nerve SEP results in more than two thirds of cases with complete C5–T1 involvement, although the SEPs were judged to have been at least "helpful" in 11 out of 18 cases. SEP indications concerning the locus of the lower root

Table 34–2. DIAGNOSTIC VALUE OF SEPs CONFIRMED BY SURGERY*

Extent of Agreement with SEP Indications	Upper Roots (C6, C7)	Lower Roots (C8, T1)
Complete lesions of C5–T1 (N = 19):		
Good	6	9
Fair—helpful	5	2
Fair—unhelpful	4	4
Poor	4	3
		(1 not assessed)
Partial lesions of C5–C7 (N = 16):		
Good	9	
Fair—helpful	2	
Fair—unhelpful	4	
Poor	1	

*From Jones, S. J.: Clin. Plast. Surg., 11:171, 1984.

lesion were slightly more accurate. This may be because the damage to these roots was generally more straightforward—either an infraclavicular postganglionic lesion or an avulsion, and less often a combination of pre- and postganglionic elements. Median nerve SEP results were more predictive in partial lesions of the upper trunk, the location being fully confirmed by surgery in 9 of 16 cases with a further 2 classified as "helpful." In one case (classified as "good" agreement) the brachial plexus was discovered to be "prefixed," with a postganglionic lesion of the C4 and C5 roots instead of C5 and C6 as anticipated.

In the larger group of 100 lesions, three cases with C5–T1 involvement were noted in which the N9 component recorded preoperatively was present but distorted, with relative enhancement of the initial positive phase and attenuation of the major negativity. Two of these were surgically explored, and in both at least one root was found to be recoiled into the supraclavicular fossa, with the ganglion lying superficially beneath the clavicle. A possible explanation for this waveform is proposed in the following Discussion.

During surgery, if one or more roots were in anatomic continuity or stumps appeared to be intact farther proximally, the exposed elements were stimulated (with parameters comparable to those of the median nerve stimulus) in order to establish whether there was functional continuity with the CNS. Nerve action potentials could often be recorded from the exposed roots and trunks, indicating the continuity of sensory fibers with their dorsal root ganglia. In many cases it was possible to confirm central continuity by recording cortical SEPs intraoperatively.[6] In other cases with roots apparently intact, no SEPs could be elicited (Fig. 34–5), indicating a failure of conduction on the proximal side of the stimulation site. When this was associated with preserved nerve action potentials, the lesion could be assumed to be proximal to the dorsal root ganglia, i.e., an intradural avulsion.

DISCUSSION

A fairly large proportion of patients with complete C5–T1 lesions have normal or near-normal SNAPs,[5] but the N9 component of the SEP is very seldom unattenuated and is usually reduced by at least 80%. Although

R.G.   ♂   Age: 21

Hand area → Fz

Stimulation
at (root)

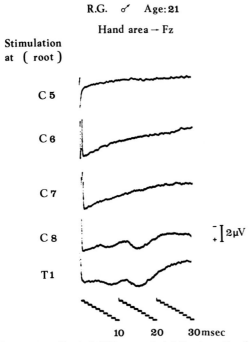

Figure 34–5. Cortical SEPs recorded following stimulation of individual exposed roots during surgery. All roots appeared to be in anatomic continuity, but only C8 and T1 gave rise to a response, in keeping with the clinical picture. The C5, C6, and C7 roots were assumed to have been damaged on the proximal side of the stimulation site, where surgical repair was not possible.

some of this may be due to the degeneration of motor axons, which takes place irrespective of whether the lesion is distal or proximal, the evidence suggests that antidromic activity in motor axons is responsible for only a very small proportion of N9 at normal stimulus intensities just above the motor threshold. If a root is violently avulsed with its ganglion attached and cannot be found in the supraclavicular fossa, the sensory fibers (which may still give rise to normal SNAPs in the distal extremities) may lie too deep for any potential to be recorded by an electrode over the midpoint of the clavicle. However, the absence of any clavicular response is likely to be interpreted as being due to a postganglionic lesion and may lead to a falsely optimistic prognosis. One can improve the diagnostic accuracy of the SEP in such cases by not considering the possibility of postganglionic involvement until N9 is reduced by at least 75% compared with the intact arm. Nevertheless, it is still felt that in patients with complete C5–T1 involvement less reliance can be placed on SEP findings than on conventional SNAP recordings,

which should indicate a proximal or distal lesion without the possibility of confusion due to the disruption of the normal brachial plexus anatomy. It has repeatedly been stressed that neither the SEP nor the SNAP technique is capable of detecting an avulsion when there is additional involvement of the same fibers on the distal side of the dorsal root ganglia, and for this reason the myelogram is still a necessary investigation, in spite of occasional false results.[3]

With less severe lesions, usually involving the upper roots down to C6 or C7, SNAPs may be more difficult to interpret, since some fibers may still be in continuity with the spinal cord. The main focus of the damage in these cases is more easily identified at surgery, with a lower incidence of missing roots, and the preoperative SEP indications were found to be considerably more accurate. One would therefore recommend routine recording of SEPs in patients with partial brachial plexus lesions, but not when there is complete denervation in the distribution of the C5–T1 roots.

A further defect of both SEP and SNAP techniques in this context is that neither appears to reflect the state of the C5 root. This root was found to have postganglionic damage, with the possibility of surgical repair, in at least 22 of 35 cases described earlier, and since C5 fibers have relatively little distance to grow in order to reinnervate the muscles of the upper arm, they are the most likely to give rise to useful functional recovery. Unfortunately, the C5 root appears to have negligible representation in the median nerve at the wrist or the ulnar nerve at the elbow, and attempts to provide assessment by recording SEPs and SNAPs in response to stimulation of the musculocutaneous nerve have proved unsuccessful.[5] One would suggest, therefore, that there is still an important role for the "axon reflex" histamine flare test employed by Bonney.[1]

Although perhaps of little diagnostic importance, there were three patients (two of them subsequently surgically explored) in whom the N9 waveform was distorted as well as attenuated on the damaged side. All three patients had relative enhancement of the initial positive deflection, whereas the main negative phase was greatly reduced. This was suggestive of a "killed end" recording, in which the action potential propagates up to but not beyond the recording electrode. In both surgically explored patients, at least one dorsal root ganglion could be identified superficially in the supraclavicular fossa, so conduction in this root at least would terminate in the vicinity of the clavicular electrode. This particular SEP pattern does seem to indicate a fairly violent avulsion, although not as violent as in the "missing root" cases.

It is probably worthwhile at this stage to reassess the value of SEP recordings in brachial plexus lesions. Clearly the technique is no more infallible than other investigations, but the success ratio in patients with upper trunk lesions is encouraging. EMG recording machines with the facility of averaging responses from two electrodes simultaneously are becoming more widely available, and one hopes that in the near future the recording of clavicular and cervical SEPs, as well as SNAPs, may become standard practice in EMG clinics.

Acknowledgments: The author is grateful to Mr A. Landi and Mr R. Birch, who performed the surgical explorations, and to Dr C.B. Wynn Parry for advice and discussion.

References

1. Bonney, G.: The value of axon responses in determining the site of lesion in traction lesions of the brachial plexus. Brain, *77*:588–609, 1954.
2. Bonney, G., and Gilliatt, R. W.: Sensory nerve conduction after traction lesion of the brachial plexus. Proc. Roy. Soc. Med., *51*:365–367, 1958.
3. Davies, E. R., Sutton, D., and Bligh, A. S.: Myelography in brachial plexus injury. Br. J. Radiol., *39*:362–371, 1966.
4. Jones, S. J.: Investigation of brachial plexus traction lesions by peripheral and spinal somatosensory evoked potentials. J. Neurol. Neurosurg. Psychiatry, *42*:107–116, 1979.
5. Jones, S. J., Wynn Parry, C. B., and Landi, A.: Diagnosis of brachial plexus traction lesions by sensory nerve action potentials and somatosensory evoked potentials. Injury, *12*:376–382, 1981.
6. Landi, A., Copeland, S., Wynn Parry, C. B., and Jones, S. J.: The role of somatosensory evoked potentials and nerve conduction studies in the surgical management of brachial plexus injuries. J. Bone Joint Surg., *62B*:492–496, 1981.
7. Narakas, A.: Indications et resultats du traitement chirurgical direct dans les lesions par elongation du plexus brachial. Rev. Chir., *63*:88–106, 1977.
8. Wynn Parry, C. B.: Rehabilitation of the Hand. London, Butterworth, 1981.

35

Electrophysiologic Intraoperative Evaluations of the Damaged Root in Tractions of the Brachial Plexus

■

L. Celli, M.D.
C. Rovesta, M.D.

In lesions of the brachial plexus caused by traction, the type and degree of traumatic force and resultant unnatural position of the upper extremity and vertebral column cause various patterns of root lesions. Sunderland[18] distinguishes a peripheral from a central mechanism when explaining how lesions with root avulsions or with total or partial intraforaminal damage can occur. The interpretation of the pathogenesis can help clarify how intraforaminal lesions with meningocele can occur with a primarily peripheral mechanism, whereas intraforaminal lesions without meningocele can be caused by a mainly central mechanism. When extraforaminal lesions occur, the transverse groove becomes a critical point for the angle formed by the roots as they move to the supraclavicular fossa (Fig. 35–1). Although this process is present in a clear and definitive manner for C5 and C6, it progressively diminishes for C7 and is absent in C8 and T1. Therefore, C5, C6, and, less frequently, C7 develop extraforaminal lesions, owing to the force of traction, which is integrally transmitted to the intraforaminal portion of the roots, whereas C8 and T1 develop lesions with root avulsion.

The anatomicopathologic aspects of root lesions can therefore be classified as follows (Fig. 35–2):

1. At the extraforaminal level:
   a. In continuity
   b. In pseudocontinuity
   c. With a stump (when the root is broken on the edge of the transverse process)
   d. With extraforaminal avulsion
2. At the intraforaminal level:
   a. In pseudocontinuity
   b. With breakage of the sensory root
   c. With breakage of the motor root
   d. With extraforaminal avulsion
3. Involving two of the intra- and extraforaminal levels in various combinations.

These different anatomicopathologic aspects require the surgeon to make a precise anatomic and functional intraoperative evaluation of the root lesion. Anatomic integrity can be ascertained only by direct surgical exploration of the extra- and intraforaminal root tract, i.e., the brachial plexus exploration would have to be combined with an earlier cervical hemilaminectomy at several levels.[17]

Even in cases in which it is possible to show an apparent anatomic continuity of the root in the extra- and intraforaminal tract, it is still necessary to evaluate the functional capacity of the nerve fibers to conduct an electrical stimulus. For this reason, we feel it unnecessary to subject patients to a traumatic surgical exploration of the roots in the intraforaminal tract. However, in surgical explo-

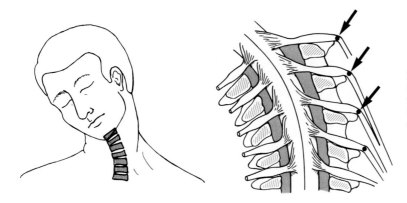

Figure 35–1. The angle formed by the roots on the edge of the transverse groove progressively diminishes from C5 to T1, while it increases as the head tilts and turns.

ration of root lesions of the brachial plexus, we do consider it essential to establish a correct intraoperative electromyographic evaluation of the functional capacity of motor and sensory roots to conduct an electrical stimulus. If correctly carried out, these evaluations can supply conclusive information for the definition of the anatomicofunctional integrity of the root in its intraforaminal tract.

CLINICAL AND INSTRUMENT PREOPERATIVE EVALUATIONS

Preoperative evaluations provide direct and nonspecific information about the level and type of intraforaminal lesion.

The *clinical examination,* based on motor, sensory, and autonomic findings, provides a general diagnosis of root lesions. The clinical parameters regarding suspected intraforaminal root lesions are as follows:

1. Paralysis of the hemidiaphragm and serratus anterior muscle for roots C5 and C6.
2. Type and nature of the pain.
3. Absent Tinel's sign.
4. Presence of Claude Bernard–Horner syndrome for roots C8 and T1.
5. Positive histamine flare test (of Bonney).

In some of our observations, however, the presence or absence of these conditions has been contradictory as far as other clinical manifestations or the anatomicopathologic and functional intraoperative pattern.

The preoperative *electromyographic examination* provides more precise indications of intraforaminal root lesion, as follows:

1. Signs of denervation in the paravertebral muscles.[1]
2. Presence of sensory action potentials (SAPs) in an anesthetic zone.
3. Absence of spinal and somatosensory evoked potentials (SEPs).

When lesions involve multiple roots, the

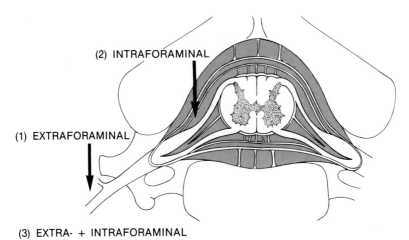

(2) INTRAFORAMINAL

(1) EXTRAFORAMINAL

(3) EXTRA- + INTRAFORAMINAL

Figure 35–2. The drawing indicates the three possible levels of lesion: (1) Extraforaminal, (2) Intraforaminal, and (3) Extra- + Intraforaminal.

EMG cannot provide information pertaining to the damage characterizing each individual root. Furthermore, the absence of SEPs may not be significant when there is a second level of a more peripheral lesion.

Cervical myelography with radiopaque contrast medium is an excellent complementary examination for detection of traumatic root lesions of the brachial plexus. In our experience, a normal myelogram indicates functional integrity of the root in 93% of cases.[2,12] Small plus or minus images due to scars or intraforaminal meningocele can show different aspects of partial or total intraforaminal lesions. A large extraforaminal meningocele almost always indicates root avulsion.

Computed tomography, with or without contrast medium, is a method that has not yet become routine for preoperative investigations but can supply further useful information regarding the suspected intraforaminal lesion.

ELECTROPHYSIOLOGIC INTRAOPERATIVE EVALUATIONS

The clinical and instrument preoperative and anatomicopathologic intraoperative evaluations of root lesions must be combined with electrophysiologic intraoperative findings if a satisfactory reconstruction is to be achieved. The entire brachial plexus must undergo careful surgical preparation in order to accomplish these tests. External neurolysis of the root in the interscalenic area and near the foraminal junction must be especially accurate. This surgical step is difficult, in that the root is often surrounded by abundant scar tissue, causing fixation of the root to the adjacent tissues (fibrotic scalene muscles, transverse groove, etc.).

We perform anterior scalenectomy in order to increase operative space in this small area and to achieve root neurolysis up to the outlet from the foramen. Having accomplished neurolysis and exposed the root lesion, instrument evaluations are made according to the following scheme: simple stimulation, recording of nerve action potentials, recording of somatosensory evoked potentials, and recording of paravertebral muscular evoked potentials. (We do not use the root stimulation and spinal evoked potential recording technique because the stimulus artifact, the brief latency, and the poor ampli-

tude of the potential do not enable us to obtain a reliable signal.)

To carry out these studies, it is necessary to use equipment for electromyography with an averager and sterile electrodes (bipolar or unipolar). For our evaluations, we used a model MS 92 Medelec electromyograph and model E220 sterilizable Medelec biopolar electrodes. When performing these studies, particular care must be taken to eliminate possible sources of interference involving the electrical signal (coagulators, monitoring equipment, etc.).

Simple Stimulation

This can be accomplished only in cases of lesions with extraforaminal continuity or when there are stumps that have retained the more proximal muscular rami. Using a bipolar electrode, we apply a direct stimulus lasting 0.1 msec (frequency of 2/second) to the root. This stimulus has a progressively increasing intensity of 0 to 40 to 50 volts, but not above 50 volts, so as to prevent diffusion. Although the determination of the response to the peripheral muscular contraction is a parameter of subjective evaluation, it can also supply indirect information concerning the partial or total integrity of the root. Besides the evaluation of muscular response to a low-frequency stimulus, one must also consider the response to a high-frequency stimulus (10 to 20/second and more). This creates tetanic contraction in the peripheral muscles, allowing movements to be more easily evaluated. The response to the resulting contraction is evaluated as minimal (+) when the response is visible and determines a limited movement, as medium (+ +) when contraction causes a movement that can be easily hindered, and as maximum (+ + +) when the contraction causes a movement against resistance. We believe that this distinction is important, as in our experience, a minimal response was often associated with lack of recovery of motor function. In these cases, evaluation must be completed by other functional methods.

In root lesions, this method gives no indication as to the integrity of the sensory fibers. Furthermore, in the absence of evident muscular contraction, it does not allow differentiation of the intraforaminal, extraforaminal, or peripheral level of the conduction block.

Recording of Nerve Action Potential (NAP)

In root lesions, NAP can only be evaluated in lesions in extraforaminal continuity. An electrical stimulus (0.1 msec duration with a frequency of 2/second) is applied directly on the root with a bipolar electrode on the previously isolated nerve, and recording is made by using a bipolar electrode at a distance of at least 6 cm from the first electrode.[14] The potential recording methods must take into account the distribution of the nerve fibers of each root in the trunks and peripheral nerves. For this reason, recordings for each stimulated root are made on the trunks and nerves leading from the root itself.

The schematic drawing (Fig. 35–3) indicates the more important peripheral recording points for each stimulated root. This schema is combined with another, indicating the amplitude, duration, latency, and distance of the recorded NAP stimulus.

A confirmation of the validity of the obtained signal, which prevents errors caused by diffusion of the stimulus, can be obtained

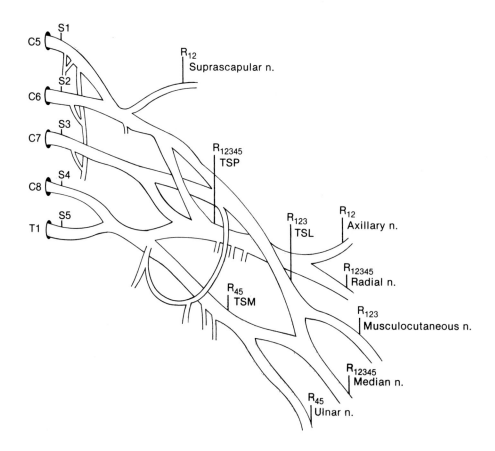

STIMUL.	RECORDING	Distance S-R cm	Intensity Stim. (V)	NAP Absent	NAP Present		
					Latency	Amplitude	Duration

Figure 35–3. The figure schematically indicates the root stimulation zones (S) and the corresponding peripheral recording (R), taking the distribution of the nerve fibers of each root into account. The data obtained are indicated in a diagram showing the stimulation and recording zones, the distance between them, and the NAP characteristics.

by reversing the position of the electrodes, stimulating the periphery and recording at the root.

The presence of NAPs confirms the integrity of the nerve fibers leading from the root in pseudocontinuity. Signal amplitude indirectly supplies information about the quantity of fibers able to conduct the stimulus.[19] The observation of each NAP obtained, leading from each examined root, permits indirect and approximate identification of the number of fibers in the root that are capable of conducting the stimulus.

There are limits to this method as regards the evaluation of root lesion in continuity.

1. The absence of NAPs can result from a second-level lesion, although one with intraforaminal root integrity.

2. The presence of NAPs can be due to a preganglionic lesion with conservation of the sensory fibers.

3. The presence of NAPs does not supply information that distinguishes between the integrity of the contingent sensory and motor fibers.

This test is, therefore, applicable only to extraforaminal lesions in continuity, with the possibility of false-positive and false-negative results. It does not differentiate motor and sensory tracts and can be of use only if compared and evaluated together with other diagnostic parameters.

Recording of Somatosensory Evoked Potentials (SEPs)

In 1947, Dawson showed that after stimulating a peripheral nerve of the upper or lower limb, it was possible to record very low amplitude potentials on the scalp overlying the contralateral cortex.[11] Studies of these SEPs proceeded with the introduction of the first compact computers used in association with electrophysiologic instruments. In 1979 Jones[13] reported on the preoperative use of SEPs, and in 1980 Jones and associates[15] described an intraoperative technique of direct root stimulation with recording in the contralateral parietal zone.

The presence of SEPs testifies to the integrity of the sensory tract proximal to the root, especially in the intraforaminal area. We have employed this method, with certain variants, for over 3 years. Using colloid and adhesive plasters, the electrodes are fixed to the scalp overlying the somesthetic cortex area con-

trolling the hand. This is found 2 cm to the rear and about 7 cm to the side of the vertex and corresponds to Calmes and Cracco's position x, x_2. It has been demonstrated that the greater amplitude neurogenic components N20 and P21 are registered here after stimulation of the median nerve.[2, 10] The passive electrode is positioned on the frontal zone, while the grounding electrode is placed at the occipital level or on the contralateral limb.

Intraoperative stimulation is accomplished by using a bipolar electrode directly on the root with a frequency of 10/second, an intensity of 40 to 60 volts, and a duration of 0.1 msec. Recording is achieved by connecting the preamplifier of the electromyograph to the surface electrode on the parietal hemisphere contralateral to the explored plexus and to the reference electrode on the frontal area.

Next, a 20 msec duration is recorded with averager of at least 1000 sweeps, using a CER filter (2 to 100 Hz). We normally obtain an initial negative peak generated by the cortex at approximately 7 to 10 msec, followed by a positive potential of great duration. The negative deflection range is variable (from about 0.3 to 2 μv). Recording is repeated at least twice for each examined root, comparing the superpositionability with the obtained signal (Fig. 35–4).

Although curare has the advantage of preventing interference by muscular contractions, we do not utilize this agent, as this would preclude the use of additional electrophysiologic examinations, which are helpful when defining root damage.[16]

Intraoperative SEP recording enables the integrity of the intraforaminal part of the sensory tract to be evaluated. However, not even indirect information can be obtained as to the condition of the anterior motor root. This limitation is important, considering that there are dissociated intraforaminal lesions of both the motor and the sensory roots. If one bases evaluation only on the presence of SEPs, it is possible to reconstruct root continuity by using only sensory fibers but nothing will be learned about motor fibers.

Recording of Paravertebral Muscular Evoked Potential (PMEP)

The necessity of using the greatest possible number of motor fibers has encouraged re-

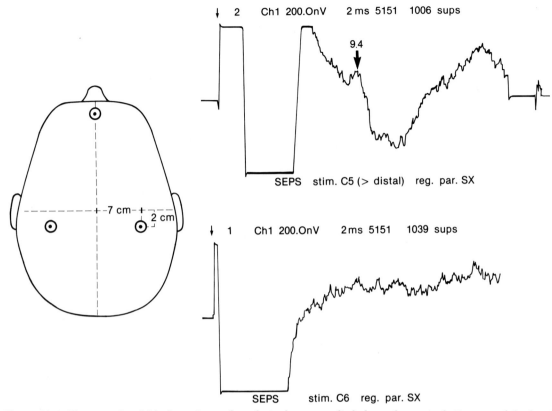

Figure 35–4. The zones in which the active surface electrodes are applied above the somesthetic areas of the hand while the passive electrodes are positioned frontally. The diagram obtained by the intraoperative stimulation of the stump of C5 and C6 in pseudocontinuity is indicated below; a satisfactory SEP is obtained in the former (C5), while SEP is absent in the latter (C6).

search to find a method of evaluating the integrity of the intraforaminal tract of the anterior motor roots.

Immediately after leaving the intervertebral foramen, the spinal nerve formed by the union of the anterior and posterior roots divides into the large anterior branch and the small posterior branch, which innervates the skin and the deep paravertebral muscles of the neck (Fig. 35–5). Our method, utilized since 1978, consists of the intraoperative stimulation of the nerve root at its outlet from the foramen by means of a sterile bipolar electrode connected to the electromyograph.[6] Muscular response (M) is recorded

by a bipolar needle electrode introduced about 0.5 cm lateral to the spinous apophysis corresponding to the root to be examined and deep in the paravertebral muscles (Fig. 35–6). The presence of this response (M) provides proof of the functional integrity of the posterior dorsal ramus and, consequently, of the anatomic and functional continuity of the anterior motor root in the spinal canal (Fig. 35–7).

We obtained the following mean values for PMEP: latency, 2.8 msec; amplitude, 4.9 mV; and duration, 6.9 msec. The sterile zone is extended to the paravertebral region in order to carry out this procedure when preparing

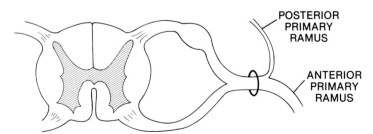

POSTERIOR
PRIMARY
RAMUS

ANTERIOR
PRIMARY
RAMUS

Figure 35–5. The spinal nerve formed by the union of the anterior and posterior roots divides into the large anterior ramus and the small posterior ramus immediately after its outlet from the foramen.

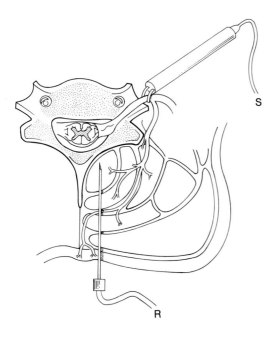

Figure 35–6. The recording electrode (R) is introduced 0.5 cm laterally to the spinous apophysis of the paravertebral muscles near the lamina, while the stimulating electrode(s) is (are) applied at the root immediately after its outlet from the foramen.

the operative zone. This enables the introduction of a needle recording electrode during intraoperative evaluation and its easy movement until the best recording level is obtained. To ensure that the applied stimulus does not spread to the adjacent roots, thus altering the evaluation, we stimulate the root above and the root below without moving the needle recording electrode. Thus obtained, the PMEPs differ as to morphology, amplitude, and latency, and this confirms that the recorded PMEP refers to the examined root only (Fig. 35–8).

The preoperative paravertebral muscle re-

cording techniques are based on the same anatomic factors but are not able to supply a precise evaluation of the damage to individual roots.[1, 20]

This simple method does not require a considerable number of stimulations and records amplitude potentials that are 10,000 times higher than those of SEPs and, therefore, are very much less influenced by possible interference. Although this method gives no indications of the continuity of the posterior sensory tract, we believe it is important to have a valid motor contingent for the reconstruction of the plexus.

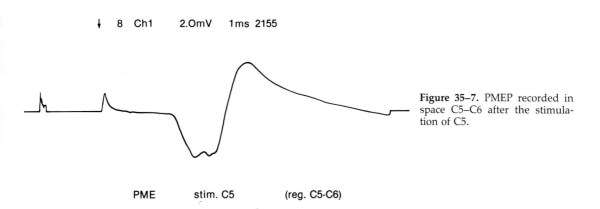

↓   8   Ch1   2.0mV   1ms 2155

PME   stim. C5   (reg. C5-C6)

Figure 35–7. PMEP recorded in space C5–C6 after the stimulation of C5.

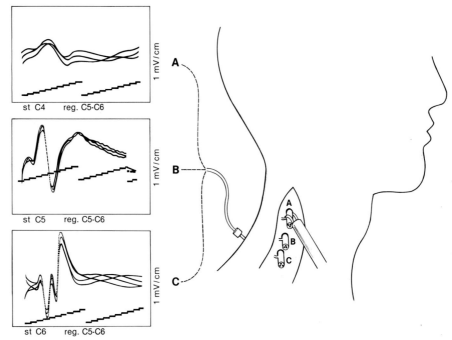

Figure 35–8. The stimulation of the root above and below that examined, without moving the recording needle, obtains PMEPs that differ as to morphology, amplitude, and latency. This confirms that the recorded PMEP depends only on the examined root.

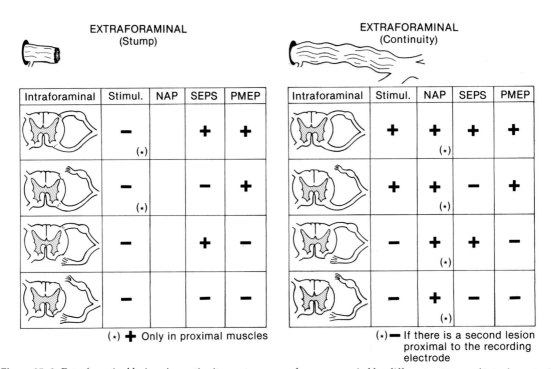

Figure 35–9. Extraforaminal lesions in continuity or stumps can be accompanied by different patterns of intraforaminal lesions, e.g., roots conserved, only one root damaged, both roots avulsed. These anatomicopathologic patterns determine the different indicated intraoperative instrument patterns.

DISCUSSION

During the years 1971 to 1982, we operated on 234 patients with traumatic lesions of the brachial plexus caused by traction. The failures of the first few years regarding the reconstruction of root lesions led us to believe that the single intraoperative evaluation of the root under the operative microscope was insufficient.[3] We have therefore been using electromyography in the operating room since 1977 and have compiled a list of intraoperative electrophysiologic investigations that, having been gradually perfected, have become an integral part of our reconstruction of root lesions of the brachial plexus. The anatomicopathologic aspects of root lesions based on various electrophysiologic evaluations are compared in Figure 35–9.

Of 96 operations on the brachial plexus accomplished during 1978 to 1982, we recorded the PMEP of 33 patients, examining 1 roots in order to évaluate the intraforaminal integrity of the motor fibers. Nineteen roots had a stump, whereas 52 roots showed extraforaminal pseudocontinuity and their stimulation did not produce a contraction of even the most proximal muscles. The examined roots were C5 (30), C6 (23), C7 (14), C8 (3), and T1 (1). The majority were therefore upper roots, and the stumps were only found at levels C5, C6, and C7.

Of the 71 examined roots, 45 showed PMEPs. In 22 roots PMEPs were absent. It was impossible to obtain a good recording for four roots because initially, before starting the operation, we introduced the needle recording electrode in an area outside the operating zone. PMEPs were present in 19 and absent in 4 of the examined root stumps and were present in 30 of the 52 roots in extraforaminal continuity. These data enable us to confirm that intraforaminal damage is rare when traction has caused extraforaminal breakage.

We recorded NAPs for roots in psuedocontinuity, observing the concomitant presence or absence of both PEMPs and NAPs in only 23 roots (frequently lesions at several levels).

We have been using the preroperative and intraoperative SEP recording since 1980.[8, 9] The combined evaluation of PMEPs and SEPs was used in the case of 47 roots. There was concordance, i.e., concomitant presence or absence of both PMEPs and SEPs, in 39 roots and discordance in 8 roots. This means that the intraforaminal findings for motor and sensory roots were the same in 83% of the cases, whereas there was a dissociation of functional data corresponding to different anatomicopathological findings in 17%.

CONCLUSIONS

The intraoperative electrophysiologic evaluation of the root in brachial plexus lesions can give reliable data on intra- and extraforaminal function. To prevent possible errors in the recording and interpretation of the obtained data, it is necessary that:

1. *The surgeon* carefully prepare the plexus and especially the root by freeing it from the scar tissue adhering up to its outlet from the foramen.

2. The *examiner* performing the electrophysiologic tests has direct knowledge of the preoperative evaluations concerning intraoperative problems and reconstruction possibilities. Furthermore, the examiner must know how to apply a precise evaluation schema according to the different aspects of the lesion.

3. The *electromyograph* be easily handled and portable but equipped with systems able to record signals of minimal amplitude and complete with adequate electrodes.

4. The *interferences* in the operating room be reduced to minimal acceptable levels.

5. The available *time* be sufficient to carry out the different evaluations, allowing the possibility of verification and comparison. This generally requires a pause in surgical activities of about 1 hour.

Compared with the preoperative clinical and instrument examinations and with the anatomicopathologic features of the lesion, the intraoperatively obtained data help determine the possibility of using the damaged root in the reconstruction of the brachial plexus lesion or establish the need to resort to neurotization by accessory (eleventh cranial) and intercostal nerves.[4, 5]

References

1. Bufalini, C., and Pescatori, G.: La elettromiografia dei muscoli posteriori del collo nella prognosi delle lesioni di plesso brachiale. Arch. Putti. Chir. Org. Mov., 23:23–31, 1968.
2. Calmes, R. L., and Cracco, R. Q.: Comparison of somatosensory and somatomotor evoked responses to median nerve and digital nerve stimulation. Electroenc. Cl. Neuroph., 31:547–562, 1971.

3. Celli, L., Mingione, A., and Landi, A.: Nuove acquisizioni di tecnica chirurgica nelle lesioni del plesso brachiale: indicazioni alla neurolisi, autoinnesti e trapianti nervosi. Comunication, LIX Congress S.I.O.T., Cagliari, 1974.

4. Celli, L., Montorsi, A., de Luise, G., and Rovesta, C.: Utilizzazione dell'XI nervo cranico e dei nervi del plesso cervicale nelle lesioni radicolari del plesso brachiale. Chir. Org. Movim., 64:365–371, 1979.

5. Celli, L., Balli, A. L., de Luise, G., and Rovesta, C.: La neurotizzazione degli ultimi nervi intercostali, mediante trapianto nervoso peduncolato nelle avulsioni radicolari del plesso brachiale. Chir. Org. Movim., 64:461–464, 1979.

6. Celli, L., Canedi, L., and Rovesta, C.: I potenziali muscolari evocati intraoperatori nel trattamento delle lesioni traumatiche del plesso brachiale. Chir. Org. Movim., 65:399–403, 1979.

7. Celli, L., Montorsi, A., Balli, A., and Luchetti, R.: Myelographic study of the traumatic radicular injuries of the brachial plexus. J. Neurosurg. Sci., 25:123–125, 1981.

8. Celli, L., Rovesta, C., and de Luise, G.: Intraoperative paravertebral muscular evoked potentials (PMEP) in treatment of traumatic root lesions of the brachial plexus. Acta Ort. Belgica, 49:564–570, 1983.

9. Celli, L., and Rovesta, C.: Intraoperative paravertebral muscular evoked potentials (PMEP) in treatment of traumatic root lesions of the brachial plexus. Communication, Brachial Plexus Meeting, London, January, 1983.

10. Cracco, R. Q.: Spinal evoked response: peripheral nerve stimulation in man. Electroenc. Cl. Neuroph., 35:379–386, 1973.

11. Dawson, G. D.: Cerebral response to electrical stimulation of peripheral nerves in man. J. Neurol. Neurosurg. Psychiatry, 10:134–140, 1947.

12. Frot, B.: La myelographie cervicale opaque dans les paralysies traumatiques du plexus brachial. Rev. Chir. Orthop., 63:64–72, 1977.

13. Jones, S. J.: Investigation of brachial plexus traction lesions by peripheral and spinal somatosensory evoked potentials. J. Neurol. Neurosurg. Psychiatry, 42:107–116, 1979.

14. Kline, D. G., and de Joung, B. R.: Evoked potentials to evaluate peripheral nerve injuries. Surg. Gynecol. Obstet., 127:1239, 1968.

15. Landi, A., Copeland, S. A., Wynn Parry, C. B., and Jones, S. J.: The role of somatosensory evoked potentials and nerve conduction studies in the surgical management of brachial plexus injuries. J. Bone Joint Surg., 62B:492–496, 1980.

16. Pelissier, J., Asencio, G., Georgesco, M., Piade, J. P., Allieu, Y., and Cadilhac, J.: Exploration électrophysiologique pré et per-operatoire des traumatismes du plexus brachial. In Plexus Brachial et Medicina de Réeducation. Paris, Masson, 1982, pp. 33–40.

17. Privat, J. M., Mailhe, D., Allieu, Y., and Bonnel, F.: Hemilaminectomie cervicale exploratrice et nevrotisation précoce du plexus brachial. In: Plexus Brachial et Medicina de Réeducation. Paris, Masson, 1982, pp. 66–73.

18. Sunderland, S.: Meningeal-neural relations in the intervertebral foramen. J. Neurosurg., 40:756–761, 1974.

19. Terzis, J. K., Dykes, R. W., and Hakstian, R. W.: Electrophysiological recording in peripheral nerve surgery: A review. Hand Surg., 1:52–66, 1976.

20. Zalis, A. W., Oester, Y. T., and Rodriquez, A. A.: Electrophysiological diagnosis of cervical nerve root avulsion. Arch. Physiol. Med., 51:708–710, 1970.

36

Rehabilitation of Patients Following Traction Lesions of the Brachial Plexus

■

C. B. Wynn Parry, M.B.E., M.A., D.M.
Victoria Frampton, M.C.S.P., S.R.P.
Alison Monteith, Dip., C.O.T., S.R.O.T.

The Royal National Orthopaedic Hospital in London has been a referral center for patients with brachial plexus lesions for approximately 40 years. The pioneering work of George Bonney[4] and Philip Yeoman[16] established the various types of lesions and devised a program of surgical management. In the early postwar years, the exploration of the plexus was abandoned, most observers reported that there was so much scar tissue that it was difficult to distinguish one structure from another, and it was rare to see frank ruptures of nerves that would be amenable to repair by grafting.[3] Brooks (personal communication) found that only 10% of patients whom he explored surgically had a rupture. Therefore, for some 30 years the management of these lesions was predominantly conservative, waiting until such time as it was clear that further recovery was not going to occur spontaneously and then instituting a program of surgical reconstruction. In some cases the totally flail arm was treated by amputation, arthrodesis of the shoulder, and fitting of a prosthesis. Some of these patients returned to work and used their prosthesis regularly. However, injuries in those days were less severe, and many such patients had good scapular control, as the C5 muscles were spared. In recent years, the situation has changed radically, as there is a far higher proportion of total lesions. Injuries are most probably more severe today because crash helmets are now compulsory, and patients who would previously have died are now surviving. Consequently, much more serious injuries are being seen.

Table 36–1 shows an analysis of the percentage of patients referred to our center who have total lesions. Moreover, these lesions involve the entire plexus, paralyzing all the C5 muscles. In such cases, patients will not be able to use an artificial limb, as there is no scapular control to effect the elbow-locking device. The pioneering work of Narakas[10] showed that a higher proportion of patients had ruptures of nerve roots than hitherto had been reported. Narakas was the first to

Table 36–1. PATIENTS WITH BRACHIAL PLEXUS LESIONS REFERRED TO THE ROYAL NATIONAL ORTHOPAEDIC HOSPITAL

Number of New Patients Seen		Total Lesions	
Year	No.	No.	%
1977	58	14	24
1978	73	17	23
1979	102	32	31
1980	117	46	40
1981	110	54	50
Pre-1975	135	181	16

explore the plexus routinely, and he found that many patients had ruptures of C5–C6 and that these were amenable to surgical repair.

During the years 1950 to 1970, we had the experience of following a large number of patients who were treated conservatively in the Military Rehabilitation Units.[14] We showed that approximately two thirds of patients with C5–C6 lesions that were complete and proved by electromyography would recover elbow flexion, whereas only one third of patients with complete C5–C7 lesions would recover elbow flexion. Not surprisingly, very few patients with total lesions recovered any function. The interesting question is why one third of our patients with C5–C6 lesions did not recover elbow flexion. It would now seem that this is because those patients suffered rupture of their nerves, and of course spontaneous recovery was impossible. This coincides nicely with the experience of Narakas,[10] who showed that on exploration some one third of his patients had rupture of C5 and C6.

Elsewhere in this book, the indications and need for surgical exploration are fully described. It is the view of our surgical team that the sooner the patient is explored, the better. Ideally this should be within a few hours or at least within 48 hours of the accident. At that time, the dissection is easier, a definitive diagnosis can be made, and a decision can be reached as to whether nerves are ruptured or merely stretched or whether there is total avulsion from the cord. This enables an accurate prognosis to be made, and a plan of rehabilitation can be established at the earliest stage. Furthermore, repair by grafting is much more likely to be successful at the earlier stage. The demonstration of avulsion of C8 and T1 at open operation will allow the use of the ulnar nerve as a vascularized nerve graft to repair the C5–C6 roots and sometimes the C7 root. The use of vascularized grafts has greatly improved the functional results. However, many patients are not suitable for early exploration because of difficulty in referral to a specialized center, or because of multiple injuries (in particular, head injuries). Thus, there will continue to be many patients who only can undergo surgical exploration some months after injury.

It is important to know at what stage exploration is futile. Based on the work of surgeons during World War II, we have been led to believe that muscles will not maintain viability for longer than 18 months after interruption of their nerve supply. However, we have seen patients who have had spontaneous and very good functional recovery of elbow flexion 5 years after injury. Clearly, a muscle is viable for a much longer period than the orthodox teaching implies. It may well be that the war injuries were associated with severe vascular damage and that the muscles may have been fibrotic as a result of damage to their blood supply. In lesions in which the blood supply is intact, it may well be that muscles will survive for much longer periods, and therefore delayed surgery may not be as disappointing as one would expect. However, our surgical team believes that surgery after the first year of onset is probably not worthwhile, and this is certainly true when damage to major blood vessels in the limb has occurred. If surgery can be undertaken in the early stages, the diagnosis is clear and there is no need for the various ancillary investigations that are required to determine the diagnosis at a later stage.

However, we are here concerned with those patients in whom surgery has not been possible in the early stage and who are referred for consultation at a few months after injury. At this stage the important need is to establish the exact diagnosis, if possible. Is the lesion in continuity (for which spontaneous recovery can be expected in time)? Is there a possibility of a rupture of one or more of the upper nerve roots, or are the nerve roots avulsed from the cord and therefore completely and irrevocably damaged? It is our practice to admit all patients to our Rehabilitation Ward for a careful and intensive assessment. At the Royal National Orthopaedic Hospital, we are fortunate in having two mini-care wards, with 16 beds for female and 16 beds for male patients. These operate on a Monday to Friday basis. During this time, patients are up and dressed and are undergoing either intensive assessment or comprehensive rehabilitation. Gathering together a number of young people with similar injuries under these circumstances is very good for their morale, and patients learn from each other and gain inspiration from each other's recovery.

PRELIMINARY INVESTIGATIONS

The first step is the institution of investigations to establish the site and nature of the lesion. A careful clinical history and examination will go far to determining these factors. Table 36–2 shows factors that indicate a poor prognosis, and Table 36–3 indicates factors that suggest that the lesion is relatively mild. The painful neuroma sign has proved helpful; i.e., if one taps the neck over the site of the nerve root and can reproduce several painful paresthesiae in the distribution of a particular nerve root, this is a strong suggestion a rupture has occurred, particularly if there is no distal Tinel's sign. Sometimes the ruptured nerve root can actually be felt through the neck.

Electromyographic investigations are then carried out. Representative muscles of each nerve root are routinely sampled to see if there are any surviving units, which would of course indicate some continuity in that root. For C5 we routinely examine the rhomboids and infraspinatus muscles and the clavicular fibers of the pectoralis major muscle; for C6, the biceps and brachioradialis muscles; for C7, the triceps and the extensors of the wrist and fingers; for C8, the finger and wrist flexors; and for T1, the intrinsic muscles of the hand. If total denervation is found in muscles of the nerve root being examined, it is clear that there has been total disruption of the axons. The next question follows—is this a rupture or an avulsion? Sensory conduction tests have virtually replaced the old histamine test to establish if the lesion is pre- or postganglionic, except for the C5 root. We routinely measure the radial sensory nerve action potential (SNAP) for C6, stimulating in the mid-forearm and recording with surface electrodes over the first dorsal interosseous space, and for C6–T1 stimulating the median and ulnar nerves at the wrist and recording with ring electrodes over the four fingers. We also stimulate the ulnar nerve at the wrist and record with surface electrodes over the nerve just above the elbow. If a SNAP is found in the presence of total anesthesia, this must indicate a preganglionic

Table 36–2. POOR PROGNOSTIC SIGNS IN BRACHIAL PLEXUS LESIONS

High speed injury
Coexistence of bony damage, particularly fracture of transverse processes
Complete lesion
Long tract signs
Positive Horner's sign
Burning pain with paroxysmal shooting pain
Paralysis of thoracoscapular muscles

Table 36–3. GOOD PROGNOSTIC SIGNS IN BRACHIAL PLEXUS LESIONS

Mild trauma
Incomplete paralysis
No pain
Progressive Tinel's sign
Sparing of serratus, rhomboid, and latissimus muscles
Absent Horner's sign
Absent sensory action potentials
Surviving motor units on EMG

avulsion lesion. The degree of attenuation of the amplitude of the response on the injured side compared with the normal side will give some indication of the degree of postganglionic damage as well.

Sensory evoked potentials (SEPs) can also be very helpful, and Jones and colleagues[6, 7] have shown that determination of SNAP and SEP in combination yields the most information. However, if facilities for determination of SEP are not available (although with the more advanced EMG machine, this can be done without computers), the study of the SNAP provides almost as much information as the use of the more sophisticated techniques.

Careful muscle charting is carried out by both the physician and the physiotherapist. Special reference is paid to the proximal scapular muscles, in particular the rhomboids, serratus anterior, latissimus dorsi, and teres major and minor, since paralysis of these muscles indicates a very high lesion with an almost uniformly poor prognosis. It is important to beware of "trick" movements that can deceive the examiner, e.g., the ability of a patient with a C7 lesion to extend the interphalangeal joint of the thumb by the use of the abductor pollicis brevis and flexor brevis, which insert into the extensor expansion. A physiotherapist skilled in muscle testing techniques is invaluable in the routine assessment of these patients.

By a careful history, clinical examination, and electrophysiologic studies, it should therefore be possible to have a good idea as to whether the lesion is pre- or postganglionic and whether a rupture is likely, which suggests the need for surgery. Myelography undoubtedly helps, but is not as reliable as is often believed. On the whole, the myelogram tends to overestimate damage. We consistently see patients in whom a myelogram suggested avulsion of the nerve root who in fact regain excellent function or who are found to have nerve roots in continuity at operation. As a result of this workup, by the end of the first week it should be possible to have a clear idea as to whether the lesion is likely to recover spontaneously or will require exploration to graft the possible rupture, or whether there is total avulsion of one or more roots with a hopeless prognosis.

When surgery is planned, the next step is to prepare the patient to be in an optimal state for the operation. This means restoring full range of passive movements (particularly of the shoulder), dealing with any trophic lesions that the patient may have sustained in the anesthetic areas, regaining as much power from the spared muscles as possible by means of intensive physiotherapy and occupational therapy, and giving the patient a clearer idea of what is expected from surgery and what the future holds. However technically demanding the surgery may be, it must be remembered that the operation is simply one step, albeit a vital one, in the total rehabilitation of the patient. Thus, whether the patient has had surgical repair or whether a conservative line has been adopted, the general management of the patient remains the same. The outstanding aim is restoration of maximal function, as soon as possible, and the return of the patient to the community and to work.

The degree to which functional return is possible of course depends on the severity of the lesion. A patient with partial paralysis, e.g., C5 and C6, will be able to use his hand, provided some form of functional splinting is employed to enable him to position his hand properly. The common patterns of involvement are as follows:

1. C5–C6 lesions: Complete paralysis with loss of shoulder abduction, elevation, and elbow function.

2. Complete C5, C6, and C7 lesions: In addition to paralysis of the shoulder and elbow, there is paralysis of extension of the wrist, fingers, and thumb, and the patient cannot release his grasp.

3. Complete paralysis of the limb, with rupture of C5, C6, and C7 and with C8 and T1 in continuity: These are the patients for whom surgery can hopefully restore elbow flexion at least.

4. Total paralysis of the arm with rupture of C5–C6 and avulsion of C7, C8, and T1: Repair of the upper trunk is even more important in these patients than in Group 3 patients, as restoration of any degree of function is worthwhile when there is total paral-

ysis. Such patients can at least adduct the arm and can hold things between the arm and the body. They can also regain some elbow flexion, which can be helpful in using the arm as a support.

5. Avulsion of all five roots with a total and permanent flail arm.

REHABILITATION

We will now consider the rehabilitation of two groups of patients: those in whom there is some residual function and those in whom there is total paralysis of the arm.

Patients with Residual Function

A patient commonly has sparing of C8 and T1 with paralysis of elbow flexion and shoulder abduction. Functional splinting is very helpful in this situation. A simple elbow lock splint, with a ratchet device, will allow the patient to position his elbow in one of four or five positions so that he can use his hand for normal functions. The splint we provide is ready made, and the patient can learn to operate it within an hour. It is light and inexpensive and is worn under the clothing so that it is not conspicuous. Figure 36–1 shows such a splint, and we now have 16 patients who regularly wear this device when working. If the C7 component is also involved, a wrist drop support with or without finger extension loops can be provided. It is emphasized that these splints are ready made. They come in three sizes and can easily be adjusted by the orthotist to suit individual patients. Such patients can be back to work within a week of fitting the splint.

Patients with a Totally Flail Arm

These patients are likely to have total paralysis of the limb, including the scapular muscles, and amputation and arthrodesis will not provide the ability to use an artificial limb.

Use of Flail Arm Splint

The question of amputation will be discussed later in this chapter. However, it should be pointed out that fitting of a flail arm splint is likely to provide just as good

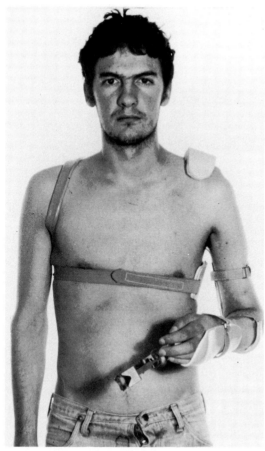

Figure 36–1. Full flail arm splint. (From Wynn Parry, C. B.: Clin. Plast. Surg., *11*:174, 1984.)

vices to suit an individual patient's needs for work or hobbies have been made. Thus, we have made devices for patients for golf, fishing, tennis, and even cricket (Table 36–4).

In patients with C8–T1 paralysis in whom C5, C6, and C7 have been spared or are no longer paralyzed, a forearm gauntlet is provided after preliminary plaster casting. This has the same arrangement as that for artificial limb appliances but can be operated by the patient's own elbow flexion and extension.

At a recent follow-up of some 200 patients fitted with a full flail arm splint, 60% are regularly using the splint for work and hobbies or both. A number of patients have used the splint for a few months and then found that they can manage without it, but it has provided a valuable means for returning to work and restoring confidence. A few patients have rejected the splint, even though it was predicted that they would find it useful. It is therefore difficult to ascertain

function as an artificial arm, since most patients use prostheses only for cosmetic purposes (if these are used at all). By far, the majority of patients prefer to keep their own arm. We have been surprised by how very few patients develop trophic lesions, for these patients learn to look after their hand well (it is, after all, part of them and of their body image). If one can provide a flail arm splint that acts as a mobile vise, these patients have the best of two worlds—some useful function with the splint and their own arm as well.

The flail arm splint comprises a shoulder support, an elbow-locking device, and a wrist support with a forearm platform into which the standard appliances of an artificial limb are fitted (Figs. 36–1 to 36–3). The patient adjusts the elbow lock himself, while the appliances are operated by the standard cable harness, controlled by the contralateral shoulder. A wide variety of appliances are available, and in many instances special de-

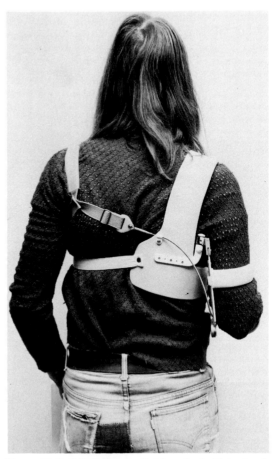

Figure 36–2. Full flail arm splint from back. Note shoulder support, shoulder "joint," and elbow lock. (From Wynn Parry, C. B.: Clin. Plast. Surg., *11*:175, 1984.)

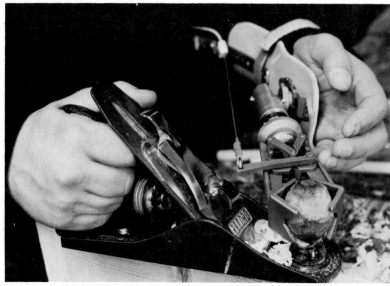

Figure 36–3. Universal tool holder in action. (From Wynn Parry, C. B.: Clin. Plast. Surg., *11*:176, 1984.)

whether a patient will or will not use the splint until he has actually tried it out under normal circumstances. However, we have had considerable success in simulating working conditions in our workshops in the Rehabilitation Department and are now much better able to judge whether a patient is likely to wear a splint or not.

We have learned that there is a right time in which to introduce the idea of wearing a flail arm splint. If one introduces this too early, the patient will object because he still feels that recovery may occur. It takes time for a patient to come to terms with the fact that he has a totally useless and irrevocably paralyzed upper limb. For example, if surgery is planned in the early stages, it is probably wiser to postpone fitting a splint until the operation clarifies exactly what the

Table 36–4. OCCUPATIONS AND HOBBIES IN WHICH FLAIL ARM SPLINTS ARE USED

Occupations	Hobbies
Gardening	Darts
Woodwork	Clay modeling
Paint spraying	Painting
Shoe making	Fishing
Operating fork lift truck	Golf
Postman	Cricket
Painting	Rifle shooting
Office Work	
Electrical repairman	
Engineering	

lesion entails. When the patient has come to terms with the fact that surgery has shown an irreversible lesion, the idea of a splint may be introduced. On the other hand, if the splint is offered some months after the injury, the patient may have become completely used to functioning with one arm and will reject it. Because there are many occupations and hobbies that are open to patients using the splints, it is a pity to deny them this opportunity, although choosing the right time in the right patient is of the utmost importance. Only by having an integrated rehabilitation team who work together all the time and have extensive experience with these lesions and with these young patients' reactions to them can one judge the suitability of splinting.

Following the fitting of a flail arm splint, it is imperative that the patient completes a period of training similar to that for upper limb amputees following fitting of a prosthesis. As the prostheses and orthoses are so similar, the training follows the same lines. This training is important not only to ensure that the patient obtains maximal use from the splint, but also to allow a period of time for psychologic adjustment to both the disability and the appliances.

Obviously, the more complex the splint, the longer the training session must be. Generally, it takes approximately 10 days to train a patient fully in the use of the complete flail arm splint, whereas training takes only 4 to 5 days for the gauntlet forearm splint, since the patient uses his own elbow and shoulder movements.

The patient visits the Occupational Therapy Department, where training begins with a simple exercise to teach use and control of the split hook, e.g., remedial games such as solitaire, using pieces of ½ inch dowel. This will build up the strength required for good operation of appliances and also improve coordination to enable the unaffected shoulder to protract, leaving the rest of the upper limb free to do the necessary work.

Control is usually learned quickly in a single morning session, in which the patient wears the splint for about 45 minutes, has a 1 hour complete break, and then continues to wear the splint for another 45 minutes. Tolerance to the splint must be built up gradually in order to prevent pressure sores. The most vulnerable site for pressure sores is the anterior part of the axilla of the unaffected side, which provides the seat for the shoulder loop.

Prior to fitting a flail arm splint, the therapist discusses the possible uses of the splint with the patient to try to ensure that the appliance will not be discarded on discharge from the hospital. Also discussed are the activities for which the patient is likely to use the splint, so that appropriate appliances may be selected. Training then continues in the use of these splints, in whichever environment is best suited to the patient's activities.

For men, use of the universal tool holder, tweezers, and quick grip pliers is taught and practiced. These patients begin with a regimen of basic exercises to illustrate methods of using such appliances, and then they undertake a project involving the techniques they have learned. The entire range of gardening is possible using various attachments. For women (and some men for that matter), training includes emphasis on domestic activities, for which the most useful appliances are the split hook, C-grip, and occasionally the universal tool holder. Activities include cooking, ironing, sweeping, and washing up.

Clerical workers and students may find the two-pronged office appliance most beneficial for stabilizing work, and practice with this is undertaken. The split hook may also be useful when the patient has to write while moving (e.g., checking stock), and a clipboard or note pad may be held.

There are also a few students with this disability who, without a flail arm splint, would be unable to partake in woodwork or metalwork classes and would have considerable difficulty with other classes, such as technical drawing and domestic science. Training, therefore, is centered on these activities.

Hobbies are not forgotten (e.g., model making and needlework), and, when necessary, specific training and practice are undertaken. For example, three of our patients use a special appliance to hold a fishing rod.

Particular emphasis is placed on the use of the splint for employment, and when possible the work situation should be simulated as part of the training process. During this time, it may become apparent that none of the existing appliances can be used, and a special one may have to be designed. Obviously, many more appliances can be used by those with good shoulder and elbow function who therefore require only the gauntlet type splint.

During this training session, any problems with the splint can hopefully be ironed out and alterations completed. These problems often become apparent only by using the splint, and they must be rectified immediately so that the patient can leave the hospital with the motivation and enthusiasm necessary to use and experiment with the splint, and, consequently, to improve his overall functional ability. During this time, a full assessment, including diagnostic tests, is made, and splintage is considered and provided when necessary. By the end of 2 weeks, the patients should be totally familiar with the management of the splint, and we should be able to tell whether or not they are likely to use it.

Return to Work

We are fortunate at the Royal National Orthopaedic Hospital, Stanmore, London, in having two rehabilitation officers as part of the rehabilitation team. These officers have had extensive experience in industry, and their role is to establish a liaison between the hospital and the employer as early as possible after the injury. If necessary, they will visit the place of work and make a careful job assessment. They can then advise the medical team as to the feasibility of the patient's return to that particular job or in what way the job may be modified to allow him to return to work.

If it is clear that the patient will never be

able to return to his former job, alternative forms of work in the same firm are explored at an early stage. If this too is impossible, vocational assessment and retraining start as early as possible and are an integral part of the rehabilitation program. Careful assessment of the work situation will also allow the surgeon to choose the correct reconstructive procedure at a later stage, based on the patient's job requirements.

Many patients who have sustained complete paralysis of the dominant arm need help in retraining to manage with only one arm. Most patients who lose function of the nondominant arm quickly learn to carry out almost everything one handed, and many patients find that there are few things that they cannot do. However, if the dominant arm is paralyzed, formal retraining may be necessary. For example, as soon as practical after the injury, the occupational therapist and the nursing staff can help the patient to overcome difficulties in dressing by stressing constant practice and also teaching new techniques. Shoe laces can be tied with one hand, once the technique has been acquired. Cuff links and buttons can be manipulated on the shirt sleeve of the unaffected arm by using the teeth or by dexterous use of the fingers of the same hand. If this is impossible, Velcro or elastic can be used. For ties, either clip-on ties can be used or the tie can be knotted first and then looped over the head and tightened by hand. A suction nail brush can be useful for washing. Most patients can manage to shave with one hand, but many of them prefer to use an electric razor.

Feeding requires the most practice, and patients may initially need to have their food cut up. Most patients prefer to use an ordinary fork in the unaffected hand rather than aids (such as the Nelson knife), which are designed for one-armed people. However, many will accept the dinafork, which is a normal-looking fork with a sharpened edge for cutting.

The patient is encouraged to continue with all household activities carried out before the injury, e.g., washing and drying up, looking after his own bedroom, making drinks, and cooking. He must expect to encounter difficulties and to be slower than normal, but with practice and perseverance the vast majority of patients manage all routine tasks with ease. Making beds can be difficult, and most patients find a quilt instead of sheets a satisfactory solution. Housewives will find the standard home aids useful. These include nonslip mats, spike boards, cutting boards, and one-handed can openers—indeed most labor-saving devices can be controlled by one hand.

Writing practice should start early, and it is surprising how quickly patients can learn to write with the nondominant hand. Magnetic writing boards and rulers are available for one-handed people.

It is generally helpful to have the patient spend a few sessions in the Occupational Therapy Department to improve dexterity and strengthen the unaffected arm. Useful activities include printing, woodwork, sewing, sanding and filing, model making, clerical work (involving collating, stapling, putting paper in envelopes, and typing), metal work, occasionally weaving on the rug loom, and remedial games such as table tennis and darts.

The physiotherapist also has a vital contribution to make. She will restore as full a range of passive movements as possible to joints that may have become stiff through disuse and will instruct the patient carefully in passive movements to be done at home, with or without the help of family members. She will also institute a program of intensive exercises to restore maximal function in spared muscles or to encourage power in recovering muscles. She will give the patient exercises to be done at home and instruct him in ways of overcoming his disability.

We do not favor regular outpatient physiotherapy because we believe that patients should return to work as soon as possible. It is very difficult, particularly at times of mass unemployment, to persuade an employer to take a patient back who requires continuing treatment. Indeed, this is quite unnecessary because the best treatment (once a full assessment and a short spell of intensive rehabilitation have taken place) is return to normal work and activities. It is our practice to review patients regularly every 4 months and periodically readmit them for an intensive program of rehabilitation. This is done to capitalize on any recovery, to check that splints still fit or need adjustment or new appliances, to make sure that passive range of movements is being maintained, and to determine whether the patient's job situation is still satisfactory. Regular, short, intensive periods of rehabilitation are, in our view, far preferable to ongoing physiotherapy, which disrupts the patient's life and may make it impossible for him to return to work.

Return to work is vital in the rehabilitation of these patients, not only in order to enable them to return to a normal life but to provide a consistent means of distracting them from severe pain, if this is present. We have referred already to our two rehabilitation officers whose sole job is to organize work. These men are an integral part of the medical team, but they have been chosen for their previous industrial experience and their understanding of the work situation. Thus, our two current rehabilitation officers have had experience in the automobile industry and in engineering. It is difficult for a physician, however experienced, to convince an employer that a patient (e.g., with one arm) is fit to go back to spray painting. However, a rehabilitation officer who has worked in industry, and knows exactly what is involved and what the dangers are, can "sell" the patient to the employer in a way that the physician cannot. On admission to the hospital, the rehabilitation officer routinely interviews the patient to find out exactly what his work was. The officer then contacts the employer immediately, explains the medical situation, and assures the employer that in due course the patient will be fit to return to work. As a result of the 2-week assessment, it should be possible to have a fairly accurate idea as to whether the patient will be able to return to his old job or whether there will be limitations that either can be overcome by adjustment of the work situation or will require a different job, preferably in the same company. It is our experience that if contact is made early, the employer does not lose interest in his employee and will be eager to take the patient back in due course. This, in turn, encourages the patient greatly, as he feels that his future is assured and he can cease worrying about problems of returning to work.

If there is the slightest doubt in the rehabilitation officer's mind as to the nature of the patient's work, he will visit the work place and discuss the requirements of the job with the employer. He will then bring this information back to the medical team, who, together with the rehabilitation officer, will be able to decide whether the patient will be able to carry out his work and whether functional splinting will be needed. A job requiring two-handed work of a heavy manual

Table 36–5. PATIENTS RETURNING TO WORK AFTER BRACHIAL PLEXUS LESIONS (1975–1980)

Patients	No.
Total referred for help and follow-up available	74
Working for original firms	35
Working for different firms	25
Total at work	60 (80%)
Total not at work:	14 (20%)
4 unemployed	
4 ill	
3 being trained	
2 in prison	
1 student	

nature will clearly be impossible for a man who has a totally and permanently paralyzed arm. It may, however, be possible for that patient to be employed in a store or in a clerical capacity.

If the patient is likely to be off for some time, suitable training can start in the Occupational Therapy and Rehabilitation Departments. This is particularly applicable when patients have multiple injuries (e.g., fractures of the leg or a significant head injury) that may require some form of psychologic reeducation. Ideally, patients who have a brachial plexus lesion without any associated injuries should be able to return to work within a few weeks of the injury. If rehabilitation is going to be a long-term process, the rehabilitation officer periodically contacts the employer to keep him informed about progress. As mentioned earlier, most employers are only too pleased to take their employees back after injury.

Finally, we cannot overemphasize the importance of considering a patient's hobbies and sports, as well as his work, particularly in periods of high unemployment, and this may be the most important factor in the patient's rehabilitation.

The success of our rehabilitation officers is shown by the fact that in a series of 74 patients with totally paralyzed arms, 80% returned either to their former work or to new work that was found for them. Follow-up is important to make sure that the patient is managing the job. If difficulties have arisen, further strenuous efforts are made to try to find alternative work for the patient (Table 36–5).

PAIN

One of the most distressing features of avulsion lesions of the plexus is the severe pain felt by the vast majority of patients. We have figures for 298 patients followed for 3 to 30 years. Of these, 167 had postganglionic lesions, but none of these patients had significant pain. There were 122 patients with proven ganglionic lesions, of whom 112 suffered severe pain. All patients with complete C5–T1 lesions suffered pain at some stage of their injury. Of these 122 patients, 48 are still suffering from severe pain 3 years or more since the onset. Another 38 patients have come to terms with their pain or the pain has abated, 10 had no pain at any stage, and 26 had severe pain that was substantially relieved by transcutaneous nerve stimulation. This pain may persist indefinitely. The natural history of severe pain is that the patients who are going to come to terms with the pain will do so within 3 years of onset. If the pain is still severe and is interfering with activities 3 years after injury, it is most likely to persist throughout the patient's life. In fact, we have 23 patients who have suffered severe pain for more than 11 years. Table 36–6 shows the time it took for the pain to become acceptable or to abate in 28 patients.

The onset of the pain may be immediate or delayed. In 40% of patients, the pain was felt immediately. In 28%, the pain developed over periods varying from 1 week to 12 weeks after injury, and in 11% of these patients, the pain developed 1 month or more after the injury. Twenty-five per cent of patients were unconscious for some time, and therefore the onset of pain could not be accurately established (Table 36–7). The pain is highly characteristic and has two distinct features. One is a constant background pain, usually described as burning (as if the arm is on fire) or as crushing (as if the arm is in a vise or is being hit repeatedly with a hammer). Sometimes the pain is described as feeling like a razor blade cutting through the skin. This pain persists throughout the day, is invariably present if waking at night, and hardly ever varies in intensity. The second feature

Table 36–6. PATIENTS WITH ACCEPTABLE OR MILD PAIN (n = 28)

Time to Become Acceptable	No. of Patients
6 months	4
9 months	2
1 year	9
2 years	7
3 years	4
4 years	2

Table 36–7. DURATION FROM TIME OF INJURY TO ONSET OF PAIN

Duration	%
Immediate	40
After 1 week	4
After 2 weeks	8
After 3 weeks	5
After 4 weeks	3
4–8 weeks	5
8–12 weeks	3
Unconscious	25
No pain	7

is pain characterized by periodic sharp paroxysms that shoot through the arm, lasting a few seconds at a time. These can sometimes be more difficult to deal with than the constant background pain, for they take the patient by surprise and may cause him to cry out or drop things. The frequency of these paroxysms varies from many shooting pains per hour to two to three per day or a few per week. Over a period of time, the paroxysms tend to become less frequent, but in a significant proportion of patients, they represent a very severe disability. Of our 122 patients, 94% had paroxysmal pain—47% several times an hour, 43% several times a day, and 10% several times a week. Table 36–8 shows factors that affect the pain. Cold weather and intercurrent illness are potent aggravating factors. Emotional stress increased the pain in half the patients.

A high proportion of patients instinctively grip their arm or move their fingers in an attempt to relieve the pain, and this can be effective temporarily. However, the single most constant feature in relieving pain or at least making it more bearable is distraction, such as being deeply involved in work or in absorbing hobbies. This is why it is so important to help these patients return to the community as quickly as possible, as this

Table 36–8. FACTORS AFFECTING PAIN IN BRACHIAL PLEXUS LESIONS

Factor	%
Cold weather	70
Intercurrent illness	70
Emotions	50
Sleep affected	65
Instinctive grasping of hand (effective in 60%)	70
Instinctive relaxation (effective in 50%)	50
Distraction effective	80

may be the only factor that helps them come to terms with their pain. Most patients say that if they are absorbed in their work, they can spend a good part of the day without distress. As soon as they return home and relax, the pain builds up and becomes severe and prevents them from undertaking social activities.

Drugs are singularly useless for this pain. The most common drugs that patients used were Distalgesic and codeine derivatives. These were only of marginal value, and 20 or more tablets were needed to have any effect. However, 40% of our patients found that alcohol was useful, probably because it helped them relax and sleep. None of our patients have become true alcoholics. Only one patient whom we have seen has become addicted to narcotics. Addiction is infrequent because patients find that any form of narcotic (e.g., cannabis) may relieve the pain temporarily, but upsets their intellectual judgment and is incompatible with holding down a job. As work is the most powerful means of reducing pain, patients would not take the risk of the drug's interfering with their performance. The effect of cannabis is interesting. We have 11 patients who have clearly stated that it significantly reduces pain. A few take cannabis over a weekend; they then find that the pain is less for some days. In addition, when it does return, they are more able to come to terms with it, as they know they can subsequently get some relief by smoking more cannabis. It might well be that if a purified form could be discovered and if it could be administered under very careful control, this could be of considerable help to these patients.

Treatment of Pain

The most valuable treatment modality that has helped our patients has been transcutaneous nerve stimulation. It is vital to use this procedure properly. Far too often we have heard of personnel in pain clinics who give a patient a stimulator with scanty instructions on how to use it. The patient then gives up the treatment after 1 or 2 hours, not having found any relief. Transcutaneous nerve stimulation needs to be given for many hours a day, for weeks on end, before it can be judged as being ineffective. The effect seems to be cumulative and technique is all important. This is one of the many reasons why

we insist that our patients be admitted to our Rehabilitation Ward, where our physiotherapists, who are very experienced in this field, will try out different positions of electrode placement and different parameters of stimulation.

The machine that we use, which we construct in the hospital, has three variables: pulse width, amplitude, and repetition rate. Most patients favor a high repetition rate (50 to 100 Hz) and an output of about half the available output on the machine, but it is common to find patients varying the different parameters from day to day, although the repetition rate tends to remain fairly constant. The electrodes are placed just proximal to the most proximal site of anesthesia. It is essential to apply the electrodes over an area where there is sensory input, as placement over anesthetic areas is obviously useless. For a total lesion, this means placing an electrode over the inner side of the upper arm, over the T2 input (which is usually spared), and over the neck or the shoulder over the C2, C3, or C4 dermatome. If C5 and C6 roots are spared, the electrodes can be placed over the upper arm.[5] Patients are encouraged to wear the stimulator for several hours a day, and if they can use it at work, we prefer to have patients wear the stimulator all day. If their work is incompatible with wearing a stimulator, we ask them to wear it as soon as they come home and until they go to bed, for this (as has been stated earlier) is often the time they suffer the most severe pain. Some patients wear the stimulator for 24 hours a day, and that is why having a rechargeable stimulator is so valuable. It does not seem to matter how long patients have experienced pain, as we have had patients who have had pain for 5 or more years in whom results of treatment have been dramatic. The most startling results occurred in a patient who had had continuous pain for 31 years and had complete loss of pain only 2 days after using the stimulator for 8 hours a day (Tables 36–9 and 36–10).

We now have a minimum 2-year follow-up of the use of electrical stimulation. Only two patients have experienced total failure of the stimulator after it originally relieved their pain, and approximately 50% of our patients use the electrical stimulator regularly, sometimes for short periods such as a week at a time or 2 or 3 hours a day. About 25% of our patients no longer need the stimulator, but we have encouraged them not to return it

Table 36–9. TIME PAIN EXPERIENCED BEFORE
TRIAL OF TRANSCUTANEOUS NERVE
STIMULATION

Time	No. of Patients
Less than 1 year	1
18 months	2
1 year	4
2 years	8
3 years	5
4 years	1
5 years	2
10 years	2
16 years	2

until they have been free of significant pain for an entire year. It is important for them to go through all four seasons before reporting that the pain has totally vanished. Most patients find that cold weather causes aggravation of pain, or it may return after having been absent for some time. However, a few patients find that hot, humid weather makes the pain worse. Interestingly, we have three patients with very severe pain that was totally relieved by a holiday in a warm climate. One patient totally lost her pain when vacationing in the mountains in Austria. The pain, however, had not disappeared when she was at a similar height in the Scottish mountains, and it occurred to us that this might be due to some ionic effect. The patient tried using an ionizing machine in her bedroom and is now totally without pain when using an ionizing apparatus throughout the night.

All patients with pain are tried on the stimulator, and we do not stop this treatment

Table 36–10. RESULTS OF TRANSCUTANEOUS
NERVE STIMULATION (TNS) FOR BRACHIAL
PLEXUS LESIONS

Factor	No. of Patients
Patients treated:	52
No help	26
Significantly helped	26
Length of time without pain or	26
substantial relief of pain to date:	
6 months	7
1 year	9
18 months	2
2 years	7
3 years	1
Still using TNS occasionally:	17
Daily	3
Weekly	6
No longer need TNS	9

until the patient has reported no change at all after a full week's trial utilizing different positions and different settings of the parameters. The stimulators are light and easily carried and indeed are compatible with wearing a functional splint. For a detailed discussion of this topic, see Wynn Parry.[14, 15]

The nature of deafferentation pain is now well established, as the experimental work of Loeser et al.[8] and Anderson et al.[2] has shown that destruction of input to the spinal cord results in the release of dorsal horn neurons to produce spontaneous firing. Such spontaneous firing does not occur for the first 8 days after deafferentation but then gradually builds up to reach a peak at 1 month after the injury. This accords well with clinical experience, in which onset of pain may not occur for a week or so after the injury but steadily builds up during the ensuing weeks.

Albe-Fessard and Lombard[1] have reproduced brachial plexus lesions in rats by cutting the C5–T1 roots, have demonstrated spontaneous firing with microelectrode pick-up in the dorsal horn, and have shown that electrical stimulation can considerably reduce the area of self-mutilation by these rats. Most interesting of all, they have shown that the area of autonomy can be significantly reduced by applying electrical stimulation *immediately* after the destructive procedures. These authors have argued that all patients with avulsion lesions of the brachial plexus should be given electrical stimulation as a prophylactic measure, and this certainly does seem logical.

However, a significant number of patients remain who become desperate with pain and whose lives become totally insupportable. Their families say that they are changed people and impossible to live with, and they may threaten or even attempt suicide. What can one do when confronted with such a tragic situation? When all other modalities have been tried, we have been referring such patients to David Thomas, Consultant Neurosurgeon at The National Hospital for Nervous Diseases, London, for Nashold's procedure. Nashold and Ostdahl[12] and Nashold et al.[11] have described an operation for destruction of the dorsal root entry zone. This destroys that area of spinal cord where the spontaneous ongoing firing of neurons, released from afferent inhibition, is taking place. This seems a logical step, far more so than division of pain-carrying tracts. It is now known that there are at least eight tracts that carry nociceptive impulses (a good example of the considerable redundancy in the nervous system), and thus division of only one of these tracts is doomed to failure. Neurosurgeons note that in patients with so-called benign intractable pain, in whom life expectancy is not affected by the disorder, the pain invariably returns months or years after destructive surgery. However, the Nashold procedure does seem logical, and we have now referred 22 patients for such procedures. In 17, there has been dramatic relief of pain, which has been maintained for 2 years or more. Long-term studies are essential before the procedure is fully appraised. It may well be that, as after so many destructive procedures, the pain will eventually return. We are therefore reserving it for desperate patients who would undoubtedly either commit suicide or become drug addicts or whose family would break up.

Thalamic stimulation has been attempted in some centers.[9] We subjected five patients to thalamic stimulation, with considerable success in two but with no effect in three.

Recently, we have become aware of the development of pain months or years after grafting of C5–C6. These patients present with the characteristic features of causalgia similar to that in partial peripheral nerve lesions. It seems therefore that severe causalgic pain may develop in a few patients in whom regeneration occurs. Such patients have responded to serial intravenous guanethidine blocks, as described by Wynn Parry and Wirthington,[5a] or to the application of transcutaneous electrical stimulation or both.

AMPUTATION

It used to be the standard procedure in a patient with a totally flail arm to offer amputation and to arthrodese the shoulder and provide a prosthesis. As stated earlier, if the scapular muscles are spared, patients will then be able to use an artificial arm. However, a review by Ransford and Hughes[13] showed that the majority of such patients abandoned their prosthesis, and only those who found it extremely difficult to change from the dominant hand and those who were athletic used their prosthesis. A more recent review by our team showed that of 24 patients who underwent amputation for brachial plexus lesions in past years and were provided with a prosthesis, 18 never used

their artificial limb at all, and of the six who did, three used it only for cosmetic reasons. Furthermore, we have seen 12 patients in whom amputation was advised elsewhere in the first twelve months following injury but who refused the procedure. Eleven of these patients developed significant functional return in the upper arm.

It used to be taught that unless one advised amputation early, patients would never use an artificial arm. Now, however, there is no need for such a regimen, as we have the functional splint already described, which can be fitted easily and quickly and allows the patient to return to work. If at subsequent stages the patient finds that the arm gets in the way or if he develops trophic and infected lesions, amputation can always be carried out at a later stage and an artificial arm applied. Approximately six of our patients have elected to have amputations subsequently, but in none of them was an artificial arm of any use. The arm was removed because it was an encumbrance or because of recurrent infection. There is thus no longer any place for amputation except in very special circumstances when patients demand it. The routine treatment should involve the fitting of a flail arm splint and regular follow-up.

One point is especially vital, i.e., amputation will have no effect at all on deafferentation pain. The pain is central and is not affected by any peripheral maneuver. It is very important to explain this carefully to the patient, for it seems logical to him that if the painful part is removed, the pain will be abolished. Indeed many surgeons still believe that amputation will relieve the pain, and it is not known widely enough that the pain is central in origin.

SUMMARY

The management of patients with brachial plexus lesions requires a multidisciplinary team. We insist on admission to our Rehabilitation Ward for a full assessment by the physiotherapist, occupational therapist, rehabilitation officer, and social worker when necessary. We confirm the diagnosis by clinical, electrophysiologic, and radiologic techniques and determine a plan of action involving either definitive surgery or a conservative program of functional splintage, relief of pain when possible, and return to work. We insist on regular follow-up visits to check that the pain is still being relieved. At subsequent reviews it may become clear that spontaneous recovery is not going to occur and a program of reconstructive surgery can be instituted. In general, 3 or more years should have elapsed before accepting that elbow flexion is not going to return. In patients with C5–C6 lesions in whom elbow flexion is permanently paralyzed, the simple elbow-locking splint may be perfectly satisfactory, but in some patients it may be wise to advise reconstructive procedures. In our experience the most satisfactory means of restoring elbow flexion is the Steindler flexorplasty, advancing the origins of the extensors and flexors of the forearm up the humerus. If present, the latissimus dorsi can be transferred to replace the biceps. The pectoralis major transfer is useful but almost always requires an external rotation osteotomy, as there is too much adduction when the patient flexes the elbow. Finally, the triceps can be transferred to the biceps, but this is an operation that we do not like to perform, as maintenance of elbow extension is so useful. For permanent paralysis of wrist and finger extension, the standard radial nerve tendon transfers are appropriate.

Table 36–11 shows the reconstructive procedures that were carried out in 130 patients before exploration grafting of ruptured nerve roots came into fashion. Obviously, if surgery can provide elbow flexion by grafting of ruptured nerve roots, this is by far the best treatment, but even so there may not be adequate functional recovery to dispense entirely with some form of functional splint or with one of the reconstructive procedures to reinforce power.

Following such reconstructive procedures, an intensive period of 2 to 3 weeks of rehabilitation is necessary in order to re-educate the transfer. Finally, one never ceases to be amazed and inspired by the way these young patients accept their disability and by their motivation to return to work and to normal life.

Table 36–11. RECONSTRUCTIVE SURGERY IN 23 OF 130 PATIENTS WITH BRACHIAL PLEXUS PALSIES (1950–1975)

Procedure	No. of Patients
Arthrodesis of shoulder	5
Arthrodesis of wrist	5
Clark's pectoralis transfer	3
External rotation osteotomy of humerus	3
Zachery's transfer: latissimus–infraspinatus	2
Steindler's procedure	2
Opponens transfer	2
Flexor transfer for finger extension	1

References

1. Albe-Fessard, D., and Lombard, M. C.: Animal models for pain due to central deafferentation methods of protection against this syndrome. To be published in Proceedings of the Third World Congress of Pain, 1981.
2. Anderson, L. S., Black, R. G., Abraham, J., and Ward, A. A.: Neuronal hyperactivity in experimental trigeminal deafferentation. J. Neurosurg., 35:444, 1971.
3. Barnes, R.: Traction injuries of the brachial plexus in adults. J. Bone Joint Surg., 31-B:10–16, 1949.
4. Bonney, G.: Prognosis in traction lesions of the brachial plexus. J. Bone Joint Surg., 41-B:4–35, 1959.
5. Frampton, V.: Pain control with the aid of the transcutaneous stimulator. Physiotherapy, 68:77–81, 1982.
5a. Wynn Parry, C. B., and Wirthington, R. H.: Painful disorders of peripheral nerves. Postgrad. Med. J., 60:869–875, 1984.
6. Jones, S. J.: Investigation of brachial plexus traction lesions by peripheral and spinal somatosensory evoked potentials. J. Neurol. Neurosurg. Psychiatry, 42:107–116, 1979.
7. Jones, S. J., Wynn Parry, C. B., and Landi, A.: Diagnosis of brachial plexus traction lesions by sensory nerve action potentials and somatosensory evoked potentials. Injury, 12:376–382, 1980.
8. Loeser, J. D., Ward, A. A., and White, L. E.: Chronic deafferentation of the human spinal cord neurones. J. Neurosurg., 29:48–51, 1968.
9. Mazars, G. J.: Contribution of thalamic stimulation to the physiopathology of pain. In Bonica, J. J., and Albe-Fessard, D. (eds.): Advances in Pain Research and Therapy, Vol. 1. New York, Raven Press, 1976, pp. 483–485.
10. Narakas, A.: Les lésions dans les élongations du plexus brachial. Rev. Chir. Orthop., 63:44–55, 1977.
11. Nashold, B. S., Urban, B., and Zorab, D. S.: Phantom pain relief by focal destruction of the substantia gelatinosa of Rolando. In Bonica, J. J., and Albe-Fessard, D. (eds.): Advances in Pain Research and Therapy, Vol. 1. New York, Raven Press, 1976, pp. 959–963.
12. Nashold, B. S., and Ostdahl, R. H.: Dorsal root entry zone lesions for pain relief. J. Neurosurg., 57:59–69, 1979.
13. Ransford, A. O., and Hughes, P. F.: Complete brachial plexus lesions. J. Bone Joint Surg., 59-B:417–421, 1977.
14. Wynn Parry, C. B.: Management of traction lesions of the brachial plexus and peripheral nerve injuries in the upper limb. The Ruscoe Clark Memorial Lecture for 1979. Injury, 11:265–285, 1979.
15. Wynn Parry, C. B.: Pain in avulsion lesions of the brachial plexus. Pain, 9:41–53, 1980.
16. Yeoman, P.: Traction injuries of the brachial plexus. Thesis for Doctorate in Medicine. Cambridge data. In Seddon, H. (ed.): Surgical Disorders of the Peripheral Nerves. Baltimore, Williams & Wilkins, 1977, pp. 184–185, 190.

OBSTETRICAL BRACHIAL PLEXUS PALSY

PART
4

37

Review of Obstetrical Palsies: Nonoperative Treatment

■

Kenneth L. B. Brown, M.D., F.R.C.S.(C)

It is the prevailing opinion that the incidence of obstetrical brachial plexus palsy (OBPP), especially that of a more severe nature, is decreasing. This has been credited to better obstetrical care, in particular to the increased cesarean section rate. As a result, practicing surgeons have little personal experience to guide their management of these difficult problems. By referring to standard orthopedic textbooks, one becomes bewildered by the confusing variety of contradictory statements. Some are overly pessimistic, such as Turek,[101] who states that: "Generally, the course is one of slow, gradual subsidence of the residual paralysis over several weeks to three or four months, after which further improvement is unlikely." Sharrard,[85] on the other hand, is quite optimistic, stating that "Some recovery occurs in nearly all cases and is complete in 75% of lesions of the upper part of the plexus and half of those with complete plexus paralysis. At the end of two years any residual paralysis may be able to be compensated by reconstructive surgery." He goes on to state that "Complete brachial plexus lesions in which no recovery occurs cannot benefit from any reconstructive procedures. Because of uselessness, loss of sensibility, and shortening of the limb, the patient may well opt for amputation when he is an adolescent." Duthie and Ferguson's textbook[23] states that "A minority of cases recover completely in three months and it is therefore impossible to determine clinically the exact extent of the lesion at an earlier

date. In all cases of the upper arm type, the prognosis is good, but in the lower arm and whole arm form the restoration of function is unlikely." Almost all standard textbooks suggest that recovery in children with minor injuries can continue until 18 to 24 months of age, whereas children with moderate to severe paralysis often are left with characteristic residual deformities. Unfortunately, these textbooks offer no guidance on how to recognize an injury that will not do well.

Successful application of microsurgical techniques for reconstructive surgery of all types has stimulated several surgeons around the world to attempt direct repair of the brachial plexus lesion itself.[11, 17, 33, 87] Unfortunately, no guidelines exist to determine which patients might benefit from surgery and when the best time for exploration is. As a complement to Gilbert and Tassin's chapter on the operative management of obstetrical brachial plexus palsies (Chapter 39), we will review all that is currently known about obstetrical palsy, what the most common residual defects are, the different classical orthopedic procedures to overcome these deformities, and the results of this type of treatment.

HISTORICAL BACKGROUND

Smellie[86] is credited as being the first to describe brachial plexus palsy as a result of birth injury. In his treatise on midwifery, which was written in 1768, he described an infant who was born with bilateral arm paralysis after a face presentation. He believed the paralysis was caused by pressure of the pelvis on the arms. Almost a century later, Danyau[21] performed an autopsy on a baby who died shortly after a traumatic forceps delivery. The infant also had a facial nerve paralysis and was found to have damage to his brachial plexus. Danyau attributed the damage to improper application of forceps.

Most of the credit for developing physician awareness of this iatrogenic problem has gone to Duchenne.[22] In his book, which was published in 1872, he described Danyau's case and added four more of his own. He was the first to publish the physical findings of an infant with obstetrical brachial plexus palsy. Typically the child has a flail arm that lies internally rotated at the side, the elbow slightly flexed, the forearm pronated, and the fingers and wrist flexed (Fig. 37–1).

In 1874 Erb[27] wrote a monograph on brachial plexus injuries in adults in which he reported his experiments on electrical stimulation of the brachial plexus. Erb discovered that the characteristic paralysis of the deltoid, biceps, coracobrachialis, and brachioradialis could be caused by disruption of C5 and C6 roots where they emerge just between the scalene muscles. Electrical stimulation at this

point (which has been named after him) resulted in contraction of all the above muscles, while all the other muscles remained relaxed.

Klumpke[51] added to our knowledge of the problem when she identified the paralysis that resulted from damage to the lower roots of the plexus C8 and T1. The sympathetic fibers are usually damaged by avulsions of these lower roots, resulting in a typical Horner's syndrome.

ETIOLOGY AND PATHOLOGY

Once the problem had been recognized and described, there was a great attempt to determine what caused the paralysis so that preventative measures could be taken. During the next 30 years there were several articles in the literature that intended to answer this question. At first there were two main theories: one group believed that compression was the cause of the paralysis, either by direct pressure of the blades of the forceps or a finger in the axilla or by pressure between the clavicle and transverse processes of the cervical spine.[21, 69, 104] A second group believed that traction was the main etiologic factor.[6, 9, 16, 19, 20, 29, 30, 79, 95, 97] This occurred while the head was abducted away from the shoulder and resulted in rupture of the nerves. There were other theories that really didn't gain any proponents. For example, Burr[15] believed that the palsy was a rare form of polio that resulted from damage in the spinal cord, and Stransky[90] felt that the common asphyxiated state of infants born after a traumatic delivery caused abnormal toxicity of the blood, therefore predisposing the plexus to damage. This particularly helped to explain bilateral palsies.

To determine the etiology more clearly, several surgeons performed experimental studies on cadavers to reproduce the damage to the brachial plexus. It was determined that longitudinal traction alone without lateral neck flexion was insufficient to cause rupture of the nerves. Sever[79] discovered that lateral neck flexion always caused rupture of the suprascapular nerve. The damage to the brachial plexus always began at C5 or C6 and worked downward. He found that very little traction was necessary to damage the plexus, and when the clavicle was fractured, injury occurred with less force. In his studies he was unable to produce any significant pres-

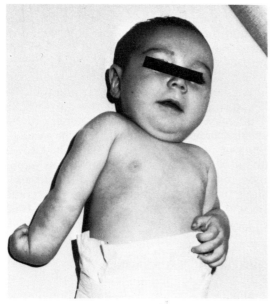

Figure 37–1. Three-month-old infant with Erb's palsy showing the classical "waiter's tip" posture of the paralyzed limb. (From Brown, K. L. B.: Clin. Plast. Surg., 11:182, 1984.)

sure on the plexus by compression between the clavicle and the first rib.

Experimental studies performed by Fieux[30] showed that Erb's point was too small to be affected by pressure alone. He believed that finger pressure was an unlikely cause of damage because there was nothing for the finger to press against. Several authors found that less force is required to rupture the lower roots than the upper roots. This is believed to be due to the straighter direction that these roots take after leaving the vertebral foramen. The traction theory of etiology was also supported by Taylor,[92] who thought that the brachial plexus fibers give way while pulling on the head during a particularly difficult delivery. He subsequently explored the brachial plexus in one patient and confirmed that it had been damaged. The child died following surgery and the plexus was studied pathologically.

In 1912 Lange[53] revived another theory that was originally proposed by Küstner.[52] Lange believed that the problem was caused by a laceration of the shoulder capsule, which upon healing produced a twist in the humerus. In 1889 Küstner wrote that the characteristic deformities seen in late childhood and early adult life were due to a primary bony injury near the shoulder rather than being secondary to brachial plexus damage. In his view this explained the paradoxical good prognosis of facial nerve palsies caused by the "hard steel of the forceps" compared with the poor prognosis of brachial plexus palsies, which he believed were due to pressure by the obstetrician's finger. Vulpius[103] and then later Thomas[98] also wrote in support of this idea. In their view any paralysis was only apparent or secondary and was unimportant, as it soon recovered spontaneously in most cases. All of these ideas were really an attempt to explain the shoulder dislocation that was often seen in the older child.

During the years from 1912 to 1920 the etiology of obstetrical brachial plexus palsy was a hotly debated issue. One group believed that the paralysis was primary and the dislocation secondary, whereas another group believed it was the dislocation that was secondary to both muscle imbalance and treatment, which we will discuss later.

Clark et al.[19] were the first to describe the pathology of brachial plexus lesions in detail. The neural damage shows all grades of severity from benign perineural swelling to hemorrhage and scar formation that follow

axonal rupture with wide separation of the ends. Experience has shown that one child may have the entire spectrum of damage. In more severe injuries the anterior cervical fascia and scalene muscles also rupture and are incorporated into the large scar mass, thus further impeding neurotization and recovery.[28, 66, 72] In 1911 Boyer[10] published a detailed autopsy examination of a woman who suffered an obstetrical brachial plexus injury 41 years earlier. He found evidence of spinal cord damage in this patient and hypothesized that in severe persistent lesions the cord may often be damaged, as well as the brachial plexus.

OBSTETRICAL FACTORS

Obstetrical brachial plexus palsy has usually been attributed to poor obstetrical technique. In the past, most of the affected children were born in families of low socioeconomic background. Many of the infants were delivered in the home without the benefit of a skilled accoucher. However, even the highly placed were not immune to this complication. Probably the most famous example is the wasted arm of Kaiser Wilhelm of Germany, who was delivered by Sir William Jenner.[19] Undoubtedly, the skill of an accoucher may be questioned when several damaged infants are delivered by the same person. The most serious charge is against a French midwife who was reported by Guillemot[41] to have delivered more than 30 affected infants. It is not uncommon in my experience and in the literature to find more than one affected child in the same family. This may be a result of delivery by the same obstetrician or excessive birth weights in succeeding children. In the series of Gordon et al.,[37] the risk of having a second affected child in a subsequent pregnancy was 14 times greater than normal. In their opinion consideration should be given to delivery of subsequent infants by cesarean section. These authors found information about possible cephalopelvic disproportion to be of much less value in predicting brachial plexus paralysis.

Contrary to popular belief, obstetrical brachial plexus paralysis is more common in multiparous than in primiparous mothers. Paralysis has been reported following 15 or 16 normal deliveries.[110] In the majority of cases there is a history of prolonged labor and the affected infants are usually of larger than normal size. However, the injury has been reported in premature infants and even those delivered by cesarean section.[25, 42, 61, 91] In one series, the incidence was higher following cesarean section than after vertex delivery.[91] It is difficult to determine from reading the literature if these cases were due to excessive vigor when removing the infant from the uterus or whether the mother had been given a trial of labor with prolonged uterine contractions without progressive descent of the baby. The actual number of paralyzed infants following vertex delivery is greater than after breech delivery. However, considering that the incidence of breech births in the normal population is about 3%, the risk of having an affected child following breech delivery is up to 175 times greater than that following vertex delivery.[74, 91]

The mechanism of injury production depends on whether the birth is breech or vertex. Damage to the upper roots of the brachial plexus usually occurs during vertex delivery, when shoulder dystocia necessitates excessive lateral flexion of the neck to free the shoulder from the pubic arch (Fig. 37-2). The right arm is paralyzed more often than the left, and this has been attributed to the more common left occiput anterior position of the descending fetus, which jams the right shoulder under the pubis.[13, 15, 16, 25, 77, 82, 84, 113]

During breech deliveries, the upper roots are also more commonly affected, usually during delivery of the arms or the aftercoming head. Damage to the lower roots can occur during breech delivery when there is arm hyperextension, but these lower injuries most commonly occur during a face presentation with hyperextension of the head. Bilateral involvement is far more common following breech birth.[1, 36, 41, 76, 91] Forceps are often implicated as an etiologic factor, but more likely they are indicative of a difficult delivery rather than being the direct instrument of damage. At least one study has shown that forceps can decrease the risk of injury during breech extraction.[91]

DISTRIBUTION

Obstetrical brachial plexus palsies have been classified according to their pattern of involvement. The majority of patients show a predominance of upper root (C5, C6) damage, which is the classic Erb's palsy. Clinically, the shoulder girdle muscles are most affected, whereas the hand is relatively normal. The next most frequent type is the complete lesion in which there is some damage to the entire brachial plexus. In Klumpke's paralysis, C8 and T1 are the sites of major damage, resulting clinically in poor hand function with a good shoulder. This classification is very crude and is based solely on the predominant clinical appearance and how carefully the patient is examined. Gjørup[35] believes that the entire plexus is affected in the majority of cases, based on measurements of grip strength. In all of his patients, the hand was always weaker on the

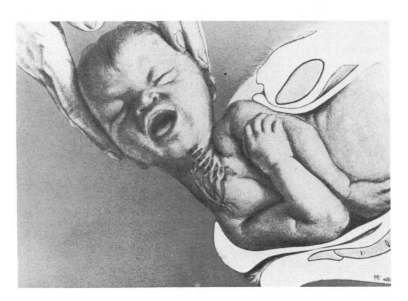

Figure 37-2. The most common mechanism of injury producing brachial plexus paralysis is lateral flexion and traction on the head to free the shoulders from the pelvis. (From Brown, K. L. B.: Clin. Plast. Surg., *11*:182, 1984.)

affected side. In many instances the difference was small and perhaps related more to the difference between the dominant vs. the nondominant extremity. This classification is also highly dependent upon the patient's age at the time of evaluation. Sever[82] preferred to wait 6 weeks before classifying the injury because many lesions appear complete at birth but after a short time are clearly only upper root injuries. In retrospective studies it is often difficult to determine the extent of paralysis that was present at birth.

DIAGNOSIS

A child with a classic Erb's palsy lies with the affected arm limp at his side, with the shoulder internally rotated, the elbow extended, the forearm pronated, and the fingers and wrist flexed. If the paralysis persists, these deformities rapidly become fixed, especially if early treatment is not instituted. This characteristic posture is usually described as the "policeman's" or "waiter's tip" position and is due to muscle imbalance. The shoulder is adducted as a result of paralysis of the deltoid and supraspinatus muscles. Activity of the pectoral and subscapularis muscles and paralysis of the infraspinatus and teres minor muscles keep the shoulder internally rotated. Elbow extension is usually due to gravity and paralysis of the forearm flexors (biceps, brachialis, brachioradialis). The pronated forearm is due to paralysis of the supinator and biceps muscles. Other physical findings are the absence of deep tendon reflexes and the possible presence of tenderness and swelling in the supraclavicular fossa. The baby's face should also be examined closely for the presence of Horner's syndrome. Detailed muscle and sensory testing in the infant is not possible, so that the degree of involvement is best determined by observations by the parents combined with frequent clinical examinations by a physician.

The differential diagnosis at birth could include cerebral palsy, poliomyelitis or cervical spine injury, and pseudoparalysis resulting from fractures or dislocations about the shoulder. In cases in which the injury is very mild and there is only partial paralysis of the upper roots, the diagnosis may be delayed for several days or weeks after birth. At this time one should also consider pseudoparalysis due to infections such as osteomyelitis of the upper extremity.

Plain x-rays should be obtained to look for associated fractures or paralysis of the diaphragm. In the past, unilateral diaphragmatic paralysis was associated with a 20 to 30% mortality and often is indicative of root avulsion. The electromyogram (EMG) can be an important prognostic tool as well. According to the experience of Eng et al.,[26] the EMG could predict the final outcome after the second or third examination. The EMG provides evidence of reinnervation at least a month in advance of the clinical examination. This study probably provides the most accurate objective evaluation of small infants.

RECOVERY

Opinions vary regarding the extent and rate of recovery following obstetrical brachial plexus palsy and are largely dependent on whether the review is a prospective or a retrospective one. In retrospective reviews it is difficult to determine the time and pattern of recovery in many cases. Most parents cannot recall the extent of paralysis at birth, when recovery began, or where it started. Many parents credit the recovery to a physician who prescribed some treatment and followed the child. It is also difficult to determine the end point of recovery, since many parents attribute the normal development of the child's psychomotor skills to improvement in the brachial plexus palsy. For example, paralysis of the arm is very obvious at the crawling stage, but when the child begins to sit and walk, he usually employs more bimanual activities. Since he is using his affected arm more, it appears that he is making some recovery. Often little information is gained from review of the patient's medical records. Usually there have been several examinations by different physicians, and the degree of detail of their notes often correlates with their interest in the problem. Since most palsies are said to improve until 18 to 24 months of age and there is little treatment to be given other than exercises until then, many physicians feel that detailed, frequent examinations are unimportant.

Prospective studies of brachial plexus palsy are usually more optimistic, i.e., stating that 70 to 80% of these patients make a full recovery. Many of these series contain patients who would never be entered in a retrospective study because they recovered very early. For example, in Vassalos' paper,[102] 36.4% of the infants improved in 10 days prior to discharge from the hospital. Similarly Hardy[42] reported that 21 of 36 patients showed improvement by the time of discharge at 10 days. Of these, six were almost normal. All arms that recovered showed some improvement within the first 1 or 2 weeks and most of these attained full function within 1 month.

Several poor prognostic signs have been identified. Ehrenfest[24] and others state that patients with lower paralysis almost never recover and that when there is total paralysis at birth, recovery is never complete. Sever[82] indicated that persistence of pupillary signs was also a poor prognostic sign. The more recent literature states that improvement will spontaneously occur until 18 to 24 months of age.[1, 109] However, most useful recovery occurs within the first year. Several authors have written that if recovery is going to occur, it will happen during the first 2 to 6 months of age.[2, 12, 35, 37, 60, 88, 91, 93] Taylor[94] dogmatically stated that if complete recovery was to occur, it would do so by 3 months of age. It is likely that these early authors followed their patients more carefully, since they were trying to determine the best time for plexus exploration.

Another problem has been the definition of recovery and whether it is functional. Forty four per cent of Wickstrom's patients never had an adequate return of motor function of the shoulder, forearm, and hand.[109] Even when the reinnervation is complete, the child may continue to ignore the limb. Whitman[106] showed that unless proper treatment was given to prevent contractures, the limb would be unable to function well even when full spontaneous reinnervation occurred. This problem is less prevalent now, since the need for early range of motion exercises is well recognized.

FUNCTIONAL LIMITATIONS

The majority of patients who do not recover completely are left with some residual shoulder paralysis. In the most common upper root type, recovery begins distally and gradually extends proximally. Most physicians consider a patient who has only limitation of external rotation of the shoulder to have made an excellent recovery. However, in many instances the patients are less than satisfied with the outcome. One of the most significant functional limitations for the patient with residual paralysis is raising the hand to the mouth.[107] Activities of daily living such as eating, dressing, and brushing the hair can be severely restricted, depending upon the degree of internal rotation contracture of the shoulder. Usually the patient compensates by abduction and forward flexion of the shoulder, which makes the elbow stick out to the side. This problem is compounded if there is also malrotation of the forearm. The patient looks very awkward, and several patients have told me that they dislike eating out, especially when they have somebody sitting on their affected side. Even when walking, the internal rotation deformity at the shoulder and flexion contracture of the elbow disrupt the natural movement of the arms during normal gait. To disguise this, many patients walk with a coat or sweater draped over their arm. Many patients are teased at school, which further adds to the psychological handicap of their condition. Often the patients with minimal disability are teased the most, since they may have no outward abnormality but appear awkward when participating in the usual childhood activities. Procedures requiring bimanual dexterity are also made more difficult. For example, several patients have trouble learning to swim and ride a bicycle.

The majority of patients adapt exceedingly well, and many do not consider themselves to be handicapped at all. Interestingly, it is often the patients with the most severe paralysis who make the best adaptations.

One outstanding patient whom I met had severe bilateral paralysis, worse on the right. She had paralysis of the entire arm on the left side and a severe Klumpke's paralysis on the right. Her paralysis was complete until about 6 months of age, when some recovery began. When I examined her, she was 28 years old, married, and had a young baby. During her childhood she did not participate in many sports, although she did a little alpine skiing. She had found riding a bicycle difficult because of poor balance and was always afraid of falling. She was able to play the piano and had made several adaptations in her activities of daily living. For example, she could not curl her hair, so she wore her hair cut short. Buttoning her blouse, doing up zippers in the back, and putting on jewelry were also more difficult (Fig. 37–3). However, she had a very positive outlook

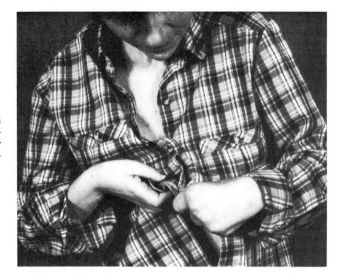

Figure 37–3. Twenty-eight-year-old patient with severe residual paralysis following bilateral obstetrical palsy. She has adapted well to her disability but has had to make many modifications in her activities of daily living.

toward her condition and attributed this to the early onset of her disability. She had never experienced "normal" function because the injury occurred at birth, so her defects felt normal for her and made adaptation easier. This is perhaps one of the greatest differences between obstetrical brachial plexus palsy and traumatic brachial plexus paralysis. The patients with acquired lesions have lost a great deal and the effects are devastating in many instances. Because patients with obstetrical brachial plexus palsy have grown up with their disability, they have very different outlooks toward their affected extremity. Thus, amputation and prosthetic fitting are never indicated for individuals with obstetrical brachial plexus palsy regardless of the severity.

Some authors have commented that a child will often ignore the affected extremity despite apparent reinnervation.[18, 25, 60, 80] I believe this problem is quite rare and is usually temporary. However, during the child's early development, one should encourage bimanual activities in order to decrease the likelihood of this occurrence.

The sensory changes in obstetrical brachial plexus palsy have never received much attention. Most authors have found the sensory deficits to be minimal.[32, 43, 54] There are several possible reasons for this. Dermatomal overlap from functioning root levels may decrease any deficit, especially in the C5–C6 region. In this region the usual two-point and moving two-point discrimination are so large and variable that a substantial deficit would have to be present before a significant change

could be measured or appreciated by the patient. Since the onset of the lesion is at birth, there may be some potential for adaptation at the cortical level. Even patients with motor involvement of the entire plexus usually have normal sensation. Those patients who do have sensory impairment usually have severe residual motor paralysis, although the deficits are rarely parallel and often the patients are unaware of them.[105] Sensory deficiencies may be more troublesome in young children, and I have seen several who had difficulty because they liked to chew their insensate fingers.[4] These problems appear to resolve as the child matures, possibly because of the factors outlined previously.

RESIDUAL DEFORMITY

The amount of deformity present depends largely upon the extent of reinnervation as well as the treatment that the patient received during his growing years. The deformities in the untreated patient are classic. The affected limb is shorter than the normal limb. All of the bones, including the clavicle and scapula, are smaller on the affected side. The shoulder is usually in the position of internal rotation and slight flexion and abduction.[45, 46] The humeral head can be subluxed or dislocated posteriorly. This is due to a combination of muscle imbalance and the smaller size of the glenoid and humeral head, which limit bony stability. The coracoid and acromion thus become hooked downward, and the scapula is usually rotated upward and forward. There is usually a fixed flexion contracture of the elbow and occasionally dislocation of the radial head. Forearm rotation is limited, with the usual position being some degree of pronation. Hand function depends upon the degree of complete involvement of the brachial plexus. The majority of patients treated today do not develop severe bony deformities. This may be due to better preventive treatment or less severe injury as a result of improved obstetrical care. It is now very rare to find a patient with the classic bony changes of the shoulder despite serious functional limitations.

A wide variety of surgical procedures have been described to treat residual problems, and there is a great potential for patients to be treated by many types of surgery without much functional benefit. However, over the last 10 to 20 years, there has been a tendency to operate less because the results of many procedures have been disappointing for the patient and the surgeon. Previously, one patient would undergo several staged procedures, whereas the trend now is to operate only in exceptional circumstances. A well-supervised exercise program decreases the chance of deformity and obviates the necessity for operation. Many of the operations for upper limb paralysis, especially tendon transfers, were developed to treat patients with residual deformities secondary to poliomyelitis. Since the nature and pattern of the paralysis are different in these disorders, the results of such operations in the treatment of obstetrical brachial plexus palsy are not as satisfactory. More can be learned about these procedures by referring to standard references on this subject.[44, 55, 85]

TREATMENT

Historical Perspective

The treatment of obstetrical brachial plexus palsy has come full circle. It is interesting to have an overview of the various treatment modalities that have been utilized during the past century. Each time a new therapy is advocated, there has been a flurry of publishing activity by the enthusiastic proponents of the new technique. Surgeons have always been stimulated to search for better methods of treatment, since the patient with a severe brachial plexus injury remains handicapped throughout life.

Once the paralysis was determined to be due to nerve injury, several surgeons attempted direct repair of the brachial plexus.[29, 47, 48, 54, 65, 66, 70, 71, 84, 89, 94, 111] Usually the neuroma was resected and the gap bridged by various materials such as catgut, fine silk, or linen. Some surgeons used Cargile membrane between the two nerve ends to help encourage direct neurotization of the distal stump. A gap of 3 cm or less could be bridged by approximating the head to the shoulder and holding it in a brace for several weeks. Sharpe[84] reported that the operation was quick and easy. The procedure took 20 to 60 minutes and anesthetic was often not required when the patient was young enough. However, the early results were dismal owing to a high mortality rate. Two of Taylor's first seven patients died (the first and fourth).[92] Detailed long-term results were never reported, but several authors made negative comments about patients they had examined.[3, 57, 83, 107] The only patient L'Episcopo had ever seen with an insensate and useless flail upper extremity had had an exploration and reconstruction of the brachial plexus.[57] The most seriously affected patient I have ever seen was a 19-year-old girl with a useless limb who had surgery on her brachial plexus at 4 months of age. Amputation had been recommended by several doctors, but she adamantly refused.

During the next several years there was a period in which little or no treatment other than massage and electrical stimulation was given.[24, 31, 59, 70, 96, 99, 100] Some physicians advocated strapping the head to the shoulder in order to approximate the nerve ends.[31] This approach was partly due to the poor surgical results and partly to the prevailing opinion among many physicians that recovery was the rule. For example, Carter[16] wrote "That the very great majority of cases get well, or practically so sooner or later, would seem to be indicated by the fact that none of the physicians connected with the nervous department of the Massachusetts General Hospital has ever seen the condition, dating from birth, in an adult patient; and so far as the writer has been able to discover only one case (Lovett's[59]) has been reported where the paralysis has persisted to adult life." This laissez-faire approach to treatment caused a large number of patients to develop severe shoulder deformities.

Between 1910 and 1920 much interest in obstetrical brachial plexus palsy was rekindled as new operations were described to treat the shoulder deformities. It was during this period that the theories of direct shoulder injury at birth were first popularized.

Prevention of deformity was also attempted. It was thought that positioning the affected arm in the "Statue of Liberty" position would eliminate the internal rotation and adduction contractures. However, it became apparent that prolonged splinting in this position resulted in abduction, external rotation contractures of the shoulder, dislocation of the radial head, and in some cases a subglenoid dislocation of the humerus.[2, 5, 57, 58] These iatrogenic deformities were very difficult to treat.

For many years, treatment has been directed toward early range of motion exercises combined with judicious splinting when indicated.[67, 68] For the majority of patients who recover, this treatment provides the greatest chance of functional return when reinnervation occurs, since the passive range of joint motion is maintained and muscle contractures are diminished.

Shoulder Deformity

In 1905 Whitman[106] described a technique of closed manipulation of the shoulder followed by prolonged casting in the corrected position. Unfortunately, in other physicians' experience, recurrence of the deformity and fracture of the humerus were common following this procedure. Bullard[13] was one of the first to correct the deformity by surgical means. In eight patients he osteotomized the acromion and tenotomized the subscapularis and pectoralis major. In an extensive article, Fairbank[29] described his technique for overcoming subluxation and internal rotation of the shoulder by incising the joint capsule, cutting the coracoacromial ligament, and tenotomizing the subscapularis, supraspinatus, and occasionally the infraspinatus tendons. Postoperatively he immobilized the arm in an externally rotated and abducted position for 3 months. Naturally, opening the joint combined with prolonged immobilization led to severe stiffness of the shoulder. To avoid this problem some surgeons advocated releasing the subscapularis from its scapular origin instead. Rogers[73] recommended osteotomy of the humerus 2 inches below the shoulder joint. This had been described in the German literature a few years earlier and

was a simple solution to the problem, but the deformity often recurred if the procedure was performed at too early an age.[53, 103]

In an excellent extensive review of all aspects of obstetrical brachial plexus palsy, Sever[79] described his procedure for treating the residual shoulder deformity. In contrast to Fairbank, he did not open the shoulder joint, and the patient was immobilized for only 2 weeks postoperatively. This helped to decrease stiffness. In addition, Sever cut the tendon of the pectoralis major. If anterior subluxation of the joint was present, he avoided cutting the subscapularis tendon, since this aggravated the condition. In those patients in whom the acromion was hooked downward, thus blocking reduction of the humeral head, he recommended osteotomy of the acromion. Sever later modified his operation to include osteotomy of the base of the coracoid, which allowed the attached muscles to retract downward. Mobilization of the shoulder was begun at 8 to 10 days.

In patients with severe secondary bony changes or severe proximal paralysis, Kleinberg[49] recommended shoulder arthrodesis. Results can be satisfactory when the trapezius, rhomboids, and serratus muscles are relatively normal. However, in the patients with severe deformity and paralysis in whom arthrodesis is most indicated, the muscles that control the scapula are rarely strong, so the results are often disappointing. Another problem is that solid bony union is often difficult to obtain; therefore, the internal rotation deformity can recur. Kleinberg[50] described another operation based on his experience with nonunion after attempted arthrodesis. He stripped the capsule and muscle insertions from the greater tuberosity, rotated the humerus externally, and then reattached them. Late results in some cases were poor owing to loss of motion. This may have been due to aseptic necrosis of the humeral head.[46]

Recurrence of deformity is common after static release operations or humeral osteotomy, especially when performed at an early age. This occurs because these operations do not correct the existing muscle imbalance. In addition, even in those cases without recurrence, these operations improved only the patient's cosmetic appearance, not his functional level.

To diminish the chances of recurrence and improve shoulder function, several tendon transfers have been described.[40, 43, 63, 64, 81] One of the most successfully utilized operations for the internally rotated adducted shoulder was developed by L'Episcopo.[56, 57] He transferred the conjoined tendons of the latissimus dorsi and teres major from the medial to the lateral aspect of the humerus after a Fairbank release. Despite the logic of the operation, the results are often not very satisfactory, since the transferred muscles function only as a tenodesis. Most often the reason for failure is insufficient strength of the transferred muscles. Saha[75] provided another explanation for the unsatisfactory results in his classic article. He showed that shoulder motion is dependent on a complex arrangement of three groups of muscles acting in harmony. He named these groups the prime movers (deltoid, clavicular portion of the pectoralis major), the steering group (supraspinatus, infraspinatus, subscapularis), and the depressor group (latissimus dorsi, teres major, teres minor, sternal head of the pectoralis major). In his opinion, the most common cause of shoulder disability is the loss of the steering muscles. When these are nonfunctional, isolated transfers about the shoulder are usually unsuccessful. For any chance of success, the well-known principles of tendon transfers must be strictly adhered to.

Elbow and Forearm Deformity

Almost all patients with obstetrical brachial plexus palsy have a fixed flexion contracture of the elbow. This occurs even when the triceps muscle is stronger than the biceps. The reason for this is not entirely clear. An elbow flexion contracture can be caused by radial head dislocation due to aggressive pronation-supination exercises or the use of splints. However, most patients do not have dislocation of the radial head or a bowed ulna. An increased range of motion can be obtained by nonoperative means such as physical therapy and corrective casts, but the gains are rarely permanent. I have not seen a successful operation to eliminate this flexion contracture. Fortunately for the patients, a flexion contracture is very functional, especially when elbow flexion power is weak.

Another common problem for patients is the loss of forearm rotation. Although the point is somewhat controversial, I believe that the most functional position for patients with obstetrical brachial plexus palsy is the

neutral position or slight supination. When the shoulder is abducted somewhat, the forearm will move to a more pronated position. Almost everyone agrees that extremes of pronation or supination are very disabling and that these patients can be greatly aided by surgery. When the contracture is fixed with no active or passive rotation, the simplest solution is a closed osteoclasis, as described by Blount.[8] Recurrence is common following this procedure, so overcorrection should be obtained. Closed osteoclasis is much simpler than osteotomy and gives similar results.[114]

When a patient has a supination contracture and some active rotation, the operation of Zancolli[112] can give good results.[78] In most cases the procedure changes the arc of rotation rather than increasing the absolute degree of rotation. Several patients have weakness of wrist extension and a pronation contracture. Good results can be obtained with a Green transfer,[39] since this procedure augments wrist extension and at the same time aids in forearm supination. Supination of the forearm and fixed flexion deformity of the elbow can be corrected by a supracondylar osteotomy of the humerus, but this leaves a bayonet deformity of the bone and is not recommended.[14]

Wrist and Hand Deformity

Most of the time wrist and hand function is not affected in the usual type of obstetrical brachial plexus palsy (Erb's). Perhaps the most common wrist problem is weak extension. Patients often cannot reach the neutral position, and as a result their grip is weakened. If passive wrist motion is good, these patients can have improved function with tendon transfers or wrist arthrodesis. I have seen the best results with arthrodesis. Very often the wrist flexors do not have normal strength, so they do not provide adequate extensor power after transfer. In addition, wrist flexion is further weakened after this procedure. One should be aware of the effects of wrist arthrodesis on forearm rotation in these patients. It is therefore useful to have the patient wear a splint or cast for a while to determine if he would benefit from repositioning the wrist.

Hand function can be severely limited in complete palsies or lower plexus injuries (Fig. 37–4). Tendon transfers to aid hand function are not commonly done for obstetrical bra-

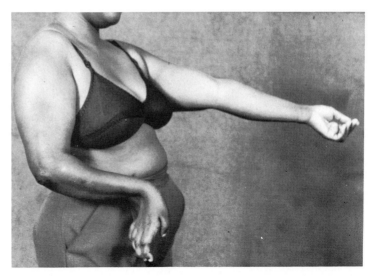

Figure 37–4. Not all patients with obstetrical palsy do well. Thirty-three-year-old patient with severe obstetrical paralysis involving her whole plexus with a predominant Klumpke's paralysis. Her right upper extremity assumes a helper function. She has absence of protective sensation in the C5 and C8 distribution with scars from previous injuries. Despite this severe handicap she is married and is raising four children.

chial plexus palsy because few patients need them and those who do often have paralysis that is too extensive for much beneficial effect.[38] Most surgeons agree that the patient should have acceptable shoulder and elbow function before reconstructive procedures on the hand are attempted.

CONCLUSIONS

For the majority of patients with obstetrical brachial plexus palsy, present-day conservative management yields good results. We now must direct our efforts toward improving results in the 10 to 15% of patients who do not do well. Presently, the role of microsurgical reconstruction of these injuries is undergoing evaluation. We must identify those patients with a poor prognosis early. To do this, a baby with this disorder should be examined at monthly intervals to document functional return, to supervise the child's exercise program, and to provide parental support. Babies who are not improving rapidly within the first 2 to 3 months should have an EMG and nerve conduction study. If such studies show evidence of a severe lesion, these patients should probably be referred to someone with a special interest in these problems.

References

1. Adler, J. B., and Patterson, R. L.: Erb's palsy. Longterm results of treatment in eighty-eight cases. J. Bone Joint Surg., *49-A*:1052, 1967.

2. Aitken, J.: Deformity of the elbow joint as a sequel to Erb's obstetrical paralysis. J. Bone Joint Surg., *34-B*:352, 1952.
3. Ashhurst, A. P. C.: Birth injuries of the shoulder. Ann. Surg., *67*:25, 1918.
4. Aston, J. W.: Brachial plexus birth palsy. Orthopedics, 2:594, 1979.
5. Babbitt, D. P., and Cassidy, R. H.: Obstetrical paralysis and dislocation of the shoulder in infancy. J. Bone Joint Surg., *50-A*:1447, 1908.
6. Bailey, P.: Brachial birth palsy. Bull. Lying In Hosp., *4*:119, 1908.
7. Bennet, G. C., and Harrold, A. J.: Prognosis and early management of birth injuries to the brachial plexus. Br. Med. J., *1*:1520, 1976.
8. Blount, W. P.: Ostoclasis for supination deformities in children: J. Bone Joint Surg., *22*:300, 1940.
9. Boorstein, S. W.: Birth injuries requiring orthopedic treatments. J.A.M.A., *85*:1866, 1925.
10. Boyer, G. F.: The complete histopathological examination of the nervous system of an unusual case of obstetrical paralysis 41 years after birth and a review of the pathology. Proc. Roy. Soc. Med., *5*:31, 1911.
11. Brown, K. L. B., Terzis, J. K., and Cruess, R. L.: Exploration and microsurgical reconstruction of obstetrical brachial plexus lesions in young children. *In* Proceedings of the Combined Meeting of the Orthopedic Associations of the English Speaking World. Capetown, South Africa, March, 1982.
12. Bruns, L.: Ueber die Verschiedenheit der Prognose der Plexus und Nervenlähmungen der oberen Extremitäten. Neurol. Zentralbl., *21*:1042, 1902.
13. Bullard, W. N.: Obstetric paralysis. Am. J. Med. Sci., *134*:93, 1907.
14. Burman, M.: Paralytic supination contracture of the forearm. J. Bone Joint Surg., *38-A*:303, 1956.
15. Burr, C. R.: Spinal birth palsies: A study of 9 cases of "obstetric paralysis." Bost. Med. Surg. J., *127*:235, 1892.
16. Carter, C. F.: Obstetrical paralysis with reference especially to the pathology and etiology. Bost. Med. Surg. J., *128*:434, 1893.
17. Celli, L.: Personal communication.
18. Chung, S. M. K., and Nissenbaum, M. M.: Ob-

stetrical paralysis. Orthop. Clin. North Am., *6*:393, 1975.

19. Clark, L. P., Taylor, A. S., and Prout, T. P.: A study on brachial birth palsy. Am. J. Med. Sci., *130*:670, 1905.

20. Darling, H. C. R.: The surgery of the brachial plexus. Med. J. Austral., 335, 1915.

21. Danyau, M.: Paralysie du membre supérieur, chez le nouveau-né. Bull. Soc. Chir., *2*:148, 1851.

22. Duchenne, G. B. A.: De l'Electrisation Localisée et de son Application à la Pathologie et à la Thérapeutique, 3rd ed. Paris, J. B. Ballière et Fils, 1872, p. 353.

23. Duthie, R. B., and Ferguson, A. B.: Mercer's Orthopaedic Surgery, 7th ed. London, Edward Arnold Ltd., 1973.

24. Ehrenfest, H.: Brachial birth palsy. *In* Birth Injuries in the Child. New York, D. Appleton and Co., 1922, p. 165.

25. Eng, G. D.: Brachial plexus palsy in newborn infants. Pediatrics, *48*:18, 1971.

26. Eng, G. D., Koch, B., and Smokvina, M. D.: Brachial plexus palsy in neonates and children. Arch. Phys. Med. Rehabil., *59*:458, 1978.

27. Erb, W.: Über eine eigenthümliche Localisation von Lähmengen im Plexus brachialis. Verhandl. Naturhist-Med. (Heidelberg), *2*:130, 1874.

28. Eversmann, J.: Beitrag zur frage der Aetiologie der Entbindings-lähmungen der oberen Extremitat. Arch. Gynäk., *68*:143, 1903.

29. Fairbank, H. A. T.: Birth palsy: subluxation of the shoulder joint in infants and young children. Lancet, *1*:1217, 1913.

30. Fieux, G.: De la pathologie des paralysies brachiales chez le nouveau-né. Paralysies obstétricales. Ann. Gynécol., *47*:52, 1897.

31. Frauenthal, H. W.: Erb's palsy. Am. J. Obstet., *65*:679, 1912.

32. Gallavardin, L., and Rebattu, J.: Paralysie radiculaire brachiale d'origine obstétrical; arrachement probable des racines sensitives. Lyon Méd., *109*:1045, 1907.

33. Gilbert, A., Khouri, N., and Carlioz, H.: Exploration chirurgicale de plexus brachial dans la paralysie obstétricale. Rev. Chir. Orthop., *66*:33, 1907.

34. Gilmour, J.: Notes on the surgical treatment of brachial birth palsy. Lancet, *2*:696, 1925.

35. Gjørup, L.: Obstetrical lesion of the brachial plexus. Acta Neurol. Scand., *42*(Suppl. 18):1, 1966.

36. Gordon, A.: An unusual form of birth palsy. J.A.M.A., *63*:2282, 1914.

37. Gordon, M., Rich, H., Deutschberger, J., and Green, M.: The immediate and long term outcome of obstetric birth trauma. Am. J. Obstet. Gynecol., *117*:51, 1973.

38. Granberry, W. M., and Lipscomb, P. R.: Tendon transfers to the hand in brachial palsy. Am. J. Surg., *108*:840, 1964.

39. Green, W. T.: Tendon transplantation of the flexor carpi ulnaris for pronation flexion deformity of the wrist. Surg. Gynecol. Obstet., *75*:337, 1942.

40. Green, W. T., and Tachdjian, M. O.: Correction of residual deformity of the shoulder from obstetrical palsy. J. Bone Joint Surg., *45-A*:1544, 1963.

41. Guillemot, Y.: Une endémie de paralysies radiculaires obstétricales. Ann. Gynécol., *47*:35, 1897.

42. Hardy, A. E.: Birth injuries of the brachial plexus. J. Bone Joint Surg., *63-B*:98, 1981.

43. Hoffer, M. M., Wichenden, R., and Roper, B.: Brachial plexus birth palsies. Results of tendon

transfers to the rotator cuff. J. Bone Joint Surg., *60-A*:691, 1978.

44. Ingram, A. J.: Anterior poliomyelitis. *In* Edmonson, A. S., and Crenshaw, A. H. (eds.): Campbell's Operative Orthopedics, 6th Ed. St. Louis, C. V. Mosby Co., 1980.

45. Johnson, E. W., Alexander, M. A., and Koenig, W. C.: Infantile Erb's palsy (Smellie's palsy). Arch. Phys. Med. Rehabil., *58*:175, 1977.

46. Kendrick, J. I.: Changes in the upper humeral epiphysis following operations for obstetrical paralysis. J. Bone Joint Surg., *19*:473, 1937.

47. Kennedy, R.: Suture of the brachial plexus in birth paralysis of the upper extremity. Br. Med. J., *1*:298, 1903.

48. Kennedy, R.: Further notes on the treatment of birth paralysis of the upper extremity by suture of the fifth and sixth cervical nerves. Br. Med. J., *2*:1065, 1904.

49. Kleinberg, S.: Arthrodesis of the shoulder for obstetrical paralysis. Arch. Pediatr., *41*:252, 1924.

50. Kleinberg, S.: Re-attachment of the capsule and external rotators of the shoulder for obstetrical paralysis. J.A.M.A., *98*:294, 1932.

51. Klumpke, A.: Contribution à l'étude des paralysies radiculaires du plexus brachial. Rev. Méd., *5*:591, 1885.

52. Küstner, O.: Ueber epiphysäre diaphysen Fraktur am Humerusende des Neugeborene. Arch. F. Klin. Chir., *31*:310, 1889.

53. Lange, F.: Die distorsion des Ochultergelenkes. Münchener Med. Vochenschrift, *59*:1257, 1912.

54. Lauwers, M. E.: Le traitement chirurgical de la paralysie obstétricale. J. Chir., *36*:161, 1930.

55. Leffert, R. D.: Reconstruction of the Shoulder and Elbow Following Brachial Plexus Injury. Philadelphia, W. B. Saunders Co., 1980.

56. L'Episcopo, J. B.: Tendon transplantation in obstetrical paralysis. Am. J. Surg., *25*:122, 1934.

57. L'Episcopo, J. B.: Restoration of muscle balance in the treatment of obstetrical paralysis. N.Y. J. Med., *39*:357, 1939.

58. Liebolt, F. L., and Furey, J. G.: Obstetrical paralysis with dislocation of the shoulder. J. Bone Joint Surg., *35-A*:227, 1953.

59. Lovett, R. W.: The surgical aspect of the paralysis of newborn children. Boston Med. Surg. J., *127*:8, 1892.

60. Mallet, J.: Paralysis obstétricales. Rev. Chir. Orthop., *58*(Suppl. 1):115, 1972.

61. Merger, R., and Judet, J.: Paralysie obstétricale du plexus brachial. Nouv. Presse Méd., *2*:1935, 1973.

62. Metaizeau, J. P., Gayet, C., and Plenat, F.: Les lésions obstétricales du plexus brachial. Chir. Pédiatr., *20*:159, 1979.

63. Moore, B. H.: A new operative procedure for brachial birth palsy–Erb's paralysis. Surg. Gynecol. Obstet., *61*:832, 1935.

64. Moore, B. H.: Brachial birth palsy. Am. J. Surg., *43*:338, 1939.

65. Osterhaus, K.: Obstetrical paralysis. N.Y. Med. J., *7*:887, 1908.

66. Parry, R. H.: Obstetrical palsy. Proceedings of the Glasgow Obstetrical and Gynecological Society. Lancet, *16*:631, 1902.

67. Perricone, G.: Lesioni Ostetriche dei Neonati. Bologna, Capelli Editore, 1963.

68. Perry, J., Hsu, J., Babber, L., and Hoffer, M. M.: Orthoses in patients with brachial plexus injuries. Arch. Phys. Med. Rehab., *55*:134, 1974.

69. Platt, H.: Clinical lecture on birth palsy. Br. Med. J., *1*:793, 1915.
70. Platt, H.: Opening remarks on birth paralysis. J. Orthop. Surg., *18*:272, 1920.
71. Prince, M.: *In* Sever, J. W.: Obstetrical paralysis—an orthopedic problem. Am. J. Orthop. Surg., *14*:473, 1916.
72. Prout, T. P.: The nature of the nerve lesion in brachial birth palsy (Erb's type). J. Nerv. Ment. Dis., *32*:118, 1905.
73. Rogers, M. H.: An operation for the correction of the deformity due to obstetrical paralysis. Boston Med. Surg. J., *174*:163, 1916.
74. Rubin, A.: Birth injuries: incidence, mechanism and end results. Obstet. Gynecol., *23*:218, 1964.
75. Saha, A. K.: Surgery of the paralyzed and flail shoulder. Acta Orthop. Scand., *97*(Suppl.):90, 1967.
76. Scaglietti, O.: The obstetrical shoulder trauma. Surg. Gynecol. Obstet., *66*:868, 1938.
77. Scaglietti, O.: Le Lesioni Ostetriche della Spalla. Capelli Editore, Bologna, 1941.
78. Seringe, R., and Dubousset, J. F.: Attitude en supination de l'avant-bras d'origine paralytique chez l'enfant. Rev. Chir. Orthop., *63*:687, 1977.
79. Sever, J. W.: Obstetric paralysis: Its etiology, pathology, clinical aspects and treatment. Am. J. Dis. Child, *12*:541, 1916.
80. Sever, J. W.: Obstetrical paralysis—an orthopedic problem. Am. J. Orthop. Surg., *14*:456, 1916.
81. Sever, J. W.: The results of a new operation for obstetrical paralysis. Am. J. Orthop. Surg., *16*:248, 1918.
82. Sever, J. W.: Obstetric paralysis. J.A.M.A., *85*:1862, 1925.
83. Sever, J. W.: Obstetrical paralysis. Surg. Gynecol. Obstet., *44*:547, 1927.
84. Sharpe, W.: The operative treatment of brachial plexus paralysis. J.A.M.A., *66*:876, 1916.
85. Sharrard, W. J. W.: Paediatric Orthopaedics and Fractures, 2nd Ed., Oxford, Blackwell Scientific Publications, 1979.
86. Smellie, W.: A collection of Cases and Observations in Midwifery, Vol. 2, 4th Ed., London, 1768, p. 446.
87. Solonen, K. A., Telaranta, T., and Ryöppy, S.: Early reconstruction of birth injuries of the brachial plexus. J. Pediatr. Orthop., *1*:367, 1981.
88. Specht, E. E.: Brachial plexus palsy in the newborn. Clin. Orthop., *110*:32, 1975.
89. Spitz, H., and Lange, F.: Orthopädie im Kindersalter. Leipzig, Vogel, 1930, p. 427.
90. Stransky, E.: Ueber Entbindungslähmungen der oberen Extremität bei kinde. Centralblatt für die Grenzgebiete der Medizin und Chirurgie, *13*:497; *14*:545, 601, 666, 1902.
91. Tan, K. L.: Brachial palsy. J. Obstet. Gynecol. Br. Common., *80*:60, 1973.
92. Taylor, A. S.: Results from the surgical treatment of brachial birth palsy. J.A.M.A., *48*:96, 1907.
93. Taylor, A. S.: Conclusions from further experience in the surgical treatment of brachial birth palsy. Am. J. Med. Sci., *146*:836, 1913.
94. Taylor, A. S.: Brachial birth palsy and injuries of similar type in adults. Surg. Gynecol. Obstet., *30*:494, 1920.
95. Thomas, J. J.: Two cases of bilateral birth paralysis of the lower arm type. Boston Med. Surg. J., *153*:431, 1905.
96. Thomas, J. J.: Obstetrical paralysis with special reference to treatment. Boston Med. Surg. J., *170*:513, 1914.
97. Thomas, J. J., and Sever, J. W.: Obstetric paralysis. J.A.M.A., *66*:2036, 1916.
98. Thomas, T. T.: The relation of posterior subluxation of the shoulder joint to obstetrical palsy of the upper extremity. Ann. Surg., *59*:197, 1914.
99. Thorburn, W.: Obstetrical paralysis. Med. Chron. (Manchester), *3*:466, 1886.
100. Thorburn, W.: Obstetrical paralysis. J. Obstet. Gynecol., *3*:454, 1903.
101. Turek, S. L.: Orthopaedic Principles and Their Application, 3rd Ed. Philadelphia, J.B. Lippincott Co., 1977.
102. Vassalos, E., Prevedourakis, C., and Paraschopoulou-Prevedouraki, P.: Brachial plexus paralysis in the newborn. Am. J. Obstet. Gynecol., *101*:554, 1968.
103. Vulpius, O.: Zur Behandlung der Lähmungen an der oberen Extremität. München Med. Wochenschr., *56*:1065, 1909.
104. Walton, G. L.: The etiology of obstetrical paralysis. Boston Med. Surg. J., *135*:642, 1896.
105. Warrington, W. B., and Jones, R.: Some observations on paralysis of the brachial plexus. Lancet, 2:1644, 1906.
106. Whitman, R.: Treatment of congenital and acquired luxation at the shoulder in childhood. J.A.M.A., *42*:110, 1905.
107. Wickstrom, J., Haslam, E. T., and Hutchinson, R. H.: The surgical management of residual deformities of the shoulder following birth injuries of the brachial plexus. J. Bone Joint Surg., *37-A*:27, 1955.
108. Wickstrom, J.: Birth injuries of the brachial plexus. J. Bone Joint Surg., *42-A*:1448, 1960.
109. Wickstrom, J.: Birth injuries of the brachial plexus. Treatment of defects in the shoulder. Clin. Orthop., *23*:187, 1962.
110. Wolman, B.: Erb's palsy. Arch. Dis. Child., *23*:129, 1948.
111. Wyeth, J. A., and Sharpe, W.: The field of neurological surgery in a general hospital. Surg. Gynecol. Obstet., *24*:29, 1917.
112. Zancolli, E. A.: Paralytic supination contracture of the forearm. J. Bone Joint Surg., *49-A*:1275, 1967.
113. Zancolli, E. A.: Classification and management of the shoulder in birth palsy. Orthop. Clin. North Am., *12*:433, 1981.
114. Zaoussis, A. L.: Osteotomy of the proximal end of the radius for paralytic supination deformity in children. J. Bone Joint Surg., *45-B*:523, 1963.

38

Our Experience in Obstetrical Brachial Plexus Palsy

■

Julia K. Terzis, M.D., Ph.D.
W. Theodore Liberson, M.D., Ph.D.
Ronald Levine, M.D.

It has been 100 years since Klumpke[6] published her celebrated description of the lower obstetrical brachial plexus palsy (OBPP) in Paris (1885). This in turn was slightly more than 100 years after the first description of a bilateral obstetrical brachial plexus palsy by Smellie[10] in London (1768). It was Duchenne de Boulogne[2] who first described the typical unilateral obstetrical brachial plexus palsy (1872), significantly, in a treatise on localized electrical stimulation. Again, it was in a paper devoted to the electrical stimulation of the brachial plexus in normal individuals and in those with OBPP that Erb,[3] 2 years later (1874), described his famous upper brachial plexus point corresponding to the lower threshold for electrical stimulation of the brachial plexus. Thus, the upper brachial plexus palsy, although described first by Duchenne, bears the name of "Erb's palsy," whereas the lower brachial plexus palsy is referred to as "Klumpke's palsy." The historical background of OBPP is discussed in greater detail in Chapter 39.

Brachial plexus palsies are among the most dramatic congenital disabilities following difficult labor. Frequently, it is only hours or days following the birth that the parents note that one of the upper extremities of their newborn baby does not move as much as the other. The physician quickly rules out other congenital abnormalities (e.g., cerebral palsy) and makes a correct diagnosis of brachial plexus involvement. In most cases, progressive improvement occurs in babies with this abnormality (50% to 80% of cases).[1] A functional restoration that starts early, within days of birth, is a very good prognostic sign. If there is no evidence of improvement of the involved extremity by 3 months, the prognosis for recovery is guarded. If 6 months elapse and improvement stops, in most cases, unfortunately, parents are told that nothing else can be done except conventional physical therapy or splinting. In the most severe cases with total paralysis, some physicians may even advise an amputation at a later date.

Fortunately, in recent years decisive progress has been made in this area owing to: (1) the introduction of microsurgical reconstruction involving interposition of nerve grafts, (2) the progress in rehabilitative secondary surgery related to tendon transfers or to muscle transfer procedures, and (3) the new developments in functional bracing and electrotherapy. Since 1978 one of us (JKT) has operated on 11 babies with OBPP. In six cases, sufficient time (more than 3 years) has elapsed from the time of the operation to evaluate the results of this surgery. In five other cases, the follow-up is not sufficient to evaluate the value of reconstructive microsurgical procedures adequately. However,

Table 38–1. TYPE OF DELIVERY IN 11
PATIENTS WITH OBPP*

Delivery	No.
Normal	2
Forceps	8
Cesarean section	1

*All 11 had cephalic pelvic disproportion.

even in these cases, important observations
can be tentatively formulated. Our findings
are reported and discussed below.

POPULATION

Among these 11 cases, two groups of patients can be distinguished: (1) those operated on early, i.e., within the first 6 months
(only two patients), and (2) those operated
on between 12 and 49 months of age. Even
though the number of observations is small,
we shall offer some suggestions concerning
the preferred time for surgery (see later discussion).

OBSTETRICAL BACKGROUND

Table 38–1 summarizes the incidents and
accidents of labor that may be related to the
genesis of OBPP. In two cases, no forceps
was used, although this was necessary in
most cases. In one case, cesarean section
followed an unsuccessful vaginal delivery.
Table 38–2 shows that head presentation was
the most frequent. Table 38–3 shows that the
weight of the babies was somewhat high.
Table 38–4 indicates that differences in sex
or side of involvement were not noted. All
11 babies had cephalic-pelvic disproportion.

The mechanism of the palsy has been recognized for a long time: i.e., the unavoidable
traction on the brachial plexus; compression
by the first rib was also considered. The
following section on Pathology may contribute to the understanding of the mechanisms
involved.

Table 38–2. PRESENTATION AT BIRTH IN 11
PATIENTS WITH OBPP*

Presentation	No.
Normal	9
Transverse	1
Breech	1

*One with umbilical cord around the neck.

Table 38–3. WEIGHT AT BIRTH IN 11
PATIENTS WITH OBPP

Baby	Weight	
	Pounds	*Ounces*
1	10	5
2	10	5
3	9	6
4	9	5
5	9	4
6	9	0
7	9	0
8	8	14
9	8	13
10	8	13
11	7	8

Mean: 9 pounds, 2 ounces

PATHOLOGY

Figures 38–1 to 38–3 show the drawings
made during surgery to illustrate the pathology found. The most striking common factor
in these drawings is the involvement of C7,
the mid-point of the origin of the plexus
(Table 38–5). In practically all cases, the lesion of C7 is associated either with that of
C5 and C6 (classic Erb's palsy) or predominantly with C8 and T1 (Klumpke's palsy). In
almost two thirds of the cases, all roots were
involved to a different degree. It is as if in
the first group of cases the traction was on
the upper part of the plexus, including C7,
whereas in the second group of cases the
traction was on the lower plexus. In the most
serious cases, almost all spinal nerves were
involved, which could result from successive
traction on the upper and then the lower
plexus. In one of these seven cases, T1 was
spared (see Fig. 38–2). The constant damage
to C7 explains why the involvement of the
long extensors of the hand and fingers is so
frequent in these babies.

To these "extrinsic" factors explaining the
frequent involvement of root C7, some "intrinsic" factors may be added (see Chapter

Table 38–4. DIFFERENCES IN SEX AND SIDE
OF INVOLVEMENT IN 11 BABIES WITH OBPP

Sex	No.
Male	6
Female	5

Side of Involvement	No.
Right	5
Left	6

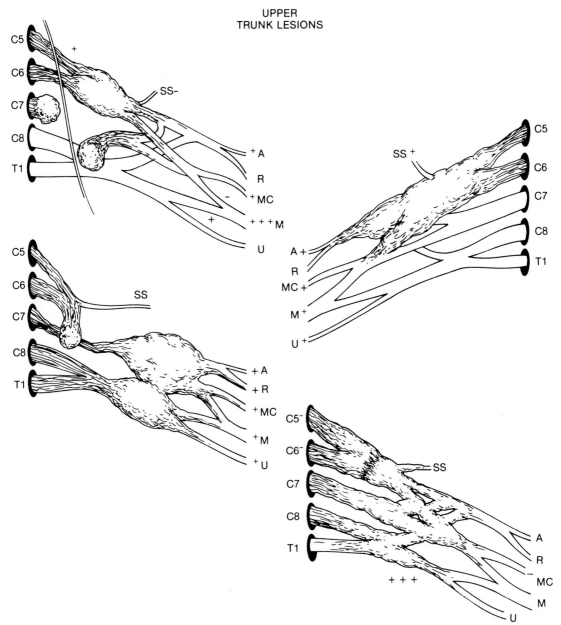

Figure 38–1. Four patients with C5 and C6 spinal nerve injuries as well as severe involvement of the upper trunk. Shoulder function in these patients will be most affected and they will have a near normal hand.

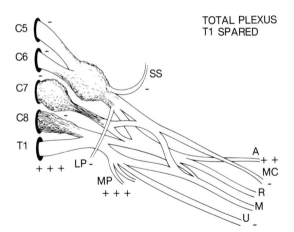

Figure 38–2. Total plexus involvement with sparing of T1. This patient showed residual hand function.

25). Frequent root involvement has been explained by the root's relative lack of protection by a connective tissue sheath. As is well known, root involvement, particularly preganglionic root involvement or avulsion of the root, is the most dreaded complication of this disability.

Table 38–6 shows the frequency of avulsion according to the involved root. No avulsion was found in roots C5 and C6, but about half of root C7 and two thirds to three quarters of roots C8 and T1 were avulsed. Incidentally, in almost all cases, deficient long extensors of the fingers and the wrist were found on electromyography (EMG), and therefore there was EMG confirmation of the constant involvement of C7 that we are reporting in this chapter. We believe that this point has not been explicitly appreciated in the previous literature.

These findings are consistent with some of the reported series (see Chapter 39). If the spinal root or nerve is involved distally to the ganglion (termed rupture instead of avulsion), the possibility of using the remaining stump of the spinal nerve as a donor for grafting is the redeeming feature of this oc-

Table 38–5. SURGICAL PATHOLOGY IN 11
PATIENTS WITH OBPP

Site	No.
C7	11 (always involved)
Upper plexus (C5, C6)	4
Total plexus:	7
T1 spared	1
C8, T1 severed	6

Table 38–6. SURGICAL FINDINGS IN ROOT
AVULSION

Root	Frequency
C5	0
C6	0
C7	3
C8	3
T1	2

currence. However, distal to the root involvement, there is frequent involvement of the trunks or other proximal structures of the brachial plexus, which appears either fibrotic or "empty" at surgery. Of course, additional intraoperative testing of these structures can be done by (1) biopsy testing for the presence or absence of ganglion cells, (2) examining the quality of the remaining fascicular structures, and (3) possibly using effective stimulation of the structures of the brachial plexus. Surgery can be better planned prior to the operation if preliminary testing is used to predict surgical findings.

Figures 38–1 to 38–3 represent the findings in all 11 of our patients. Figure 38–1 shows those cases in which the major involvement is of the upper brachial plexus. There are four such patients, whose findings are characterized by the preservation of a functional or a near functional hand. To this group we must add the one patient in whom only one of the lower roots (C8) was severely damaged, with some hand function preserved because of sparing of T1 (Fig. 38–2). The other six patients (Fig. 38–3) show what can be called a global involvement of the plexus, in which the upper, middle, and lower structures or roots are affected, the degree of damage being much more severe in the lower plexus structures (C7, C8, and T1). Obviously, these findings offer a poorer prognosis for hand function.

PRE- AND POSTSURGICAL TESTING

Thermography

The distribution of temperature changes (cooling) may pinpoint involved dermatomes. Figure 38–4 shows an example of such testing. Thermography is, however, difficult in babies, as it is essential to immobilize both hands for comparison.

Inasmuch as the presence or absence of root involvement, in particular of root avul-

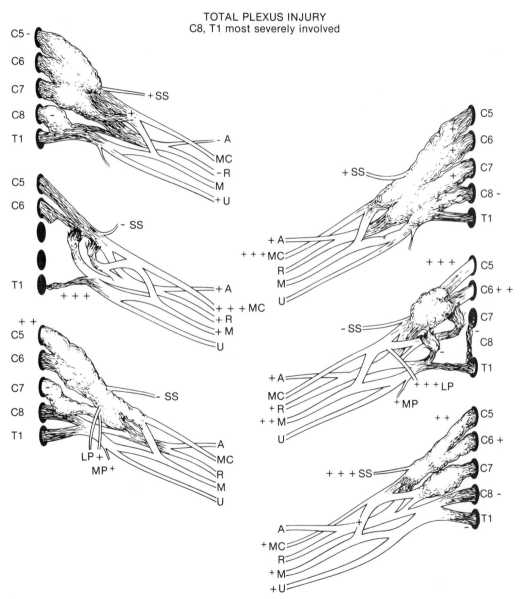

Figure 38–3. Six patients demonstrated a global plexus involvement with C7, C8, and T1 spinal nerves most severely damaged. These patients have movement in the shoulder but have very little function in the hand.

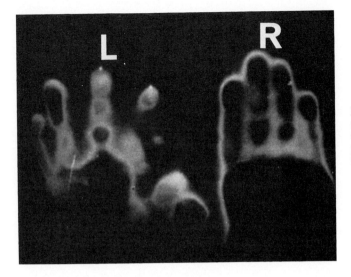

Figure 38–4. Thermogram of one patient showing abnormal pseudomotor function in the involved left hand. Note diminished temperature (light color) over the radial side of the hand.

sion, is of considerable prognostic significance, the tests that may contribute to such determination will be considered first.

Myelography

Myelograms indicate the presence of an avulsion of the root either by showing leakage of the opaque material in the empty space left by the avulsed root or by demonstrating a meningomyelocele. Figure 38–5 depicts positive myelograms and Figure 38–6 indicates whether or not the myelographic pathologic prediction was verified at surgery. There was a positive correlation in eight (80%) of the cases, and the myelogram was incorrect in two cases (20%).

Electrodiagnosis and Electromyography

Classic electrodiagnostic tests are discussed in Chapter 40 of this volume. These tests are directly related to electrotherapy,

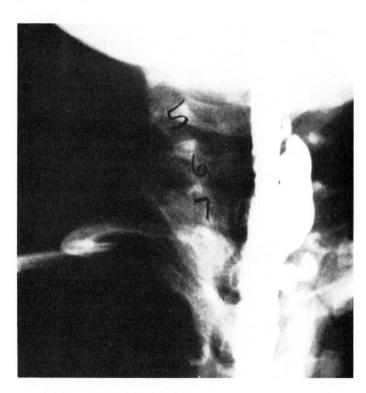

Figure 38–5. Myelogram showing meningomyelocele on the left. This suggests root avulsion.

SURGERY

MYELOGRAPHY		AVULSION	NO AVULSION
	AVULSION	4	1
	NO AVULSION	1	4

Figure 38–6. Correlation between surgery and myelography in 10 patients with obstetrical brachial plexus palsy.

8/10 GOOD CORRELATION

2/10 NO CORRELATION

which is so essential for rehabilitation of these patients.

Electromyography and other electrodiagnostic procedures are among the most valid techniques for assessing a brachial plexus lesion. These studies predict the reinnervation of a muscle far earlier than any other test. It may therefore be helpful to review the contributions of electromyography to this field. Obviously, in a case of denervation of the muscle or when recording voluntary potentials, it is impossible to determine the site of the lesion by testing a single muscle. Indeed, the same kind of fibrillations and positive sharp waves will be recorded whether the lesion is at the level of the peripheral nerve, the cord, the division, the trunk, the spinal nerve, the root, or the spinal cord segment. Likewise, the same degree of reduced (or absent) voluntary activity may be expected in each of the above-mentioned sites of the lesion.

It is the combination of findings related to several myotomes that may give a hint as to the localization of the lesion; however, this will always be a probability and not a certainty. For example, if all the muscles supplied by the nerves arising proximally to the spinal cord are preserved while the muscles supplied by the nerves arising more distally show EMG abnormalities, the electromyographer may conclude that the lesion is a distal one. The combination of myotomes involved may give another clue as to localization.

A slowing of conduction velocity may be observed in (1) a focal compression or an injury to axons and (2) the presence of an initial phase of reinnervation. For example, in certain cases when slow conduction velocity for the median nerve is observed by

stimulating Erb's point and not by stimulating the arm or forearm, one may conclude that the focal lesion is in the supraclavicular area.

The difficulties of interpreting the EMG examination and conduction velocity determination are paramount, and it is surprising to what degree electromyography is actually helpful in diagnosing cases of brachial plexus palsy (see later discussion). One can only be impressed by the concordance of EMG results with the results of intraoperative stimulation (Fig. 38–7). It should be kept in mind that the results of stimulation during the operation may be different from those prior to the operation because of a possible dissociation of excitability and conductibility of the examined structures. Indeed, axons may be embedded in the scar tissue, which prevents the stimulating current from reaching them, and yet the axons are viable, as witnessed by the preoperative EMG or muscle testing as well as by the successful intraoperative stimulation of more distal structures (Fig. 38–7).

Obviously, the more time one can devote to preoperative EMG testing, the more consistency one may expect from this investigation. EMG testing is very difficult in babies because of a violent reaction of the child to the stimulation and the introduction of needles. In order to render this test more efficient, we have been wrapping the child in a sheet to immobilize his normal extremities. We have found that, under these conditions, some babies soon realize that their agitation is futile and therefore their suffering is reduced by this procedure. We have abandoned use of sedatives, which are often ineffective and render the child unable to be-

PREOPERATIVE % OF EMG INTERFERENCE PATTERN (IP)

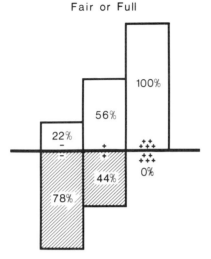

FINDINGS AT SURGERY
Fair or Full

100%

56%

22%

44%

0%

78%

///// No or Poor IP

- No Response

+ Fair Response

.+. Good Response

Figure 38–7. Graph showing the correlation between intraoperative stimulation of the plexus by the surgeon and the preoperative EMG. Note that the height of the white bar (percentage of interference patterns found preoperatively) increases with increasing success of stimulation at surgery, while the striped bars (poor I.P.) decrease correspondingly in amplitude.

have normally for several hours following the test.

The presence of "denervation" potentials (fibrillations and positive sharp waves) in the cervical erector spinae indicates the involvement of the roots or the cervical nerves prior to the emergence of the posterior ramus supplying the paraspinal muscles. Inasmuch as each posterior ramus usually distributes among three consecutive myotomes, this observation does not permit a precise delineation of the involved root. However, the presence of denervation potentials in either the upper or the lower segment of the erector spinae may provide some suggestions as to localization. The presence of such potentials does not, however, indicate whether the root is damaged pre- or postganglionically, distal to the ganglion but proximal to the take-off of the dorsal ramus. Absence of denervation potentials in the paraspinal muscles indicates

a lesion distal to the emerging posterior ramus.

One of the most elegant contributions of electroneurography to the diagnosis of a preganglionic lesion is the presence of normal sensory potentials in one or several fingers of the hand although the patient has no digital sensory perception or distal motor function. Indeed such a finding indicates the integrity of sensory axons extending from the bipolar cells in the spinal ganglion down to the digital nerves. In our patient population, such a diagnosis was made in two cases and was correct in both.

However, it would be erroneous to conclude that the *absence* of sensory potentials in the fingers signifies the absence of a preganglionic lesion in a patient who had lost hand sensibility. A preganglionic lesion may *coexist* with one or many postganglionic lesions, and in such cases an absence of sensory potentials will still be observed despite the presence of a preganglionic lesion.

It is also important to realize that the finding of a good sensory potential indicates continuity of the corresponding mixed nerve pathways. In the case of a mixed nerve, the continuity of sensory fibers also suggests the probability of the integrity of the motor pathways, unless they are interrupted at the proximal root level. This is important when one considers use of interposition grafting. As a matter of fact, the finding of motor potentials of good amplitude distally, along with a good interference pattern, also indicates continuity of a great number of fibers of the corresponding nerve, from the anterior horn to the corresponding muscle (see Chapter 40).

One additional consideration must be mentioned. One should not forget that the idea of neurotmesis associated with fibrillations and positive sharp waves was formulated before the important advance was made concerning axoplasmic flow. It is now generally accepted that fibrillations and positive sharp waves may be observed when this flow is dramatically slowed down without any actual anatomic sections of the axon. This is why fibrillations are seen in hemiplegics and paraplegics (with thoracic lesions).[5, 12] Liberson and Yhu[8] found that in these patients, the number of fibrillations is increased with increasing distance from the spinal cord.

Electromyography is also used in following the child who either has or has not had surgery. Electromyography contributes to assessing the muscle to be transplanted or to following the onset of reinnervation of an already transferred muscle.[5] In those children who may cooperate with the examiner, introduction of the stimulating needle electrode at different levels of the extremity may provide information as to the most distal point at which sensory fibers have regenerated (see Chapter 40).

When correlating EMG and intraoperative findings in patients with OBPP, we found that only 10 of 11 cases could be effectively analyzed, as the EMG recorded prior to surgery was inadequate in one case.

Correlations of EMG with surgical findings have been tested by another method (see Fig. 38–7).

It is the usual practice for the surgeon to electrically stimulate different structures of the brachial plexus intraoperatively and to score the observed responses as + + +, + +, +, or − (JKT).[11] In cases in which the surgical report indicated the effectiveness of intraoperative stimulation of the distal structures (as recorded by these symbols), one finds that the EMG reports corresponding to these same muscles correlate with the surgical findings. Thus, there were seven instances in which the surgeon classified muscle responses to stimulation of the distal plexus structures as + + or + + +. In such cases, the electromyographer reported a "good interference pattern" in five cases, whereas in the two remaining cases the electromyographer reported the presence of a "reduced interference pattern." In no case was there an EMG report of "only single motor unit potentials" or of the "absence of any voluntary potentials." In most cases, when the surgeon found an absence of any response to stimulation of the distal structures, there were generally concordant reports from the electromyographer who examined the patient prior to surgery. Nine such instances were mentioned by the surgeon. The electromyographer reported a "normal interference pattern (IP)" in only one case. The report mentioned "reduced IP" in one case. In three instances, "poor IP" was reported; in one case, "good motor units" were recorded; and in one instance, "single motor units" were present. In two cases, no voluntary potentials were found. Thus, the correlation between these reports is expressed by obvious differences between the electromyographer's findings in the instance of "double or triple pluses" indicated by the surgeon or the findings by the latter

of "no response." One must, of course, take into consideration the fact that in some cases the absence of the response at surgery could be due to difficulties of intraoperative stimulation. It must also be stressed that the correlations are positive only with distal nerve trunk stimulation. In the proximal structures, stimulation results are more difficult to interpret because of extensive scarring.

In those numerous cases in which muscle response to the intraoperative stimulation was characterized by a single plus, less clear correlation was found (as expected). There were 18 instances in which the same muscle was tested either by the surgeon during the operation or by the electromyographer before the operation. In four instances, "good IP" was reported by the electromyographer; in three cases, "fair IP" was reported; in three cases, a "reduced IP" was recorded; in two cases, a "markedly reduced IP" was reported; in two cases, only "many units" were mentioned; and in two cases, only "isolated units" were reported. Only in two cases did the electromyographer report the absence of any voluntary potentials.

To summarize, in seven instances when + + or + + + notations were made intraoperatively, some type of IP was found in each instance by the electromyographer prior to the operation. In 18 cases classified by the surgeon as "+ response only," four cases with "no IP" were found by the electromyographer prior to the operation. In only two cases were "no voluntary potentials" mentioned by the electromyographer. Finally, in nine instances when intraoperative results of stimulations were negative, the electromyographer found "single MUP" (motor unit potential) in two cases, "poor IP" in three cases, and "no voluntary potentials" in two additional cases. There were only two recordings of "normal or reduced IP" among these nine cases. Again, the IP was observed in 100% of the cases classified as + + or + + + by the surgeon, in 56% of the cases characterized by a single + only, and in 22% of cases in which the muscle did not respond to stimulation intraoperatively. Thus, there is no doubt that a strong relationship exists between the EMG and the intraoperative findings in light of this analysis. This finding is all the more remarkable in that it is based on reports of four electromyographers who examined these patients at different times (see Fig. 38–6).

Sensory Testing

Two-point discrimination is very difficult to conduct in babies; therefore, this study is not reliable. We have no definitive data to report at this time.

Skin Galvanic Reaction

The skin galvanic reaction on the palm of the hand is a function of the preservation of the cervical sympathetic ganglion and was introduced into the field of electrodiagnosis by Liberson.[7] It is obvious that this reaction is affected in patients with Horner's syndrome (see Chapter 40).

SURGERY

Reconstructive Microsurgery

One of us (JKT) contributed in the past to the development of microsurgical techniques of interposition grafting.[11] Essentially, the following proximal nerve "sources" should be mentioned: (1) nonavulsed root stumps, (2) preserved brachial plexus components, and (3) nerves of cervical or intercostal origin.

In all cases, these structures are used as "donors," "motors," or "sources," to ensure at least partial restoration of the most essential functions of the extremity. To these donors are grafted (1) sural nerves (most often) and (2) ulnar nerves (in the case of the impossibility of restoring their own function, as in C8 and T1 avulsions). The distal ends of these grafts are sutured to the affected nerve structures according to the following order of importance:

1. As the upper extremity is "floating" around the thorax unless connected to the shoulder joints by active muscles, the stability of the shoulder is the first aim of reconstructive microsurgery. This indicates the significance of reactivation of the supraspinatus and deltoid muscles. In this series, the supraspinatus was successfully restored in most cases. However, the deltoid was more difficult to revitalize.

2. Even when it is preserved in cases of upper plexus lesions, the hand is useless unless it can be brought toward the object of prehension by the elbow flexors. Therefore,

restoration of the biceps is the second priority of reconstruction.

3. In cases of a nonfunctional hand, the presence of hand sensibility is a precondition for future secondary reconstruction. Therefore, restoration of the median nerve is the third important goal of reconstructive microsurgery.

These principles of reconstruction are illustrated in Figures 38–8 and 38–9. The clinical outcome of these two exemplary cases is depicted in Figures 38–10 and 38–11.

In many cases, shoulder abduction, elbow flexion, and finger flexion achieve rewarding degrees of recovery. In both of the cases illustrated here, muscle grading was greater

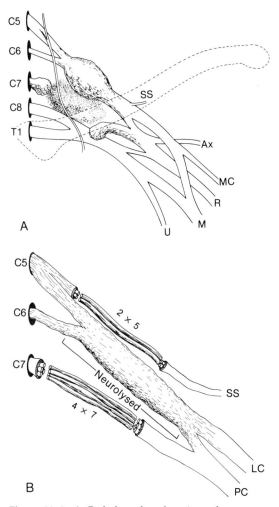

Figure 38–8. *A,* Pathology found at time of surgery, a neuroma in continuity of the upper trunk and rupture of C7. *B,* Reconstruction. Sural nerve grafts from C5 to the suprascapular nerve, neurolysis of the upper trunk, sural nerve grafts from C7 to the middle trunk.

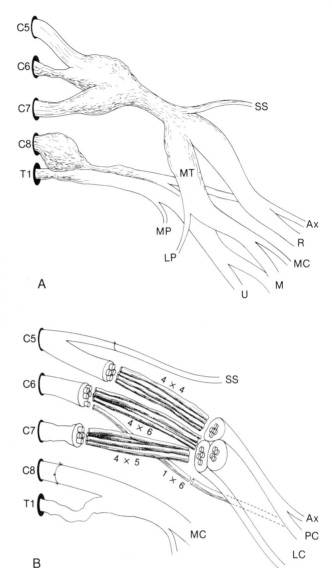

Figure 38–9. *A*, Pathology found at surgery corresponded to findings of global plexus injury with all roots and trunks involved. *B*, Reconstruction involved end-to-end repairs of suprascapular nerve and C8 spinal nerve. Interposition sural nerve grafting of C5, C6, and C7 with secondary plexus trunks and neurolysis of T1 was also done.

than M3. Table 38–7 shows the progression of improvement for some of these children. Muscle grading is limited to M3 because of the difficulty of communication between the examiner and the patient. It appears from the gradings that a definite, although not complete, improvement was achieved in each of these cases.

Table 38–8 summarizes our results; the best improvement was seen for the supraspinatus; the "next best" for the biceps, and the next for the deltoid. Flexors of the hand and fingers also improved in some cases. The poorest recovery was achieved by the extensors of the hand.

Secondary Reconstruction in Obstetrical Brachial Plexus Palsy

General. Secondary reconstructions are procedures to obtain useful function in patients with chronic OBPP not amenable to microsurgical reconstruction. These include tendon transfers, fusion, and free muscle transfers. Secondary reconstruction has been used in two ways in patients with OBPP. (1) In patients who have had a previous brachial plexus palsy reconstruction with nerve grafts and who may still lack certain functions after waiting an appropriate period for return of function. At this time, a secondary recon-

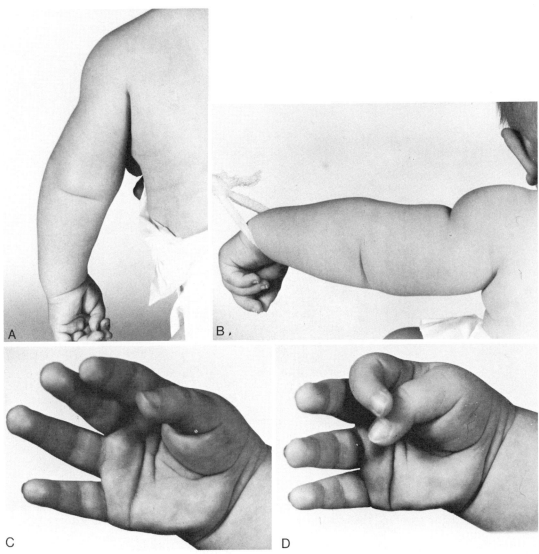

Figure 38–10. *A* and *B,* Preoperative total shoulder and elbow paralysis in 5-month-old patient. *C* and *D,* Hand function is limited to slight flexion in the index finger and thumb.

Illustration continued on opposite page

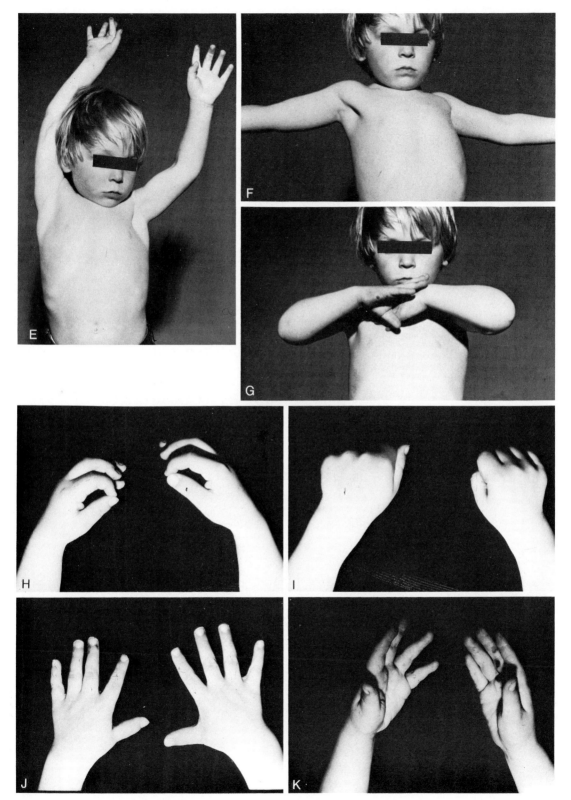

Figure 38–10 *Continued. E to G,* Three years postoperatively. Note shoulder abduction and elevation and elbow flexion. *H to K,* Hand function at 3 years following microsurgical reconstruction.

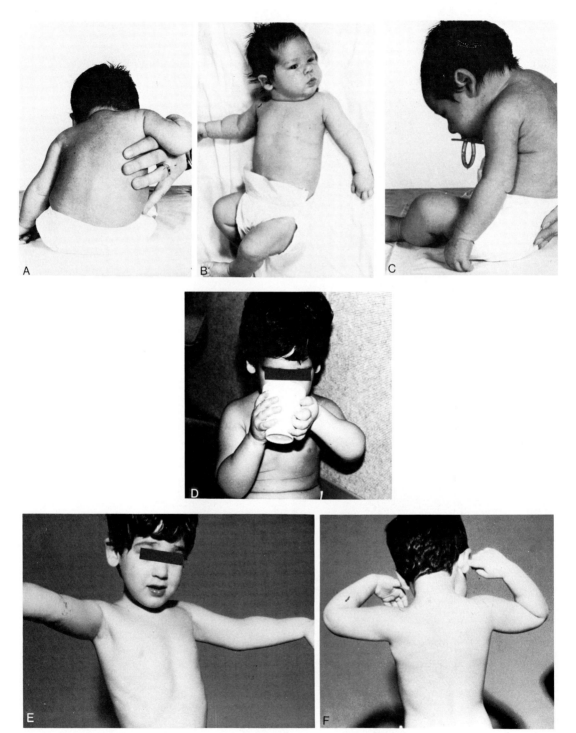

Figure 38–11. *A* to *C*, Preoperative total paralysis of left upper extremity in 6-week-old patient. *D* to *F*, Three years subsequent to left brachial plexus exploration and reconstruction. Note restoration of shoulder function and elbow flexion.

Table 38–7. MUSCLE GRADING IN PATIENTS
WITH OBPP

Patient	Preop.	Postop.	Patient	Preop.	Postop.
PG			DA		
Shoulder	2	+3	Shoulder	0	3
Elbow	+1	3	Elbow	0	3
Flexor	0	3	Flexor	+2	3
Extensor	0	0	Extensor	0	3
MD			MK		
Shoulder	0	+2	Shoulder	0	3
Elbow	0	3	Elbow	0	3
Flexor	+1	3	Flexor	0	3
Extensor	−2	3	Extensor	0	0
RW			TA		
Shoulder	0	+2	Shoulder	1	−3
Elbow	0	3	Elbow	2	3
Flexor	+1	3	Flexor	0	3
Extensor	−2	3	Extensor	0	3

struction to supplement function should be considered. (2) In patients who have been referred to the surgeon too late to consider a primary brachial plexus nerve reconstruction with nerve grafts. At this time, a secondary procedure should be done in order to improve function. In doing tendon transfers in these patients, one has to determine the functions that are missing and the existing motors that are present and that can be sacrificed. The existing motors are selected by clinical and EMG examinations. In preparing for tendon transfers in these patients, the motors that are to be used can be strengthened by electrical stimulation. We trend to delay fusion in our patients with OBPP until they have finished growing. Free muscles are considered when there are no other motors present. Many different transfers and reconstructions have been described. We will discuss here the more common ones that we (JKT and RL) have used in our patients with OBPP.

As stated earlier, each case is studied preoperatively, and each must be considered individually because of the complexity of the brachial plexus injury. Often there are only a few motors present to provide the desired functions.

Shoulder. Procedures at the shoulder are often done in conjunction with procedures by orthopedic surgeons. We commonly use one of two procedures: (1) Transfer of the trapezius to the position of the deltoid muscle to provide abduction or (2) transfer of the latissimus dorsi placed around the back of the arm and reinserting it to the bicipital groove in order to provide external rotation.

Elbow. The common procedure done at the elbow is the transfer of the latissimus dorsi from its position in the back to the position of the biceps in order to provide flexion at the elbow.

Hand. Many different procedures have been described, and surgery must be individualized according to existing motors and the lack of function. The more common procedures utilized in our patients are:

1. Opponensplasty—We commonly use the flexor digitorum sublimis to the ring finger.

2. Extension of the fingers and wrist—Many different procedures have been described. Again, these have to be individualized, depending on the existing motors. The motors that we have used are the pronator teres, brachioradialis, and either the flexor carpi ulnaris or the flexor carpi radialis.

3. Flexion of fingers—We perform a profundoplasty in which the missing portion of the flexor digitorum profundus is connected to the portion of the flexor digitorum profundus that is functioning.

4. Fusion of the wrist—This is done when the child's growth has been completed.

DISCUSSION

In this paper, we summarize our experience of the past 5 years during which one of us (JKT) has operated on 11 babies with OBPP. We are aware of the fact that this is a small series compared with the larger ones that are being published (see Chapter 39), but we feel that some of our approaches to diagnosis and therapy are novel and deserve to be reported. One important point must be discussed:

Time of Surgery. In our experience, several babies with OBPP show improvement beyond the age of 3 to 4 months. In view of the additional therapies that we use, both by electrical stimulation and by behavioral ma-

Table 38–8. RESULTS FOLLOWING
RECONSTRUCTIVE SURGERY IN PATIENTS
WITH OBPP

Best return of function:
Supraspinatus
Biceps
Deltoids
Long flexors

Poorest return of function:
Extensors

nipulation (see Chapter 40), the statistics reported in the other centers may not apply to our population. On the other hand, we cannot ignore the claim that the prognosis following surgical intervention is less favorable if the surgery is done after 9 months of age. One must be aware of the fact that, with surgery done at an earlier time, surgical statistics report improvement of the biceps or deltoid only to the level of M3 after 2 or 3 years (see Chapter 39). The rule of thumb that one of us (JKT) has been using is to follow each baby preoperatively (behaviorally, with video tapes, and with EMG) and to schedule surgery when clinical improvement stops progressing. The *time of surgery* should be the target for further investigations. It is deplorable that despite the recent progress of microsurgery in this area, thousands of babies with OBPP have not been considered for this type of surgery.

CONCLUSIONS

Eleven children with OBPP were studied before and after surgery. Sufficient time has elapsed from the operation to allow us to judge results in only six of these patients. It appears that:

1. No child was further impaired by surgery.

2. Generally, a partial but definite improvement (at least M3 or greater on muscle strength testing and electromyographically by studying interference patterns) was found for shoulder function, elbow flexion, and flexion of the fingers. This confirms the importance of the effectiveness of interposition grafts. However, improvement in extension function (elbow, wrist, and fingers) was most often unobtainable.

3. Although video tapes appear to be the best method to follow the progress in these children, EMGs also proved to be useful. A myelogram may predict the site of avulsion lesions prior to surgery in the majority of cases. The EMG has a good predictive diagnostic value, but has its well-known limitations in predicting root avulsion. Further-

more, EMGs allow evaluation of the anatomic, if not the functional, effectiveness of the success of this surgery.

4. Review of the findings at surgery shows a constant involvement of C7, whether in patients with Erb's palsy (four cases in our series) or in patients with global involvement of all the roots (seven cases in our series; in one case, T1 was spared). Possible mechanisms of the etiology of OBPP were discussed in light of these findings.

5. Review of the obstetrical factors shows the frequency, but not constancy, of the use of forceps. One other factor contributing to cephalic-pelvic disproportion seems to be the relatively high weight of these newborn babies.

References

1. Bennett, C. C., and Harrold, A. J.: Prognosis and early management of birth injuries to the brachial plexus. Br. Med. J., 1:1520, 1976.
2. Duchenne, G. B. A.: De l'Electrisation Localisée et de son Application à la Pathologie et à la Therapie, 3rd Ed. Paris, J. B. Balliere, 1872.
3. Erb, W.: Über eine eigenthümliche Localisation von Lähmengen in Plexus brachialis. Verhandl Naturhist Med. (Heidelberg), 2:130, 1874.
4. Jones, S. J.: Diagnostic value of peripheral and spinal somatosensory evoked potentials in traction lesions of the brachial plexus. Clin. Plast. Surg., 11:167, 1984.
5. Komp Gold, O.: EMO and nerve conduction studies in 116 patients with hemiplegia. Phys. Med. Rehabil., 48:59, 1967.
6. Klumpke, A.: Contribution à l'etude des paralysies radicularies du plexus brachial. Rev. Med. (Paris), 5:591, 1885.
7. Liberson, W. T.: Le reflexe psychogalvanique et l'âge. Biotypologie, 18:117, 1957.
8. Liberson, W. T., and Yhy, H. L.: Proximal distal gradient in the involvement of the peripheral neurons in the upper extremities of hemiplegics. EMG Clin. Neurophys., 17:281, 1977.
9. Millesi, H., and Terzis, J. K.: Nomenclature in peripheral nerve surgery. Clin. Plast. Surg., 11:3, 1984.
10. Smellie, W. A.: Collection of Cases and Observations in Midwifery, Vol. 2, 4th Ed. London, 1768.
11. Terzis, J. K.: Personal communication.
12. Zalis, A. W., Lafratta, C. W., Fauls, L. B., and Oester, Y. T.: Electrophysiological studies in hemiplegia: lower motor neurone findings and correlates. EMG Clin. Neurophys., 16:151, 1976.

39

Obstetrical Palsy:
A Clinical, Pathologic, and
Surgical Review

■

Alain Gilbert, M.D.
J.-L. Tassin, M.D.

HISTORICAL BACKGROUND

As discussed in Chapter 38, the term obstetrical paralysis or palsy was introduced by Duchenne de Boulogne[8] in 1872 in his treatise on localized electrical stimulation, in which he described four cases of upper brachial plexus paralysis that occurred during childbirth. However, the first clinical description was made in 1768 by Smellie,[30] who observed a bilateral paralysis that resolved in a few days. Doherty,[7] in 1844, and Jacquemier,[18] in 1846, also published observations on transient upper brachial plexus paralysis. The first anatomic description was made in 1851 by Danyau,[5] who carried out the autopsy of a newborn presenting with birth paralysis. In this case the plexus was filled with blood but was not ruptured.

Other isolated cases were described by Gueniot,[15] and Depaul[6] (1867) several years before the authoritative description by Duchenne. A short time later, Erb[10] (1874) added the classic description of paralysis of the upper roots, and Seeligmuller[26] (1877) described three patients with total paralysis of the plexus associated with Horner's syndrome. It was Flaubert,[13] who, in 1827, described this type of paralysis for the first time in the adult.

It was also at the end of the 19th century that interest in the etiology and pathologic findings increased and the first experiments

attempting to reproduce the lesions were made. The work of Trombetta[35] (1880) provides interesting figures for the forces developed during delivery, and that of Duval and Guillain[9] (1898) should also be noted. These authors studied the anatomy and connections of the intra-arachnoid segment of the plexus. They calculated the angle between the roots and the spinal cord and deduced the possible lesions resulting from traction. They also remarked that if the shoulder is lowered, the intra-arachnoid portion of C5 and C6 usually breaks at its junction and that this lesion is often associated with a stretching of the intramedullary roots. At the same time, Fieux[12] (1897) discussed the pathogenesis based on his experiments.

During the second half of the 19th century, birth paralysis provoked interest, and cases were recorded and presented. The obstetrical etiology of the lesion was generally accepted as being caused, according to Duchenne, by direct traction on the roots, or, according to others (e.g., Erb), by compression by the first rib. This traumatic theory was not questioned until later.

Surgery specifically for these lesions was introduced at the beginning of the 20th century, more or less exclusively in the United States, where this type of surgery was recommended for some years. Kennedy,[20] in 1903, described the first three patients whom he operated on, who had lesions in the upper roots C5 and C6. He resected the neuroma and directly sutured the ends. Kennedy proposed that the period for attaining spontaneous recovery should be limited to 2 months and demonstrated a satisfactory result in a child operated on at the age of 2 months.

The work of Clark et al.[4] (1905) soon followed. These authors repeated experiments concerning the site and mode of rupture and described seven patients who were operated on using the same technique. They decided to wait a year before operating. It should be noted that two of the children in this series died as a result of the operation. Other cases were published by Lange[21] (1912), Fairbanks[11] (1913), and Spitz and Lange[31] (1915), although it was not until 1916 that surgery appears to have become widespread. In that year, Wyeth and Sharpe[36] published a report concerning 81 patients operated on for birth paralysis. They gave no results, although they specify that the operation should be carried out at 1 month of age in patients with total paralysis and at 3 months in patients with partial paralysis.

In 1920, Taylor[33] described his experience with 200 patients with birth paralysis, 70 of whom were operated on. The technique was the same, although the mortality was now low (three patients). Results were satisfactory, although no details were given. A short time later, Harrenstein[17] (1927) carefully studied the anatomico-pathologic lesions caused by experimental traction.

In 1930, Lauwers[22] wrote a very good review of the problem and proposed neurotization when the roots were avulsed (nerve transplants) with nerves preserved in alcohol for transplants. He described nine patients, the majority of whom he treated personally by neurolysis. After this, reports of this type became scarce in the world literature, and surgical treatment was not regarded favorably, perhaps because results were unconvincing and morbidity was high. For the next 50 years a "wait and see" policy predominated. The traumatic origin of these lesions, so clearly demonstrated earlier, was now criticized in favor of medullary theories (Thomas[34]) or congenital theories (Ombredanne[25]). It was not until the development of microsurgery, and particularly surgery of the adult brachial plexus (Millesi, Narakas) that physicians showed renewed interest in the surgical treatment of obstetrical palsy.

Some surgeons continued to operate on these lesions, and Janec et al.[19] (1968) operated on 29 patients in 10 years using mainly neurolysis. However, their technique and results were unconvincing. These authors proposed surgery during the sixth week of life in patients with infra-ganglionic lesions.

During the last few years, renewed interest in the treatment of these lesions involved the use of microsurgery and improved anesthesia. It is now possible to make a preliminary evaluation of these operations, to compare results with results of similar patients treated conservatively, and to formulate the conditions necessary for surgery.

DEVELOPMENT

The spontaneous evolution of obstetrical palsy lesions has been described in many articles, but the conclusions are often contradictory. Duchenne[8] had already realized their severity in 1872 and stressed the significance of their sequelae. Most recent work confirms his observations. Gjørup,[14] in 1966, carried out a remarkable long-term study on a very large number of patients. The study followed 103 patients for 33 years. It showed the significance and the social repercussions of the sequelae and the difficulty of judging the results of treatment. For example, when replying to the question "Are you handicapped?" 22 of the patients with "good results" replied yes. The study of Gjørup is a major contribution and provides valuable information about the fate of these patients.

Adler and Patterson[1] (1967) are even more pessimistic. According to them, only 7% of brachial paralysis patients recover completely. In this study, 88 adult patients surveyed seemed to have a satisfactory social life despite many handicaps, including a nonfunctional elbow, which is the most serious disability according to the authors. In 1971, Sharrard[29] noted that in his experience only 10% of patients recovered completely. However, in 1976, Bennet and Harrold[2] asserted that, on the contrary, 75% of patients recovered spontaneously and that when recovery was complete, this occurred between 5 days and 5 months of age. The contrast is even more remarkable in the series studied by Hardy[16] (1981), in which the fate of 36 babies with obstetrical palsy was investigated. The extraordinary conclusion was that 80% of the children recovered completely and that none of the remaining 20% had any major functional defect.

How can one reconcile such differences of opinion? It is probable that different conditions were discussed in the different reports. Most patients with mild paralysis, with recovery in a few days, are not seen by the orthopedist, who will consequently treat only serious cases and will therefore have a pessimistic view of the frequency of recovery. However, patients with severe paralysis are quickly transferred from the care of the neurologist or pediatrician to that of the surgeon, and the former no doubt remain too optimistic.

Other difficulties are also involved in the evaluation of these patients. The main difficulty, which is the weak point of large series such as those of Gjørup and Adler, is the lack of information about the initial clinical picture and the evolution of the paralysis. This prevents formulation of a prognosis. The second problem is the general lack of uniform clinical testing of these children and the very different significance given by each author to the appraisal of clinical results. For most authors, a good result corresponds to excellent function of the hand limited in abduction and external rotation of the shoulder. However, as will be discussed, the lower roots are not injured in 75% of patients, and these patients all have excellent function of the hand, even if the shoulder remains paralyzed. Gjørup recorded only two "lower" forms of paralysis among 104 patients but nevertheless found 44 "weak" hands! It therefore appears necessary to establish a strict scale for evaluating muscle strength in these patients based on the British Research Council classification but simplified to account for the difficulty when examining infants:

M0 = no contraction.
M1 = contraction without movement.
M2 = slight or complete movement with weight eliminated.
M3 = complete movement against the weight of the corresponding segment of extremity.

The analysis should also provide a functional evaluation of these patients, who may lack coordination and function despite considerable recovery. Mallet[23] proposed a functional evaluation based on simple gestures (Fig. 39–1). However, this has two disadvantages. It may be carried out only after 3 or 4 years of age, when specific voluntary movements are possible on command, and it does not correspond completely with the use of a limb (e.g., too much importance is attached to the internal rotation of the active shoulder). Surgeons who treat children must, however, establish a standard evaluation procedure in order to best compare results of different treatments.

CLINICAL STUDIES

Forty-four children suffering from obstetrical brachial plexus palsy were followed for more than 10 years at the Saint-Vincent de Paul Hospital in Paris. The group was limited to those patients with a complete medical record, who could therefore be followed from birth. All these children were followed prior to the introduction of brachial plexus microsurgery. Any recovery therefore evolved spontaneously and the results are reported in detail by Tassin.[32]

1. Complete recovery, 14 patients: These patients are characterized by their speed of recovery. The M3 stage on muscle testing is reached by the second month for the deltoid and the biceps and by the third month for the external rotators. The triceps and the extensors of the digits and wrist recover in 1½ months. These cases all involve the upper roots (C5, C6, and sometimes C7). If the lower roots are involved, this is only very transient.

2. Near-complete recovery (stage IV of Mallet), 11 patients: In these cases the biceps and the deltoid reached stage M1 by the third month and the M3 stage 5 months later. The external rotators never recovered spontaneously and this group of children had eight disinsertions of the subscapularis, two transplantations (teres major or latissimus dorsi), and one disinsertion plus transplantation. Pronation and supination are normal in eight patients. The hand is always normal or nearly so. Extensors C5, C6, and C7 are involved (eight patients), and the extensors of the digits and wrist reach stage M1 by 4½ months at the latest and M3 at 10 months.

3. Others, 19 patients: Results are much poorer in these patients, in whom the biceps reaches stage M1 only after 3½ months and M3 after 5 months. According to Mallet's classification, the shoulder was designated as III in 12 patients and as II in 7 patients. Patients in whom biceps reached stage M1 before 3 months but whose recovery evolved slowly (M3 at 7 months) are also included in this category. Often recovery of the biceps

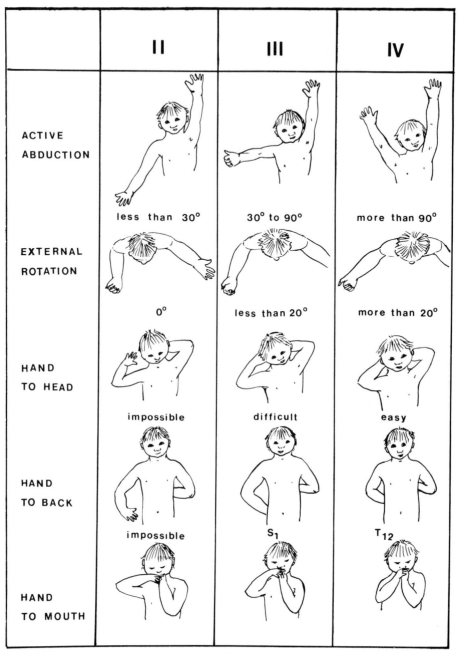

	II	III	IV
ACTIVE ABDUCTION	less than 30°	30° to 90°	more than 90°
EXTERNAL ROTATION	0°	less than 20°	more than 20°
HAND TO HEAD	impossible	difficult	easy
HAND TO BACK	impossible	S_1	T_{12}
HAND TO MOUTH			

Figure 39–1. Functional assessment of the shoulder (after Mallet). We have not taken in account the internal rotation, which is always diminished but is rarely a functional problem.

only appears after 10 months; it always recovers, however. After the key dates, there is no relation between the final shoulder value and the date of appearance of recovery of the biceps. There are frequent co-contractions between the biceps and the triceps. Recovery of the external rotators never occurs. Problems in pronation and supination

are considerable, with an absence of active mobility in half the patients.

The hand was normal in six patients and the shoulder was designated as III (Mallet's classification). In these patients, initial lesions are C5–C6 or C5–C7. In eight patients the hand was "rigid," almost spastic. Initial paralysis was total with early recovery of the hand muscles (M3 before 10 months). In five patients recovery of the hand was poor, with paralytic or trophic problems and deformities with muscle retractions. These patients had complete initial forms of the disorder with very long and incomplete recovery. The M3 stage is never reached before 15 months of age.

Taken together, these results show that complete recovery is possible only when the biceps and deltoid reach M1 by 2 months. If 3½ months are required to reach M1, the result, even if still good, is incomplete. However, if the biceps is not at M3 by the fifth month, the result will necessarily be unsatisfactory. Conditions requiring surgery are apparent from these results, and the decisive period is between 2 and 3½ months. For practical reasons, the majority of conditions that may require surgery are evaluated at 3½ months.

From October 1977 to October 1982, 230 patients with obstetrical brachial plexus palsy were examined at the Trousseau Hospital. Thanks to the participation of pediatricians and obstetricians it was often possible to see these children during the first days and almost always during the first month after injury. The large number of patients reflects the national and even international population (20% of patients came from outside France).

During this period, 114 of these patients were operated on. Their ages ranged from 2 to 6 months for the majority, although some patients who were seen later were older (Fig. 39–2). Several patients were operated on much later (7 to 9 years old). However, the results were so unsatisfactory that we have decided not to continue this late surgery. One hundred records were re-examined to eliminate all those that were incomplete. Two patients also died later of an intercurrent disorder.

Obstetrical Findings

The right side was predominantly affected (59 cases); 37 cases involved the left side and 2 were bilateral. This was the same proportion as that found by Sever[27] and Bentzon,[3] but differs from that of Gjørup,[14] who found a majority of left-sided injuries. Birth weight varied from 2000 to 6000 gm, although most newborns weighed more than 4000 gm. Vertex presentation was observed in most cases (67), with 47 recorded cases of dystocia of the shoulder. Breech presentation occurred 14 times and there was one cesarean section. The presentation was not recorded in 19 cases. One interesting fact should be noted: vertex presentations were associated with a heavy birth weight, whereas breech presentations were more often associated with a lighter birth weight (between 2000 and 4000 gm). Therefore, if a heavy birth weight increases the risk of dystocia and paralysis, breech presentation also incurs the same risk, even at low birth weight. A cesarean section does not totally eliminate the chances of injury to the plexus; an unknown mecha-

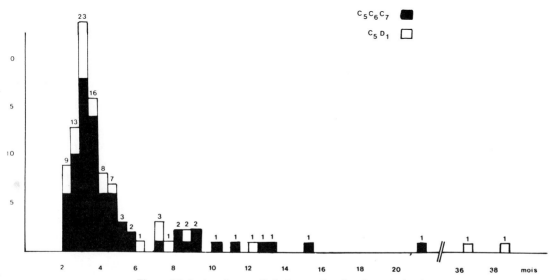

Figure 39–2. Age (in months) at operation for obstetrical palsy.

nism, probably traction, is responsible. Our observations differ markedly from those of Sever[27] and Gjørup,[14] who found a majority of breech presentations. Perhaps this is due to modern modifications in obstetrical procedures.

Preoperative Evaluation

Clinical evaluation should begin with the first consultation. Often the child is only a few days old and detailed examination is difficult. Clinical testing of the newborn requires patience and only a few simple aids (a toothbrush and a few keys). With these tools alone, the examiner should try to stimulate active movement by the baby. At the same time he should palpate the muscles between two fingers in order to feel the slightest muscular contraction. This examination is difficult and requires a calm atmosphere, a relaxed child, and a certain amount of experience. One should be wary of "tricks" that the child uses, in particular, bending the elbow when lying down. Rotation of the joints, particularly the shoulder, should also be noted.

Only an approximate examination of sensitivity may be made in a baby (reaction when pinched, trophic problems, nail and hair growth, color of fingers). Symptoms of Horner's syndrome, signifying serious injury of root T1, should also be looked for. Finally, radiography of the thorax shows if there is an associated fracture (clavicle, humerus) and if the diaphragm dome is in place, demonstrating the integrity of the phrenic nerve. This study also eliminates the only other differential diagnosis of the paralysis, i.e., epiphyseal separation of the humeral head. Radiography is only useful after 1 or 2 weeks of age, when calcification is apparent. Examination of the four limbs and the hips should be complete. Bilateral abnormalities should be looked for with particular care. Neurologic examination of the lower limbs should look for paralysis that is symptomatic of obstetrical tetraplegia. We have observed two cases of this condition, which is not always obvious because of the persistent reflex movements of the lower limbs.

This examination allows the injury to be localized. The diagnosis of C5–C6 paralysis is evident from the position of the limb, i.e., in internal rotation without abduction. Total paralysis is revealed in the same way by a limp limb associated with closed fingers and ocular symptoms (Horner's syndrome).

If the child is seen during the first days of life, an electromyogram (EMG) at this time is useless, as it provides full information only after 20 days. The limb is left to rest, without therapeutic exercises or splints, for the first 3 weeks.

The child is re-examined during the third week and recovery is often obvious; the hand has become normal, the elbow has started to bend, and the shoulder has begun to function. In these cases, stretching has occurred without axonotmesis and recovery will be complete. A few gentle manipulations may speed recovery.

In other cases there is no recovery. If paralysis is complete and is associated with Horner's syndrome, the prognosis is gloomy and a date for surgery should be settled with the parents. Surgery should be carried out as soon as possible, usually around the second month. If the hand has recovered but the shoulder has remained paralyzed, there is still a chance of spontaneous recovery, although the family should be prepared for an operation. A first electromyogram may now be carried out. Further evaluation will be made during the third month, and this may or may not be followed by an operation. All these clinical evaluations and the results of electrical tests are recorded on a special card to enable the course of the disorder to be followed at a glance.

After the third week, gentle manipulations are performed with the limb in traction. There is no reason to prescribe splints in abduction or external abduction-rotation at this stage. As shown by Sever,[28] Milgram,[24] and Adler and Patterson,[1] splints are useless and are often harmful, as they may cause stiffness in abduction.

The final evaluation will be the preoperative evaluation and should include muscle testing, electromyography, and myography.

Muscle Testing. We have already discussed the difficulties of testing young infants. However, such tests are fundamental at this stage, for if biceps function reappears at 3 months, surgery should not be carried out. One should also not hesitate to ask for a second opinion.

Electomyography. This is also a difficult study to perform in the child. For the last 5 years of our series, all the examinations have been carried out by the same electromyographer (Dr. G. Raimbault). The electromy-

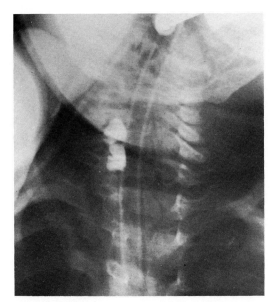

Figure 39–3. Myelography. Pseudomeningocele at level of the C5–C6 roots.

ogram should include a certain number of test muscles, which are re-examined every time. An electromyogram of the diaphragm is also carried out with an esophageal probe. The interpretation of these electromyograms is difficult and there are few correlations with the clinical picture. Results of the electrical examination are often more optimistic than the clinical situation warrants. Negative results are the most interesting, as a total absence of reinnervation at 3 months demonstrates an almost certain avulsion of the corresponding root.

Myelography (Figs. 39–3 and 39–4). We perform this examination systematically. Among 118 patients, 108 had a myelogram at a mean age of 124 days. The examination is usually performed under general anesthetic, sometimes under a preanesthetic with a single injection of metrizamide (Amipaque). The child should rest for 48 hours after myelography. Complications are not serious: one patient had nonfatal aseptic meningitis and two patients experienced convulsions.

Results and correlations were made based on 79 useful medical records, reporting results of only good quality, unquestionable examinations. Fourteen false-positive results were recorded: four pseudo-meningoceles with visible roots and no clinical injury, interpreted as physiologic pseudo-meningoceles; nine pseudo-meningoceles with no vis-

ible roots and clinical injury, proof of avulsion not obtained at the time of surgery; and one case in which there was no pseudomeningocele but in which the root was not seen. We found three false-negative results among 495 roots studied. In these cases myelography was normal and the roots were avulsed.

To conclude, the examination is reliable and the absence of meningocele practically confirms the extraforaminal injury. It is for this reason that we use myelography systematically.

Decision to Operate

This decision is made in conjunction with the parents on the basis of the results of the preoperative evaluation. The clinical examination is the most important, and if the biceps is totally paralyzed, even if the electrical signs are encouraging, surgery is recommended. The existence of meningoceles does not modify this decision. The presence of false-positive results justifies the systematic examination of all the affected roots.

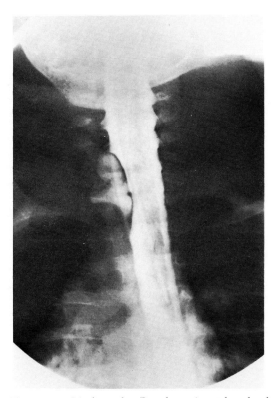

Figure 39–4. Myelography. Pseudomeningocele at level of the C8–T1 roots.

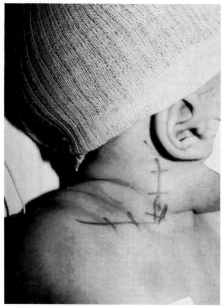

Figure 39–5. The surgical approach for upper root lesions.

OPERATIVE TECHNIQUE

The child is operated on a few days after myelography. After intubation and halothane induction, anesthesia is continued by injections of phenoperidine and continuous infusion of alfaxalone with an automatic syringe. Curare is not used.

The child lies on his back, with his head turned to the side opposite the lesion. A small cushion is used to raise the spine. Cephalic electrodes for recording stimulated potentials are placed, and the apparatus is tested by stimulating a large distal trunk (usually the median nerve). The two lower limbs, neck, shoulder, and affected limb are prepared. The operative region and the two calves are infused with a solution of diluted (1 ampule/30 ml serum) vasopressin. Because of the use of this vasoconstrictor, no patient has ever required a blood transfusion.

A supraclavicular incision is made first (Fig. 39–5) and is sufficient for C5, C6, and C7 lesions. It is the classic incision, with a vertical limb on the posterior edge of the sternocleidomastoid muscle and a horizontal limb on the clavicle. The platysma is lifted with the cutaneous flap. A second lymphatico-adipose flap is then lifted. The omohyoid is sectioned, and often the ascending cervical vein and artery are sectioned as well. The phrenic nerve is located and is often included

in the fibrosis surrounding the scalenus anterior muscle. In nearly every case there is an anastomosis with C5 and one must be careful not to injure this nerve when the scalenus anterior muscle is separated. We have observed several temporary postoperative phrenic paralyses. The spinal nerve of C5 first appears, followed by C6. Soft silicone loops are placed around these nerves to aid dissection, and an adherent and very fibrous neuroma is usually found at their junction. When C7 is affected, it is also adherent within this neuroma (Figs. 39–6 and 39–7).

The trunks are identified in the uninjured zone, usually under the clavicle. The suprascapular nerve should also be identified coming from the neuroma, either from C5 or from a more distal location. When all the nerves have been identified, the cervical spinal nerves are stimulated and the evoked potentials are recorded, confirming the quality of their connection with the spinal cord (Figs. 39–8 to 39–10). We have never found evidence of an obvious lesion or rupture with medullary avulsion.

Generally, a neuroma in continuity is found and the question of possible neurolysis arises. The results of the few neurolyses carried out by us and other colleagues (Narakas [37]) are not encouraging.

In nearly every case we have preferred resection of the neuroma followed by nerve grafts. Serial histologic sections of 20 resected neuromas have shown the almost total absence of nerve fibers at the distal end of the neuroma. Resection of the neuroma should be carried out prudently, taking care to preserve the branches of the nerve to the serra-

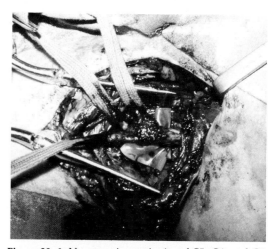

Figure 39–6. Neuroma in continuity of C5, C6, and C7.

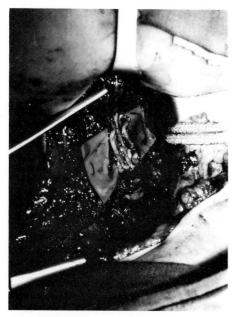

Figure 39–7. After resection and grafting of the neuroma shown in Figure 39–6.

tus, which often originate very high on the nerve roots and are intact.

In the case of total paralysis, exploration should continue in the subclavicular region. An incision opens the delto-pectoral groove toward the medial side of the pectoralis major, which is disinserted from the clavicle. The cords are identified and tagged with silicone loops. Then the clavicle is sectioned, leaving intact the two anterior and posterior periosteal flaps. This cut is made obliquely with an oscillating saw. The section of the subclavian muscle and the separating of the two ends of the clavicle open this region widely. The plexus may be followed from the cord level to the intervertebral foramen, taking care to avoid injury to surrounding blood vessels and, on the left side, to the thoracic duct. In this series the subclavian artery was damaged once and was immediately repaired. The thoracic duct was injured twice without effect. When fibrosis is extensive and widespread in the subclavian region, one should expect to find one or two curled-up avulsed roots, and the spinal ganglion is easily recognized (Fig. 39–11).

A difficult problem is the identification, either on C8 or T1, or particularly on C5 or C6, of nerves and trunks that are without fibrosis but are slightly slack and are associated with total paralysis. Meningoceles may be found, but their presence is not pathog-nomonic and their identification is difficult. Sometimes the evoked potentials may be useful, although they demonstrate only the integrity of the posterior root and partial avulsions are known to occur. If the clinical, operative, and electrophysiologic findings do not agree in these cases, it is best to close the incision without any therapeutic action and to wait for further progression. When the information correlates, the affected roots are immediately neurotized.

When the plexus has been explored and the neuromas are resected, an evaluation is made before deciding what to repair. This decision is easy for ruptures of C5, C6, and C7, as two ends are present that may simply be joined with a graft. In cases of complete paralysis, the possibilities for repair depend on the lesions.

C8 and T1 have usually been avulsed, sometimes in association with C7 and C6. We have never found avulsion of all the roots. If C5, C6, and C7 have simply been broken, the stumps of these three roots may be used to directly reinnervate the three cords and the suprascapular nerve.

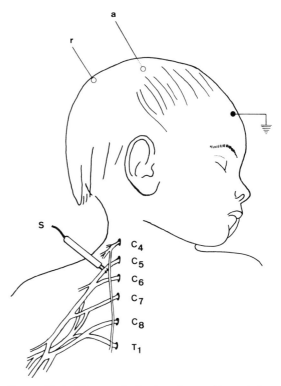

Figure 39–8. Diagram indicating the position of the recording electrodes in evaluating somatosensory evoked potentials and the position of the stimulating electrodes on the roots of the brachial plexus.

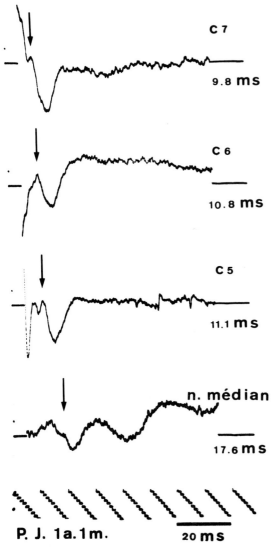

P. J. 1a.1m.   **20 ms**

Figure 39–9. A 13-month-old child suffering from deficits of C5, C6, and C7 secondary to an obstetrical injury. Somatosensory evoked potentials: From below to above, percutaneous stimulation of the median nerve at the wrist prior to operation; somatosensory evoked potentials with a normal latency of 17.6 msec.; direct successive intraoperative stimulation of the C5, C6, and C7 roots. Evoked potentials are of normal shape and latency.

If only C5 and C6 remain, a choice must be made concerning the type of surgery. This choice varies from one school to another, although we think it fundamental to recover the mobility of the hand, which is possible in the newborn. For this reason we neurotize the lateral cord (median and musculocutaneous nerves) and the ulnar nerve with C5 and C6. The posterior cord is sacrificed. If possible the suprascapular nerve is reinner-

vated. The stability of the shoulder will later be established by a transfer of the trapezius.

If only C5 remains, the prognosis is grim. This root is used to graft the musculocutaneous and the suprascapular nerves and sometimes the lateral root of the median nerve. The intercostal nerves T2 and T5 are used to graft the medial root of the median nerve or the entire median nerve (Fig. 39–12). The grafts used are sural nerves, taken by continuous incision to prevent rupture. Sometimes the cervical plexus or the medial brachiocutaneous nerve is used. A special problem is posed by the isolated avulsion of roots C5 and C6, as there is no possibility of direct repair. In these cases the musculocutaneous nerve is neurotized by the medial nerve of the pectoralis major muscle. It is possible to suture these two nerves directly. In some cases we have tried to reinnervate either the suprascapular or the axillary nerve by a cross neurotization from the contralateral plexus. A graft is sutured on the lateral nerve of the opposite pectoralis major muscle, passed under the skin of the thorax and out again at the level of the plexus. The distal suture will be carried out 6 or 12 months later to prevent fibrosis.

After repair, if the clavicle has been sec-

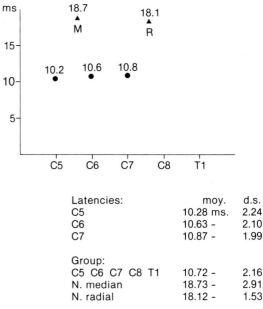

Latencies:		moy.	d.s.
C5		10.28 ms.	2.24
C6		10.63 –	2.10
C7		10.87 –	1.99
Group:			
C5 C6 C7 C8 T1		10.72 –	2.16
N. median		18.73 –	2.91
N. radial		18.12 –	1.53

Figure 39–10. Graph of the mean latencies of somatosensory evoked potentials recorded from 33 subjects by direct intraoperative stimulation of the C5, C6, and C7 roots. The upper part of the graph shows the median (M) and radial (R) nerve latencies stimulated at the upper arm and at the elbow, respectively.

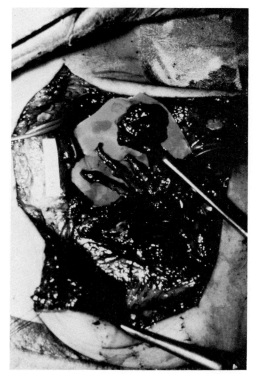

Figure 39–11. Rupture to the upper trunk and avulsion of C7, C8, and T1.

tioned, it is sutured with absorbable thread. The skin is closed along two planes and the arm is immobilized in a Mayo sling. The child is then placed in a plaster body cast, molded the evening before the operation, for 20 days.

ANATOMIC LESIONS

The lesions observed during the surgical operations were variable, but could be classified into distinct categories, corresponding to typical clinical pictures.

Injury to the Upper Roots: C5, C6, and at Times C7. These are the most frequent injuries (51 patients with lesions of C5 and C6 and 25 patients with lesions of C5, C6, and C7). Avulsions of the roots C5 and C6 are rare (11 patients) and more often the nerve root or the upper trunk and its divisions are ruptured. The more distal the lesion on the upper trunk, the more frequent are the associated lesions at other levels (Figs. 39–13 and 39–14). If the divisions of the upper trunk are affected, there is nearly always rupture or avulsion of C7. However, the rare cases of lesions of spinal nerves C5 and C6 are always isolated (Fig. 39–15).

A special situation occurs with isolated avulsions of C5 and C6 (11 patients) or of C5, C6, and C7 (Fig. 39–16). These avulsions are never associated with lesions of the lower roots and always followed breech presentation in an infant of low birth weight.

The clinical picture is usually of a neuroma involving the C5–C6 junction, the upper trunk and its divisions, and, in particular, the suprascapular nerve. Sometimes the nerve ends are separated without a neuroma (Fig. 39–17). This is a particularly serious sign and often indicates very widely distributed lesions.

Total Paralysis. Twenty-four patients with

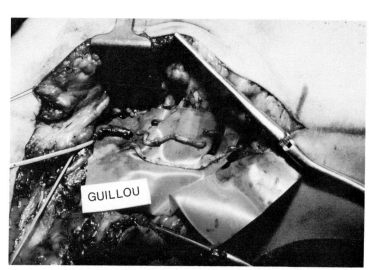

Figure 39–12. Neurotization of the median nerve by intercostal nerves.

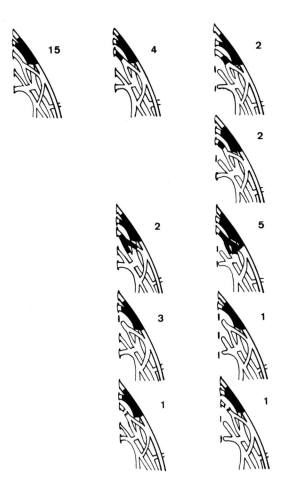

Figure 39–13. Pathologic anatomy. The most frequently encountered lesion was a neuroma in continuity involving C5, C6, the upper trunk, and its branches. Associated lesions include neuroma, rupture or avulsion of C7, and avulsion of C8 and T1.

Figure 39–14. Neuroma in continuity not involving the divisions of the upper trunk was only rarely associated with lesions of C7, C8, and T1.

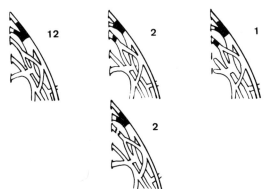

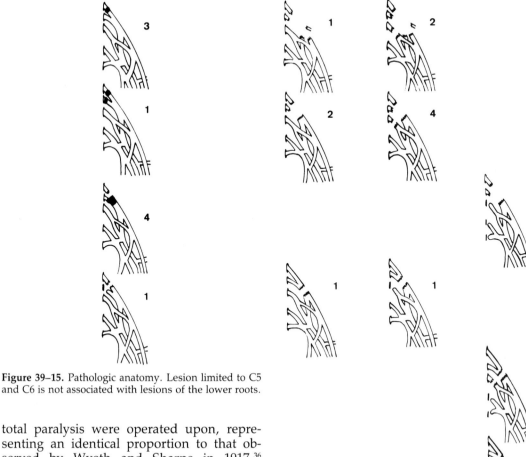

Figure 39–15. Pathologic anatomy. Lesion limited to C5 and C6 is not associated with lesions of the lower roots.

total paralysis were operated upon, representing an identical proportion to that observed by Wyeth and Sharpe in 1917.[36] Among 81 patients who underwent surgery, 62 had lesions of C5 and C6 and 19 had lesions of C8 and T1 (slightly more than 23%). The anatomico-pathologic findings of these lesions are not always obvious because for the study to be precise, a complete exploration of the spinal nerves C8 and T1 up to the intervertebral foramen is required. This exploration is possible only after section of the clavicle and is not without danger. Sometimes the spinal nerves are continuous, although slack and thin. The presence of myelomeningoceles and total paralysis and the absence of response to stimulation are signs

Figure 39–17. Pathologic anatomy. Complete rupture of roots and trunks.

that point to avulsion, but proof can be provided only by posterior laminectomy, which is impossible in a baby. The study of somatosensory potentials may be deceptive because, when positive, they show only the continuity of the sensory root and do not provide information about the motor root. Only progression of the disorder will sometimes permit retrospective diagnosis. This explains why so many surgeons prefer to operate directly on roots C8 and T1 when a lesion at this site is strongly suspected. However, surprises often occur with direct surgery, and we have always tried to follow the rule of complete exposure of the plexus before repair.

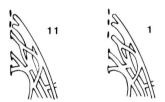

Figure 39–16. Pathologic anatomy. The operative findings of upper root avulsions and the frequency of occurrence.

One aspect of brachial plexus injuries in children is fundamentally different from adult plexus trauma, i.e., complete avulsion of all five roots is never observed. One intact root always remains that may be used. Direct surgery is therefore always helpful to redistribute the axons of the plexus.

In more than two thirds of cases, roots C5, C6, and C7 are ruptured and allow complete repair of the plexus. We believe that this reconstruction is possible and desirable in the very young, who have a good chance of the reinnervation of the hand.

We have never found a lower Klumpke type paralysis without injury to the upper roots. It is probable that the cases described in the literature were total lesions with subsequent successful recovery of the upper roots (Figs. 39–18 and 39–19).

To conclude, this anatomico-pathologic investigation demonstrates the following characteristics:

1. Lesions of C5, C6, and C7 are nearly always extramedullary ruptures and may therefore be repaired (Fig. 39–20).

2. These lesions are always above the clavicle and may therefore be repaired by limited surgery.

3. Lesions of roots C8 and T1 are always avulsions.

4. In cases of total paralysis, there is always at least one root that may be repaired and therefore justifies systematic surgical intervention (Fig. 39–21).

POSTOPERATION TREATMENT

The child is immobilized in a plaster cast for 20 days, after which physical therapy resumes. This gentle therapy is given every day, accompanied by electrical stimulation. Although electrical stimulation has never been proved to be of any value, our impression has been favorable. Also, the appearance of muscular contractions during stimulation precedes active contractions by several weeks and is often a good prognostic sign.

Clinical monitoring with testing is carried out every 3 months and electromyography every 6 months. The date of appearance of muscular contractions is noted, as this is of great prognostic value. Particular attention should be given to screening for signs of joint stiffness and, in particular, reduction of external rotation of the shoulder, extension of the elbow, supination, and pronation. This diminution of mobility should be treated by energetic physiotherapy, although one should not hesitate to operate if mobility does

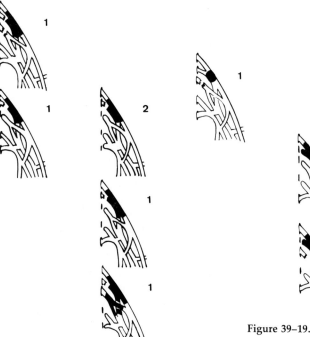

Figures 39–18 and 39–19. A more extensive lesion of the upper trunk is always associated with involvement of C7 and sometimes of C8 and T1.

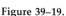

Figure 39–19.

Figure 39–18.

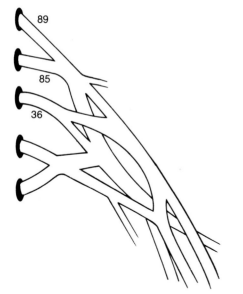

Figure 39–20. Anatomic lesions on the upper roots.

not improve. Fifteen of 100 patients studied had subscapular disinsertion for contraction of the internal rotators of the shoulder. The result in all cases was excellent with no instances of recurrence.

Sequelae and treatment by various muscle transfers are not dealt with in this chapter.

RESULTS

The results in the baby are classified M0 to M3, as described earlier. Only an analytical

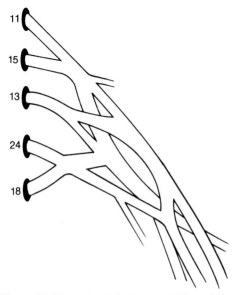

Figure 39–21. Anatomic lesions in total paralysis.

classification can be made, as complex voluntary movements are difficult to obtain before 4 years of age.

Isolated Avulsion of the Upper Roots

The clinical picture in isolated lesions is typical, with total paralysis in the field of action of the injured roots and clear-cut muscle atrophy. Even after 3 months there is no sign of recovery, and the electromyogram shows complete denervation.

Intraoperative diagnosis is often easy if the nerve root ganglion is found outside the intervertebral foramen. In other cases diagnosis is difficult or even impossible. In these cases spontaneous evolution is the only proof of avulsion.

We have studied 12 cases of spontaneous recovery (Fig. 39–22). The deltoid recovered in seven cases: three times with a good result (M1 before 9½ months, M2 before 13 months) and four times with incomplete recovery (M1 at a maximum of 41 months). Five patients experienced total lack of recovery of the deltoid. The external rotators recovered spontaneously six times: two with good results (M3 at 18 months) and four with insufficient results. The biceps recovered spontaneously four times. These recoveries occurred early (M2 at 7 months). The supinators recovered poorly in general and three remained at M0.

Muscles innervated by C7 have a variable fate, depending on the lesion. When the lesion of C7 was incomplete and was associated with an avulsion of C5 and C6 (eight cases), recovery was complete. When avulsion of C5, C6, and C7 was proved (one case), the triceps recovered completely in 2 years; however, the wrist and the finger extensors are at M1 at the date of this writing.

The direct treatment of these avulsions is unequivocal. Only neurotization is possible (Fig. 39–23). In cases of paralysis of the deltoid, the axillary nerve was neurotized once by the lateral nerve of the pectoralis major muscle, once by intercostal nerves, and twice by the lateral nerve of the contralateral pectoralis major muscle, extended by a nerve transplant along the front of the thorax. Results are disappointing: two results are classified as M0 at 8 and 12 months and one as M1 at 10 months, a result too premature to be judged.

Paralysis of the external rotators has never

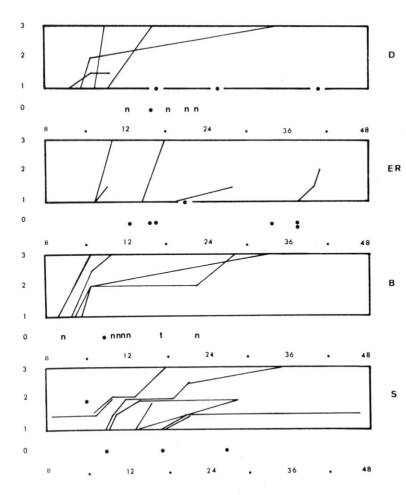

Figure 39–22. Level of spontaneous muscle recovery after medullary avulsion of upper roots C5 and C6. The curve indicates the initial and current strength of deltoid (D), external rotators (ER), biceps (B), and supinator (S) muscles. The assessment is indicated on the vertical axis and the age of the child in months on the horizontal. The large dots indicate the date of the last examination and the muscle grade attained in those patients without functional recovery. The letter "n" indicates the date of neurotization of the musculocutaneous or axillary nerve. The letter "t" indicates the date of muscle transfer.

Figure 39–23. A review of spontaneous muscle recovery in 11 cases of avulsion of C5 and C6 and in one case of avulsion of C5, C6, and C7. Each case is represented by one horizontal line, and the muscles evaluated include deltoid (D), external rotators (ER), biceps (B), and supinator (S). The length of follow-up (FU) is expressed in months. The letter "R" indicates partial or complete recovery of the muscles, and the associated number indicates the muscle grade at the last examination. Complete absence of muscle recovery is indicated by the shaded area. The letter "N" or "T" indicates either neurotization of the motor nerve (N) or muscle transfer (T) to replace the action of a paralyzed muscle.

C5 C6

D	ER	B	S	FU
R_3	R_3	R_3	R_3	44
R_1+	R_3	R_3	R_2	10
N	R_1+	R_3	R_2	29
R_3	R_1+			9
R_1	R_2	N	R_1+	46
R_3		R_3		34
N		N	R_2	13
N		N	R_1+	38
		N	R_2	16
N		N	R_3	38
R_1		N		17
R_1	R_1	T	R_2	26

C5 C6 C7

been treated by neurotization but sometimes has been managed by tendon transfer. Paralysis of the biceps was treated six times by neurotization, using a nerve from the pectoralis major muscle. Results were variable. One result was excellent (M3 at 4 months), one was a failure (M0 at 18 months, treated by transfer of the latissimus dorsi), and four results are too early to judge. In cases of avulsion of C5, C6, and C7 when the latissimus dorsi was paralyzed, we have also transferred the gracilis with vascular anastomoses and innervation by a graft from the contralateral plexus. This operation was performed very recently and cannot be evaluated yet.

These avulsions are often difficult to diagnose and spontaneous recovery sometimes occurs. Neurotizations should be attempted, although their result is often disappointing. It should be mentioned that the spinal nerve should not be used to neurotize the upper roots, as the trapezius is the best transplant to stabilize the shoulder.

Assessment of Recovery of Other Lesions

Recovery has been studied by muscle testing at several intervals and especially at two years postoperatively. For some muscles (biceps, external rotators, deltoid), the grading of muscle recovery has allowed us to trace a curve from M1 to M3, according to the time elapsed. These curves have been compared and fall into several distinct forms or shapes. The areas circumscribing the curves of a certain shape have been traced and are termed "zones." The muscles whose curves fit within one of these zones undergo the same type of recovery. It is then possible, after a follow-up of only a few months, to know in which zone the curve of recovery will fall and therefore to predict the ultimate result.

Recovery of the External Rotator Muscles (Fig. 39–24)

Grafts of the suprascapular nerve were studied when the nerve was grafted directly to a root (37 cases) or when the graft originated from the upper trunk (32 cases).

Recovery usually occurs between 12 and 24 months after surgery: 7% of cases are at M3 at 1 year (three curves are in zone I) and 53% of cases are at M3 at 2 years (26 of 56 curves are in zones II and III). Two years

after the repair of 28 suprascapular nerves, 50% are at M3, 25% are at M2, and 25% are at M0 or M1. Too few 3-year results are available for statistical study; however, the zone system provides the following evaluation: M3, 61%; M2, 16%; M1, 16%; and M0, 7%.

Factors Affecting Recovery

1. Extent of the paralysis: The prognosis is better in the upper root lesions (M3, 60 to 75% at 2 to 3 years) than in global paralysis (M3, 25 to 30% at 2 to 3 years).

2. Nature of the lesion: The graft of a C5–C6 neuroma in continuity shows better results (M3, 64% at 2 years) than results following avulsion or rupture of roots C5 and C6 (M3, 33% at 2 years).

3. Type of repair: It seems preferable to directly graft the suprascapular nerve (M3, 78% at 2 years) rather than the entire upper trunk (M3, 41% at 2 years). However, this impression is contradicted by the analysis of recovery zones, which shows roughly equal chances for both types of repair.

Secondary Surgery. Stiffness of the internal rotation of the shoulder developed in 14 patients. This stiffness usually occurred a short time (4½ to 18½ months) after the operation. In all cases disinsertion of the subscapular muscle from the scapula was carried out by axillary surgery. Passive external rotation, which was zero before surgery, was 65° immediately after surgery and 70° after approximately 1 year. In all except two patients, external rotators showed active recovery after disinsertion. This indicates that it is not necessary to transfer the teres major and the latissimus dorsi at the same time as the disinsertion, as was carried out in one patient. It is therefore sufficient to place the rotator muscles in a better position to allow active recovery.

Recovery of the Biceps (Fig. 39–25)

Overall results concerning the recovery of the biceps are usually judged during the first 2 years. After one year, 34% of patients are already at M3 and 11% are still at M0. After two years, 67% of patients have reached M3 and 11% remain at M0. After 3 years, 72% of patients are at M3. However, this final result is not accurate owing to the small number of patients.

A more exact result is given by the analysis of zones at 3 years: 50 curves at M3 (82%), 8 curves at M1 (11%), and 3 curves at M0 (7%).

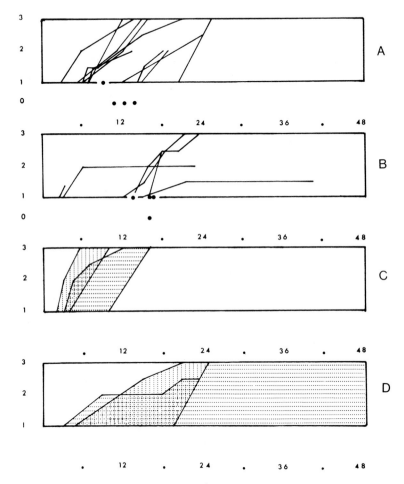

Figure 39–24. Level of postoperative recovery of the external rotators. The large dots indicate the muscle grade at the last examination in those patients who have recovered little or no function to date. *A*, Level of recovery after nerve grafts directly to the suprascapular nerve after resection of a neuroma in continuity. *B*, Level of recovery after nerve grafts between C5 and C6 and the upper trunk above the level of the suprascapular nerve after resection of a neuroma in continuity. *C*, Zone I (vertical lines), Zone II (horizontal lines). *D*, Zone III (vertical lines), Zone IV (horizontal lines).

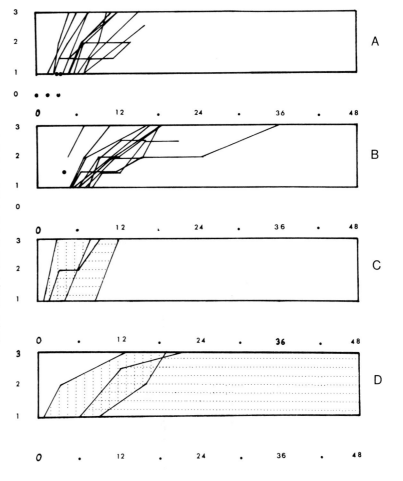

Figure 39–25. Postoperative recovery of the biceps. The muscle grade from 0 to 3 is indicated on the vertical axis and the postoperative follow-up in months on the horizontal. The large dots mark the muscle grade attained at the last examination for those patients who had little or no recovery at the time of examination. *A,* Level of biceps recovery in those patients who had nerve grafts placed between C5 and C6 and the anterior and posterior division of the upper trunk. *B,* Level of recovery with graft placed between C5 and C6 and the upper trunk. *C,* Zone I (vertical lines), Zone II (horizontal lines). *D,* Zone III (vertical lines), Zone IV (horizontal lines).

The overall recovery of the biceps is therefore good, as it reaches 82% at 3 years. The percentage of patients who are at M0 stays the same at 1, 2, or 3 years.

Factors Affecting Recovery

1. Extent of the lesion: The smaller the extent of the lesion, the earlier the recovery. At 1 year, 45% of patients with C5–C6 lesions were at stage M3, compared with 25% of those with C5–T1 lesions. Zone analysis confirms this effect and shows that 90% recovery to stage M3 at 3 years may be predicted for patients with C5–C6 lesions. Patients with C5–C7 and C5–T1 lesions recover more slowly and less completely.

2. Nature of the lesion: This has only a small effect, as zone analysis shows that 29% of the curves are in zone IV for neuromas and 35% for ruptures and avulsions.

3. Type of repair: Grafts of the upper trunk have a much better prognosis than those of the lateral cord or of the musculocutaneous nerve.

Secondary Surgery. In eight patients secondary surgery (muscle transfer of the latissimus dorsi or neurotization) was carried out to restore flexion of the elbow. In two patients, co-contractions with the triceps have required elongation of the triceps tendon.

Recovery of the Deltoid (Fig. 39–26)

Results show that the percentage of patients reaching M3 were 22% at 1 year, 46% at 2 years, and 64% at 3 years. The distribution of zones confirms these percentages and their chronology. The amplitude of active abduction is parallel to the speed of recovery: 40% of patients will have abduction greater than 40°, 40% will have abduction between 90 and 120°, and 20% will have at least 80% active abduction.

Factors Affecting Recovery

1. Extent of the paralysis: This, as always, is the most important factor, as in the C5–C6 lesions, M3 is reached in 100% of patients by 3 years (75% at 2 years). However, recovery is less satisfactory in patients with C5–

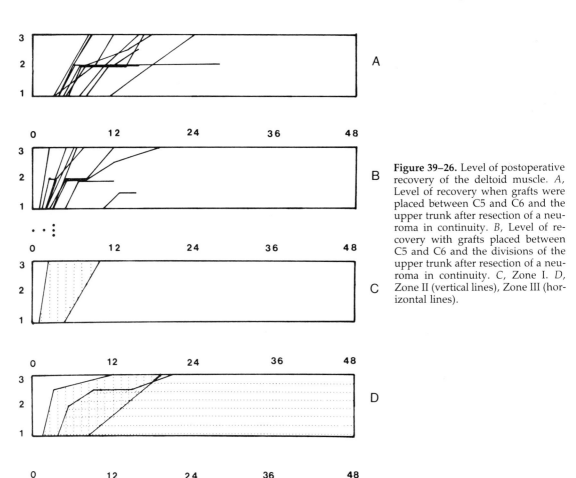

Figure 39–26. Level of postoperative recovery of the deltoid muscle. *A*, Level of recovery when grafts were placed between C5 and C6 and the upper trunk after resection of a neuroma in continuity. *B*, Level of recovery with grafts placed between C5 and C6 and the divisions of the upper trunk after resection of a neuroma in continuity. *C*, Zone I. *D*, Zone II (vertical lines), Zone III (horizontal lines).

C7 and C5–T1 lesions, as the M3 stage is reached at 2 years in only 30% of the former and 17% of the latter patients.

2. Nature of the lesion: This has a much clearer effect, as neuromas recover much better than ruptures or avulsions.

3. Type of repair: Results are much better in grafts of the trunks and their branches than in those of the cords or the axillary nerve.

Secondary Surgery. These give mitigated results: transfer of the latissimus dorsi on the rotator cuff, transfer of the trapezius on the infraspinatus, transfer of the trapezius on the trochanter, and tenotomy of the teres major.

Recovery of the Supinators
(Fig. 39–27)

Recovery is not very good, as only 12% of patients reach the M3 stage at 2 years and 25% at 3 years. The C5–C6 lesions recover better than the C5–C7 injuries. In general there is always some improvement, with a deficit in supination of about 30°. For the C5–T1 lesions the problem is the opposite, as there is a passive supination. Zancolli's operation was performed five times with immediate improvement each time and no passive supination. It was necessary to carry out radial osteotomy for pronation three times.

Recovery of the Triceps, Wrist Extensors, and Extensors of the Digits (C7)

The triceps always recovers (M3 at 2 years), whatever the type or extent of the lesion or the type of repair (Fig. 39–28). Recovery is very fast (3 to 5 months) for the C5–C7 lesions (influence of C8) and slower after repair of the cords (M3 at 1 year) or neurotization (M3 at 15 to 20 months).

Supination of the radial wrist extensors differs from that of the triceps, and at 2 years only 25% of patients have reached the M3 stage. No factor in particular seems to affect these results. These mediocre results are balanced by the fact that improvement is still possible after 2 years and that secondary surgery gives excellent results.

The recovery of the extensors of the digits varies mainly according to the level of the lesion (Fig. 39–29). For the C5–T1 lesions, the results are poor (no result at M3). The C5–C7 lesions, however, have more satisfactory results. Of 19 patients, 10 are at M3 at 1 year and 9 have average results (M2 or M3 at 2 years). Here, too, tendon transfer (when possible) provides good functional results.

Final Results

The final overall function was studied 2 years after surgery using Mallet's classifica-

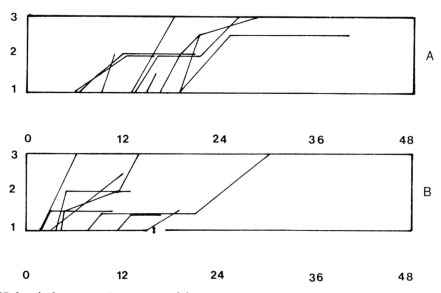

Figure 39–27. Level of postoperative recovery of the supinator. *A,* Recovery of the supinator with graft between C5 and C6 and the upper trunk after resection of a neuroma in continuity. *B,* Recovery with grafts placed between C5 and C6 and the primary divisions of the upper trunk after resection of a neuroma in continuity.

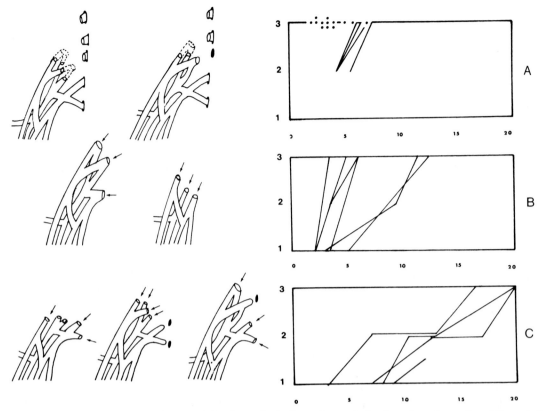

Figure 39–28. Level of recovery of triceps. Muscle grade (1–3) on the vertical axis and postoperative follow-up (in months) on the horizontal axis. The configuration of the plexus as explored or repaired is sketched adjacent to each graph. *A,* Early recovery in those instances when the C8 and T1 roots are intact. *B,* Maxium recovery in total lesions when three trunks or three cords could be grafted. *C,* Late recovery when certain elements of the plexus could not be grafted.

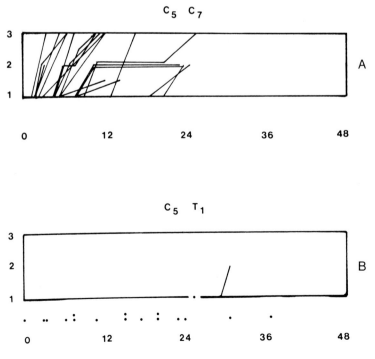

Figure 39–29. Level of recovery of the digital extensors. Muscle grade (0–3) on the vertical axis and postoperative follow-up (in months) on the horizontal axis. The large dots indicate the date of the last examination in patients who were either seen only one time postoperatively or who had little or no recovery to date. *A,* Recovery of the extensors with injuries of C5 to C7. *B,* Recovery of the extensors when the lesion involved C5 to T1.

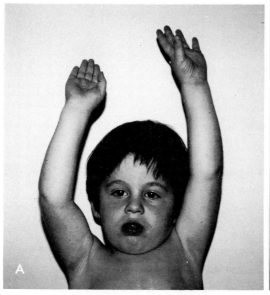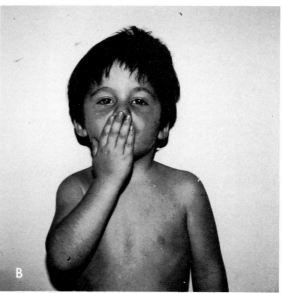

Figure 39–30. Boy with right brachial palsy operated at 3 months. Graft of C5–C6. *A,* Abduction at 18 months. *B,* Flexion of the elbow with good external rotation control.

tion. In this classification a shoulder at stage IV is more or less normal, stage III is an average result, and stage II is an unsatisfactory result.

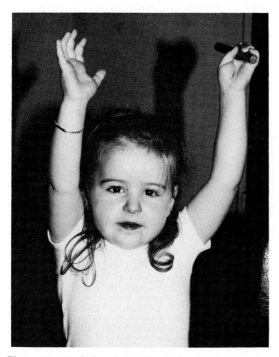

Figure 39–31. Girl with left brachial palsy operated at 3½ months. Graft of C5–C6. Abduction at 2 years.

Results of C5–C6 Grafts. Avulsions of the roots were eliminated, as the results depend little on the surgical technique.

After 2 years, we found the following results among 14 patients: six shoulders at stage IV or more (i.e., near-normal) (Figs. 39–30 and 39–31), three shoulders between stage III and stage IV, and five shoulders at stage III.

Results of C5–C7 Grafts. Only 10 cases can be evaluated at this time after 2 years: three shoulders are at stage IV (Fig. 39–32), five shoulders are at stage III, and three shoulders are at stage II. We believe that these results are not nearly as good as for the lesions discussed above. It is possible that this observation is due to the much more extensive lesions, as the violence of the trauma required to break three roots is much greater.

Results of C5–T1 Grafts. Three years are required to judge a result, and as only five patients have reached this point, the results cannot yet be evaluated. Among these five patients, three shoulders are at stage III and two are at stage II. The important point is that in three of these five patients the hand is functional and is used. This fact is fundamental if one considers the unfavorable prognosis of C8–T1 avulsions and the consistent poor spontaneous results.

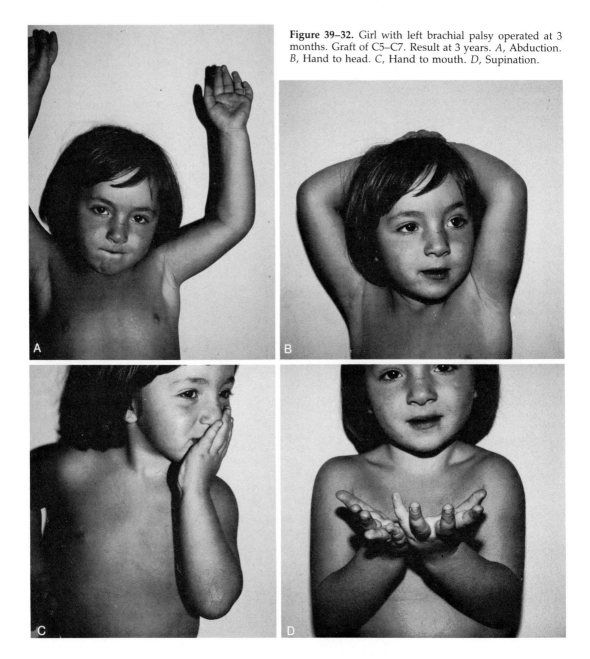

Figure 39–32. Girl with left brachial palsy operated at 3 months. Graft of C5–C7. Result at 3 years. *A*, Abduction. *B*, Hand to head. *C*, Hand to mouth. *D*, Supination.

CONCLUSIONS

To conclude this study and to summarize the first results of reconstructive surgery for obstetrical brachial plexus palsy, certain fundamental points must be clarified:

1. The obstetrical pathology of the brachial plexus is that of a traumatic lesion caused by a forced lowering of the shoulder during delivery.

2. The lesions may affect all the roots; however, the upper roots are usually ruptured, whereas the lower roots are always avulsed.

3. Spontaneous recovery is possible but its quality depends on how early it begins. If the biceps has not started to recover by 3 months, the final result will not be good. After this time interval, surgery is advisable.

4. Surgical repair is always possible, usually by grafting, although this is sometimes difficult after avulsion.

5. The results of this repair are much better than the spontaneous recovery in patients having reached the age of 3 months.

Therefore, the systematic approach at the start of our experiment has been confirmed by the quality of the results. For example, more than half the patients had a nearly normal shoulder after C5–C6 grafts, whereas none of the patients in the same population achieved this result spontaneously. It is, however, important to make the decision to perform surgery as quickly as possible before the child's body image is fixed and articular retractions occur. Patients operated on after 9 months do not have as good results as children operated on earlier.

References

1. Adler, J. B., and Patterson, R. L.: Erb's palsy. Long-term results of treatment in eighty-eight cases. J. Bone Joint Surg., 49-A:1052, 1967.
2. Bennet, G. C., and Harrold, A. J.: Prognosis and early management of birth injuries to the brachial plexus. Br. Med. J., 1:1520, 1976.
3. Bentzon, P. G. K.: De Obstetriske Lammelser af Plexus Brachialis. Disputats. Levin og Munksgaard Kbenmavn, 1922.
4. Clark, L. P., Taylor, A. S., and Prout, T. P.: A study on brachial birth palsy. Am. J. Med. Sci., 130:670, 1905.
5. Danyau: Paralysie du membre supérieur, chez le nouveau-né. Bull. Soc. Cher., 2:148, 1951.
6. Depaul: Gaz. des Hôpitaux, 1867, p. 90
7. Doherty: Nervous affections in young infants. Dublin J. Med. Sci., 25:82, 1944.
8. Duchenne, G. B. A.: De l'Electrisation Localisée et de son Application à la Pathologie et à la Thérapeutique, 3rd Ed. Paris, J. B. Baillière, 1872, pp. 357–362.
9. Duval, and Guillain: Pathologie des accidents nerveux consécutifs aux luxations et traumatismes de l'epaule. 2:143, 1896.
10. Erb, W. H.: Über eine eigenthümliche Localisation von Lähmungen im Plexus brachialis. Verhandl. Naturhist Med. (Heidelberg) 2,:130, 1874.
11. Fairbanks, H. A. T: Birth palsy: subluxation of the shoulder joint in infants and young children. Lancet, 1:1217, 1913.
12. Fieux, G.: De la pathologie des paralysies brachiales chez le nouveau-né. Paralysies obstétricales. Ann. Gynécol., 47:52, 1897.
13. Flaubert: Cité par Clark Taylor Prout.
14. Gjørup, L.: Obstetrical lesion of the brachial plexus. Acta Neurol. Scand., 42(Suppl. 18):1, 1966.
15. Gueniot: Bull. Soc. Chir., 13:34, 1867.
16. Hardy, A. E.: Birth injuries of the brachial plexus. J. Bone Joint Surg., 63-B:99, 1981.
17. Harrenstein: Experimental and Practical Experience with Paralysis of Arm. Nedernt Sydschr. V Gencesk, 1927, pp. 828–846.
18. Jacquemier, Manuel des Accouchements, 2nd Ed. 1846, p. 785.
19. Janec, M., Siman, J., and Majesky, I.: Ergebnisse der chirurgischen Revision perinataler Schadigungen des Plexus brachialis. I. Z. Kindechirurg. Grenzgbiete, 1968.
20. Kennedy, M.: Suture of the brachial plexus in birth paralysis of the upper extremity. Br. Med. J., 1:298, 1903.
21. Lange, F.: Die Entbindungslahmung des Armes. Munch. Med. Wochenschr., 1912, p. 1421.
22. Lauwers, M. E.: Le traitement chirurgical de la paralysie obstétricale. J. Chir., 36:161, 1930.
23. Mallet, J.: Paralysie obstétricale du plexus brachial. Traitement des séquelles. Rev. Chir. Orthop., 58(Suppl. I):166, 1972.
24. Milgram: Discussion of presentation by l'Episcopo: Restoration of muscle balance in the treatment of obstetrical paralysis. NY State J. Med., 39:357, 1939.
25. Ombredanne: Preécis de Cirurgie Infantile. 1925, pp. 784–788.
26. Seeligmuller: Deutsch Arch. Klin. Med, 20:101, 1877.
27. Sever, J. W.: Obstetric paralysis—its etiology, pathology, clinical aspects, and treatment, with report of four hundred and seventy cases. Am. J. Dis. Child, 12:541, 1916.
28. Sever, J. W.: Obstetric paralysis. Report of eleven hundred cases. J.A.M.A., 85:1862, 1925.
29. Sharrard, W. J. W.: Paediatric Orthopaedics and Fractures. Oxford, Blackwell Scientific Publications, 1971.
30. Smellie, W. A.: Collection of preternatural Cases and Observations in Midwifery Complicating the Design of Illustrating this First Volume on that Subject, Vol. III. London, 1768, pp. 504–505.
31. Spitz, H., and Lange, F.: Chirurgie und Orthopadie un Kindersalter. Leipzig, Vogel, 1915, p. 384.
32. Tassin, J. L.: Thèse, Paris, 1983.
33. Taylor, A. S.: Brachial birth palsy and injuries of similar type in adults. Surg. Gynecol. Obstet., 30:94, 1920.
34. Thomas, A.: Les paralysies obstétricales du membre supérieur. Gynécol Obstét., 2:76, 3:175, 1946.
35. Trombetta: Sullo Stiramento dei Nervi. 1880.
36. Wyeth, J. A., and Sharpe, W.: The field of neurological surgery in a general hospital. Surg. Gynecol. Obstet., 24:34, 1917.
37. Narakas, A.: Discussion at the Brachial Plexus Symposium. Lausanne, September, 1982.

40

Contribution of Clinical Neurophysiology and Rehabilitation Medicine to the Management of Brachial Plexus Palsy

■

W. Theodore Liberson, M.D., Ph.D.
Julia K. Terzis, M.D., Ph.D.

In Chapters 25 and 38 we showed that microsurgery proved to be useful in a number of patients with brachial plexus palsies (BPPs) in whom no other effective treatment has been offered for the past 200 years (since the recognition of the nature of this devastating trauma). There are reasons to believe that microsurgery will be useful in treating other catastrophic nervous system diseases as well.[17] In this chapter, we discuss the contribution of clinical neurophysiology and rehabilitation medicine to the total management of patients with BPPs.

CLINICAL NEUROPHYSIOLOGY

In Chapters 25 and 38, we discussed the contributions of electromyography (EMG) to the diagnosis and follow-up of patients with BPP treated by microsurgery. We provided evidence that EMG is helpful in predicting the localization and extent of the lesion found at surgery. However, this test has two limitations:

1. EMG can predict avulsion of a root only in the absence of other postganglionic lesions corresponding to the same root. This is done by finding a good sensory evoked potential on a finger, following the stimulation of the median, ulnar, or radial nerves at the wrist, in the absence of subjective sensory perception or corresponding voluntary movements. Such a finding invariably signifies integrity of the postganglionic sensory pathways and avulsion of the dorsal root proximal to the spinal ganglion. Unfortunately, this is found rarely because of masking of the preganglionic lesions by the postganglionic ones, with the resulting suppression of the sensory potential.

2. Needle EMG (collecting information in restricted areas of the muscle) may show a complete interference pattern, testifying to good local electrogenesis during the postsurgery restorative process. Yet the mechanical function of the muscle still may be gravely compromised. It is true that by using skin electrodes with an integrated EMG the total electrogenesis of the muscle may be expressed with the aid of modern computers. This would, however, significantly prolong the EMG test, whereas a simple manual muscle test requires only a few minutes, and no special instrumentation is necessary.

One wonders whether this dissociation between electrical and mechanical activity has a pathophysiologic significance that should be investigated further. Indeed, the axons are not only conducting electrical impulses from the cells of the anterior horn but are also transporting crucial biochemicals by axoplasmic flow. These chemicals were found to be essential for such aspects of muscle contractility as its tonic or phasic characteristics (see review of a related problem in Vrbova et al.[25]). No wonder that after an interruption of this flow for years the mechanical properties of the muscle may be changed. In addition, the *number* of active axons is dramatically reduced in muscles innervated by axons grafted to an unusual source. A great number of the proximal axons are diverted into the sensory channels and ungloriously die. In addition, there may be a reduced number of donor axons to begin with, some of which cannot be voluntarily activated by the untrained patient. In this case, there is a biochemical mismatch between the donor cells and the muscle fibers. Finally, the gliding of the tendon may be compromised after years of inactivity. Unfortunately, these explanations do not help the patient, who requires a mechanical (not electrical) performance from his muscle.

Additional electrodiagnostic tests have also been used.

Evoked Potentials

The possibility of recording cortical somatosensory evoked potentials from the scalp was discovered by Dawson in 1947,[3] and the first recording of the potentials originating from the brain stem, roots and spinal cord was done by Liberson and his associates in 1963 and 1967.[18, 20] In 1979 Jones[7, 8] introduced the use of these potentials in patients with BPPs.

Recording of the evoked potentials contributes to the exploration of more proximal portions of the brachial plexus, including spinal nerves and roots. This is helping to determine whether or not the latter conduct messages to the brain. The damage to the roots is important to predict, inasmuch as a well-preserved root is a good source for nerve grafts.

Jones' technique involves the stimulation of the peripheral nerves (median or ulnar) at the wrist, although the stimulation of the fingers themselves would seem to be more appropriate for dermatomal identification. In the case of the median nerve, four different dermatomes are involved. The situation is better for the ulnar nerve, in that information is derived from two dermatomes only.

Technique Involving Referred Subjective Perception

After trying different techniques, we found a better solution than recording evoked potentials prior to surgery, at least for adults. We introduce stimulating needle electrodes down to the vertebral laminae, according to the technique of MacLean for peripheral EMG recordings (Fig. 40–1). Then we simply

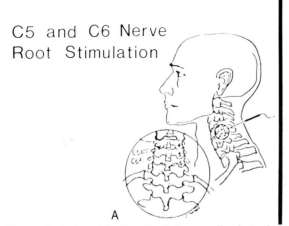

C5 and C6 Nerve Root Stimulation

A

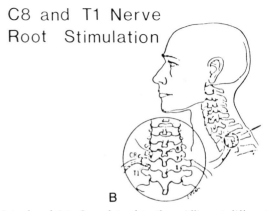

C8 and T1 Nerve Root Stimulation

B

Figure 40–1. *A* and *B*, The stimulating needle electrode is introduced 1 to 2 cm lateral to the midline at different levels of the cervical spine until it hits the lamina. As the current is progressively increased (brief stimuli, 0.5 m sec duration), the patient refers his/her perception to one particular finger or fails to do it. Once the finger is named, the needle is moved to another segment. (Drawing after MacLean, I. C., and Taylor, R. S.[21])

ask the patient to identify the fingers with referred sensory perception. We repeat this procedure at progressively higher cervical levels. If, for example, the patient identifies the little finger, the integrity of C8 or T1, or both is ascertained. If the patient identifies the index and/or long fingers, the integrity of roots C7 and/or C6 is proved. If a thumb is identified, the integrity of C5 or C6 is evident. If the patient identifies the top of the shoulder, C5 may be considered to be intact, particularly if the area of the axillary nerve is identified. If no referred sensation in the fingers is identified, all roots are severely involved. If sensation is perceived in only one finger, there is severe damage to most of the roots.

We have started to use this technique only recently and so far can confirm its usefulness in only four patients.

Its limitations are (1) the difficulty of ascertaining the veracity of the patient's reports, (2) the presence of pluridermatomal innervation, and (3) the aversion to simple solutions of clinical scientists immersed in computer research. Indeed, the advantage of this technique is its simplicity.

"Electrical Tinel Sign"

One of us (WTL) wrote in 1966: "For the classical electrodiagnosis (EMG) the growing nerve which has not yet reached its destination is desperately silent. It would be of considerable practical interest to be able to detect the activity of a growing nerve *before* it reaches the muscle."[11] Since most of the sensory axons travel together with the motor axons in a mixed nerve, their regeneration also suggests that of the motor axons.

Reconstructive surgeons (such as JKT) use the Tinel sign to detect a growing nerve endpoint by local percussion proceeding in a disto-proximal fashion. Normal nerve fibers have a very high mechanical threshold. However, the terminal sprouts of the growing nerve have a relatively low threshold for mechanical stimulation, and thus the Tinel sign is useful.

This test has three limitations:

1. Foremost, the Tinel sign is a very difficult clinical sign to elicit properly and its interpretation requires a deep understanding of nerve regeneration mechanisms.

2. In inexperienced hands, the test does not permit precise localization, as the waves of mechanical vibration may reach the nerve endings well above the level of percussions.

3. It identifies abnormal nerve fibers only, which may or may not reach their final destination.

An "electrical Tinel sign," as developed by one of us (WTL), is a local excitation of the growing nerve by a stimulating needle electrode introduced into its vicinity. The needle insertion is made progressively more and more distally along the trajectory of the nerve until the stimulus ceases to elicit the referred distal perception. The referred distal effect indicates the location of normal nerve fibers, as the abnormal terminal sprouts prove to be insensitive to single brief electrical stimuli. This is why the Tinel sign elicited from the growing nerve is always distal to that revealed by the "electrical Tinel sign."

Galvanic Skin Response

Liberson introduced "galvanic skin responses" into electrodiagnosis in 1949 and again in 1979 (Fig. 40–2).[10, 14] The interest of this test for the diagnostic work-up of pa-

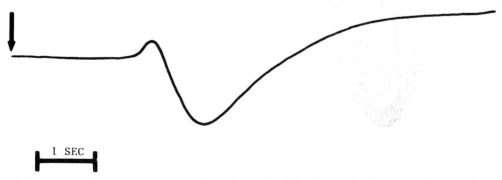

1 SEC

Figure 40–2. A normal skin galvanic response (the palmar skin) following a stimulus (*arrow*). The stimulus may be applied anywhere, or may be an auditory click. Recording by an EEG machine. Note the latency of almost 1 second. (After Liberson, W. T.[10])

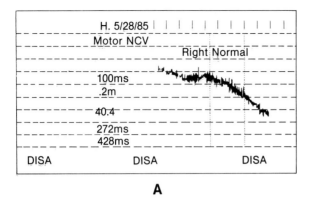
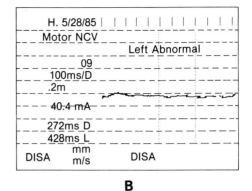

A   **B**

Figure 40–3. A skin galvanic response recorded from the right normal hand (upper trace) in a patient (H) with a left brachial plexus lesion with avulsion of the C8 and T1 roots (lower trace). Note change of potential occurring about ½ second after chest stimulation. Note that the baseline shows small amplitude muscle potentials corresponding to the muscle tone (*A*). On the left side there is no galvanic skin response and no muscle tonic potentials (*B*).

tients with BPP is obvious: when the sympathetic nerve fibers degenerate, the galvanic skin response is abolished.

Sympathetic nerve fibers travel with root T1 to reach the cervical sympathetic ganglia. Some of these fibers may also travel in root C8. When these roots are damaged, there is no galvanic skin response.

The technique of galvanic skin response recording is quite simple (Fig. 40–3). We place large electrodes over the palmar and dorsal aspects of the hand, respectively. Then we apply a strong electrical stimulus to the normal thoracic or abdominal skin. We then compare the response (reflex) to brief stimuli on the normal and abnormal sides. The galvanic skin response appears after a latency of about ½ second following the stimulation of thoracic or abdominal skin. It

is essential to use amplifiers with a very long time constant (over 1 second) in order to record this reflex (Fig. 40–3).

Thermography

The use of this test for diagnosis of radiculopathies has been proposed by many authors. It would therefore seem that thermography should be applied for diagnosing the location of lesions in patients with BPPs. We have used this test so far only on the hand, and in many cases the findings are significant in peripheral nerve palsies. However, the analysis of our data has not as yet been completed (Fig. 40–4).

The temperature of the skin is a function of several factors. In a patient with a transection of either the ulnar or the median nerve, the local coolness of the skin is characteristic, although not fully understood.

Sympathetic nerve fibers are traveling within the peripheral nerves. Section of the sympathetic nerve fibers should lead to vasodilation and therefore to the warming of the skin. The suppression of perspiration should also result in warming of the skin. In fact, however, the skin becomes cooler after nerve transection. This could be explained by the suppression of the vasodilating effects (Fig. 40–4).

Standard thermography therefore expresses a balance between the effects of nerve lesions in different directions either compensating each other or adding to each other. *Functional thermography*,[15] as introduced by Liberson,[15] is a recording of the cooling effects on the skin, expressing reflex stimulation of sympathetic nerve fibers. This effect is suppressed in

Figure 40–4. Patient with bilateral ulnar palsy secondary to bilateral cubital tunnel syndrome. Note dark regions over the fourth and fifth fingers on the right and to a lesser degree on the left hand, indicating lower skin temperature.

areas where sympathetic nerve fibers are cut, and therefore no effect is observed in a lesion of root T1 (Fig. 40–5).

Classic Electrodiagnosis

Classic electrodiagnosis has been replaced by EMG because the former was not helpful in disorders in which the latter is very proficient (e.g., in discogenic radiculopathies, primary muscle diseases, or myasthenic syndromes). Classic electrodiagnosis is, however, very helpful in traumatic neuropathies and may have some advantages compared with electromyography (e.g., it may be useful at a much earlier date).

Briefly, the main principles of classic electrodiagnosis may be summarized as follows. *Innervated muscles* are almost equally well excitable by long stimuli (above 100 msec) as by brief stimuli (below 100 μsec). They are most excitable at the motor point projecting on the skin the intramuscular fibers of the motor nerve. They are not excitable by progressively increasing current below 2.5 rheobases. The induced single muscle twitch is fast.

Denervated muscles are more easily excitable by long stimuli and may be inexcitable by brief stimuli. They are equally excitable by progressively increasing currents as by the square waves. Denervated muscles are much more excitable by longitudinal stimulation, when the electrodes are placed above and below the muscles, than by stimulation in the region of the motor point (which ceases to exist with denervation). The induced muscle contraction (single twitch) is slow, particularly the decontraction.

Classic electrodiagnosis can therefore easily identify denervated muscles by the absence of motor points, the slow electrically induced contractions, and the inexcitability by brief stimuli. These factors are important for electrotherapy (to be discussed).

Intraoperative Electrodiagnosis

One of us (JKT) has contributed to the study of intraoperative fascicular electrodiagnosis (see Chapter 38). The nerve structures during surgery are systematically stimulated and the presence or absence of peripheral responses is then noted. Recent analysis of the data, however, shows that stimulation of the proximal structures, which are embedded in fibrous tissue, may be less reliable than stimulation of the distal structures of the brachial plexus (see Chapter 38). In the latter cases, stimulation effects are positively correlated with the preoperative EMG (see Chapters 25 and 38).

Obviously, intraoperative stimulation and recording of muscle responses of the key muscles by using a multichannel electroencephalograph as well as the simultaneous recording of cerebral evoked potentials may facilitate the diagnosis at surgery. We are now developing this technique and will report the results at a later date. We are also developing an intraoperative brief pulse stimulator. The stimulator that is now routinely used during surgery is a DC stimulator. With such a stimulator, the intensity of the applied current has to be limited because of possible nerve damage.

Microelectrodiagnosis

Potentially, percutaneous microelectrical recordings from the sensory and sympathetic nerve fibers in the hand may provide important diagnostic information in the future.

Other Tests

Of course, the classic techniques of goniometry, manual muscle testing, recording of perspiration, and two-point sensory discrimination testing may be very useful. As we noted in Chapter 38, the manual muscle test permits follow-up of the patient's progress and also reveals some extremely important data related to the repair of the brachial plexus.

Serial video taping of active range of motion is another important technique, as is myelography.

REHABILITATION

As noted in Chapters 25 and 38, the analysis of the manual muscle test, repeated after increasing time has elapsed following surgery, reveals an important aspect of recovery. No matter how significant and helpful the use of nerve grafts may be, in most cases they do not permit the muscle to regain its normal strength even 4 years after surgery.

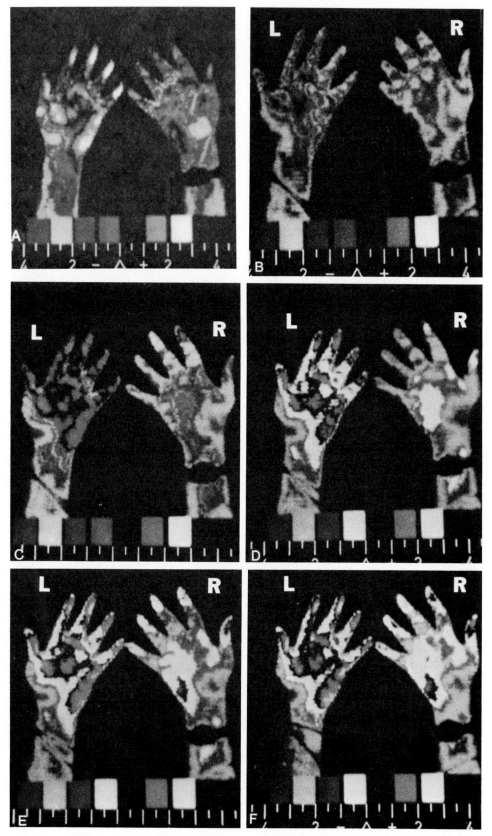

Figure 40–5 *See legend on opposite page*

This is mostly because all the channels of the distal peripheral nerve cannot successfully accept the regenerating motor axons and therefore complete functional recovery cannot occur. This is generally not true for grafting peripheral nerve gaps.

Our responsibility is therefore to promote maximal use of rehabilitative techniques to make the involved extremity functional. The routine techniques of physical therapy, such as range of motion exercises, massage, and application of cold and heat will not be discussed in this chapter, although they are of vital importance for the functional survival of the extremity. Nor will the static splinting and static bracing covered in a recent article by Wynn Parry[27] be discussed (see Chapter 36 of this volume). We have, however, been investigating another type of ratchet elbow brace, but this is still in a trial stage.

The remaining part of this chapter will be devoted to electrotherapy and motorized braces, as well as to the importance of psychological (cosmetic) factors.

Electrotherapy

Electrotherapy is applied in a completely different fashion, according to whether denervated or reinnervated muscles are involved.[16]

Denervated Muscles

As stated in the section devoted to classic electrodiagnosis, denervated muscle fibers must be stimulated by slow pulses of current (above 100 msec) with progressive onset[13] if these are mixed with innervated muscle fibers and with electrodes applied below and above the muscle (longitudinal stimulation) (Figs. 40–6 and 40–7). This latter circumstance permits simultaneous stimulation of practically all the muscles of the upper extremity by placing one electrode on the shoulder and the other on the palmar aspect of the fingers and/or on the dorsal skin of the base of the thoracic cage.

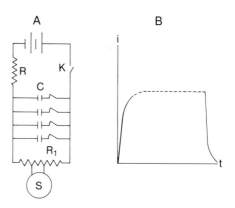

Figure 40–6. *A*, Schematic diagram of progressive current stimulator with "exponential" onset and ending. *B*, Shape of the stimulus.

Although the wisdom of stimulation of denervated muscles has often been challenged, let us state unequivocally that we now have undeniable proof that this does not apply to human denervated muscles. Indeed we have observed one patient who was stimulated daily for 5 hours every 10 seconds, with subsequent reinnervation of the transplanted gracilis muscle. Inasmuch as this was a muscle transplanted from the lower to the upper extremity, its total denervation was unquestionable. On the other hand, the common experience in brachial plexus palsy is that nonstimulated intrinsic muscles of the hand have not been reinnervated following repair at the level of the plexus precisely because their atrophy in the absence of systematic stimulation leaves no muscle tissue to be reinnervated.

One of us (WTL) was impressed some 20 years ago by an experiment on a rabbit carried out by Dr. Smith of the Detroit Rehabilitation Institute. Both the rabbit's sciatic nerves were sectioned. The gastrocnemius on one side was left unstimulated, while that on the other side was stimulated every minute around the clock. After 1 year the stimulated muscle retained more than 90% of its bulk, whereas that on the unstimulated side was atrophied. This effect was already noted by Debedat in 1894, when he found an increased volume in rabbit muscles following

---

Figure 40–5. Reflex effect of nerve stimulation (R, median nerve) on skin's temperature. *A*, Resting condition. Note cooler left hand, which is frequently observed in right-handed individuals (white areas are cooler). *B*, During 9-minute stimulation. Note cooling of the right hand. *C*, Cooling persists during the stimulation. *D*, Stimulation stopped. Right hand cooling persists. There is some cooling of the left hand also. *E*, Cooling persists. *F*, At 12 minutes after end of stimulation left hand begins to warm up while cooling of the right hand persists. Note that despite the reflex value of this effect, ipsilateral action predominates. (After Liberson, W. T.[16])

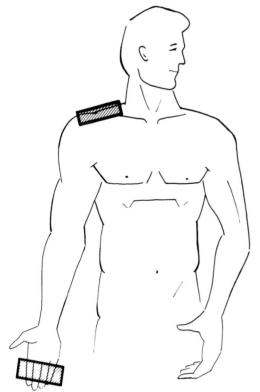

Figure 40–7. Positioning of electrodes for slow pulse stimulation.

electrical stimulation of denervated muscle. In 1939, Fisher found that when electrical stimulation of the denervated muscle was applied as soon as possible, there was a marked arrest of atrophy. Jackson measured the limb volume in 161 subjects, 54 of whom had complete ulnar nerve palsy. He gave direct current stimulation 6 days a week and found good results.

The question "to stimulate or not to stimulate" in brachial plexus palsy is superfluous. If one does not stimulate the distal muscles, nothing will be left after 2 years of denervation.

In many hospitals through the United States, the patient's muscles are stimulated by galvanic current, closed and opened by a manual switch operated by the patient himself. The patient is usually told to place the stimulating electrode (generally very small) on the region of the motor point of each muscle (as if it existed) for several minutes for each muscle. Then the electrode has to be moved to another denervated muscle (of which there may be a dozen in extensive brachial plexus palsy).

Under the best circumstances, the patient uses this technique for 30 minutes daily,

without ever realizing to what degree the muscles are stimulated. Thus he stimulates each particular muscle for only a few minutes per day. Sometimes, the patient's muscles are stimulated in the same fashion by the therapist, also for 30 minutes per day but only three times a week.

These practices of stimulation are unacceptable for the following reasons. The stimulating current flows as long as the subject keeps the switch closed. This means that the current is applied for an additional period beyond the time of its stimulating effectiveness, which is on the order of a tenth of a second—a duration that cannot be limited by hand. During this extra time, the current acts unnecessarily on the skin, which then becomes irritated. In addition, such a needlessly long duration of stimulation may be painful. For this reason, the patient decreases the amplitude of the current, which then becomes ineffective. If the denervated muscle fibers are mixed with the reinnervated ones, the latter may also become unnecessarily stimulated.

Therefore, the current techniques of stimulating the denervated muscle fibers are grossly inadequate. No wonder that electrotherapy fell into disrepute. Faced with this observation, one of us (WTL) has developed a "slow pulse stimulator" that permits the rational technique of treating denervated muscle.

First, the slow pulses are calibrated as to their duration so that the latter may be chosen for each individual patient according to his needs. The pulses are delivered automatically at a rate that may be harmless. We are now satisfied with the fact that stimuli succeeding each other at a rate of one during each 10 seconds do not harm the skin if applied for a period of 20 to 30 seconds. The stimulator has a timer that limits each session to 20 minutes or so. The alternative technique is to stimulate every minute or so all day long. In addition, a "contracurrent" is built into this stimulator, reducing the polarization of the skin to a minimum. Indeed, the charge brought by this "contracurrent" is distributed over 10 seconds at least and therefore its amplitude is only 1/100th of that of the stimulating current. In this fashion the polarization induced by the stimuli is counterbalanced by the current delivered between pulses.

Finally, inasmuch as the denervated fibers are sometimes mixed with the normal ones or a denervated muscle is sometimes found next to an innervated one, the diffusion of the current may cause the contraction of the innervated muscles. Thus, the contractions of the involved muscles may be masked by those of the normal muscles. This undesirable effect may be minimized or eliminated by the use of progressive onset of the stimulating pulses. A time of onset on the order of 100 to 200 msec may indeed suppress the contraction of the innervated muscles. We limit now the total time of stimulation to 5 hours for adults and 3 hours for children. The treatment sessions are 20 minutes each, with an interval of 1 hour in between. The patient is warned never to restimulate an area that remains red following the previous session of stimulation.

It is premature to assess the effects of these electrotherapy techniques for the rehabilitation of the patient quantitatively, as these were introduced only a few months ago and the repair of BPP needs years for follow-up. We have, however, every reason to believe that this new technique will contribute to the functional result in patients with BPPs.

Reinnervated Muscles

About 25 years ago, Offner and Liberson[23] developed a brief pulse stimulator to excite normal nerves and muscles. The duration of these pulses was somewhat below 100 μsec and their frequency of occurrence was 30 to 40 cycles/sec. The device was used for functional electrical stimulation,[19] which was first applied to the peroneal electrophysiologic brace and later to the muscles of upper extremities for their activation and for inhibition of pain and spasms. The stimulator was developed 5 years prior to the publication of Melzak and Wall[22] describing their gate theory of pain and the publication of Liberson's English edition of Beritoff's book[1] reporting his stimulating therapy for patients with causalgia. Only later did Wall and Sweet[26] publish their technique of transcutaneous electrical nerve stimulation (TENS), which of course was used for a century prior to their publication. A few years later Liberson modified the Offner/Liberson stimulator by introducing pauses between the trains of stimulating pulses (2½ seconds on and 2½ seconds off).

The brief pulse stimulator has been used for three purposes in patients with BPPs:

1. To increase the strength of the innervated muscle.

2. To bombard the centers with musculocutaneous feedback stimuli and therefore contribute to restoration of both the muscle and sensory perceptions.

3. To reduce pain.

Liberson introduced a brief pulse stimulator for brain stimulation in 1945[9] and for neuromuscular stimulation in 1961.[19] The TENS stimulator introduced later retained the pulse duration and pulse frequency of the Offner/Liberson stimulator.

In the Staodyne muscle stimulator, built on Liberson's request, pauses of variable duration were introduced. This was also done later in another commercial stimulator ("Respond"). The amplitude of the stimulating current is higher in Liberson's stimulator than in commercial TENS stimulators.

Many investigators have used brief pulse stimulators of the same type for increasing strength and decreasing fatigability of the innervated muscles.

For all these reasons we introduced brief stimulus therapy for patients with BPPs for treatment of those muscles that either remain innervated or are reinnervated and therefore are now responding to brief stimuli. The advantages of an electrically induced contraction over voluntary activity is the avoidance of psychological fatigue due to monotony and boredom caused by repeated voluntary muscle contractions and the elimination of distractions by the environmental stimuli. However, whenever possible, patients are advised to "help the current" by adding a voluntary effort to the electrically induced contractions. It seems as if the electrical "pacemaker" helps in reducing psychological fatigue.

We first applied brief stimulus therapy to babies with obstetrical brachial plexus palsies (OBPPs) prior to eventual surgery. We did not want to experiment with these unfortunate babies by having a control group deprived of stimulation. Invariably, the parents reported that after only a few weeks of stimulation the extremity became at least partially functional. Although the increase in strength is a common experience after the introduction of brief stimulus therapy, a positive effect of a barrage of afferent muscle stimuli bombarding the spinal cord and the brain may be the explanation for this welcome phenomenon.

Obviously, not all muscles respond to this therapy. However, we personally observed a return of sensation following brief stimulus therapy in a few patients with trigeminal lesions with focal anesthesia.

At least two babies have recovered upper extremity function following this therapy despite the fact that, initially, surgery seemed inevitable. It is true that both of these babies also underwent the "behavioral therapy" to be described next. Liberson's peroneal electrophysiologic brace was manufactured in Europe, using a ministimulator that was particularly small and effective. Therefore, Liberson modified this stimulator in such a way that it may automatically induce contractions alternating with periods of "pause." The ministimulator is now being used for many of our patients with facial palsy, "traumatic" neuropathy, and BPPs, as well as for pain.

We have no data with which to prescribe a specific duration of daily brief stimulus therapy. It is essential that this be done at home every day and that the patient actively participate in these exercises. "One thousand exercises a day" is our present formula for both children and adults.

Behavioral Therapy

The behavioral therapy just mentioned stems from the early observations of some babies with "Erb's palsy" whose deltoid muscles, although inactive voluntarily, showed normal electrical patterns. These findings were easily "explained" by the following hypothesis. Since these children obviously had early disruption of peripheral nerve conduction during the period of development of motor behavior at an early age, these muscles were "forgotten" by the brain. After repair, the brain continued to ignore these muscles. We therefore advise the parents not only to immobilize the normal extremity for a number of hours during the day (and therefore induce the use of the affected limb), but also to insert a "pacifier" or a lollipop into the involved hand, so that the child can be increasingly stimulated to use the partially involved or reconstructed muscles of the extremity (Fig. 40–8).

Myoelectrical Control

Unexpectedly, we found that EMG recovery may be more complete than the mechanical performance of the muscles after microsurgical repair. If all the previously men-

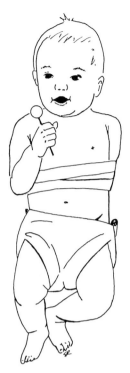

Figure 40–8. Use of behavioral therapy.

tioned electrotherapeutic effects fail in some patients, there is now a promise that microsurgically induced improvement in electrogenesis will contribute to the functional performance of the involved extremity. Indeed, the development of the electrical upper extremity prosthesis ("Russian hand") is now nearly perfected. Electrogenesis, properly amplified, may thus successfully control the action of an electric motor that can induce lacking movements of the corresponding segments of the extremities. About 20 years ago Liberson used a small DC electric motor to flex and extend paralyzed fingers (Fig. 40–9). The electric motor is activated by a switch closed either by a shoulder movement or by the myoelectrical signal. The same muscle may be used for both: the first contraction elicits flexor motion and the second elicits extension. In an otherwise normal individual, this is easily done by forcibly contracting first one and then the other pectoralis or abdominal muscles or by contracting the platysma. One may design a system so that only forced contractions of these muscles are effective. In this way, the normal contractions occurring during daily activities are unable to activate these motors.

The advent of microsurgery favorably changed the situation. Now one may activate the electromechanical system so that the elec-

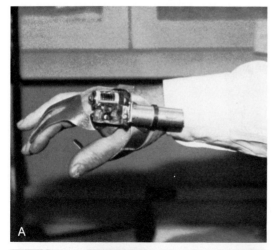

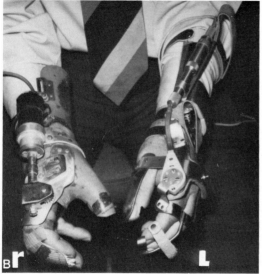

Figure 40–9. *A,* Original motorized brace. *B,* Original brace on the right hand. Modern myoelectrical brace on the left hand.

This seems to be the "wave of the future." Yet one must be aware that, just as in the case of the myoelectrical prosthesis, patients will resist wearing these braces. There appears to be a psychological aversion in young men and women to a dependence on "gadgets." However, this is not a reason to stop development of these devices. Someday, perhaps in the privacy of their homes or in their work place, these patients will use the brace. One must, however, respect the psychological needs of these patients and discuss them with sympathy.

Electrotherapy for Pain

One of us (WTL) published recently a chapter[16] summarizing his technique for control of pain and painful spasms by brief stimuli. The same technique was used in our patients with pain due to avulsed roots, in which one electrode was applied to one axilla and the other electrode to the other axilla (Fig. 40–10).

An effort should be directed toward implanting electrodes for intractable chronic pain, as the technology for this is already available (as is well known).

PREVENTION

Since "one ounce of prevention is better than one pound of therapy," it is the responsibility of physicians treating patients with BPPs to promote the design of preventive braces in certain specific individuals prior to injury, e.g., motorcyclists, in whom BPPs are frequently observed (see Chapter 25).

Indeed, abduction and elevation of the arm with consequent traction appear to be the universal mechanisms for these lesions. A brace that would limit these movements beyond 100° (possibly integrated in a jacket) may offer effective protection and yet permit the person to bring his hands to protect his face if needed or to make useful hand signals during the motorcycle ride. Such a brace should be attached to the thorax and the arms. Because the latter attachment should be very solid, the possibility of fractures of the humerus may be the price to pay for the avoidance of BPPs. However, such fractures are infinitely preferable to BPPs.

trogenesis of the microsurgically restored muscles may be sufficient to control it. In other words, when electrogenesis is restored by microsurgery but mechanical action is lacking, this electrogenesis may be sufficient to power the needed movements of the extremity. To cite another example, the supraspinatus is easily restored microsurgically; the deltoid less often. By capting the electrogenesis of the supraspinatus, one may power the abduction of the arm despite the deficiency of the deltoid. Of course the muscle contraction is always preferable to the electromechanical solution. The latter will be used only if "secondary surgery" is not able to compensate for the motor deficit.

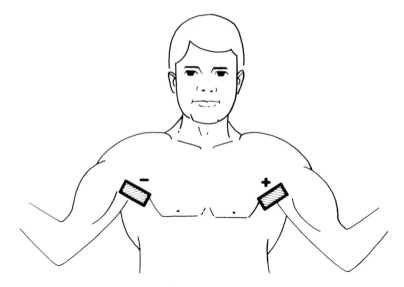

Figure 40–10. Bilateral stimulation for pain.

SUMMARY

Electrodiagnostic tests are described, including EMG, skin galvanic reactions, functional thermography, "electrical Tinel sign," and direct root stimulation, which refers subjective perceptions to the intact dermatomes and reveals the damaging nonconducting roots. Emphasis was placed on the principles of classic electrodiagnosis, as these constitute the basis for rational electrotherapy. Indeed, the modern development of electrotherapy (by revising classic notions), as well as the development of behavioral therapy, contributes significantly to the management of patients with BPPs, including pain. The development of myoelectrical control of prostheses and braces provides new hope for better performance with a partially restored extremity. It is also hoped that the patients' reluctance to use these "gadgets" will abate when they are miniaturized to such an extent that the self-image of the patient will not be violated.

New research is needed to speed up the mechanical recovery of muscles following microsurgical grafting, after years of being deprived of the usual axoplasmic flow in the axons that innervate them. Perhaps new therapeutic procedures will be developed to compensate for this deprivation.

Finally, attention is called to the necessity for developing preventive braces for motorcyclists, who are frequent victims of BPPs. General principles of such preventive bracing are described.

References

1. Beritoff, J. S.: Neural Mechanisms of Higher Vertebrate Behavior. Boston, Little, Brown and Co., 1965 (edited and translated by W. T. Liberson).
2. Buller, A. J., Eccles, J. C., and Eccles, R.: Interaction between motor neurons and motoneurons in respect to the characteristic speeds of their responses. J. Physiol., *150*:417, 1960.
3. Dawson, G. D.: Cerebral responses to electrical stimulation of peripheral nerves in man. J. Neurol. Neurosurg. Psychiatry, *10*:134, 1947.
4. Debedat, X.: Influence des different formes d'électricité en électrothérapie. Bordeaux, 1894.
5. Fisher (1939): Quoted by Licht, S.: *In* History of Electrotherapy, Therapeutic Electricity, Physical Medicine Library, Vol. 4. Baltimore, Waverly Press, 1959.
6. Jackson (1939): Quoted by Licht, S.: *In* History of Electrotherapy, Therapeutic Electricity, Physical Medicine Library, Vol. 4. Baltimore, Waverly Press, 1959.
7. Jones, S. J.: Investigation of brachial plexus traction lesions. Peripheral and spinal somatosensory evoked potentials. J. Neurol. Neurosurg. Psychiatry, *42*:107, 1979.
8. Jones, S. J.: Diagnostic value of peripheral and spinal somatosensory evoked potentials in traction lesions of the brachial plexus. Clin. Plast. Surg., *11*:167, 1984.
9. Liberson, W. T.: Time factors in electric convulsive therapy. Yale J. Biol. Med., *17*:571, 1945.
10. Liberson, W. T.: Research on the skin galvanic response in mental patients. EEG Clin. Neurophysiol., *1*:251, 1949.
11. Liberson, W. T.: Application of computer techniques to EMG and related problems. Proceedings of the 1st Caribbean Congress of Physical Medicine and Rehabilitation. San Juan, 1966, pp. 25–29.
12. Liberson, W. T.: Electrophysiological and electromechanical devices for handicapped individuals. Presented at the International EMG Meeting, Glasgow, 1967.
13. Liberson, W. T.: Progressive and Alternating Cur-

rents. *In* Licht, S. (ed.): Electrodiagnosis and Electromyography, 3rd Ed. Baltimore, Waverly Press, 1971, pp. 272–285.

14. Liberson, W. T.: Conduction velocity index in sympathetic nerve fibers. Presented at the International EMG Meeting, Stockholm, 1979.

15. Liberson, W. T.: Effects of peripheral nerve stimulation on the thermogram of the hand. Presented at the 10th International Congress of EEG and Clinical Neurophysiology, Kyoto, 1981.

16. Liberson, W. T.: Electrotherapy. *In* Ruskin, A. F. (ed.): Current Therapy in Physiatry. Philadelphia, W. B. Saunders Co., 1984, pp. 161–191.

17. Liberson, W. T.: Clinical neurophysiology and rehabilitative microsurgery (editorial). EMG Clin. Neurophysiol., 25:83, 1985.

18. Liberson, W. T., Gratzer, M., Zalis, A., and Grabinski: Comparison of conduction velocity of motor and sensory fibers determined by different methods. Arch. Phys. Med. Rehab., 47:17, 1966.

19. Liberson, W. T., Holmquist, A., Scott, B., and Dow, C.: Functional electrotherapy: Stimulation of the peripheral nerve synchronized with the swing phase of the gait in hemiplegic patients. Arch. Phys. Med. Rehab., 42:101, 1961.

20. Liberson, W. T., and Kim, K. E.: Mapping evoked potentials elicited by stimulation of median and peroneal nerves. EEG Clin. Neurophysiol., 15:721, 1963.

21. MacLean, I. C., and Taylor, R. S.: Nerve root stimulation to evaluate brachial plexus conduction. Abstracts of Communication of the 5th International Congress of Electromyography, Rochester, Minnesota, 1975, p. 47.

22. Melzack, H., and Wall, P. D.: Pain mechanisms: A new theory. Science, 150:971, 1965.

23. Offner, F. F., and Liberson, W. T.: Method of Muscular Stimulation in Human Beings to Aid in Walking. U.S. Patent 3.344.792, October 3, 1967.

24. Publicover, N., and Terzis, J. K.: Experimental electrophysiologic records. Interpretation of the compound action potential. Clin. Plast. Surg., 11:39, 1984.

25. Vrbova, G., Gordon, T., and Jones, R.: Nerve Muscle Interaction. London, Chapman and Hall, 1978.

26. Wall, P. D., and Sweet, W. H.: Temporary abolition of pain in man. Science, 155:108, 1967.

27. Wynn Parry, C. B.: Rehabilitation of patients following traction lesions of the brachial plexus. Clin. Plast. Surg., 11:173, 1984.

COMBATING FACIAL
PARALYSIS

PART
5

41

Surgical Anatomy of the Facial Musculature and Muscle Transplantation

■

Sean G. L. Hamilton, M.B., B.S., F.R.A.C.S.
Julia K. Terzis, M.D., Ph.D.
James T. Carraway, M.D.

Synchronous facial animation and appropriate emotional expression are essential in our ability to function effectively in today's society. Facial palsy seriously handicaps the individual, both socially and psychologically. Surgical efforts to restore function to the paralyzed face have been many, but a totally appropriate functional reconstructive result still eludes our skills. The introduction of microsurgical techniques has provided a further approach to achieve an improved result in facial reanimation. Free neurovascular muscular transplantation provides an opportunity for replacement of the atrophic and denervated facial musculature. The necessary scientific data concerning the basic morphofunctional characteristics of the facial musculature have not been fully investigated with respect to the component neuromuscular units. Likewise, the characteristics of the available donor muscles have not been accurately defined. Therefore, a recommendation for the more suitable muscle for transplantation based on scientific facts cannot be provided. To make an appropriate recommendation about a free neurovascular muscle transfer, the effect of denervation and revascularization at a distant site and the method of attachment to the facial musculature need to be considered.

This chapter will discuss the gross, functional, and surface anatomic characteristics of the face. It will then contrast the normal facial muscles with the characteristics of facial palsy. The evolution of muscle transplantation techniques will be related to the results achieved and correlated with laboratory studies. This evolution will be explored further and the results of laboratory studies detailed. This, in turn, will provide additional information with which to make a considered judgment of free muscle transfers, particularly as related to the face.

NORMAL ANATOMY

Gross Anatomy

The facial muscles extend from the occipitalis to the platysma. They can be divided into four regions, of which the central two are responsible for the characteristics of facial movement (Fig. 41–1). The muscles relating to the eyelids and brow act in a totally different fashion from those affecting the lips and cheeks. All the facial muscles have an origin on bone or fascia and an insertion into muscle. The separate muscles of the upper and lower face have been dissected (Figs. 41–2 and 41–3), and this discrete anatomy of the facial musculature is well documented.[12] The nomenclature varies marginally between texts.[11, 15]

571

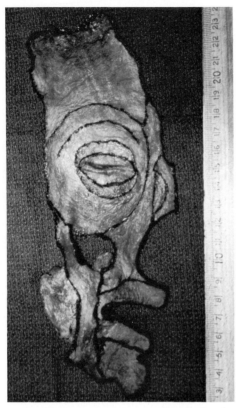

Figure 41–1. Dissection of upper and lower facial muscles.

In the upper face, the relevant muscles include the frontalis and the orbicularis oculi. The latter may be subdivided into orbital, preseptal, and pretarsal components. The corrugator supercilii and procerus may be regarded as accessory muscles. The lower facial muscles can be grouped according to their direction of action and their insertion. The origins of the radiating muscles are around the perimeter of the middle and lower third of the facial skeleton. They insert into the circular orbicularis oris. The elevators of the upper lip are the levator labii superioris alaeque nasi, levator labii superioris, and zygomaticus minor. The depressors of the lower lip are the depressor labii inferioris and the mentalis (an accessory muscle). The muscles inserting into the orbicularis oris just lateral to the angle of the mouth at the modiolus radiate in four diverging directions. The levator anguli oris is more peripherally and superficially placed than the elevators of the upper lip. The zygomaticus major is the longest and most peripherally placed of the lower facial muscles. The depressor anguli oris is less discrete in its origin and insertion

with the depressor labii inferioris than its contrasting levator equivalents. The large buccinator not only inserts into the modiolus but also interdigitates with the remainder of the upper and lower orbicularis oris and takes its origin from the pterygomandibular raphe and adjacent bone. The muscles of secondary importance are the platysma and risorius.

The superficial musculature aponeurotic system (SMAS) is of importance in draping the skin over the underlying muscles.[1] There is no direct attachment between the aponeurotic element and the deeper facial muscles. There is an indirect effect through the platysma and the junctional area in the region of the modiolus.

The blood vessels of importance to the facial musculature are the superficial temporal artery and the facial artery. These vessels travel in the subfascial and submuscular plane.

The facial nerve is a complex structure in the central two thirds of its distribution. The branches at the extremes are more isolated. In the central region, the facial nerve has an extensive anastomosis within the parotid gland.[4] Less commonly recognized is the extensive plexus within the buccal fat pad (Fig. 41–4). Although there is usually a dominant marginal mandibular branch, there are usually two or three minor branches to sup-

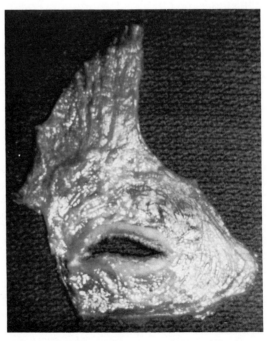

Figure 41–2. Dissection of upper face.

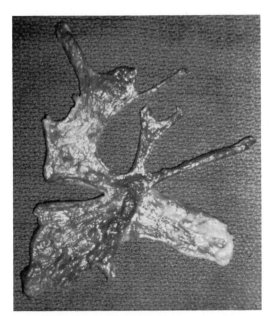

Figure 41–3. Dissection of lower face.

ply the depressors of the lower lip in addition.[14, 18, 19] All muscles are supplied on their deep surface. This generalization includes the submucosally placed buccinator (the forgotten facial muscle of the cheek), which is also innervated on its deep aspect when viewed this way.

The discrete anatomy, which is well documented, provides a two-dimensional approach to the facial muscles. Adding the third dimension provides a clearer concept of the organization of the facial muscles. To demonstrate this, four full-thickness sections were taken, as shown in the outlined diagram (Fig. 41–5). In the vertical section through the brow and eyelid region (Fig. 41–6) the thin pregaleal frontalis muscle can be seen extending into a hypertrophic area beneath the brow. It inserts into the orbital part of the orbicularis oculi muscle. The orbicularis oculi muscle can be easily dissected into three sub-areas, the orbital, preseptal, and pretarsal components.

In the section through the upper outer aspect of the lower face (Fig. 41–7), the zygomaticus major muscle can be seen. The nasolabial fold is also shown at right angles to the skin. The fold tends to drape over the facial musculature. There are no apparent attachments between the overlying skin and radiating muscle (Fig. 41–7). The skin is adherent to the underlying sphincter muscles.

The section through the modiolus and through the angle of the corner of the mouth (Fig. 41–8) shows the thickness of the buccinator compared with the zygomaticus major muscle. The arrow shows the nasolabial fold, and again there is no direct insertion of muscle into this fold. With regard to the lower lip (Fig. 41–9), there is considerably more fat in these muscles than in the other facial muscles.

Functional Anatomy

Although the basic anatomic structures are reasonably well defined, it is worthwhile considering the facial muscles from a functional viewpoint. The upper facial muscles have three essential vector movements: (1) elevation of the brow, (2) orbital sphincter function, and (3) pretarsal and preseptal eyelid closure (Figs. 41–10 and 41–11). The lower facial vector movements are: (1) elevation and depression of the lip, (2) elevation and depression of the modiolus, (3) sphincter function, and (4) retraction of the angle and cheek control in the lower face (Figs. 41–12 and 41–13). The areas in this region of the face that have tended to be ignored are the

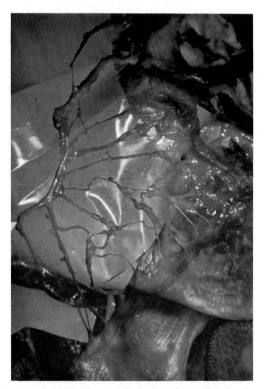

Figure 41–4. Facial nerve dissection shows the plexiform arrangement and deep innervation of the muscles.

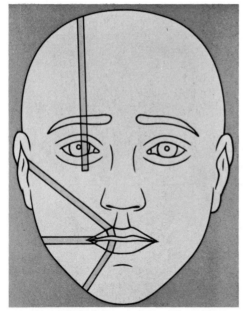

Figure 41–5. Diagram of the full-thickness facial sections to show the organization of the facial musculature (see also Figures 41–6 to 41–9).

buccinator and lower lip. The constant relationship between the buccinator ridge and the occlusal plane appears important.[2]

Muscle weight is a very important parameter depicting the functional capacity of the muscle unit.[22] The data in Table 41–1 are from a cadaver dissected for all the facial muscles. The upper facial muscle weight is only 6.4 gm, and there is almost three times as much muscle in the lower face. Within the lower facial muscles, the buccinator accounts for over one third of the total muscle bulk. Muscle fiber counts and myelinated nerve fiber counts were obtained from histologic studies, and a ratio depicting the density of innervation was calculated (Table 41–2). The

Table 41–1. WEIGHTS OF MUSCLES OF FACE

Muscle	Weight (gm)
Upper face:	
Elevators	3.2
Orbicularis oculi	3.2
Total:	6.4
Lower face:	
Elevators, lip	2.8
Elevators, angle	1.6
Orbicularis oris	2.0
Depressor, angle	1.6
Depressor, lip	1.8
Buccinator	6.2
Total:	16.0

Table 41–2. DENSITY OF INNERVATION OF ZYGOMATICUS MAJOR MUSCLE

No. of myelinated nerve fibers	822
No. of muscle fibers	6559
Ratio	1:8

facial muscles have a relatively high ratio. For subsequent comparison, the zygomaticus major muscle has a ratio of 1:8.

Surface Anatomy

Nasolabial Fold. The nasolabial fold does not appear to be related to muscle insertion to the skin. It is due to the draping of the skin over the muscles inserting around the orbicularis oris and the interrelationship of their axis radiating from the upper lip, modiolus, and lower lip (see Figs. 41–5 and 41–12).

Facial Movement. The lines of the face are complex and are related to underlying muscle movement, gravitational drag, and contour lines.[10] Following standardized photography of the face at rest (Fig. 41–14) and comparison with the photographic appearance with

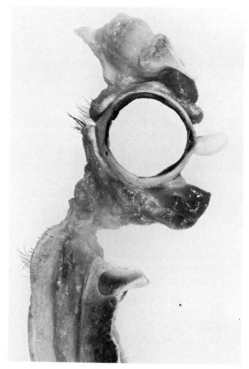

Figure 41–6. Vertical section through the upper face, showing the hypertrophic ridge at the fronto-orbital muscular junction.

Figure 41–7. Upper oblique section through the lower face, showing the thin zygomaticus major muscle and the nasolabial fold.

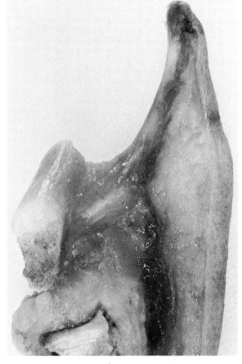

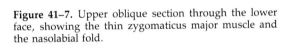

Figure 41–8. Transverse per-modiolar section of the face, showing the nasolabial fold.

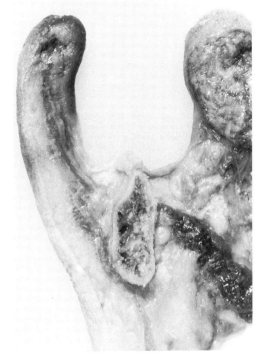

Figure 41–9. Lower oblique section through the lower face.

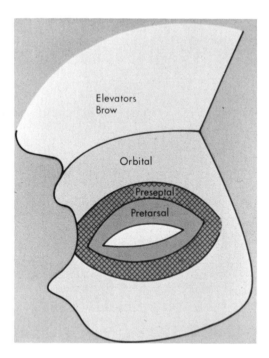

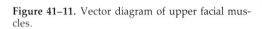

Figure 41–10. Diagram of upper facial muscle components.

Figure 41–11. Vector diagram of upper facial muscles.

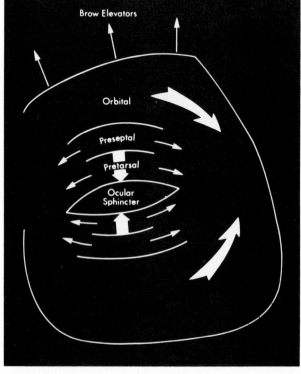

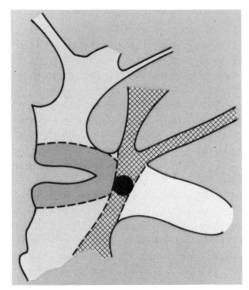

Figure 41–12. Diagram of lower facial muscle components.

Table 41–3. UPPER FACIAL EXCURSION
MEASUREMENTS

Excursion	Measurement (mm)
Brow elevation	10.1
Approximation	10.3
Eyelid separation	10.9
Upper lid	9.7
Lower lid	1.2

movement (Fig. 41–15), the computerized and digitized tablet allowed a noninvasive measure of excursion. In the upper face, the range of excursion of the forehead in the horizontal and vertical direction was approximately 1 cm (Table 41–3). The orbicularis oculi movement confirmed previous results of upper and lower eyelid function. In the lower face, there was nearly 2 cm of movement vertically, nearly 2.5 cm of movement horizontally, and about 1 cm of movement in forward projection (Table 41–4).

ABNORMAL FACIAL ANATOMY

The classic denervation effect of the facial nerve is well known (Fig. 41–16). The areas

of the eyebrow, buccinator, nose, and lower lip have been largely ignored, whereas further attention needs to be directed toward the eyelids and lower face. Although patients with facial palsy may have minimal facial deformity, some have extreme unilateral and contralateral changes in the face. In the more severe cases, paralysis of the facial muscles has a direct effect on facial movement together with secondary changes in relationship to the SMAS and overlying skin.[1] There are also secondary changes in the contralateral side of the face from overactivity. The surface characteristics of the face are therefore significantly altered.

FREE MUSCLE TRANSPLANTATION

Many muscles have been used for transplantation. Initially, devascularized and denervated muscles were transferred.[23] Subsequently, devascularized reinnervated muscles were used. This has now progressed to transfer of free neurovascular muscular units.[13, 15, 20, 21] The ultimate success of muscle transplantation depends on (1) the transfer of an appropriate muscle to replace the nonfunctioning unit; (2) the reliability of the procedure (this is really related to the choice

Figure 41–13. Vector diagram of lower facial muscles.

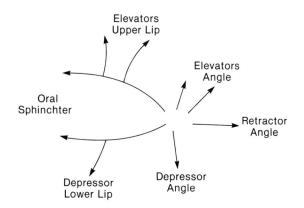

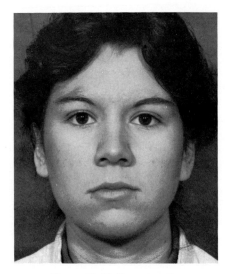

Figure 41–14. Face at rest.

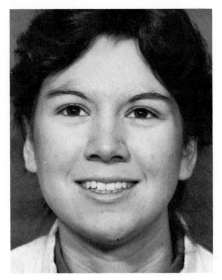

Figure 41–15. Face with movement.

of an appropriate neurovascular pedicle and other general factors related to free flap surgery); (3) the strength and excursion of the transplanted muscle so as to construct appropriate muscle movement[3, 22] (this has to take into account the denervation atrophy effect); and (4) the origin and insertion of the muscle (the muscle must have an origin and insertion appropriate to the line of action intended to be reconstructed) (see Figs. 41–12 and 41–16).

The muscles that have been transferred to the face include the palmaris longus, extensor digitorum brevis, tensor fascia lata, gra-

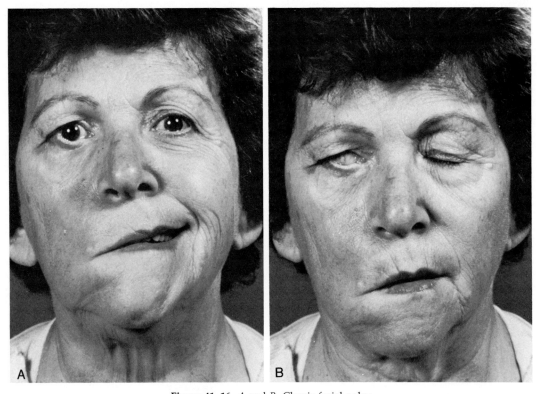

Figure 41–16. *A* and *B*, Classic facial palsy.

Table 41–4. LOWER FACIAL EXCURSION MEASUREMENTS

Excursion	Measurement (mm)
Elevation	12.6
Depression	5.6
Smile	3.4
Retraction	8.8
Sphincter	13.4
Pucker	
Upper	11.3
Lower	7.8

Table 41–5. FACIAL MUSCLE PARAMETERS

Muscle	Measurement
Palmaris Longus	
Muscle length	10.3 cm
Muscle weight	3.2 gm
Nerve length	4.4 cm
Vessel length	—
Tendon length	14.5 cm
Extensor Digitorum Brevis	
Muscle length	5.4 cm
Muscle weight	3.6 gm
Nerve length	3.3 cm
Vessel length	3.0 cm
Tendon length	7.0 cm
Tensor Fascia Lata	
Muscle length	18.5 cm
Muscle weight	28.8 gm
Nerve length	10.8 cm
Vessel length	7.8 cm
Fascia length	40.6 cm
Gracilis	
Muscle length	32.0 cm
Muscle weight	58.0 gm
Nerve length	10.2 cm
Vessel length	8.5 cm
Tendon length	10.0 cm
Pectoralis Minor	
Muscle length	6.9/13.9 cm
Muscle weight	29.7 gm
Nerve length	4.2 cm
Vessel length	4.9 cm
Tendon origin	1.5 cm
Fascia insertion	Slips
Latissimus Dorsi	
Muscle length	38.0/43.0 cm
Muscle weight	147.0 gm
Nerve length	13.7 cm
Vessel length	8.9 cm
Tendon origin	5.0 cm
Fascia insertion	Broad
Serratus Anterior	
Muscle length	16.2/19.2 cm
Muscle weight	68.2 gm
Nerve length	4.2 cm
Vessel length	9.0 cm
Tendon origin	<1.0 cm
Rectus Abdominis	
Muscle length	31.2/34.7 cm
Muscle weight	83.5 gm
Nerve length	3.0/15.0 cm
Vessel length	5.8 cm
Tendon length	2.0 cm
Platysma	
Muscle length	10.5/14.5 cm
Muscle weight	6.4 gm
Nerve length	2.2 cm
Vessel length	—
Tendon length	—

cilis, pectoralis minor, latissimus dorsi, and the lower four segments of the serratus anterior. These muscles have all been assessed in the laboratory together with two additional muscles, the rectus abdominis and the platysma. The muscles were assessed with regard to their basic parameters and their intramuscular neurovascular topography. Table 41–5 presents these basic data.

In an attempt to correlate the donor and facial muscles from several total body studies, the muscle weights have been expressed as a percentage of the heaviest muscle in the body, i.e., the latissimus dorsi, and the results were then averaged (Table 41–6). The weight of the total facial musculature is only 20 per cent of the weight of the latissimus dorsi muscle. Perhaps the whole muscles that are comparable to the facial muscles are the tensor fascia lata, pectoralis minor, and segments of gracilis, serratus anterior, latissimus dorsi, and rectus abdominis.

This basic information will be discussed further in relation to the extra- and intramuscular neurovascular topography for each muscle.

Extra- and Intramuscular Neurovascular Topography

The neurovascular supply was investigated by direct muscular dissection under magnification combined with intra-arterial angiography from a fresh cadaver specimen using a total body lead-latex injection technique. The relevance of these investigations to other studies will be highlighted for each muscle individually.

Palmaris Longus Muscle. This muscle has an unpredictable vascular pedicle, a random intramuscular pattern, and minimal weight (Table 41–5 and Fig. 41–17). It is interesting to consider the initial encouraging reports

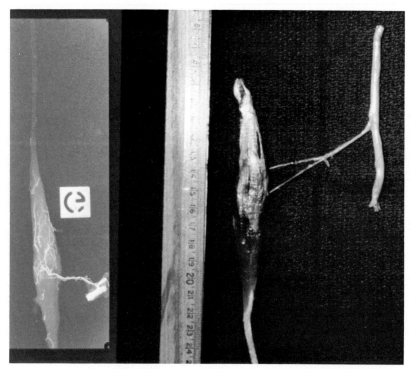

Figure 41–17. Palmaris longus muscle and angiogram.

using this muscle as a free devascularized denervated transfer.[24] However, these reports have not been substantiated. The reason for this is demonstrated in the cross section of an orthotopic palmaris longus muscle transplant in the monkey.[7] The outer muscle survived as a free transfer. Just beneath the surface are bundles of regenerating muscle fibers as a result of the ischemic episode. These surround a central core of dense fibrous connective tissue as a result of ischemic necrosis. The formation of the central core of connective tissue indicates that preservation of the whole muscle would be an indication for the use of microvascular anastomoses. If this central core of necrosis does not occur, the vascular anastomoses are probably not necessary.[7]

Extensor Digitorum Brevis Muscle. This muscle has a long and predictable neurovascular pedicle, a random intramuscular pattern, and minimal muscle bulk (Table 41–5 and Fig. 41–18). The experience with transfer of this muscle has demonstrated the progression of transfer from a preliminary denervated and subsequently devascularized unit[24] to the revascularization of the whole muscle unit.[20] Preliminary denervation does not appear to offer any significant advantage for a muscle of this bulk. Initially, the extensor

digitorum brevis appeared to suffer the same fate as the free palmaris longus muscle transfer. Reinnervation and revascularization of the extensor digitorum brevis have provided less than encouraging results as there is insufficient bulk and excursion of this muscle.[2] The inadequate situation is shown in Figure 41–19.

Tensor Fascia Lata Muscle. This muscle has a predictable neurovascular pedicle, and the nerve and vascular pedicle approach the muscle from either side. There is a random intramuscular pattern, adequate bulk, and a

Table 41–6. AVERAGED COMPARATIVE WEIGHTS FOR DONOR AND FACIAL MUSCLES (EXPRESSED AS PERCENTAGE OF LATISSIMUS DORSI MUSCLE)

Donor Muscles	Weight (gm)	Facial Muscles	Weight (gm)
Palmaris longus	3.4	Upper face	7.5
Extensor digitorum brevis	1.9	Lower face	12.6
		Total	20.1
Gracilis	37.7		
Pectorialis minor	20.2		
Latissimus dorsi	100.0		
Serratus anterior	37.1		
Tensor fascia lata	23.5		
Rectus abdominis	60.5		
Platysma	8.6		

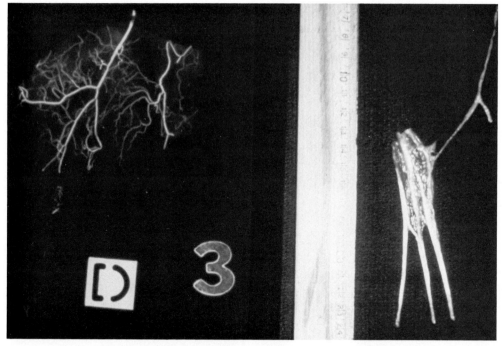

Figure 41–18. Extensor digitorum brevis muscle and angiogram.

long fascial extension (Table 41–5 and Fig. 41–20).

Gracilis Muscle. This muscle has a predictable and adequate neurovascular pedicle and a longitudinal intramuscular neurovascular pattern. There is adequate bulk but excessive length (Table 41–5 and Fig. 41–21). The range of excursion of this muscle can be tailored to the amount resected and left for subsequent use. When part of the muscle is transferred to the face,[13, 20] the results are more encouraging. The excessive bulk and length can be seen (Fig. 41–22). This muscle has been designed and inserted as a dynamic sling and therefore has advantages over the static fascia lata suspension sling. The gracilis muscle is not without problems. Because of its longitudinal architecture and therefore, of necessity, its limited origin and insertion, its direction of pull can provide no alternative to dynamic elevation of the lower face. The gracilis muscle is too bulky for eyelid reconstruction.

Pectoralis Minor Muscle. This muscle has an ideal shape for reanimation of the upper part of the lower face. It has a predictable but complex neurovascular pedicle. There is a dominant vessel supplying the whole muscle but two independent nerves. The pectoralis minor muscle has adequate weight and length (Table 41–5 and Fig. 41–23). Its inser-

tion into the lateral side of the nose, upper lip, and angle of the mouth is similar to normal facial muscles. The results are therefore encouraging.[23]

Latissimus Dorsi Muscle and Serratus Anterior Muscle (Lower Four Segments). These two muscles have a predictable external neurovascular pedicle and a longitudinal intramuscular topography (Fig. 41–24). The nerve

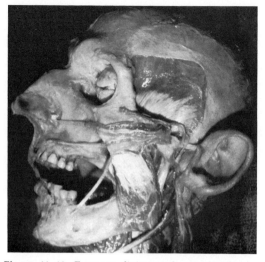

Figure 41–19. Extensor digitorum brevis muscle on a dissected face. (From Hamilton, S. G. L., and Terzis, J. K.: Clin. Plast. Surg., *11*:199, 1984.)

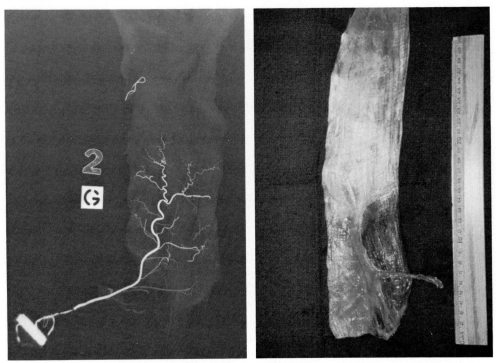

Figure 41–20. Tensor fascia lata muscle and angiogram.

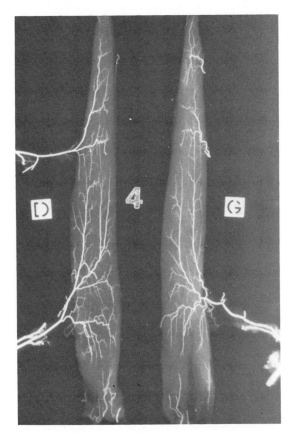

Figure 41–21. Gracilis muscle angiogram. (From Hamilton, S. G. L., and Terzis, J. K.: Clin. Plast. Surg., *11*:199, 1984.)

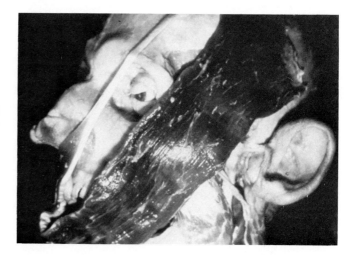

Figure 41–22. Gracilis muscle on a dissected face. (From Hamilton, S. G. L., and Terzis, J. K.: Clin. Plast. Surg., *11*:200, 1984.)

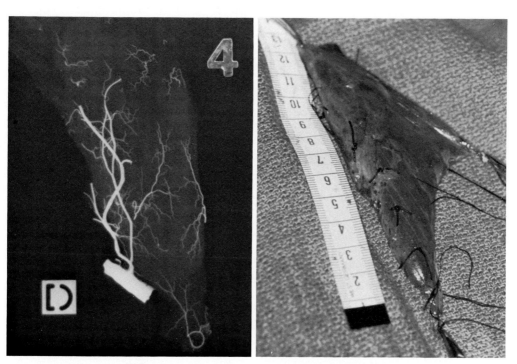

Figure 41–23. Pectoralis minor muscle and angiogram.

Table 41–7. DENSITY OF INNERVATION OF
GRACILIS MUSCLE

No. of myelinated nerve fibers	1945
No. of muscle fibers	100,080
Ratio	1:50

to the serratus is short unless denervation of the upper segments is undertaken. The muscle is sparsely innervated (Table 41–7). The latissimus dorsi muscle has a predictable external neurovascular pedicle and a longitudinal segmental intramuscular topography similar to a "flattened" gracilis muscle. Both muscles are too bulky and require segmental separation, which would then reduce their overall density of innervation (Table 41–5).

Rectus Abdominis Muscle. The overall length and bulk of this muscle are too large for transfer to the face. However, like previously mentioned muscles, segments can be transferred. This muscle has a predictable and long external vascular pedicle. There is a longitudinal intramuscular pattern with transverse segmental elements (Table 41–5 and Fig. 41–25). The nerve supply is laterally based and segmental. Within the muscle segment there is a longitudinal supply, splitting the muscle into medial and lateral compo-

nents. The range of contraction is up to 4 cm and the minimum recorded is 2 cm. This is sufficient for facial muscle reanimation (Tables 41–3 and 41–4).

Platysma Muscle. This is a very thin facial muscle that is innervated and vascularized by the facial artery and nerve (Table 41–5). Its weight makes it a potential donor for the upper face only. The platysma muscle may be suitable for free devascularized reinnervated transfer and survival as a free graft because of its lack of bulk.

Other Factors

When doing a reconstruction, it is critical to be able to transfer a known volume and weight of muscle and to be confident that a functioning volume of tissue will be present following the transfer and reinnervation.[8, 22] This must allow for up to 50 per cent denervation atrophy, providing appropriate length and tension are supplied to the muscle at the site of transfer.[3, 17, 22] The muscle transferred must act in an appropriate fashion. The limitations of the muscles so far used have been related to a disproportionate bulk and to inappropriate attachments of origin and in-

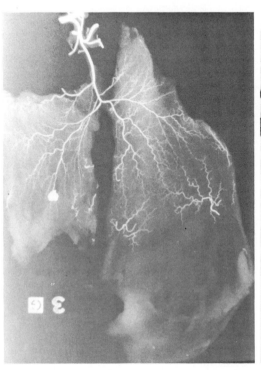
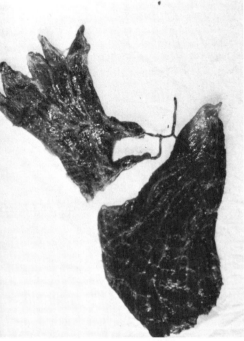

Figure 41–24. Latissimus dorsi muscle and serratus anterior muscles and angiogram (lower four segments).

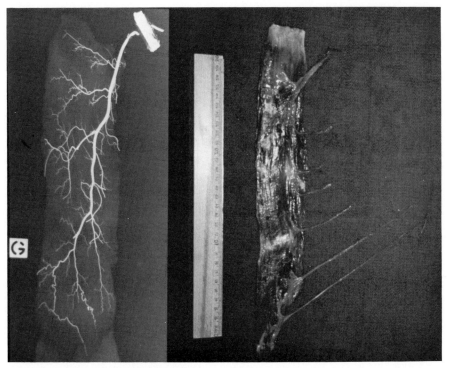

Figure 41–25. Rectus abdominis muscle and angiogram. (From Hamilton, S. G. L., and Terzis, J. K.: Clin. Plast. Surg., *11*:200, 1984.)

sertion.[13, 20] More finesse in these areas is required. The rectus abdominis muscle appears to offer a unique situation. It is a midline structure, as are the facial muscles, and the overall appearance allows for a more appropriate reconstruction by segmental transplantation and territorial manipulation than by the dynamic suspension procedures discussed earlier. The platysma muscle is the only available thin muscle comparable to the pretarsal and preseptal orbicularis oculi muscle.

To further contrast the smartness of the facial muscles to the donor muscles, the ratio of the number of myelinated nerve fibers to the number of muscle fibers supplied by that nerve was investigated (Tables 41–2 and 41–7). To highlight an example, the zygomaticus major muscle has a ratio of 1:8. It is at least six times smarter than the gracilis muscle, with a ratio of 1:50.

The method of neurotization is critical to the functional capacity of the muscle, hence the limitations of local muscle transfer techniques using masseter and temporalis muscles and the limitations of neurotization of the facial nerve using crossover techniques. When combining the transfer of a skeletal muscle with a nerve crossover technique, the results are less satisfactory than when using a successful generous two-stage cross-facial nerve graft to neurotize the skeletal muscle. An interesting finding with significant functional implications was noted on histologic study of the myelinated nerve fibers. The number of myelinated nerve fibers within the facial nerve actually increased toward the periphery, whereas the number in the hypoglossal nerve remained static. Therefore, combined with the plexus arrangements of the facial nerve, sacrifice of part of the facial nerve is a safe and justifiable procedure.

CONCLUSIONS

The optimal muscle unit to reconstruct the eyelids and brow should be thin and placed in the pretarsal/preseptal plane and the pregaleal plane, respectively. This muscle should be reinnervated by appropriate nerve anastomosis. Revascularization should occur without fibrosis by vascularized or nonvascularized transfer. The optimal muscle to reconstruct the lower face should be bulky and therefore would definitely require revascularization. The intraoperative manipulation requires a territorial and segmental neurovascular pattern. The muscle should be attached to bone around the periphery of the middle and lower thirds of the face and inserted into the musculocutaneous segment of the lip to allow for a radiating form of contraction. The range of excursion should be up to 2.5 cm in overall length.

Consideration in all these muscle transfers requires knowledge of the predicted weight and volume reduction following denervation and transfer.*

*Acknowledgements:
1. Microsurgical Research Center, Eastern Virginia Graduate School of Medicine, Norfolk, Virginia—for cadavers, facilities (in part), and clinical cases.
2. Academie de Paris, Université Rene Descartes Biomedicale Laboratoire d'Anatomie; Director: Professor J. Hureau. In association with Dr. A. Gilbert, Trousseau Hospital, Paris—for cadavers and facilities (in part).
3. American Association of Plastic Surgeons, Research Grant for financial support (in part).

References

1. Balch, G. R.: Superficial musculoaponeurotic system suspension and buccinator plication for facial nerve paralysis. Plast. Reconstruct. Surg., 66:769–771, 1980.
2. Berry, D. C.: The buccinator mechanism. J. Dent., 7:111–114, 1979.
3. Brand, P. W., Beach, R. P., and Thompson, D. E.: Relative tension and potential excursion of muscles in the forearm and hand. J. Hand Surg., 6:209–219, 1981.
4. Celesnik, F.: Surgical anatomy of the intraglandular portion of the facial nerve. J. Maxillofac. Surg., 1:65–73, 1973.
5. Clodius, L.: Reconstruction of the nasolabial fold. Plast. Reconstr. Surg., 50:467–473, 1972.
6. Edgerton, M. T.: Surgical correction of facial paralysis. Ann. Surg., 165:996, 1967.
7. Freilinger, G., Holle, Jand, Carlson, B. M.: Muscle Transplantation. New York, Spring-Verlag, 1981, Fig. 4.
8. Gilbert, A.: Free muscle transfer. Int. Surg., 66:33–35, 1981.
9. Gordon, L., and Buncke, H. J.: Heterotopic free skeletal muscle autotransplantation with utilization of a long nerve graft and microsurgical techniques: A study in the primate. J. Hand Surg., 4:103–108, 1979.
10. Grabb, W. C., and Smith, J. W.: Plastic Surgery, 2nd Ed. Boston, Little Brown & Co., 1973, p. 5.
11. Grant, J. C. B., and Basmajian, J. V.: Grant's Method of Anatomy, 7th Ed. Baltimore, Williams & Wilkins, pp. 540–542.
12. Gray's Anatomy, 36th British Edition, edited by Williams, R., and Warwick, P. L. Philadelphia, W. B. Saunders Co. pp. 529–534.
13. Harii, K., Ohmori, K., and Torii, S.: Free gracilis muscle transplantation with microneurovascular anastomoses for the treatment of facial paralysis. Plast. Reconstr. Surg., 57:133, 1976.
14. Kempe, L. G.: Topical organization of the distal portion of the facial nerve. J. Neurosurg., 52:671–673, 1980.
15. Kubo, T., Ikuta, Y., and Tsuge, K.: Free muscle transplantation in dogs by neurovascular anastomoses. Plast. Reconstr. Surg., 57:495, 1976.
16. Last, R. J.: Anatomy, Regional and Applied, 6th Ed. Edinburgh, Churchill Livingstone, 1977, pp. 379–382.
17. Manktelow, R. T., and McKee, N. H.: Free muscle transplantation to provide active finger flexion. J. Hand Surg., 3:416–426, 1978.
18. Moffat, D. A., and Ramsden, R. T.: The deformity produced by a palsy of the marginal mandibular branch of the facial nerve.
19. Nelson, D. W., and Gingrass, R. P.: Anatomy of the mandibular branches of the facial nerve. Plast. Reconstr. Surg., 64:479–482, 1979.
20. O'Brien, B. McC., Franklin, J. D., and Morrison, W. A.: Cross-facial nerve grafts and microneurovascular free muscle transfer for long established facial palsy. Br. J. Plast. Surg., 33:202–215, 1980.
21. Tamia, S., et al.: Free muscle transplants in dogs with microsurgical anastomoses. Plast. Reconstr. Surg., 46:219, 1970.
22. Terzis, J. K., Sweet, R. C., Dykes, R. W., and Williams, H. B.: Recovery of function in free muscle transplants using microneurovascular anastomoses, J. Hand Surg., 3:37–59, 1978.
23. Terzis, J. K.: On pectoralis minor muscle for facial reanimation. Personal communication.
24. Thompson, N.: Autogenous free grafts of skeletal muscle, preliminary experimental and clinical study. Plast. Reconstr. Surg., 48:11, 1971.

42

Management of Acute Extratemporal Facial Nerve Palsy

■

Kenneth K. Lee, M.B.B.S., F.R.A.C.S.
Julia K. Terzis, M.D., Ph.D.

The facial nerve is the most frequently paralyzed peripheral nerve of the body. Acute palsy of this nerve is one of the most devastating, although by themselves nonlethal, medical conditions. Facial nerve paralysis is associated not only with loss of normal function of the mouth and eyelid but also with loss of ability to form facial expressions. This results in a major handicap, as it interferes with the patient's normal interrelationships with others. Depending on the cause and management, many of these paralyses will be permanent.

For centuries, physicians have worked to find ways to reverse the acute palsy or reduce deformity and morbidity of the established palsy. With advances in the understanding of peripheral nerve function and the benefit of microsurgery, the diagnosis and management have improved considerably, particularly in the last 20 years. Advances have been made in both early repair and late reconstruction. The latter topic is discussed in Chapters 44, 45, and 46. Early repair of the facial nerve is divided by region into intratemporal and extratemporal segments. As plastic surgeons, we are primarily concerned with the extratemporal segment, which begins at the exit of the facial nerve at the stylomastoid foramen to its termination either directly or via a plexus with branches of the trigeminal nerve into the facial muscles of expression.

In this chapter, the anatomy and physiology of the facial nerve are outlined. The history of facial nerve surgery is then described, leading to the present state of the art. Finally, the management of acute extratemporal facial nerve palsy is discussed in light of present-day procedures.

ANATOMY AND PHYSIOLOGY OF THE FACIAL NERVE

The facial nerve (seventh cranial nerve) has the longest and the most tortuous course of any cranial nerve.[1] The motor root of the facial nerve emerges from the pons between the olive and the inferior cerebellar peduncle. It is accompanied by the vestibulocochlear nerve along with the intermediate nerve (sensory root of the facial nerve containing efferent preganglionic parasympathetic fibers for the submandibular and lacrimal glands and glands of the nasal, palatal, and pharyngeal mucosa as well as central processes of the unipolar cells of the geniculate ganglion). These three nerve roots enter the porus of the acoustic meatus. Here the facial nerve runs in the internal auditory canal obliquely in an interior-lateral direction. This segment is approximately 8 to 10 mm long. All these nerves are initially enclosed by a common sheath of meninges. The sensory roots join the motor roots in this segment. Communication between the seventh and eighth cranial nerves also occurs here. At the fundus of the internal meatus, the facial nerve leaves the vestibulocochlear nerve, pierces the dura, and enters the fallopian canal (facial canal), which is situated at the anterior-superior corner. This canal is approximately 30 mm long and is usually divided into three sections: the labyrinthine, the tympanic or horizontal, and the mastoid or vertical.

1. The labyrinthine segment of the facial nerve is about 4 mm long. The facial nerve runs laterally between the vestibule and the cochlea to the hiatus of the facial canal, where it is expanded by the geniculate ganglion, which contains the unipolar cells of sensory roots. The peripheral processes of these cells consist of some efferent taste fibers by way of the chorda tympani and greater petrosal nerves and some efferent somatic fibers from the skin around the concha. The greater and lesser petrosal nerves join the facial nerve here. Communication with the sympathetic plexus of the middle meningeal artery also occurs here.

2. The tympanic or horizontal segment is approximately 12 mm long and extends from the ganglion, where the nerve makes an abrupt posterior bend of almost 90° in the medial wall of the tympanum through the lateral semicircular canal distally. This bend is often referred to as the genu of the facial nerve. This segment is inferior to the lateral semicircular canal and superior to the oval window and stapes.

3. The mastoid or vertical segment is approximately 15 mm long and begins with a gentle curve (the pyramidal turn) to descend through the mastoid to the stylomastoid foramen. The branch to the stapedius muscle occurs here. The chorda tympani branch comes off at the lower portion of the mastoid segment. This segment also communicates with the vagus by the external petrosal nerve and innervates a small area of skin over the conchal cartilage.[2]

4. Variations in the intratemporal course of the facial nerve occur infrequently. The most common anomaly is dehiscence in the bony fallopian canal. The most frequent site involved is the tympanic segment.[3] Variation in the course of the vertical segment is the next most common anomaly.[4] Other anomalies include variations in the course of the facial nerve.[5] The facial canal may be absent.

Gross variations may also occur in a congenitally deformed ear.[6]

The extratemporal segment of the facial nerve (Fig. 42–1) begins at the stylomastoid foramen, which is situated where the digastric ridge joins the posterior bony wall of the external auditory canal. It is lateral to the styloid process and curves inferiorly and laterally through the retromandibular fossa into the parotid gland. Two branches are given off: (1) the posterior auricular nerve to the occipital belly of occipitofrontalis and posterior auricular muscles and (2) a branch to the posterior belly of the digastric and stylohyoid muscles. At the neck of the mandible, the extratemporal segment divides into two main branches: the temporal-facial and the cervical-facial trunks. The temporal-facial trunk continues upward across the lower edge of the inferior margin of the mandible. The cervical-facial trunk goes down and parallel to the inferior edge of the mandible. These trunks then split into numerous branches, which anastomose with each other and with branches from the trigeminal nerve to form the parotid plexus. At the superior, anterior, and inferior borders of the parotid gland, five terminal branches are usually identified: temporal, zygomatic, buccal, marginal mandibular, and cervical. Communications occur between the glossopharyngeal, vagus, and great auriculotemporal nerve at the stylomastoid foramen and with the lesser occipital and sensory branches of the cervical plexus in the neck and posterior auricular regions.

The anatomy of the extratemporal facial nerve is interesting because of the variable pattern of ramifications in the substance of the parotid gland. Detailed knowledge of the anatomy is required for repair and for surgery of surrounding structures, particularly the parotid gland.

Dissection and identification of the extratemporal facial nerve and its branches are prerequisite for the repair of a damaged facial nerve and surgery in its region. The use of an electrical nerve stimulator has provided help in cases in which the nerve is intact or damage occurred within 72 hours of the initial trauma. However, this is not always applicable. Depending on the clinical situation, the facial nerve trunk and/or the facial nerve branches may need to be identified and dissected first. Full knowledge of various methods of dissection is important in surgery of the facial nerve. Various methods of identification of the facial nerve and branches

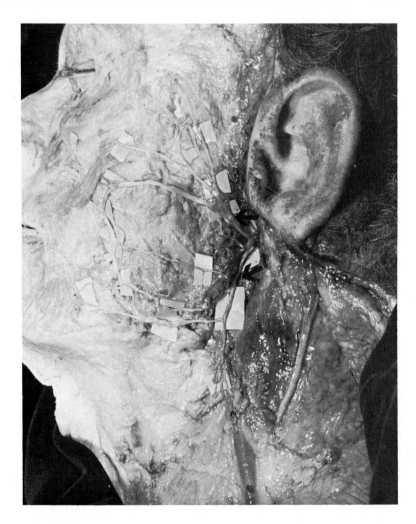

Figure 42–1. The anatomy of the extratemporal facial nerve. Note the division of the nerve into its two main branches (*arrows*). (From Lee, K. L., and Terzis, J. K.: Clin. Plast. Surg., *11*:204, 1984.)

have been described in the past. Blair,[7] in 1912, was the first surgeon to emphasize preservation of the facial nerve and branches during surgery of the parotid gland. He advocated a method of dissection of the branches and another direct approach to the facial nerve trunk using the posterior belly of the digastric muscle as a landmark. Subsequent to that, Janes[8] in 1940 described in detail the dissection of the facial nerve trunk using landmarks such as the styloid process, the posterior belly of the digastric muscle, and the first cervical vertebra. This has become the basis for surgery of the facial nerve by many surgeons, e.g., Martin,[9] Conley,[10] Maxwell et al.[11] and Lathrop.[12] Other surgeons, i.e., Byars[13] and Kidd,[14] identified the submandibular and cervical branches of the facial nerve at the lower pole of the parotid gland in relation to the posterior facial vein deep to the platysma fascia. Dissection was then carried out in a retrograde fashion until the trunk of the facial nerve was identified.

An entirely different approach was advocated by Bailey,[15] who identified the facial nerve branches at the anterior margin of the parotid gland. An approach similar to that of Bailey was used by Sistonk[16] and Riesner,[17] who identified the zygomatic branches on the zygomatic arch and then progressed proximally. The close proximity of Stensen's duct to the buccal branch of the facial nerve was used as the landmark for dissection of this nerve by surgeons such as McNealy and McCallister.[18] Finally, there is the otosurgical approach described by Hogg and Kratz,[19] which utilized the fact that the facial nerve trunk is 6 to 8 mm medial to the tympano-mastoid fissure.

Plexiform Variations of the Facial Nerve

In the substance of the parotid gland, the facial nerve begins to divide into its terminal branches. Each branch divides and forms interconnections between each other, forming a plexiform structure. This plexiform structure of the facial nerve branches has been divided into six basic patterns by Shapiro.[20] Based on dissection of 350 specimens, Davies et al.,[21] in 1956, provided an introduction to the six basic patterns. It is important to note that in their description, 67% of specimens show communication between the temporal-facial and cervical-facial trunks. According to this plexus arrangement, a facial muscle group can be supplied at the periphery by several branches of the facial nerve. This fact explains the clinical findings that facial nerve injuries to the mid-face branches anterior to the vertical line at the lateral margin of the orbit will result in little, if any, deformity. However, branches with little communication, i.e., the frontal and the marginal mandibular branches, are more prone to permanent partial paralysis as a result of injury.

Miehlke et al.,[22] in 1979, excised the extratemporal course of 100 facial nerves during surgery and classified them according to the type of nerve and the anastomosis. In contrast to Davies, they found no anastomosis in nearly 50% of their dissections. Thirty-seven per cent of their dissections had anastomoses between the branches of the temporal-facial portion and 12% between the branches of the cervical-facial region. Only 18% had connections between the temporal and cervical-facial trunks. Based on this, Miehlke et al. advocated the use of the ipsilateral facial nerve in combination with the hypoglossal nerve or facio-facial nerve anastomosis.

Intraneural Pattern and Topography of the Facial Nerve

The intraneural pattern of the facial nerve has been described by Sunderland.[24] He characterized the facial nerve as consisting of one large fascicle from the internal auditory meatus to the general area of the mid-mastoid segment. This fascicle divides into two and subsequently more fascicles at a variable distance between the lateral semicircular canal and the stylomastoid foramen. Meissl and Millesi[25] studied the extratemporal segment of the facial nerve by microscopic dissection. They found the facial nerve to be arranged in three fascicle groups at the stylomastoid

foramen. A few millimeters distally, these fascicles fuse to form one single fascicle again. At the middle third of the extratemporal segment of the facial nerve, the single fascicle again splits into a polyfascicular pattern. These fascicles continue to divide, so that the temporal-facial and cervical-facial trunks both have a polyfascicular pattern.

Mapping of the internal topography of the facial nerve has been attempted by many investigators in the past. For the intratemporal segment of the facial nerve, the presence of a regular somatotopic pattern of nerve fibers to different muscle groups has been suggested by May[26, 27] and Miehlke[28] based on documentation of clinical observations. May further presented experimental evidence that the facial nerve has an orderly arrangement from the facial nucleus all the way down the facial muscles. However, May and Miehlke proposed different configurations of nerve pattern to each muscle group. Meissl and Millesi[25] studied extratemporal facial nerves by serial sectioning and came to the conclusion that in spite of the plexiform arrangement, the changing fascicular pattern, and the fiber exchange between individual fascicles, there are areas within the cross section of the facial nerve in which the nerve fibers supplying a certain muscle group are predominant.

On the other hand, Sunderland and Cossar,[29] in 1953, performed microscopic dissection and documentation of 13 facial nerves of the frog and could not detect any regular intraneural topography. This finding therefore suggests that a diffuse distribution of nerve fibers supplies a particular muscle over the cross section. This idea was supported by Fisch and Esslen,[30] who in 1971 performed systemic stimulation of peripheral facial nerve branches on more than 50 patients and showed that the individual branches contain fiber components for very different facial muscles as far as the distal segments. More recent studies using horseradish peroxidase to trace axons from specific muscles again showed conflicting results. Thomander[31] suggested a random mixing of fibers, whereas a study by Crumley[32] indicated a precise anatomic topography. To date, there have been no definitive topographic studies performed on the human facial nerve.

The significance of the spatial orientation in the facial nerve is that, if this is present, fascicular repair and multiple single fascicle nerve grafts for facial nerve injuries will be indicated. This may reduce the severity of synkinesis, facial spasm, fractures, and disorders of lacrimation in patients who had repair of the facial nerve performed following section. At present there is general agreement that fibers collect into groups supplying regional muscles in the facial nerve distal to the stylomastoid foramen. This is supported by Fisch,[33] who showed that lacerations or surgical transections of the nerve distal to the pes anserinus will minimize synkinesis. In conclusion, intrafascicular nerve repair is indicated at least for injuries to the distal extratemporal segment of the facial nerve.

Facial Nerve Sheath

As the facial nerve leaves the brain stem, it has a delicate layer of pia mater only. In the internal acoustic meatus, the dura mater and periosteum blend together and become the covering of the facial nerve in the fallopian canal. In this canal, the sheath is a combination of bony periosteum and a condensation of loose connective tissue with blood vessels. This layer of nerve covering merges with the perineurium, which is the continuation of the pia mater. This has been referred to as epineurium[34] or perineurium,[35] depending on the author. As the facial nerve descends to the vertical segment of the fallopian canal, the sheath thickens to become more distinct as epineurium. At the stylomastoid foramen, the classic triple layers of epineurium, perineurium, and endoneurium become quite distinct and continue their termination into the facial muscles.

Blood Supply

The blood supply to the facial nerve, in particular the intratemporal segment, has been a point of focus because of the hypothesis that ischemia, primary or secondary, is the cause of many types of acute facial palsy. In the intratemporal segment, the facial nerve is supplied by three arteries, which overlap and anastomose with each other.[36] They also anastomose with the marrow spaces of the surrounding bone and middle ear mucosa.[37] The three arteries are: (1) the anterior inferior cerebellar artery in the posterior cranial fossa and its branch, the internal auditory artery, which accompany the facial nerve in the internal auditory canal to the geniculate ganglion; (2) the petrosal branch of the middle meningeal artery, which gives off ascending and descending branches, including the facial nerve at the geniculate foramen; and (3) the stylomastoid branch of the posterior auricular artery, which enters the facial nerve canal from the stylomastoid foramen. The venous drainage in general follows the arterial pattern. The extratemporal portion of the facial nerve is well supplied by branches from the stylomastoid, posterior auricular, superficial temporal, and transverse facial arteries.

CLASSIFICATION OF NERVE INJURIES

Based on the histology of the nerve trunk, Sunderland[111] (1951) classified nerve injuries into five grades. However, the simpler classification of Seddon[112] (1943) is more useful, as it tends to correlate both clinical and anatomic aspects. Seddon's three grades of nerve injuries are:

1. Neurapraxia: This condition occurs when the injury to the nerve results in a conduction block. Loss of function, particularly paralysis of the motor unit, occurs without any peripheral degeneration. More severe cases can be associated with myelination of the nerve axons. Remyelination occurs within a few days, and recovery of function can be expected in 3 weeks. Typical lesions are moderate forms of ischemic injuries, such as pressure palsy in Bell's palsy.

2. Axonotmesis: This condition occurs when damaged nerves result in complete peripheral degeneration with minimal disruption of the epineurium and the supportive structures of the nerve. The internal architecture or endoneural sheaths are preserved. Chances of functional recovery are excellent because the regenerating axons are guided into their proper path by their original sheath. Expected time of recovery varies from 6 weeks to 6 months. Examples of lesions causing axonotmesis of the facial nerves are severe ischemia, compression, crushing, and hypothermia.

3. Neurotmesis: In this case there is complete loss of anatomic continuity. Sharp lacerations and severe trauma are examples of such injuries.

The effects of injuries to the facial nerve and changes occurring to the neuron cell body, proximal nerve fibers, and distal nerve fiber stump, as well as effects on neuromuscular function and muscles, are discussed in Chapters 2, 4, and 5.

HISTORICAL PERSPECTIVE

The history of facial nerve surgery has been a process of continuous improvement over a relatively short time. Its progress parallels advances in peripheral nerve surgery and has been the result of clinical and experimental work of many specialists, i.e., plastic surgeons, neurosurgeons, and otolaryngologists. The motor function of the facial nerve was first demonstrated by Bell.[38] The first recorded facial nerve repair was performed by Drobnik[39] and consisted of an accessory facial nerve cross-over anastomosis. Ballance[40] in 1924 and Manasse[41] in 1900 independently reported further cross-over repair using hypoglossal and glossopharyngeal nerves, respectively.

The unsatisfactory results of these procedures led to the development of end-to-end anastomosis of damaged facial nerves. To achieve this after excision of scars, rerouting of the facial nerve was required to bring the ends together. This was first performed by Bunnell[42] in 1927 and successful results were published. The problem of rerouting was that after such a procedure the facial nerve was left unsupported in the middle ear and the vascular connections to the nerve in the ear were disturbed. Martin[43] achieved end-to-end anastomosis by intratemporal stretching of the nerve ends. However, with Martin's stretching procedure, traction injuries and scar formation were promoted. At the same time, extensive experimental work had been performed on monkeys by Ballance and Udel,[44] which led to the use of autogenous nerve grafts in 1931.

The next major advance was the introduction of magnification with the use of an operating microscope by Cawthorne.[45] Better exposure and prudent access to the intratemporal support structure of the facial nerve were described by Wullstein[46] in 1957, with respect to the mastoid segment (House and Crabtree, 1965[47]) and to the petrous segment of the fallopian canal. Further advances in exposure of the nerve were developed by Pulec[48] and Fisch and Esselen.[49]

Advances in extratemporal facial nerve reconstruction were initiated by Duel[50] and Bunnell,[51] who performed nerve grafting following segmental loss. Cardwell[52] first attempted direct neurotization into facial muscles. Significant work has been done by Maxwell et al.[53] on reconstruction following parotid tumor excision and by Lathrop[54] on repair following traumatic injuries. Finally, the continuous efforts and experience of Conley and Miehlke[55] helped to bring extratemporal facial nerve surgery to the present level of development.

ETIOLOGY OF ACUTE FACIAL PALSY

Acute facial palsy can be caused by either upper or lower motor neuron lesions. By far, the most common cause is idiopathic or Bell's palsy, the etiology of which may be multifactorial and has not yet been proved. The immediate management of acute Bell's palsy may be surgical or medical. The excellent review of various forms of treatment by Huizing et al.[56] casts doubt on all present forms of treatment. This may remain so until the etiology is better understood and the prediction of prognosis is more reliable. Furthermore, once facial palsy is established in patients with Bell's palsy, the management is the same as in patients with long-standing facial palsy.

The causes of acute extratemporal facial palsy include trauma, neoplasm, and inflammation. Depending on the region and the level involved, paralysis may be complete but most commonly is incomplete, i.e., partial.

Trauma. This is the most common cause of acute extratemporal facial palsy. It can be the result of an accident or of surgery (both iatrogenic injuries and therapeutic excision). The causative agent may be sharp or blunt, of high or low velocity, due to an extreme in temperature, and so forth. Two forms of presentation are usual: open (e.g., a facial laceration) or closed (e.g., a fractured mandible). In closed injuries of the head and neck presenting with acute facial palsy, differentiating the extratemporal from the intratemporal and intracranial injury is important, although at times difficult. Extratemporal facial palsy resulting from mandibular fracture can be caused by different mechanisms.[57] Similarly, temporal bone fracture may cause injuries at different sites.[58] Although far less common than intratemporal trauma, iatrogenic injuries to the extratemporal segment of the facial nerve do occur.

The visualization of the facial nerve is the

key to parotid surgery without complications. Therapeutic excision of the facial nerve and its branches may occur as a result of tumor surgery.

Neoplasm. Neoplastic involvement of the facial nerve is rare. Acute extratemporal facial palsy as a result of tumor involvement is rarer still. As a rule, these tumors are malignant and the onset is progressive. Involvement can be destructive or infiltrative but is usually secondary to compression, particularly in the tight spaces of the mastoid. Neoplasms can derive from the facial nerve itself or more commonly from the surrounding structures. Those arising from the nerve itself are invariably of Schwann cell origin, i.e., neurofibromas and neurilemomas. Most neuromas are benign and are found intratemporally, but they may be found in the extratemporal region and may be misdiagnosed as a parotid tumor.[59, 60] Fifty per cent of these neuromas are found in the facial nerve trunk and 50% in the peripheral branches.[59, 61] Paralysis is usually caused by pressure and therefore is extremely rare in the extratemporal region. When malignant, 50% of the neuromas are associated with von Recklinghausen's disease.[59]

Histologically, the neurilemoma lies eccentrically away from the nerve fibers, whereas the axons run through the neurofibroma. Preservation of the nerve during surgery is therefore difficult. However, attempts should be made to secure the proximal stump for reconstruction.

The facial nerve can also be involved by surrounding primary and secondary tumors. Parotid tumors are the most common lesions involving the facial nerve owing to the position of the nerve and its branches in the substance of the parotid gland. Although malignant neoplasms are found in most cases of paralysis due to parotid tumors, benign tumors have also been reported.[62] Management of the facial nerve in a parotid tumor has been very well described.[63, 64] As a guide, radical total parotidectomy with the sacrifice of the facial nerve is indicated in high-grade cancer of the superficial lobe, all malignant tumors of the deep lobe, all cancers with preoperative facial nerve paralysis, and all recurrent malignant tumors.

Inflammation. Acute facial palsies secondary to inflammation (e.g., bacterial, viral, and metabolic) are extremely rare. Inflammatory lesions are, as a rule, always intracranial and intratemporal. The former is a result of involvement of the neurons and the latter is caused by secondary pressure and ischemia.

INVESTIGATION OF ACUTE FACIAL PALSY

All patients with acute facial palsy should undergo a full and thorough investigation to confirm diagnosis, to identify the site of the lesion, and to determine if surgery is indicated. These steps begin with a full history and physical examination. A specific medical history concerned with the palsy will assist in diagnosing the extent and site of the lesion. The duration and nature of onset, the time interval since onset, and any associated symptoms such as pain, hyperacusis, and disorders of lacrimation are important factors. A past history of injury, paralysis, or illness and a pertinent family history may contribute to the work-up and management. A complete and thorough examination should then be performed. General examination should be followed by examination of both the normal and the abnormal facial nerves and their muscles.

With the face in repose, motor function is examined for symmetry and deformity, e.g., the height and width of the palpebral fissure and the position of the mouth, particularly the commissure of the mouth. The brow and nasolabial landmarks are checked. This step is followed by dynamic movement of the basic facial muscles individually and in unison. The range and excursion of movement are checked by observation and palpation. Signs of atrophy, fasciculation, fibrosis of muscles, and so forth are noted.

Sensory testing follows and is usually confined to taste only. Special investigations for acute facial palsy are then carried out. Most of these tests have been used primarily for Bell's palsy but are also essential in all other forms of facial palsy. They are divided into two groups: (1) topographic tests of facial nerve function and (2) electrodiagnostic tests.

Topographic Tests

Lacrimation. Schirmer's test is used to compare the normal and the paralyzed side. A decrease of 25% or less in tear production compared with tear production on the normal side is regarded as significantly abnormal. While this test may vary with the amount of the degeneration of the affected facial nerve, palsy from traumatic injuries shows significant unilateral reduction of tear flow.[65] This test is complicated by lesions such as acoustic neuroma, which may have an irritative effect leading to increased lacrimation.[66]

Stapedius Reflex Tests. An impedance bridge is sealed in the external canal of the ear being tested and a sound is presented to the opposite ear until a level sufficient to elicit reflex contraction for both stapedius muscles is reached. If the facial nerve is intact proximal to the stapedius branch, the muscle will contract. This test, however, depends on intact conduction hearing of both ears. The stapedius reflex can be measured by altered acoustic impedance followed by strong acoustic stimulation. If perceptive deafness is present, a nonacoustic reflex can be elicited by unilateral electrical stimulation to the external auditory canal. According to Koike et al.,[67] this test is totally objective and allows good correlation between prognosis of palsy and time of stapedius reflex recovery.

Electrogustometry. If the facial nerve is intact down to and including the level at which the chorda tympani comes off, taste on the anterior two thirds of the affected side will be intact and can be tested chemically or electrically. This procedure was developed by Krarup[68] and Pulec and House[69] and involves the application of a small anodal galvanic current to the surface of the tongue. The minimal current, detected subjectively by the patient as a metallic taste, is called the electrogustometric threshold. An increase of 100% or more is considered pathologic.[70]

Salivary Flow and pH Test. Wharton's ducts on both sides are cannulated and saliva is collected over a fixed period of time. A flow of 25% is indicative of damage and, according to May et al.,[71] predicts a poor prognosis and is an indication for surgical exploration. Saito et al.[72] claimed that the pH is directly proportional to the volume of saliva. A low pH is consistent with a decrease or the absence of activity of the chorda tympani. This test is valuable only in the first few days, before electrical testing becomes abnormal in Bell's palsy. After that, the results of salivary flow testing should not be relied upon. With these tests it is possible to determine accurately whether the lesion of an acute facial palsy is extra- or intratem-

poral. In addition, the site of an intratemporal lesion can be identified.

Electrodiagnostic Tests

Electrodiagnostic tests study the function of neuromuscular structure. They will assist in determining if an affected nerve is completely or partially degenerated, if the injury is reversible, and if surgery is indicated. The tests include the following:

Nerve Excitability Test. This procedure involves stimulation of the facial nerve percutaneously at the angle of the jaw. Short-duration current is used with increasing intensity until a threshold contraction is seen. Both the affected and the normal sides are tested and compared. A facial nerve undergoing Wallerian degeneration will lose its conduction after 72 hours, whereas a nerve with neurapraxia will continue to conduct with high intensity. A difference of 3.5 mA or more is regarded as abnormal and warrants daily repeated testing until recovery begins. An increase of 20 mA or more indicates that definite degeneration has occurred and that complete recovery is unlikely.[73] This test should be performed on day one of the injury. A modification by May, called the maximal excitability test, uses maximal rather than minimal stimulation and was reported to be a more reliable guide to prognosis.[74] In extratemporal lesions, stimulation of the nerve proximal to a divided nerve will not conduct and the nerve should be explored and/or repaired. The point of stimulation can be moved distally past the site of the lesion in other instances of extratemporal nerve injury.

Electromyography. A needle electrode is introduced into the affected muscle and a signal is recorded. The pattern will distinguish a muscle that is normal from one that is denervated. Myopathies affecting the muscle can also be detected. The limitation of this test is that denervation patterns will only appear 14 to 21 days after injury. It also gives no quantitative indication of the amount of degenerated muscle. However, it is a good test for follow-up and for determining signs of regeneration. Granger[75] used it to predict prognosis in Bell's palsy.

Nerve Conduction Study. This test combines electromyography (EMG) and nerve stimulation and calculates the conduction time or velocity. With Wallerian degeneration, the conduction time is seldom delayed unless degeneration is severe. However, with neurotmesis, no conduction is seen. This test is particularly helpful in extratemporal lesions, as it can be used to test each facial muscle group in turn. The test has been modified by Esslen[76] to be used as electroneurography, i.e., supramaximal stimulation and registration of summation potential by an electrode, to predict prognosis for Bell's palsy and as an indication for decompression.

Trigeminal–Facial Nerve Reflex. This test is useful in acute facial palsy to predict prognosis. In particular, study of the blink reflex has been standardized by Kimura et al.[77] The earlier the blink reflex returns to normal in Bell's palsy, the more complete the recovery of facial nerve function.

Radiology

The use of radiology is particularly important in lesions of the intracranial or intratemporal segment of the facial nerve. For extratemporal lesions, radiologic studies can be used to exclude intratemporal causes as well as to identify acute facial palsy secondary to a fractured mandible. As a general rule, plain x-rays of the skull will demonstrate lesions such as acoustic neuroma and meningoma and will outline the bony canal and destructive lesions involving bone that may lead to facial paralysis. Special views such as Towne and 20° oblique are useful for areas around the geniculate ganglion and the horizontal segment of the facial nerve canal.[78] Tomography is more accurate in locating the exact pathologic site and in defining fractures. In particular, coronal tomography is used for transverse fractures and lateral tomography is used for longitudinal fractures of the temporal bone. Other indicated radiologic studies may include mandibular views such as panoral and oblique views of the mandible and angiography and computed tomography for intracranial lesions.

Documentation

An essential part of assessment is that of documentation of the exact deficit in acute facial palsy, which should be performed during the first assessment of the patient if possible. For a traumatic situation, brief documentation is done preoperatively and again during the postoperative period. If nerve repair is not done, documentation can be performed immediately postoperatively when the patient's general condition is stable and permits the procedure. If, however, nerve repair has been carried out, documentation is done about 3 weeks postoperatively. Two weeks are allowed for the site of nerve repair to consolidate, and 1 week is allowed to mobilize the muscle that was not damaged but was kept at rest during the preceding 2 weeks. Documentation will assist in progress assessment, as well as comparison of results and long-term evaluation of different methods of treatment.

Since 1955, various attempts have been made to standardize the reporting of facial palsy results. Jenssen[79] used a point percentage system, which includes symmetry as well as the three regions of the face in dynamic function, i.e., forehead, eyes, and mouth. This system has been the basis of many later studies, e.g., Jonkees.[80] Determination of the strength grade of muscle was advocated by Granger,[81] but this is difficult and not practical. May[82] suggested a more complete system based on the dynamic motion of main facial muscle groups and division of the groups into ten facial functions. In addition, Adour and Swanson[84] used minus points for complications and compiled a Facial Paralysis Recovery Index. Miehlke et al.[85] suggested a system based on a paralysis score as well as a secondary defect score. This system is essentially the basis of our documentation. In addition, we use life-sized photographic documentation of the paralysis and the defect. We have also started to make video tape recordings of the patient. However, the future may be in three-dimensional computerized documentation.

In addition to preoperative and postoperative documentation, intraoperative records are made. At exploration, the damaged nerve or nerve branches are identified and carefully mapped out using an electrodiagnostic stimulator. A complete view of the damaged nerve and branches and the method of repair are recorded by color photography as well as by diagrams.

TREATMENT

Before starting specific treatment, the patient must first be treated as a whole. Any other injuries are assessed and treated according to a plan of priority, e.g., a head injury will be treated before a facial nerve injury. The cause of the acute facial palsy must be confirmed and treated medically if possible. This step is followed by proper diagnosis of the facial nerve problem and planning of surgery if indicated. The timing of surgery is critical.

1. Immediate surgery: It is now recognized that facial nerve repair should be performed immediately if possible. This is particularly true following trauma and tumor excision. If surgery is not delayed, there is no scar and the nerve stumps are easily identified with a good possibility of realignment of the corresponding fascicles. Minimal shortening and resection of the nerve are required, making end-to-end anastomosis more likely. Immediate repair can be carried out only if there are no complicating factors, e.g., a patient who is a poor general risk or who has a contaminated wound, extensive tissue destruction, high velocity injuries, and so forth.

2. Delayed repair: Delayed surgery should be considered in patients with extensive injuries and wound contamination. An interval of 3 weeks will enable more accurate evaluation of the amount of nerve and tissue damage and will also allow control of infection. At the same time, fibrosis is still not prominent, and neuroma formation is only just beginning. After 3 weeks, repair should be carried out as soon as possible. The quality of the result deteriorates in proportion to the period of delay because of contraction of the distal nerve tubules, thickening of the muscle membrane, proximal neuroma formation, fibrous tissue, Schwann cell proliferation, and loss of regenerating neurofibral elements from the proximal stump. Twelve months is usually the time limit for repair of the facial nerve if good results are to be expected because of end stage fibrosis of the muscle. Provided some innervation is present, good results can occasionally be seen as late as 2 to 3 years after loss of facial movement.[83] Study of degenerative changes in the severed human facial nerve confirmed that the distal stump collagenization was not greater after 30 months' degeneration than after 3 months' degeneration.[86]

Three main factors involving extratemporal facial nerve repair should be considered, as they have a major influence on results of this repair.[87]

1. The level of injury: The more distal the injury, the better the functional return and the less the secondary defect. This fact has been discussed earlier in regard to intraneural topography. Proximal injury will also decrease the number and the quality of the regenerating axons.

2. The prevailing biologic condition: The biologic condition is related to many factors that apply to the specific nerve to be repaired. These include the cause of the paralysis, the level of injury, the amount of damage and tissue loss, the vascularity of the bed where repair is carried out, and the age, general health, and nutritional condition of the patient. Also important are factors such as previous or impending postoperative radiotherapy. The effect of radiotherapy is still controversial. Conley[88] and Miehlke et al.[89] concluded that the effect of radiotherapy on nerve grafting is negligible. On the other hand, Lathrop,[90] McQuirt and McCabe,[91] and Pillsbury and Fisch[92] showed significantly poorer results following radiotherapy and concluded that a nerve graft is not indicated in areas where radiotherapy is planned.

3. Technique of repair: Advances in surgery have resulted from use of magnification and atraumatic technique and avoidance of factors causing fibrosis. Nerve repair is divided into three aspects: (a) Preparation of the nerve end or graft end and adequate excision of the proximal and distal stumps— Tension is avoided at all times, and the epineurium is excised. (b) Coaptation—This technique involves the careful and proper alignment of nerve ends and the use of a nerve graft of adequate quantity to provide a sufficient amount of nerve tissue as a graft. The use of tubes and adhesives has not been shown to be beneficial. (c) Suture material— The use of a minimal number and thickness of suture material is important. Postoperative care is essential if such minimal fine sutures are used so that the fibrin seal between the nerve ends will adequately consolidate and maintain the anastomotic site in position.

All three principles have been extensively investigated and summarized by Millesi.[93] The value of perineurial sutures and the applicability of interfascicular repair for the facial nerve have been studied by Rouleau et al.,[94] Crumley,[95] and Hagan,[96] and favorable results have been reported in perineurial repair.

Method of Repair

Direct End-to-end Anastomosis. If applicable, this method gives the best result. It is particularly effective with a sharp, clean division that is repaired immediately.

Nerve Graft. When loss of a segment of nerve occurs as a result of injury, a nerve graft will be the procedure of choice. Conley[97] has shown that some degree and quality of improvement will occur in 95% of optimal cases following the procedure. This graft could be interpositional from the proximal nerve end on the same side, as is commonly used, or from a contralateral cross-facial nerve graft, as described by Scaramella,[98] Smith,[99] and Anderl.[100]

Cross-over Nerve Graft. An extensive series by Conley and Baker[101] has shown that this procedure is useful in cases of acute facial nerve palsy. However, because of the resulting mass movement, abnormal inappropriate features, absence of spontaneous affective expression, and sacrifice of normal function of the muscles supplied by the donor nerve, this procedure should be reserved as a back-up in cases in which multiple stage surgery is contraindicated.

Direct Neurotization. This method has not had any definitive proof of advances since Cardwell[52] first carried out direct neurotization in 1938. However, it is used in cases in which the distal nerve stumps are not available (to be discussed).

Nerve-Muscle Pedicle Graft. This procedure has problems similar to those of crossover nerve grafts and is suitable for cases in which multiple long procedures are contraindicated.[102]

No Repair. In the last 30 years, many authors have reported spontaneous return of movement after resection of the facial nerve.[103–107] At present, this phenomenon is still unexplained. Various theories exist, including open field regeneration, cross innervation from trigeminal nerve branches, contralateral innervation, myoneurotization, and other accessory pathways. It is interesting to note that most of the reported cases followed resection of the facial nerve in extratemporal regions without interfering with the intracranial or the intratemporal region. The results of Martin and Hapster[104] showed that approximately 28.5% of their patients had some return of motion. However, this figure is not sufficiently high to justify not doing a repair in view of the excellent results achieved with facial nerve grafting.[108]

Clinical Situations

1. Both proximal and distal nerve stumps are available for repair: In such a situation, direct anastomosis of the injured nerve ends should be carried out if possible. However, with loss of a segment, nerve grafting should be used. The facial nerve proximal stump should be available for repair in most cases of extratemporal facial palsy. Every effort should be made to identify and secure this proximal stump, as it will provide better results than any other alternative. This may require the help and cooperation of an otolaryngologist for the intratemporal dissection or a neurosurgeon for the intracranial segment of the facial motor nerve.

2. Only the distal nerve stump is available: In these cases, a cross-facial nerve should be considered first. In cases in which multiple prolonged surgical procedures are contraindicated, a crossover nerve or pedicle transfer should be considered.

3. Only the proximal nerve stump is available: An attempt should be made to neurotize the facial muscles directly, using nerve grafts. If no result is obtained, the same nerve grafts can be used later to innervate new motor units, i.e., free vascularized muscle to reanimate facial movement.

Postoperative Care

Following repair of the extratemporal facial nerve, postoperative care begins in the operating room at the time of repair or reconstruction. Millesi has shown that a significant number of nerve graft failures have been the result of improper handling of the graft site in the immediate postoperative period. Therefore, all manipulation, torsion, and shear forces around the repair site must be avoided. Proper measures should be taken to prevent hematoma and infection. The patient should be brought out of anesthesia gently, without undue movement, coughing, or struggle. Once the patient awakes, the movement of the face is avoided by sedation in a quiet, dark room. Oral functions, such as talking or food intake, should not be carried out for at least 48 hours, and only a minimal amount of movements should be allowed until 5 days later. All these factors will have to be carefully explained to the patient in the preoperative assessment period.

After 2 weeks, massage of the skin incision or wound, as well as the site of repair and anastomosis, is begun to soften the area and discourage excessive scar formation and adhesions. Nerve stimulation has not been proved to be of benefit to axonal growth, although direct muscle stimulation may retard the degeneration atrophy of striated muscle.[109] It also has a psychological benefit, as the patient sees the muscles move under stimulation. Each case should be assessed individually concerning the use of postoperative nerve stimulation. Regular follow-up is important and a repeat EMG is performed when the nerve has progressed clinically to the muscles. This can be identified using the Tinel sign.

Once the muscles have been innervated, intensive physical therapy consisting of facial muscle exercise,[22] neuro re-education of facial muscles, and biofeedback[110] should be carried out to stimulate and control movements of the reinnervated muscles. Finally, documentation that had been decided preoperatively is carried out.

The total follow-up period should be at least 2 years for assessment of results. Present evidence shows that the facial nerve continues to improve for many years following repair procedures.

References

1. Diamond, C., and Frew, I.: The Facial Nerve. New York, Oxford University Press, 1979, p. 3.
2. Hollinshead, W. H.: Anatomy for Surgeons. Vol. 1. The Head and Neck. New York, Hoeper-Harper, 1954.
3. Baxter, A.: The lesions of the fallopian canal: an anatomical study. J. Larynogol., 85:587, 1971.
4. Wright, J. W., and Taylor, Z. E.: Trigeminal facial nerve abnormalities revealed by polytomography. Arch. Otolaryngol., 95:426, 1972.
5. Fowler, E. P.: Variation in the temporal bone course of the facial nerve. Laryngoscope, 71:937, 1961.
6. Crabtree, J. A.: The facial nerve in congenital ear surgery. Otolaryngol. Clin. North Am., 7:505, 1974.
7. Blair, V. P.: Surgery of the Mouth and Jaws. 1st Ed. St. Louis, C. V. Mosby Company, 1912.
8. Janes, R. M.: Surgical treatment of tumors of salivary gland. Surg. Clin. North Am., 23:1429, 1943.
9. Martin, H.: Operative removal of tumors of the parotid salivary gland. Surgery, 31:670, 1952.
10. Conley, J. J.: Surgical treatment of tumors of the parotid gland with emphasis on immediate nerve grafting. West. J. Surg., 63:534, 1965.
11. Maxwell, J. H., Buxton, R. W., and French, A. J.: The surgical treatment of parotid gland tumors. Am. Acad. Ophthalmol., 57:711, 1953.
12. Lathrop, F. D.: Management of the facial nerve during operation on the parotid gland. Ann. Otol., 62:780, 1963.
13. Byars, L. T.: Preservation of the facial nerve in operations for denying conditions of the parotid area. Ann. Surg., 136:412, 1952.
14. Kidd, H. A.: Complete excision of the parotid gland with preservation of the facial nerve. Br. Med. J., 1:989, 1950.
15. Bailey, H.: The treatment of tumors of the parotid gland with facial reference to total parotidectomy. Br. J. Surg., 28:336, 1941.
16. Sistonk, W. E.: Mixed tumors of the parotid gland. Minn. Med., 4:155, 1921.
17. Riesner, D.: Surgical procedures in tumors of the parotid gland. Arch. Surg., 65:831, 1952.
18. McNealy, R. W., and McCallister, J. W. M.: Parotid gland tumors and their surgical management. J. Surg., 83:648, 1952.
19. Hogg, S. P., and Kratz, R. C.: Surgical exposure of the facial nerve. Arch. Otolaryngol., 67:560, 1958.
20. Shapiro, H. H.: Maxillo-facial Anatomy. Philadelphia, J. B. Lippincott Company, 1954.
21. Davies, R. A., Anson, B. J., and Budinger, J. M.: Surgical anatomy of the facial nerve and parotid gland based upon 350 cervical facial halves. J. Surg. Gynecol. Obstet., 1:385, 1956.
22. Miehlke, A., Stennart, E., and Chilla, R.: New aspects in facial nerve surgery. Clin. Plast. Surg., 6:451, 1979.
23. Miehlke, A., and Stennart, E.: New techniques for optimum reconstruction of the facial nerve in its temporal course. Acta Otolaryngol., 91:497, 1981.
24. Sunderland, S.: Some anatomical and pathophysiological data relative to facial nerve injury repair. In Fisch, U. (ed.): Facial Nerve Surgery. Birmingham, Ala., Aesculapius Publishing Company, 1977, pp. 47–61.
25. Meissl, G., and Millesi, H.: Nerve suture and grafting to restore extratemporal facial nerve. Clin. Plast. Surg., 6:335, 1977.
26. May, M.: Facial paralysis peripheral type: A proposed method of reporting. Laryngoscope, 80:331, 1917.
27. May, M.: Anatomy of the facial nerve (spatial orientation of fibers in the temporal bone). Laryngoscope, 82:1311, 1973.
28. Mihelke, A.: Normal and anomalous anatomy of the facial nerve. Trans. Acad. Ophthalomol. Otolaryngol., 68:1013, 1964.
29. Sunderland, S., and Cossar, D. F.: Structure of the facial nerve. Anat. Rec., 116:147, 1953.
30. Fisch, U., and Esslen, E.: The Acute Facial Palsies. Berlin, Springer-Verlag, 1977, p. 8.
31. Thomander, L.: The topographic organization of the facial nerve. In Graham, M., and House, W. (eds.): Disorders of the Facial Nerve. New York, Raven Press, 1982.
32. Crumley, R. L.: Spatial anatomy of the facial nerve fibers—a preliminary report. Laryngoscope, 90:274, 1980.
33. Fisch, U.: Facial nerve grafting. Otolaryngol. Clin. North Am., 7:517, 1974.

34. Sunderland, S.: Nerve and Nerve Injuries, Vol. 1. Edinburgh, Churchill Livingstone, 1968, p. 35.

35. Karnes, W. E.: Diseases of the 7th Cranial Nerve. *In* Dyck, P., Thomas, P. K., and Lambert, E. H. (ed.). Peripheral Neuropathy, Vol. 1. Philadelphia, W. B. Saunders Company, 1975, p. 573.

36. Blunt, M. J.: Blood supply of the facial nerve. J. Anat., *88*:520, 1954.

37. Anson, B. J., Donaldson, J. A., Warpeha, L., and Rensink, M. J.: The facial nerve sheath blood supply in relation to the surgery of decompression. Ann. Rhinolaryngol., *79*:710, 1970.

38. Bell, C.: The anatomy of the facial nerve. Philos. Trans. R. Soc., 1927.

39. Drobnik: Beschrieben durch S. Bromias. *In* L'Ethe Actuel de la Chirurgie Nerveus II. Paris: J. Ruess, 1902.

40. Ballance, C.: Results obtained in some experiments in which the facial and recurrent laryngeal nerves were anastomosed with each other. Br. Med. J., *2*:349, 1924.

41. Manasse, P.: Uber Vereinigung des N. facialis mit den N. accessorius durch die Nervenpsropfung [Gresse nerveuse] Arch. Klin Chir., *62*:805, 1900.

42. Bunnell, F.: Suture of facial nerve within the temporal bone, with report of very successful case. Surg. Gynecol. Obstet., *45*:7, 1927.

43. Martin, R. C.: Intratemporal suture of the facial nerve. Arch. Otolaryngol., *13*:259, 1931.

44. Ballance, C., and Udel, A. B.: The operative treatment of facial palsy by introduction of nerve grafts in the fallopian canal and by other intratemporal methods. Arch. Otolaryngol., *15*:1, 1932.

45. Cawthorne, T. Quoted from Shambauth, G. E.: History of facial nerve surgery. *In* Fisch, U. (ed.): Facial Nerve Surgery. Birmingham, Ala., Aesculapius Publishing Company, 1977, p. 2.

46. Wullstein: Quoted from Miehlke, A.: A history of the facial nerve. *In* Miehlke, A. (ed.): Surgery of the Facial Nerve, 2nd Ed. Philadelphia, W. B. Saunders Company, 1973, p. 6.

47. House, W. F., and Crabtree, J. A.: Surgical exposure of the petrous portion of the seventh nerve. Arch. Otolaryngol., *81*:506, 1965.

48. Pulec, J. L.: Total decompression of the facial nerve. Laryngoscope, *76*:1015, 1966.

49. Fisch, U., and Esselen, E.: Total intratemporal exposure of the facial nerve. Arch. Otolaryngol., *95*:335, 1972.

50. Duel, A. B.: Advanced methods in surgical treatment of facial paralysis. Ann. Otorhinol. Laryngol., *43*:76, 1934.

51. Bunnell, F.: Surgical repair of the facial nerve. Arch. Otolaryngol., *25*:235, 1937.

52. Cardwell, E. T.: Direct implantation of free nerve grafts between facial musculature and facial trunk. Arch. Otolaryngol., *27*:469, 1938.

53. Maxwell, J. H., Buxton, R. W., and French, A. J.: The surgical treatment of the parotid gland tumors. Trans. Acad. Ophthalmol. Otolaryngol., *57*:711, 1953.

54. Lathrop, F. D.: Management of traumatic lesions of the facial nerve. Arch. Otolaryngol. *55*:410, 1955.

55. Conley, J., and Miehlke, A.: Quoted from Techniques of extratemporal nerve surgery. *In* Miehlke, A. (ed.): Surgery of the Facial Nerve, 2nd Ed. Philadelphia, W. B. Saunders Company, 1973, pp. 147–174.

56. Huizing, E. H., Mechelse, K., and Staal, A.: Treat-ment of Bell's palsy and analysis of the available study. Acta Otolaryngol., *92*:115, 1981.

57. Goin, D. W.: Facial nerve paralysis secondary to mandibular fracture. Laryngoscope, *19*:1777, 1980.

58. Lindeman, R. C.: Temporal bone trauma in facial paralysis. Otolaryngol. Clin. North Am., *12*:403, 1979.

59. Conley, J., and Janecka, I.: Neurilemmona of the facial nerve. Plast. Reconstr. Surg., *52*:55, 1973.

60. Ruthoos, D., Byars, L. T., and Ackermann, L. T.: Neurilemonas of facial nerve presenting as neurotic gland tumor. Ann. Surg., *144*:258, 1956.

61. Hingorani, R.: Neurilemmona of facial nerves. J. Laryngo-Otolaryngol., *84*:1275, 1970.

62. Lavenuta, F., Flynn, W., and Moore, J.: Facial nerve paralysis secondary to benign parotid tumor. Arch. Otolaryngol., *88*:603, 1969.

63. Conley, J.: Technique of extratemporal facial nerve surgery. *In* Miehlke, A. (ed.): Surgery of the Facial Nerve, 2nd Ed. Philadelphia, W. B. Saunders Company, 1973, p. 147.

64. Eneroth, C. M.: The parotid tumors in facial nerves. *In* Miehlke, A. (ed.): Surgery of the Facial Nerve, 2nd Ed. Philadelphia, W. B. Saunders Company, 1973, p. 109.

65. Fische, U.: Lacrimation. *In* Fisch, U. (ed.): Facial Nerve Surgery. Birmingham, Ala., Aesculapius Publishing Company, 1977, pp. 147–153.

66. Morrison, A. W.: Management of Sensorineural Deafness. London, Butterworth, 1975, p. 68.

67. Koike, Y., Ohojo, K., and Iwasaki, E.: Prognosis of facial palsy based on the stapedial reflex tests. *In* Fisch, U. (ed.): Facial Nerve Surgery. Birmingham, Ala., Aesculapius Publishing Company, pp. 159–164.

68. Krarup, B.: Electro-gustometry: A method for clinical case examination. Acta Otolaryngol., *49*:294, 1958.

69. Pulec, J. L., and House, W. F.: Facial test in the early diagnosis of acute acoustic neuromas. Laryngoscope, *74*:118, 1964.

70. Morgen, F.: Electrically evoked case threshold. Ann. Otolaryngol. *85*:359, 1976.

71. May, M., Lucente, F. E., Harvey, J. E., et al.: Salivation test in traumatic facial paralysis. Ann. Otolaryngol., *82*:17, 1973.

72. Saito, H., Higashitsuji, J., Kishimoto, S., Miya-moto, K., and Kitamura, H.: Mandibular salivary pH as a diagnostic aid for prognosis of facial palsy. Laryngoscope, *88*:663, 1978.

73. Jongkees, L. B. W.: Nerve excitability test. *In* Fisch, U. (ed.): Facial Nerve Surgery. Birmingham, Ala., Aesculapius Publishing Company, 1977, pp. 83–86.

74. May, M., et al.: The prognostic accuracy of the maximal stimulation compared with that of the nerve excitibility test in Bell's palsy. Laryngoscope, *81*:931, 1971.

75. Granger, C. B.: Towards an earlier forecast of recovery in Bell's palsy. Arch. Phys. Med. Rehab., *48*:273, 1967.

76. Esslen, E.: Electromyography and electroneurog-raphy. *In* Fisch, U. (ed.): Facial Nerves Surgery. Birmingham, Ala., Aesculapius Publishing Company, 1977, pp. 93–100.

77. Kimura, J., Giron, L. T., and Young, S. M.: Electrophysiology study of Bell's palsy. Electrically elicited blink reflex in assessment of prognosis. Arch. Otolaryngol., *102*:140, 1976.

78. Potter, G. B.: Radiologic assessment of the facial

nerve. Otolaryngol. Clin. North Am., 7:343, 1974.

79. Jenssen, S. O.: Over be postoperatieve facialis-berlamming, Thesis, University of Amsterdam, 1963.

80. Jongkees, L. B. W.: Decompression of the facial nerve. Arch. Laryngol. (Special Section), 1967, pp. 473–478.

81. Granger, C. B.: Towards an earlier forecast of recovery in Bell's palsy. Arch. Phys. Med. Rehab., 48:273, 1967.

82. May, M.: Facial paralysis, peripheral type: A proposed method of reporting. Laryngoscope, 86:331, 1970.

83. Conley, J., et al.: Longstanding facial paralysis rehabilitation. Laryngoscope, 84:2155, 1974.

84. Adour, K. K., and Swanson, P. J. Jr.: Facial paralysis in 403 consecutive patients. Emphasis on treatment response in patients with Bell's palsy. Am. Acad. Neuro-Otolaryngol., 75:1284, 1971.

85. Miehlke, A., Stennart, E., and Chilla, R.: New aspects in facial nerve surgery. Clin. Plast. Surg., 6:451, 1979.

86. Ylikoski, J., Hitfelberger, W. E., House, W. S., and Sanna, M.: Degenerative changes in the distal stump of the severed human facial nerve. Acta Otolaryngol., 92:239, 1981.

87. Conley, J.: Panel discussion No. 5: Factors influencing results in extratemporal facial nerve repair. Moderator, J. Conley. In Fisch, U. (ed.): Facial Nerve Surgery. Birmingham, Ala., Aesculapius Publishing Company, 1977, p. 216.

88. Conley, J.: Facial nerve grafting. Arch. Otolaryngol., 73:322, 1961.

89. Miehlke, A., Stannart, E., Schuster, R. F. O., et al.: Ueber die Regeneration derpher Nerven nach Einwilkung ionisieibender Strahlen. ORL, 98:88, 1972.

90. Lathrop, F. D.: Management of the facial nerves during operation of the parotid gland. Ann. Otolaryngol., 72:780, 1963.

91. McGuirt, W. F., and McCabe, B. F.: The effect of radiation therapy on facial nerve cable autogram. Laryngoscope, 87:4154, 1977.

92. Pillsbury, A. C., and Fisch, U.: Extratemporal facial nerve grafting in radiotherapy. Otolaryngol., 105:441, 1979.

93. Millesi, H.: Nerve suture and grafting to restore extratemporal facial nerve. Clin. Plast. Surg., 6:333, 1979.

94. Rouleau, M., Crepeau, J., Tetreualt, L., and Lamarche, J.: Facial nerve suture at the epineural versus perineural sutures. Otolaryngol., 10:338, 1981.

95. Crumley, R.: Interfascicular nerve repair. Arch. Otolaryngol., 106:313, 1980.

96. Hagan, W. H.: Microneuro techniques for nerve grafting. Laryngoscope, 91:1759, 1981.

97. Conley, J.: Facial nerve grafting In Fisch, U. (ed.): Facial Nerve Surgery. Birmingham, Ala., Aesculapius Publishing Company, 1977, pp. 206–208.

98. Scaramella, L.: L'anastomostosi tra i due ner i facial i. Arch. Otolaryngol., 82:209, 1971.

99. Smith, J. W.: A new technique of facial animation. Transactions of the Fifth International Congress of Plastic Reconstructive Surgery. Chadswick, New South Wales, Australia, 1971. London, Butterworths, 1971.

100. Anderl, H.: Cross facial nerve transplantation in facial palsy (principal and further experience). Transactions of the Sixth International Congress of Plastic and Reconstructive Surgery, Paris, 1975. Paris Manson, 1975.

101. Conley, J., and Baker, D. C.: Hypoglossal facial nerve anastomoses for rehabilitation in facial paralysis. Plast. Reconstr. Surg., 63:66, 1979.

102. Tucker, H. M.: Restoration of selective facial nerve function by the nerve-muscle pedicle technique. Clin. Plast. Surg., 6:293, 1979.

103. Conley, J., Papper, E. M., and Kaplan, N.: Spontaneous return and facial nerve grafting. Arch. Otolaryngol., 77:89, 1963.

104. Martin, H., and Helsper, J.: Spontaneous return of function following surgical section or excision of the seventh cranial nerve in the surgery of parotid tumor. Ann. Surg., 146:715, 1957.

105. McCoy, E. G., and Boyle, W. F.: Reinnervation of the facial muscle following extratemporal nerve resection. Laryngoscope, 81:1, 1971.

106. Trojaborg, W., and Siemssem, S.: Reinnervation after resection of the facial nerve. Arch. Neurol., 26:17, 1972.

107. Norris, C. W., and Proud, G. O.: Spontaneous return of facial motion following seventh cranial nerve resection. Laryngoscope, 91:211, 1981.

108. Conley, J., and Baker, D.: The surgical treatment of extratemporal facial paralysis: An overview. Head Neck Surg., 1:12, 1978.

109. Post, C. F.: Value of galvanic muscle stimulation immediately after paralysis. In Rubin, L. R. (ed.): Reanimation of the Paralyzed Face. St. Louis, C. V. Mosby Company, 1977, pp. 194–200.

110. Brown, D. M., Nnahai, F., Wolf, S., and Basmagian, J. V.: Electromyographic biofeedback in the reeducation of facial palsy. Am. J. Phys. Med., 57:13, 1978.

111. Sunderland, S.: Function of nerve fibers whose structure has been disorganized. Anat. Rec., 109:503, 1951.

112. Seddon, H. J., Medawar, P. B., and Smith, H.: Rate of regeneration of peripheral nerves in man. J. Physiol., 102:191, 1943.

43

Cross-Facial Nerve Grafting
■
Marcus Castro Ferreira, M.D.

The surgical treatment of the facial palsy remains a challenging issue despite the number of techniques devised to obtain reanimation of the facial muscles. One technique, that of cross-facial nerve grafting, was first described in the last decade[1, 10, 11] and has given rise to some controversy. We have used cross-facial nerve grafts in 38 patients since 1975, [3, 4] and an account of this experience will be reviewed here.

OPERATIVE TECHNIQUE

Cross-facial nerve grafting can be performed in one or two stages (Fig. 43–1). Although no conclusive data have been reported showing significant differences in the final result, most authors prefer the two-stage procedure. We agree that there are some advantages to this latter technique:

1. The one-stage operation is much longer and accuracy may decrease at the end of the procedure, when matching the nerve stumps on the paralyzed side is performed.

2. The distal stump of the graft can be observed directly at the second stage, and a more precise evaluation of its condition can therefore be made.

3. The decision whether to suture the nerve graft to the facial nerve or to use it to reinnervate a muscle transfer can be postponed until the second stage, when another evaluation of the state of the denervated facial muscles can be made.

First Stage

One incision is made on the skin of the nonparalyzed side lateral to the nasolabial fold in order to obtain good exposure of the

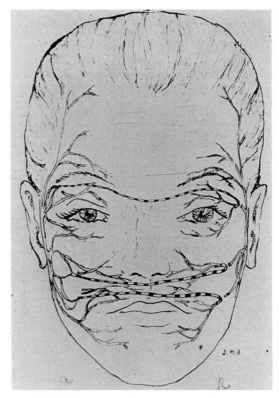

Figure 43–1. Cross-facial nerve grafting. (From Ferreira, M. C.: Clin. Plast. Surg., *11*:212, 1984.)

fat pad of Bichat, which is a point of reference for finding the buccal plexus of the facial nerve (Fig. 43–2). (The anatomy of this plexus was studied by Le-Quang,[8] who showed that the plexus was formed by the buccal branches of the facial nerve and that there are a number of anatomic variations.) We have found that a nerve stimulator is very useful for identifying the distal divisions of the upper and lower buccal branches and separating them by their area of innervation. There are often two or three buccal branches going upward, supplying the muscles connected to the upper lip and the external aperture of the nose. The branch situated more cranially also supplies muscles on the zygomatic branch, such as the orbicularis oculi and the corrugator. This branch is the one we usually select, as its cross-section size is similar to that of the sural nerve graft.

It should be noted that the division of this branch does not produce a significant paralysis on the "normal" side. If a selective neurectomy is desirable,[2] as is often the case with long-standing palsies, other distal branches should be interrupted. Even then, significant weakness may not be achieved, as a few intact nerves could remain that were not recognized during surgery.

The lower buccal branch also has two or three subdivisions and receives communicating branches from the upper buccal branch and from the marginal mandibular nerve. Two subdivisions are usually selected to be sutured to another segment of the sural nerve.

In early cases, when reinnervation of the paralyzed orbicularis oculi can still be expected, another incision can be made over the lateral part of the orbit. The zygomatic and temporal branches are then dissected and sutured to a third nerve graft.

More often, only the two grafts on buccal branches are performed. A whole sural nerve is taken, divided, and pushed through a subcutaneous tunnel across the upper lip up to the paralyzed side, where it is anchored to the dermis as close as possible to the ear.

Meticulous microsurgical approximation of the facial branch stumps and the nerve grafts should be made in order to assure the best reinnervation possible on the nerve graft (Fig. 43–3). A good end-to-end neurorrhaphy is obtained with the upper branch, and the two lower divisions should be accommodated with the other segment of sural nerve.

Second Stage

Four to six months later, a modified rhytidectomy approach is used on the paralyzed side in order to expose the nerve graft stumps. Although there is often scarring around the grafts, it is not difficult to dissect the scars out.

The neuromas are then inspected under the surgical microscope and transected. In the great majority of cases, the pattern suggests a normal nerve (Fig. 43–4). Histologic study reveals nerve fibers surrounded by a proliferation of connective tissue. Information about the number and form of the regenerated fibers, as compared with the nor-

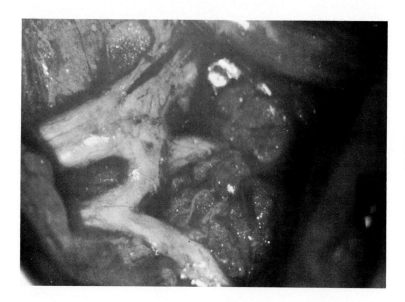

Figure 43–2. View of the buccal plexus of the facial nerve. Magnification about 10 ×.

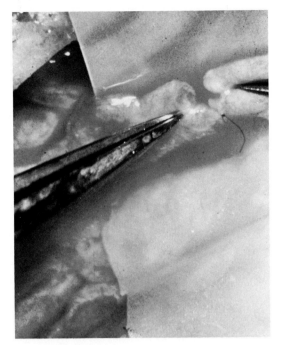

Figure 43–3. Microsurgical suture of the facial nerve branch to the graft.

mal sural nerve pattern, is scarce. Our preliminary studies showed a reduced number of fibers with individual variations, but the nerve graft connected with the upper buccal branch usually repopulates better than the other grafts.

If suture to the facial nerve is decided, the buccal and zygomatic branches are dissected where they leave the parotid gland. They are divided and their distal part is sutured to the nerve graft using microsurgical technique. If a muscle transfer is preferred, the nerve grafts are sutured either to the motor nerve of the transplanted muscle or directly to the muscle itself (neurotization).

INDICATIONS

Facial palsy can be classified according to several criteria, but from the point of view of the surgeon, three factors are important in deciding the type of operation and the prognosis: (1) whether the paralysis is complete or incomplete, (2) whether or not the facial nerve can be reconstructed, and (3) depending upon the time elapsed since the onset, whether the palsy is recent or long-standing. Of course, a combination of these factors may occur, and each case should be decided individually.

Injuries to the facial nerve are usually amenable to microsurgical reconstruction unless a long time has elapsed since the beginning of the palsy. This time has been considered to be 2 years at most, but there are considerable individual variations.

Cross-facial nerve grafting may be indicated for all palsies that cannot be treated by reconstruction of the facial nerve. However, a complete procedure may not be possible in long-standing cases, as regeneration of the facial nerve and muscle reinnervation and reactivation may be compromised.

We reviewed our experience during the

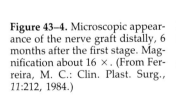

Figure 43–4. Microscopic appearance of the nerve graft distally, 6 months after the first stage. Magnification about 16 ×. (From Ferreira, M. C.: Clin. Plast. Surg., 11:212, 1984.)

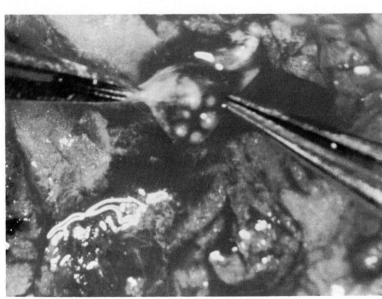

period 1975 to 1978[3] and found that those patients with palsy of less than 6 months' duration had better results in terms of voluntary activation of the face than the group with long-standing palsies. In the latter group, cross-facial nerve grafting was unable to achieve good reanimation of facial movement, although muscular contraction and weak motion could be observed.

We can now see more clearly that the procedure can reinnervate the facial nerve and has the advantage of providing brain control to make possible satisfactory re-education of the patient. In the cases rated good, involuntary motion is regained and the results sometimes resemble those of nerve reconstruction (with some mass movement) (Fig. 43–5).

We are uncertain why the good results are not more consistent with cross-facial nerve grafting. One reason may be reduction of the number of fibers, made more severe by a possible loss of regeneration on these long grafts and the two suture lines. The recipient bed may also play a role and there are many technical problems to be dealt with.

Results are poorer in patients with high palsies, such as those caused by the resection of acoustic neurinomas. However, the reasons for this are unknown.

Nevertheless, we think that the procedure is still useful for palsies of less than 6 months' duration. When a good result is obtained, reanimation is much better than that obtained by any other cross-over nerve operation.

Ways to improve the results include good microsurgical technique and perhaps better assurance of vascularity of the nerve grafts by use of microvascular nerve transplantation. Determining a reliable way of keeping the mimetic muscles free of denervation effects would be another important measure.

Management of partial palsy, as may occur following Bell's palsy and some types of temporal trauma, is another field to be ex-

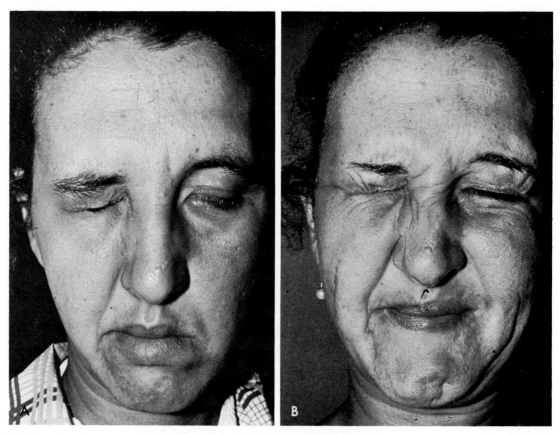

Figure 43–5. *A* and *B*, Complete facial palsy caused by removal of a cholesteatoma; cross-facial nerve grafting done after 4 months. (From Ferreira, M. C.: Clin. Plast. Surg., *11*:213, 1984.)

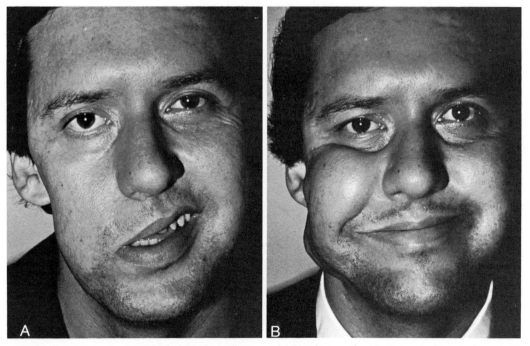

Figure 43–6. *A* and *B*, Long-standing facial palsy. Microvascular gracilis transfer to reanimate the mouth area. Nerve coaptation was performed between a cross-facial nerve graft and the obturator nerve.

plored. In some instances the weakness of the facial muscles is significant and very distressing to the patient. We have operated on several of these patients, and cross-facial nerve grafting seemed to improve symmetry of the face.

Unfortunately, a significant number of patients have long-standing palsies. At the present time, we treat these patients with a two-stage procedure. In the first stage, two cross-facial nerve grafts are sutured to the buccal branches, passed through the tunnels up to the paralyzed side, and anchored on the dermis. In the second stage, these grafts are a source of axons to either neurotize a local muscle[5] (in our experience the temporalis had better results than the masseter) or reinnervate a microsurgical muscle transplant.

Since the first report of a gracilis transfer to the face,[6] several other muscles were transplanted to the face by microvascular anastomoses. These included the extensor digitorum brevis, latissimus dorsi, pectoralis minor, and serratus anterior. The gracilis has so far had the most consistent results,[7, 9] but results are not yet ideal (Fig. 43–6).

Finally, the transfer of part of the muscle instead of the whole muscle is one of the procedures being investigated in order to ameliorate long-standing facial palsies.

References

1. Anderl, H.: Reconstruction of the face through cross-face nerve transplantation in facial paralysis. Chir. Plast., 2:17, 1973.
2. Clodius, L.: Selective neurectomies to achieve symmetry in partial and complete facial paralysis. Br. J. Plast. Surg., 29:43, 1976.
3. Ferreira, M. C.: Microsurgical procedures in the treatment of facial palsy. Transactions of the Eighth International Congress on Plastic and Reconstructive Surgery, Rio de Janeiro, Cargraf, 1979 p. 92.
4. Ferreira, M. C., Marchese, A. T., and Spina, V.: Injertos transfaciales de nervio en el tratamiento de la paralysis facial observaciones iniciales. Chir. Plast. Ibero Lat. Am., 3:301, 1977.
5. Freilinger, G. A.: A new technique to correct facial paralysis Plast. Reconstr. Surg., 56:44, 1975.
6. Harii, K, Ohmori, K., and Torri, T: Free gracilis muscle transplantation with neuro-vascular anastomoses for the treatment of facial paralysis. Plast. Reconstr. Surg., 57:133, 1976.
7. Harii, K.: Microneurovascular free muscle transplantation for reanimation of facial paralysis. Clin. Plast. Surg., 6:361, 1979.
8. Le-Quang, C.: Le plexus génien du nerf facial. Anatomie et conséquences cliniques. Ann. Chir. Plast., 21:5, 1972.
9. O'Brien, B. McC.: Management of facial paralysis. Presented at the Annual Meeting of the American Society of Plastic and Reconstructive Surgeons, New Orleans, 1980.
10. Scaramella, L.: L'anastomosis tra i due nervi faciali. Arch. Otol., 82:209, 1975.
11. Smith, J. W.: A new technique of facial animation. Transactions of the Fifth International Congress on Plastic and Reconstructive Surgery, Melbourne, Butterworths, 1971.

44

Free Muscle Transplantation for Facial Paralysis

■

Ralph T. Manktelow, M.D., F.R.C.S.(C)

The surgical reconstruction of an established facial paralysis is one of the most demanding tasks of the reconstructive surgeon. The 16 mimetic muscles on each side of the face are controlled by the facial nerve. These muscles act independently and in concert to provide three different functions: production of facial tone, voluntary facial movement, and involuntary facial expression.

Facial muscle tone preserves symmetry at rest and provides functional support of the eyes, nose, and mouth. Without this tone, the face on the affected side sags and the lower half is displaced to the normal side. Paralysis of the eyelid musculature results in epiphora and conjunctival irritation. The person has a staring appearance with sclera showing below the cornea. Loss of tone about the mouth results in drooling and pocketing of food in the cheek.

Voluntary facial movements are under the person's conscious control and include blinking the eyes, pursing the lips, eating, drinking, speaking, and consciously smiling. One of the most important functions is the ability to smile voluntarily and thus allow emotional communication.

Involuntary facial expressions are reflex facial movements that are associated with emotional communication. Of the many emotions that these muscles convey, the portrayal of a spontaneous smile is the one missed most by the facial paralysis patient.

HISTORY OF FACIAL PARALYSIS SURGERY

The history of reconstructive procedures began with operations designed to reconstruct facial tone function. Static slings to the eye and mouth were partially successful in replacing tone function. Subsequent procedures were designed to produce voluntary facial movements. Masseter and temporalis muscle transfers and hypoglossal to facial nerve transfers provided not only tone functions but a controlled voluntary closure of the eye and elevation of the mouth to simulate a smile and produce some voluntary movements. Patients with procedures of this type learned to smile by voluntary effort of clenching their teeth or pressing their tongue in their mouth. Since the smile was voluntary and not spontaneous, it could not become a reflex unconscious act. Unfortunately, necessary chewing and tongue movements during eating and speech produced unwanted facial movements.

Presently, we are attempting to reconstruct the third function, reflex facial expression. Two processes are necessary in reconstructing this third facial function capability, i.e., neurotization and muscle transplantation.

Neurotization must be through the facial nerve, as this is the only means of providing the impulses that produce involuntary facial movements. Viable stumps of the facial nerve on the paralyzed side are present following tumor resection or injury and may be employed to control movement, or impulses from the opposite normal side may be utilized. Neurotization can be by neural or muscular methods. The most satisfactory is neurotization by nerve microsuture technique. When the facial musculature has been paralyzed recently, it may be neurotized from the opposite normal side using cross-facial nerve grafts. However, in many cases, this does not provide satisfactory reanimation and is certainly never useful in long-standing cases of facial paralysis.

Since the first *muscle transplantation* by Zielonko in 1874, there have been many attempts to transplant functioning skeletal musculature.

Muscle transplantation with revascularization by the ingrowth of vessels from surrounding tissues was popularized by Thompson[11] and Studitsky.[10] There are many experimental series that have established the feasibility of muscle transplantation in the animal model.[2, 5, 10, 11] It appears likely that muscle fibers about the marginal layer of the muscle survive, whereas central fibers break down and then regenerate.[1] This process is not as clearly defined in humans. However, there is clinical evidence that a functioning muscle can be transferred in this manner and that it can survive and continue to function by means of muscular neurotization.[12]

The technique of muscular neurotization of the extensor digitorum brevis and the palmaris longus for reconstruction of the eyelid and sphincter function of the mouth has been described by Thompson. Although Thompson has reported good results with these procedures, one would have expected more widespread acceptance.

A similar type of muscle revascularization with neural neurotization from the opposite unparalyzed facial nerve has also been done to provide elevation to the corner of the mouth and simulate a smile. Muscle contraction has been produced by using the extensor digitorum brevis with nerve suture of the anterior tibial nerve to the buccal branches of the opposite facial nerve. Although good movement has been reported by Thompson,[11] Nicolai and Robinson[8] and Miyake[7] were unable to obtain any muscular function with this procedure.

In 1976, Harii et al.[3] reported the successful transplantation of the gracilis muscle to the face in order to provide elevation of the corner of the mouth. Their technique involved microvascular anastomoses between the muscle's artery and vein and an artery and vein in the face. For reinnervation of their first case, the motor nerve to the temporal muscle was used. Subsequent cases employed a first stage cross-facial nerve graft for eventual reinnervation. A powerful muscle contraction was obtained, and in some cases the contraction was actually more powerful than necessary.

Subsequent series have been reported involving transfer of the extensor digitorum brevis with microvascular anastomoses and cross-facial neurotization.[6, 9, 13] It was hoped that this procedure would provide a muscle that was of a more suitable length and cross-sectional area with a number of separate bellies that could replace several of the muscles of facial expression. All of these series have concluded that this procedure did not provide as strong and reliable a lift of the corner of the mouth as was necessary. The likely reasons for failure are the small size of the muscle units, their variable vascular anatomy, and the mixed motor and sensory structure of the anterior tibial nerve.

With reports of Harii et al.[3] and O'Brien et al.[9] of successful, powerful muscle transplantation using the gracilis muscle, we entered a new era of transplantation capability. A solution to the problem of the too large gracilis has been either to shave it down following reinnervation (Harii) or to insert only a portion of the muscle (see Case Presentation).

The success in transplanting this muscle has prompted a search for muscles that could be reliably transplanted with microneurovascular anastomoses and would have the functional capabilities required by various recipient sites within the face. Terzis has recommended the pectoralis minor, Buncke has suggested the serratus anterior, and Manktelow and Zuker have recommended the single fascicle muscle territory of the gracilis and other muscles.[4]

The variables associated with muscle transplantation are outlined in Table 44–1.

TECHNIQUE OF MUSCLE TRANSPLANTATION FOR FACIAL PARALYSIS USING MICRONEUROVASCULAR ANASTOMOSES

The technique of muscle transplantation can be utilized for any one of the muscles that are available for transplantation by microneurovascular techniques. There are three parts to any muscle transplantation: preparation of the muscle for transplantation, preparation of the recipient site, and the actual muscle transplantation. Frequently, the first two parts may be done simultaneously by two teams, thus shortening the overall length of the procedure.

Table 44–1. VARIABLES IN MUSCLE
TRANSPLANTATION

A. Vascularization
  1. By ingrowth from surrounding tissues
  2. By microvascular anastomoses
B. Innervation
  1. Facial nerve
    a. Stumps on paralyzed side
    b. Opposite side
      (1) Nerve graft with nerve suture or
          implantation
      (2) Nerve pedicle with nerve suture
      (3) Muscular neurotization
  2. Nonfacial nerve
    a. Motor branches of the trigeminal nerve
    b. Hypoglossal nerve
C. Choice of muscle
  1. Extensor digitorum brevis
  2. Gracilis
  3. Palmaris longus
  4. Serratus anterior
  5. Latissimus dorsi
  6. Pectoralis minor

Choice of Muscle

The choice of muscle should depend upon
the dynamic requirements. A muscle should
be selected that will provide a range of excursion equal to the opposite normal side.
Muscle transplantation can be done to provide eye closure, oral sphincter control, or
elevation of the angle of the mouth. The
most common use of a muscle for microneurovascular transplantation is for elevation of
the corner of the mouth to create a smile.
The muscle must have a reliable vascular and
nerve pattern that is suitable for microneurovascular repairs. The location of the vessels
and nerve on the muscle after it is transplanted to the face should approximate the
location of the vessels and nerve within the
face. Multiple points of innervation providing independent functioning muscular units
within the muscle may be desirable. Removal
of the muscle should leave no functional
disability. Preferably, the muscle should be
located at a site distant to the face so that
two teams can work simultaneously without
being in each other's way. The muscles that
have been used successfully for facial reanimation have included the gracilis, pectoralis
minor, serratus anterior, and latissimus
dorsi.

Preparation of the Muscle

The muscle is identified by an appropriate
incision that allows ready access to the neurovascular bundle. The origin and insertion
of the muscle are identified and cleared. The
vascular and nerve pedicles are identified
and dissected free from the surroundings
with ligation of the side branches. Nerve
stimulation may or may not be done, depending upon the need to identify independent functioning territories within the muscle.
The muscle is not removed from its site until
the face is prepared to receive it in order to
minimize the ischemia time.

Preparation of the Face

The incision should allow good exposure
of all areas. A face lift–type preauricular incision with an inferior extension will provide
adequate exposure and is cosmetically acceptable. There must be access to the donor
nerve, the recipient vessels, the corner of the
mouth, the orbicularis oris, and the intended
site of muscle origin.

The usual vessels for repair are the facial
artery and common facial vein. Alternative
vessels are the superficial temporal artery
and vein and occasionally a transverse facial
vessel. Neck vessels, because of their distant
site from the muscle transplantation, are the
least preferable.

The nerve to be used depends upon the
cause of the facial paralysis. In an old facial
nerve injury, distal to the mastoid or following a resection of a parotid or other facial
tumor, the stump of the facial nerve may be
used. If the paralysis is due to an intracranial
nerve lesion, a cross-facial nerve graft from
the opposite nonparalyzed site will be employed. The cross-facial nerve graft should
be inserted at a preliminary operative procedure 6 to 12 months prior to the muscle
transplantation.

Cross-Facial Nerve Grafting

Exposure of the nonparalyzed side is
through a preauricular face lift–type incision.
The branches of the facial nerve are identified
at their point of exit from the parotid gland.
At this anatomic level, the facial nerve has
undergone many divisions, and at least 10
branches can easily be found. A nerve stimulator with both frequency and voltage control will allow identification of the function
of each branch. At the time of surgery, a
sketch is prepared that identifies the function

of each branch. Branches that have the same function desired in the transplanted muscle are then identified, and half of them are divided and used to innervate the cross-facial nerve graft. For example, if the objective is to create a smile, branches that control the risorius, zygomaticus, and levator labii should be used. Care should be taken to leave the marginal mandibular branch, as there may be only one nerve supplying the lower lip.

If the muscle transplantation is to provide both eye and mouth reanimation, two cross-facial nerve grafts are required. Each graft will supply innervation to the portions of muscle that are inserted into the eye and mouth, respectively. We have frequently removed 50% of the branches of the facial nerve at this distal level without any observable weakness in the face.

The sural nerve grafts should be placed high in the upper lip from the normal side to the paralyzed side. The suturing to the buccal branches should be done with interrupted 10–0 or 11–0 nylon sutures using a fascicular technique. The cross-sectional surface of the sural nerve should be matched by an equal surface area of facial nerve branches in order to obtain optimal reinnervation of the entire graft. The terminal stump is placed on the paralyzed side in a preauricular position, where it can easily be identified at the time of muscle transplantation. After the Tinel-like sign has advanced to the distal end of the nerve graft, the muscle can be transplanted.

Muscle Transplantation

The location of the insertion and origin of the muscle should be selected with care. Preoperative planning studies of the shape of the patient's smile will indicate the direction and distance that the commissure moves on smiling. This is frequently at a 30° angle to the horizontal but varies from patient to patient, and a simulation of the patient's normal side should therefore be attempted. Intraoperative traction with forceps on the orbicularis oris in the region of the commissure allows selection of the most appropriate location for the muscle insertion to match the shape of the smile on the other side. Double-armed sutures are placed through each traction location about the orbicularis musculature. This allows simulation of the effect of

the muscle transplant by pulling on all the sutures at once. The muscle is frequently inserted into the commissure, a portion of the upper and lower lip, and, in some cases, the base of the nose and nasal labial fold. The site of the muscle's origin will depend upon the angle of pull desired. This should be between the zygomatic arch and the tragus of the ear. The muscle should be inserted inferior to the zygomatic arch so as not to produce a bulge over the prominence of the arch.

The muscle is inserted into the desired location with interrupted mattress sutures and is lightly tacked to the approximate origin prior to neurovascular repairs. Revascularization should be done with an artery and a vein that lie in a comfortable position relative to the muscle without undue tension. An end-to-end anastomosis is usually preferable. Patency depends upon good technique, the repair of undamaged vessels, and a good perfusion pressure. A single artery and vein are usually adequate. Revision of a vascular thrombosis in the postoperative period will not be possible, not only because of the difficulty in recognizing the thrombosis but also because of the ischemic damage that would likely occur before the anastomosis could be revised. Therefore, there should be no compromise in the selection of vessels or the technique of their repair.

A fascicular nerve repair should be done with interrupted 10–0 or 11–0 nylon sutures, with the repair placed as close as possible to the neuromuscular junction in order to minimize denervation time. All of the muscle's fascicles should be satisfied with fascicles from the facial nerve or facial nerve graft.

The technique for determining the correct tension at which the muscle should be inserted has not been refined. Although the technique in muscle transplantation to the extremities involves placing the muscle at considerable tension in order to obtain maximum muscle contraction, the significance of this practice in facial nerve reanimation is not yet clear. The author's technique consists of placing the muscle in enough tension so that under anesthesia it is tight enough to place the paralyzed corner of the mouth in balance with the other side. Following revascularization and the nerve repair, the exact position of the muscle origin is determined, depending upon the tension and the angle of lift required. Closure of the skin should be done in such a manner as to avoid compression of the vascular pedicle. Drains should be placed judiciously so that they cannot obstruct the vascular pedicle. The patient must not lie on the involved side during the postoperative period, and movements of the mouth are discouraged.

CASE PRESENTATION

A 33-year-old woman had been treated 9 years previously for a fibrosarcoma of the left cheek by an excision of all the soft tissues from the ear to the commissure. Most of the lower division of the facial nerve and facial musculature to the left side of her mouth had been removed. Reconstruction had been accomplished with a neck flap. She subsequently had partial facial paralysis with normal eye function and good oral sphincter function. Her only problem was the inability to move the upper lip and commissure when smiling. In addition, there was a significant soft tissue depression from the inferior margin of the zygoma to the angle of the mandible (Fig. 44–1).

It was decided to transplant a portion of the gracilis muscle, which would provide a functioning length of approximately 5 cm and a cross-sectional area sufficient to lift the corner of her mouth approximately 1 cm. On the basis of our experience with gracilis muscle transplantation to the forearm and our observations in patients with facial paralysis in whom larger and smaller muscles were used, we felt that approximately one third of the cross-sectional area of the normal gracilis would provide this function.

A two-team procedure was done, with one team preparing the face while the other team prepared the muscle. In previous cases of muscle transplantation, we had done intraoperative single fascicle nerve stimulation, and J. Fish has carried out cadaver gracilis nerve examination in our laboratory. There are usually two to seven fascicles present in the gracilis muscle, and each of these fascicles usually supplies a different longitudinal portion of the muscle. Thus, it is possible to separate the muscle longitudinally into independently functioning neuromuscular units. Each of these units has been termed a single fascicle muscle territory.

When the gracilis was exposed in the leg, the vascular and neural pedicles were separated, and

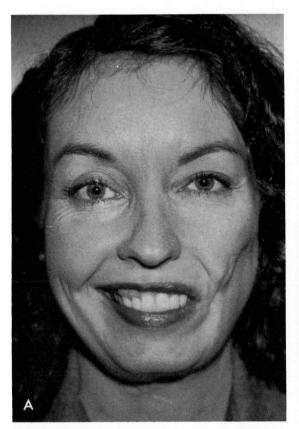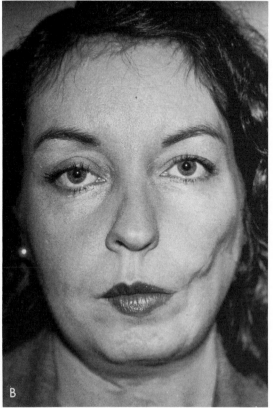

Figure 44–1. Preoperative appearance. *A*, Smiling, showing inability to elevate the corner of the mouth and soft tissue defect in left cheek. *B*, Face at rest, showing deviation of upper lip and nose to normal side. (*A*, From Manktelow, R. T.: Clin. Plast. Surg., *11*:219, 1984.)

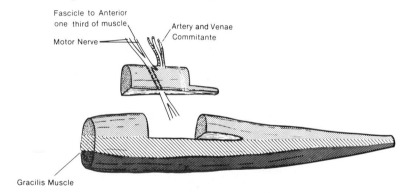

Fascicle to Anterior
one third of muscle

Motor Nerve

Artery and Venae
Commitante

Gracilis Muscle

Figure 44–2. Artist's rendering illustrates the three different longitudinal fascicular motor territories on the gracilis. An 8 cm length of the anterior territory containing the dominant neurovascular pedicle has been removed for transplantation. (From Manktelow, R. T.: Clin. Plast. Surg., *11*:218, 1984.)

fascicular nerve stimulation was carried out (Fig. 44–2). One fascicle supplied the anterior one third of the gracilis and the other two fascicles supplied the posterior two thirds of the muscle. This allowed an 8-cm length of the anterior one third of the muscle to be removed with the neurovascular bundle attached (Fig. 44–3). The fascicle supplying this portion was labeled with a microsuture. Although it is possible to neurotize the entire nerve, if there is a shortage of good motor fascicles in the face, we can increase the chance of strong reinnervation by using the limited motor fascicles available to reinnervate only the fascicle that supplies the muscle being transplanted.

The muscle was transplanted using microvascular techniques. Revascularization was accomplished using the facial artery and vein with end-to-end anastomoses. A branch of the lower division of the facial nerve, which had been divided at the time of tumor resection, was found anterior and inferior to the lobe of the ear. One fascicle from this branch was sutured to the single fascicle that governed the motor territory (Fig. 44–4). A significant soft tissue deficit below the muscle was filled with vascularized subcutaneous fat that was

transferred attached to the muscle. By draping this fat flap like an apron from the muscle down to the angle of the mandible, this soft tissue defect was also corrected.

At 3 months, the patient noted the beginning of muscle contraction. There was a gradual increase in the range of contraction for 6 months, after which function ceased to improve. She now has a balanced position of her mouth at rest (Fig. 44–5A) and a natural, spontaneous, and symmetrical smile (Fig. 44–5B). Not only is she able to move the position of her mouth at will (Fig. 44–5C and 5D) but she also has normal reflex expression of emotion transmitted through the facial nerve to the muscle transplantation.

DISCUSSION

Free muscle transplantation without vascular anastomosis has major limitations. There have been few reports of obtaining satisfactory muscle function unless revascularization is done. Without revascularization,

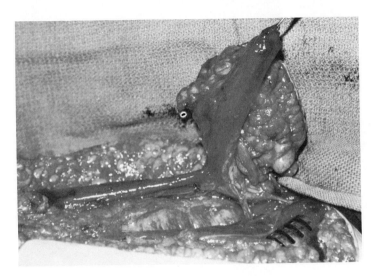

Figure 44–3. The anterior fascicular motor territory is being separated from the remainder of the gracilis muscle. Attached vascularized subcutaneous fat can be seen behind the muscle against the drape.

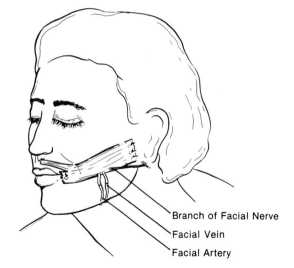

Figure 44–4. Insertion of muscle within the face. The vascularized fat flap is omitted from illustration. (From Manktelow, R. T.: Clin. Plast. Surg., *11*:219, 1984.)

Branch of Facial Nerve

Facial Vein

Facial Artery

most of the transplanted muscle fibers appear to undergo degeneration and replacement with collagen.[5] Very small muscles and the surface of large muscles undergo neovascularization, whereas portions of the muscle further removed from the recipient bed undergo fibrous replacement. In the experimental animal, there may be some regeneration in small muscles.[1, 10] With vascular anastomoses it is possible to have complete survival of the transplanted muscle. The function of the muscle will then depend upon the amount of muscle transplanted, the adequacy of reinnervation, and the position and tension in which the muscle is inserted into the face. There are 16 separate muscles on each side of the face that function independently and in groups to provide expression to the eyes, nose, and mouth. It is impossible to replace all of these functions with a single muscle. Therefore, shades of expression within a single movement, such as a smile, will be impossible to create in balance with the normal side.

The surgeon and patient must have realistic objectives. A realistic expectation would be to have voluntary closure of the eye and continence at rest so that there is no conjunctival irritation. Another realistic objective would be to have the mouth in balance at rest and to have active elevation of the corner of the mouth, which can occur as a voluntary or as a reflex movement. The direction and extent of movement of the corner of the mouth should be close to that of the normal side.

Our present problem is determining the amount of muscle to be transplanted to obtain the desired dynamic result. The solution to this will be to try different muscles with different cross sections at different tensions and improve the reliability of the innervation. By means of careful recording of the procedures and the results, we will refine the specific technique that is most likely to be productive in a given patient.

It is difficult to obtain independent facial movements in the eye and mouth. A possible solution is to use muscles that have separate functioning units, such as the serratus anterior, pectoralis minor, or the separate motor territories of the gracilis. Separate motor neurotization will be necessary using either two cross-facial nerve grafts or separate branches of the damaged facial nerve on the paralyzed side. Another alternative is to employ a different procedure for the eyes and use the muscle transplantation for the mouth.

Patients who have a bilateral facial paralysis, such as the Möbius syndrome, present a particularly difficult problem. Bilateral muscle transplantations can be done; however, neurotization with facial nerve impulses is impossible. We have split the hypoglossal nerve using only a portion of its cross-sectional area to innervate separate muscle transplantations on each side of the face. We have also used the motor nerve to the masseter muscle for reinnervation of the muscle transfer. This allows the possibility of voluntary facial expressions, but will not provide reflex involuntary expressions.

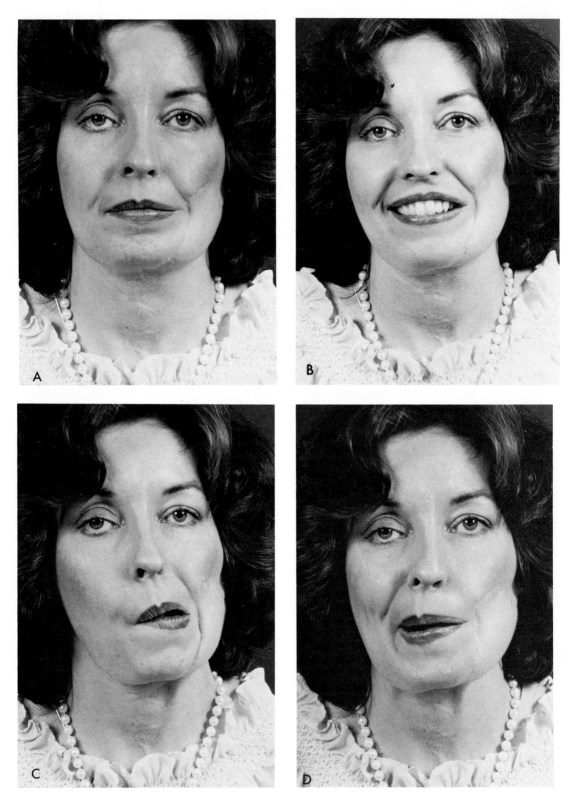

Figure 44–5. *A,* Postoperative appearance of face at rest. *B,* Postoperative appearance, smiling. *C,* Voluntary movement of previously paralyzed side of mouth using muscle transplantation that matches. *D,* Movement of opposite normal side. (From Manktelow, R. T.: Clin. Plast. Surg., *11:*219, 1984.)

References

1. Carlson, B. M.: The biology of muscle transplantation. *In* Freilinger, G., Holle, J., and Carlson, B. M. (eds.): Muscle Transplantation. New York, Springer Verlag, 1981.
2. Frey, M., Gruber, H., Holle, J., Klein-Peter, G., and Freilinger, G.: Experimental studies on factors influencing muscle transplantation. *In* Freilinger, G., Holle, J., and Carlson, B. M. (eds.): Muscle Transplantation. New York, Springer Verlag, 1981.
3. Harii, K., Ohmori, K., and Torii, S.: Free gracilis muscle transplantation with microneurovascular anastomoses for the treatment of facial paralysis. Plast. Reconstr. Surg., *57*:133, 1976.
4. Manktelow, R. T., and Zuker, R. M.: Muscle transplantation by fascicular territory. Plast. Reconstr. Surg., *73*:751, 1984.
5. Markley, J. M., Jr., Faulkner, J. A., and Carlson, B. M.: Regeneration following transplantation of skeletal muscles in monkeys. Plast. Reconstr. Surg. *62*:415, 1978.
6. Mayou, B. J., Watson, J. S., and Harrison, D. H.: Free microvascular and microneural transfer of the extensor digitorum brevis muscle for the treatment of unilateral facial palsy. Br. J. Plast. Surg., *34*:362, 1981.
7. Miyake, I.: Experience with Thompson's free muscle grafts. *In* Freilinger, G., Holle, J., and Carlson, B. M. (eds.): Muscle Transplantation. New York, Springer Verlag, 1981.
8. Nicolai, J.-P. A., and Robinson, P. H.: Negative experiences with free muscle grafts to the cheek in patients with facial paralysis. *In* Freilinger, G., Holle, J., and Carlson, B. M. (eds.): Muscle Transplantation. New York, Springer Verlag, 1981.
9. O'Brien, B. M., Franklin, J. D., and Morrison, W. A. Cross facial nerve grafts and microneurovascular free muscle transfer for long established facial palsy. Br. J. Plast. Surg., *33*:202, 1980.
10. Studitsky, A. N.: Dynamics of the development of myogenic tissue under conditions of explantation and transplantation. *In* Rose, G. G. (ed.): Cinemicrography in Cell Biology. New York, Academic Press, 1963.
11. Thompson, N.: Autogenous free grafts and skeletal muscle. A preliminary experimental and clinical study. Plast. Reconstr. Surg., *48*:11, 1971.
12. Thompson, N., and Wynn Parry, C. B.: Restoration of emotional expression to the unilateral paralyzed face. *In* Freilinger, G., Holle, J., and Carlson, B. M. (eds.): Muscle Transplantation. New York, Springer Verlag, 1981.
13. Tolhurst, D. E., and Boss, K. E.: Free vascularized muscle grafts in facial palsy. Plast. Reconstr. Surg., *69*:760, 1982.

45

Surgical Correction of Lagophthalmos

■

Ian T. Jackson, M.D.

In the normal situation, the upper eyelid position results from a constant state of balance between the actions of the levator palpebrae and the orbicularis oculi muscles. During the day, levator tone is prominent, but at night this relaxes and the lids close owing to the action of the orbicularis. In facial palsy, the orbicularis is nonfunctional, and the palpebral fissure remains open when the patient is awake or asleep. Fortunately, because of Bell's phenomenon, the eyeball rotates upward and the cornea comes to lie under the upper lid. Thus, the cornea is protected from trauma and desiccation. There is also a condition known as reversed Bell's phenomenon in which the globe rotates inferiorly and the cornea is covered and protected by the lower lid (Fig. 45–1).

One further physiologic reflex to consider is levator relaxation, which is important in relation to the success of certain therapeutic modalities that we employ. At the moment of initiation of blinking, there is total relaxation of the levator for an instant. This then allows the orbicularis to close the palpebral fissure.[37] The same reflex occurs in the patient with facial palsy, which explains why lid loading procedures are effective.

CLINICAL FINDING IN LAGOPHTHALMOS

As stated, in the patient with lagophthalmos the eye remains open under all conditions, and the palpebral fissure is wider than the fissure on the nonparalyzed side. As a result of orbicularis tone, the lower lid may sag and even evert. The lacrimal punctum falls away from the globe and no longer functions for drainage. Because of this, tears accumulate in the lower fornix, well over the lid edge, and run down the cheek. This is further aggravated by excess tear production due to the ever-open fissure, especially when the eye is irritated (e.g., by wind or a dusty atmosphere).

Conjunctivitis with redness, irritation, and pain can occur from time to time as a result of these adverse conditions. Drying of the cornea with ulceration and scarring can also occur, but is unusual unless the eye is anesthetic or if Bell's phenomenon is inadequate or is not present.

TREATMENT OF LAGOPHTHALMOS

General Measures

These are directed at making the eye comfortable. When the patient is outdoors, spectacles are advised (sometimes with a side screen to keep out the wind). If the eye commonly becomes irritated overnight, ophthalmic ointment or artificial tears are inserted before going to sleep. If this situation is severe, a plastic dome shield may be used to provide a moist atmosphere around the eye. If conjunctivitis is severe, it is advisable to consult an ophthalmologist.

617

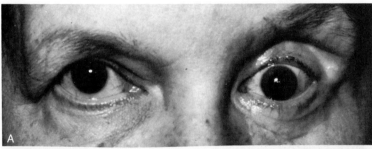
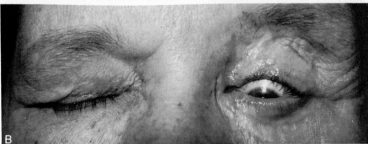

Figure 45–1. *A* and *B*, Patient showing the reversed Bell's phenomenon.

Lagophthalmos Associated with Acute Facial Palsy

This can be very disturbing, especially in the young patient. In patients under 30 years of age, reassurance is the order of the day, as there is virtually 100% recovery. In older patients, recovery may be delayed, and a temporary measure may be used if the eye is very uncomfortable and this cannot be controlled by the general measures suggested earlier.

Surgical treatment should be considered temporary and capable of being reversed; however, if recovery does not occur, surgery should also be capable of providing permanent correction. The procedures advised are (1) lateral tarsorrhaphy, a central procedure should *never* be done unless the eye is anesthetic; and (2) lid loading procedures, e.g., gold weight, spring, or magnets. These will be described fully in the following section.

Lagophthalmos Associated with Established Facial Palsy

Nerve Suture

When there has been a division of the main trunk or its branches, direct suture is obviously the method of choice. Careful technique and use of magnification give a high proportion of good results.

Nerve Graft

When a portion of the nerve or one of its branches has been resected and this defect can be repaired with a graft of suitable dimensions, this procedure should be performed. Again, the results may be very satisfactory (Fig. 45–2).

Cross-Facial Nerve Graft

This technique is discussed in Chapter 43. However, technical improvement has made the procedure quicker and easier. The graft is taken in three strands across the upper lip and is sutured to the second branches of the normal nerve and onto similar branches on the affected nerve. In this way, larger nerve diameters can be coapted. The results of this procedure are mixed, ranging from little or no return of function to good, if not normal, eyelid closure (Fig. 45–3).[1, 3, 27, 29, 30]

Tarsorrhaphy

The best type of tarsorrhaphy is undoubtedly by the lateral overlap technique of McLaughlin.[21, 22]

Technique. The conjunctiva of the upper lid is removed over what is thought to be the required lateral area. A similar amount of skin is removed from the lower lid. The lids are then sutured in an overlapping fashion. The lower lid is held up in good position by nylon pullout sutures tied through fine rub-

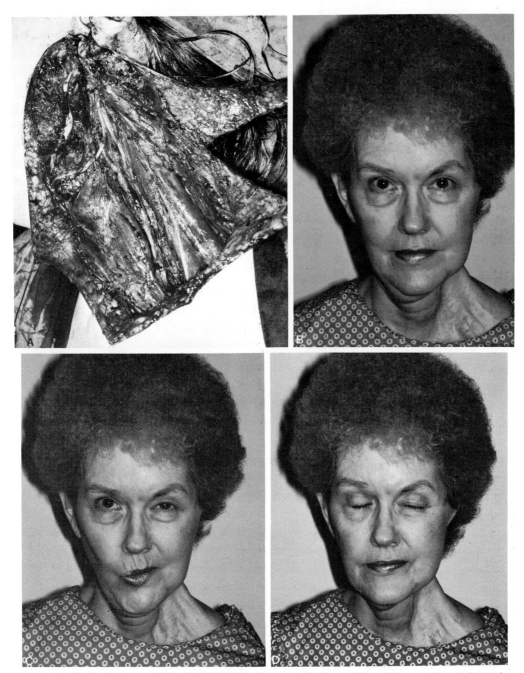

Figure 45–2. Immediate nerve grafting. *A,* Resection of recurrent adenocystic carcinoma of parotid together with subtotal petrosectomy and neck dissection. Immediate nerve grafting and free groin flap cover. *B* to *D,* Result after 4 years.

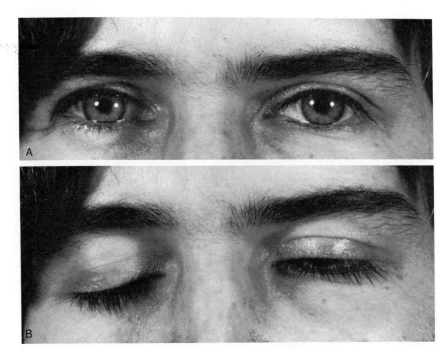

Figure 45–3. Cross-facial nerve grafting. *A* and *B* Pre- and postoperative results of patient whose lagophthalmos was treated with a cross-facial nerve graft.

ber tubing (Fig. 45–4). These are left in situ for 7 to 10 days.

Results. This procedure gives a good cosmetic and functional result because the eyelashes are maintained. The lower eyelid is tightened and epiphora is reduced. An additional benefit is protection of the lateral area of the eye, which lessens conjunctival irritation. There is absolutely no place in this situation for a central tarsorrhaphy unless it is an emergency procedure to save an eye or if there is a possible or an established exposure keratosis in an anesthetic eye.

Lid Loading Procedures

As stated earlier, these all depend on the momentary relaxation of the levator as the patient initiates the blinking reflex. With the lid in this toneless situation, the load, together with gravity, allows the lid to close. Lid loading procedures can be very successful, but each has specific problems.

Full Thickness Skin Graft. For mild cases of lagophthalmos, Tessier et al.[33] described a technique of excising an ellipse of skin of the upper lid and resurfacing the resulting defect with thicker skin from behind the ear. They maintain that this will give good results, since approximately 0.6 gm is added to the weight of the upper lid provided the skin is 6 cm square and 1 mm thick.

Results. Based on our own experience, we would agree with these findings but state that this procedure is useful only in very mild cases and thus is rarely indicated.

De-epithelialized Flaps. In many patients the drooping eyebrow is a severe esthetic disability. This can be corrected by simply excising an ellipse of skin from above the eyebrow in order to position it on the same level on the other side. The excised skin can be used to load the upper lid in mild to moderate cases of lagophthalmos.

Technique. The required amount of skin to be excised is drawn out and that area is de-epithelialized. This area is then elevated down to the periosteum and to the full extent of the lateral and medial skin excision. The bipedicled flap is divided in the midline, and the supraeyebrow skin is closed with hitching up of the eyebrow to the periosteum of the supraorbital ridge. A tunnel is then made from the undersurface of the flap pedicles through the upper lid between the skin and the tarsal plate. Nylon sutures are placed in the tips of the flaps, threaded onto a straight needle, and pulled through the tunnel and out through the lid skin. These sutures are tied over small gauze bolsters, which provides an arrangement of overlapping flaps and moderate lid loading (Fig. 45–5).

Results. These are good in mild or moderate cases. Covering gold weights with these

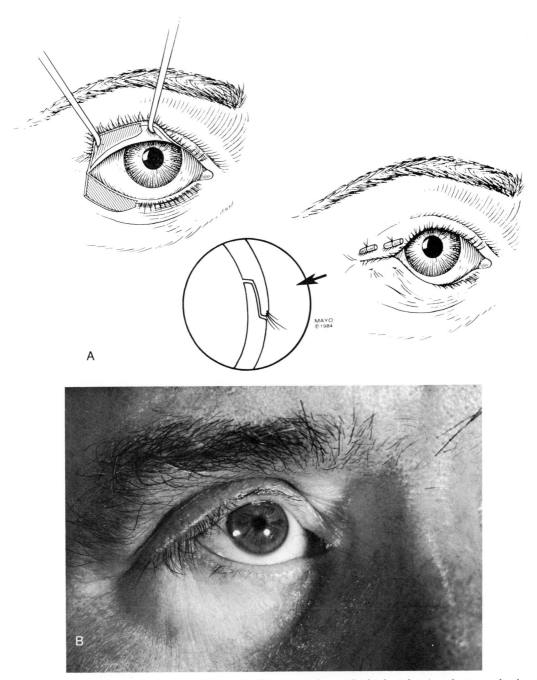

Figure 45–4. McLaughlin tarsorrhaphy. *A,* Diagram illustrating the method of performing the tarsorrhaphy. *B,* Postoperative result. Note the satisfactory esthetic appearance.

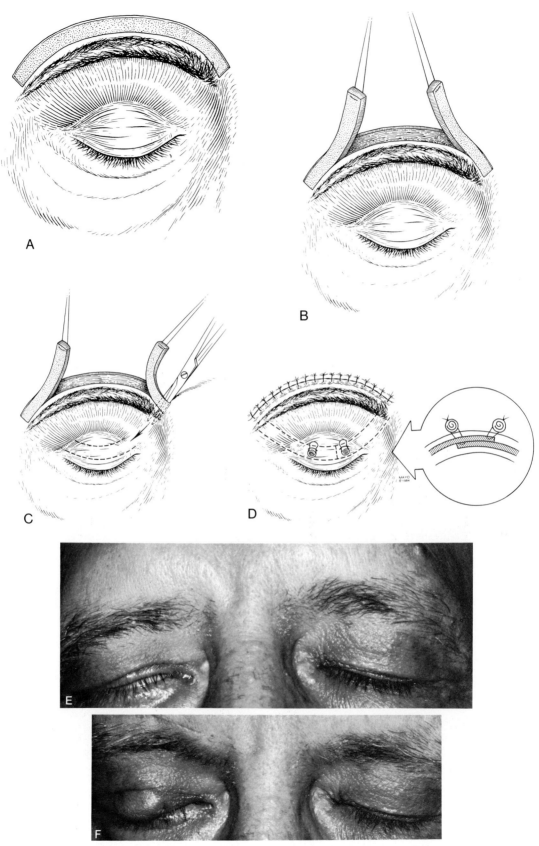

Figure 45–5. De-epithelialized flap technique. *A* to *D,* Diagram illustrating the technique of this method of lid loading. *E* and *F,* Pre- and postoperative results.

flaps is useful if there is an associated skin problem. De-epithelialized flaps are used only when supraeyebrow skin is being sacrificed.

Morel-Fatio Spring. The load in this procedure is provided by the tension of the spring, which if correct will close the palpebral fissure synchronous with levator relaxation.[24]

Technique. Using three incisions (lateral canthal, just above the lid margin, and just above the supraorbital rim), two tunnels are created between the skin and tarsal plate. The first tunnel runs just above the upper lid margin from the lateral incision to beyond the midpoint of the upper lid. The second runs from the lateral incision just beyond the midpoint of the supraorbital rim. The spring is then inserted through the lateral canthal incision, with each limb being introduced into a tunnel. It is possible to modify the tension slightly by bending the wire at the spring coil. The spring is fixed to the periosteum of the lateral orbital rim and supraorbital rim by using nonabsorbable suture material. It is also advisable to fix the spring to the tarsal plate with a similar suture (Fig. 45–6).

Results. If all goes well, the results can be excellent.[38] Unfortunately, there is a high rate of spring extrusion, which was experienced even by the originator of the technique.[12, 23, 39] Fortunately, extrusion is usually through the skin and thus the eye is rarely damaged. Other complications include spring breakage and reduction in spring tension. There are now few proponents of this method.

Lid Magnets. This technique was introduced by Muhlbauer et al.[25] and involves placing small magnets* in the upper and lower lids. When the polarity is correctly arranged, the load on the upper lid is the attracting force between the magnetic poles.

Technique. From a small lateral canthal incision, tunnels are created between the skin and the tarsal plate to beyond the midline of the lid. The distance beyond the midline is determined by the length of the magnet, which must be positioned so that its midpoint is in the center of the lid. The magnet is placed and held in position with a suture through the skin and onto the tarsal plate tied on the skin; this suture obliterates the lateral extent of the tunnel (Fig. 45–7).

Results. As with the previous method, the results can be very good. Unfortunately, the extrusion rate is again unacceptably high, even in the experience of Muhlbauer and colleagues.[3] Therefore, lid magnet correction has not become a widely used method.

Silicone Sling. In 1969 and 1972, Arion[4, 5] described a method of loading the upper lid using the tension induced by the placement of a specially constructed silicone sling or band in the lids.

Technique. Through a lateral canthal incision, tunnels are created along the full length of the lids between the skin and the tarsal plates. The procedure is done under local anesthesia. The upper lid tunnel is 1 cm above the lid margin; the lower 0.5 cm below the lower lid margin. These measurements are critical, as a tunnel too close to the margin may produce entropion and one too far away may result in ectropion. A small medial canthal incision allows identification of the medial canthal ligament, and the tunnels are joined through the ligament. The 2- to 3-mm solid silicone band is now introduced through the upper tunnel, through the medial canthal ligament, and then through the lower tunnel. By pulling on the band and asking the patient to open and close the lids, the correct tension can be judged. At this point, the lateral ends of the band are sutured to the periosteum of the lateral orbital margin with nonabsorbable suture material. A special range of instruments together with the silicone sling is available for this procedure* (Fig. 45–8).

Results. Silicone is a material that does not wear well. It tears easily under stress and absorbs lipids. Because of absorption of lipids, its mechanical characteristics change and silicone becomes more brittle and even less resistant than usual to shear stress. For this reason, virtually every sling will break. In addition, because silicone is a foreign material, it will gradually pull through body structures, and in some patients the medial canthal ligaments have been disrupted and the entire sling apparatus slackens. Use of this technique has therefore dwindled, although the rare enthusiastic report may appear.[39]

Gold Weight. Perhaps the simplest and most useful method of lid loading is the gold weight. The weight is calculated preoperatively and the results are predictable.[6, 15, 17, 28]

Text continued on page 628

---

*Magnet Service München, 8035 Gautnig b. München, Ammersee Strasse 28.1/3, West Germany.

*Chas. F. Thackray (USA) Ltd., P.O. Box 6435, Bridgewater, NJ 08807.

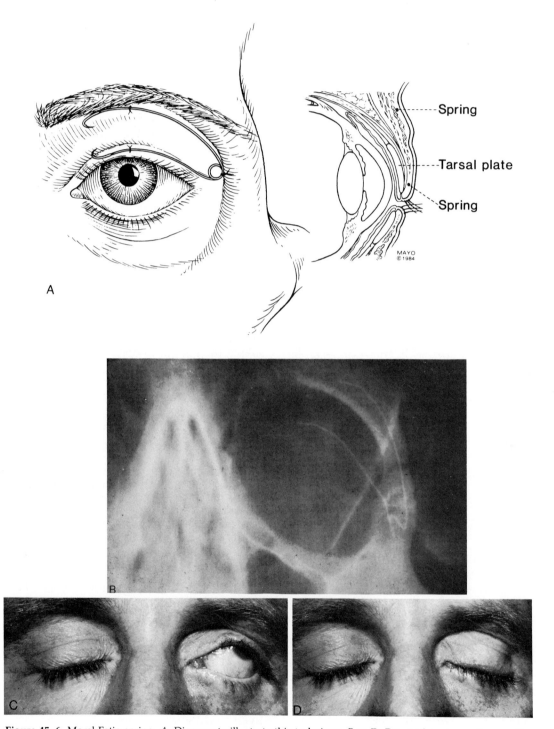

Figure 45–6. Morel-Fatio spring. *A*, Diagram to illustrate this technique. *B* to *D*, Pre- and postoperative results.

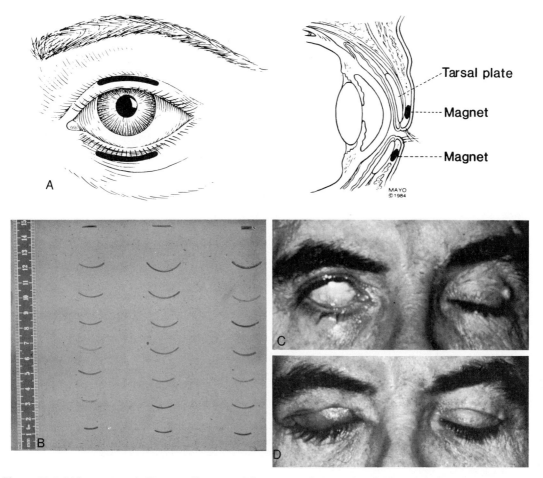

Tarsal plate

Magnet

Magnet

Figure 45–7. Lid magnets. *A,* Diagram illustrating lid magnet technique. *B* to *D,* Pre- and postoperative results.

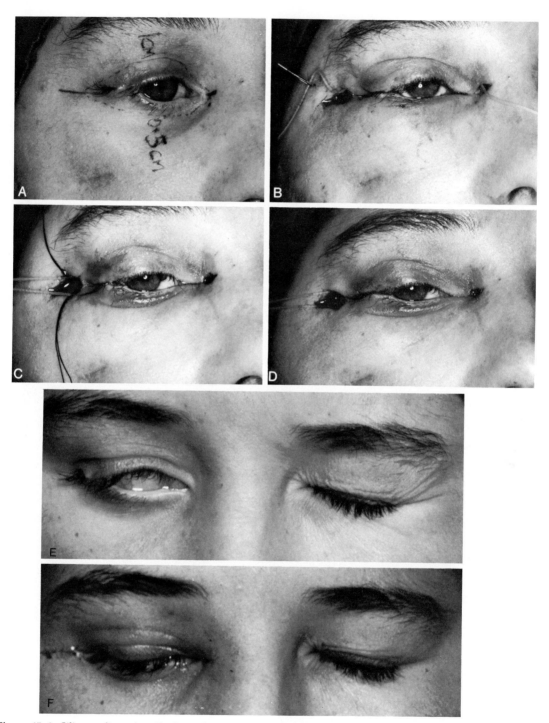

Figure 45–8. Silicone sling. *A* to *D*, Operative steps in the insertion of the sling. *E* and *F*, Pre- and postoperative results.

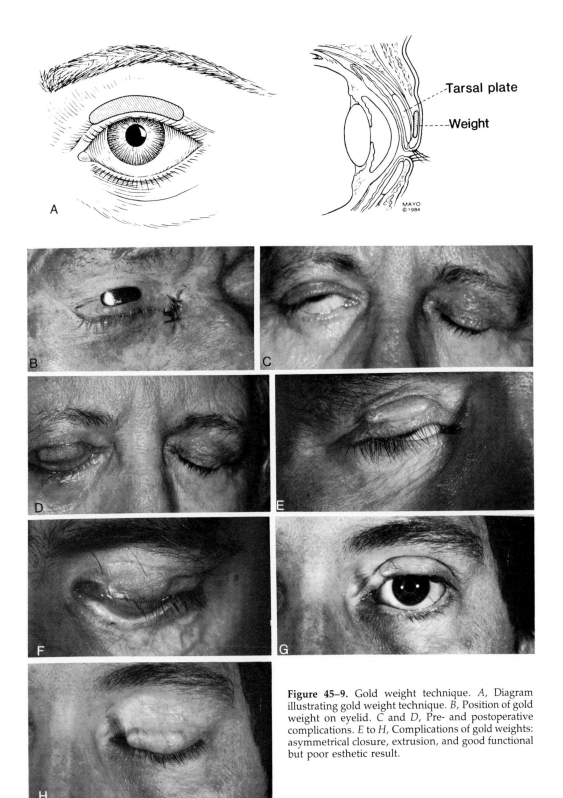

Figure 45–9. Gold weight technique. *A*, Diagram illustrating gold weight technique. *B*, Position of gold weight on eyelid. *C* and *D*, Pre- and postoperative complications. *E* to *H*, Complications of gold weights: asymmetrical closure, extrusion, and good functional but poor esthetic result.

The gold weight may be purchased pre-formed* or it can be made from the gold strips used in dental prosthetics. The gold is shaped to conform to globe convexity. A wide range of weights should be available; however, the most commonly used is 1.5 to 1.75 gm. To assess the required load, a series of weights are taped to the eyelid in succession until closure can be obtained normally. The weight that provides normal closure is inserted in the upper lid.

Technique. Under local anesthesia, a small incision is made in the lateral canthal area. A tunnel is created in the upper lid between the skin and the tarsal plate. The weight is then inserted into the tunnel, the midpoint being placed over the center of the lid. Because the weight may become displaced, nylon sutures are placed through the skin and onto the tarsal plate to immobilize the gold. These sutures are left in position for 4 to 6 weeks (Fig. 45–9).

Results. These have been satisfactory in reported series and in our own cases. The complications of this procedure are insufficient loading of the lid, infection in relation to the implant, extrusion of the implant, and asymmetrical lid closure. Of a total of 63 cases, it has been necessary to remove one implant for infection, one for exposure, and one for patient dissatisfaction; in addition, two implants had to be repositioned. Three patients referred to us from other institutions who had extrusion of the gold weights had them replaced using de-epithelialized flaps (as described earlier) for protection over the implant. The commercially available implants have holes in them to allow fixation and obviate the use of stabilizing sutures. Unfortunately, it is then difficult to remove the implant if anything goes wrong. This contravenes one of the rules of implants: easy to insert and easy to remove.

Muscle Transfer. As opposed to the somewhat static measures of the previous procedures, this is a more active approach in which the temporalis muscle is used to power the lids. Muscle transfer has been very popular for the treatment of lagophthalmos associated with leprosy.[11, 19, 26, 34]

Technique. The temporalis fascia is exposed through a vertical temporal incision over the temporalis muscle. A strip of fascia 1.5 to 2 cm is outlined and detached inferiorly from the zygomatic arch. The fascia is then lifted up to just below the insertion of the muscle into the temporal bone. At the fasciomuscular junction, it is stabilized with several interrupted nylon sutures. The fascia is divided vertically in the midline. The strip of temporalis muscle to which the fascia is now attached is dissected out and elevated from the underlying temporal bone. A wide tunnel is made from the temporal area to the lateral canthal region. Additional tunnels are made in the upper and lower lids; these are placed 1 cm from the margin of the upper lid and 0.5 cm from the margin of the lower lid. Through a small medial incision the medial canthal ligament is dissected out. The temporalis fascia is now introduced into the tunnels, pulled tight to give partial lid closure, and sutured to the medial canthal ligaments (Fig. 45–10).

Results. These depend on whether the tension in the fascia is correct and whether the patient learns to synchronize the blink with the temporalis contracture. If these two criteria are met, the results can be very good. If the fascia is too slack, this can be tightened later.

Temporalis Reinnervation. A variation of the preceding procedure has been described by Freilinger.[10]

Technique. The temporalis transfer is performed as just described. In addition, a crossfacial nerve branch from the frontal branch of the uninvolved nerve is taken across the forehead, and its free end is buried in the transposed temporalis muscle. As axons sprout from the end of the nerve graft, the temporalis is innervated from the uninvolved nerve. Thus, eyelid movement is more symmetrical.

Results. Although the originators of the technique have reported good results, our experience in using this method in the lower face for establishing oral movement has been disappointing. This has been the case even when the nerve graft has been totally successful in terms of axon regeneration.

Free Muscle Grafting. In 1971, Thompson[35, 36] described the initial technique of free muscle grafting. It was based on the concept that denervated muscle is less susceptible to ischemia and thus free grafting of muscle is more feasible. In addition, if a muscle graft is placed on healthy muscle, there will be ingrowth of nerve fibers from the healthy muscle into the empty endoneural tubes; reinnervation subsequently occurs as motor end plates are formed.[9] Thompson initially

---

*Meddev Corp., P.O. Box 1352, Los Altos, CA 94022.

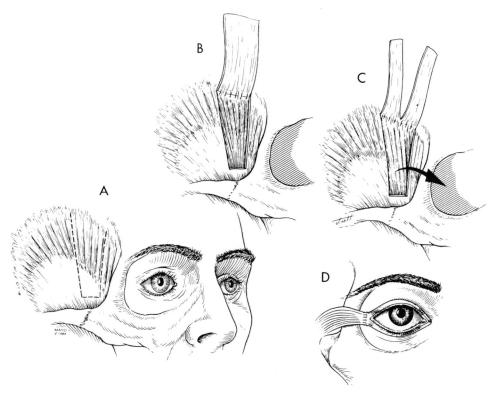

Figure 45–10. Temporalis transfer. *A* to *D*, Diagram of temporalis transfer for lagophthalmos.

employed this procedure to restore oral competence and later to treat lagophthalmos.

Technique. The muscle chosen is the extensor digiti minimi. The nerve to the muscle is divided through an incision along the edge of the dorsalis pedis vascular territory on the dorsum of the foot. At the same time, Thompson removed the nasal pyramid through a vertical midnasal bridge incision while preserving the nasal mucosa. He next placed a silicone rod across the bridgeline and replaced the pyramid after suitable defects had been created to accept the silicone rod. Stranc[31] modified this by simply drilling holes in the nasal bones, dissecting down the nasal mucosal domes, and making a hole in the bony septum; again a rod was inserted. Two weeks later the extensor digitorum and the full extent of its tendons are removed.

On the nonparalyzed eyelids, an incision is made through the midpoint of the lid parallel with the lid margin, and the orbicularis is exposed. On the lower lid a lateral canthal and subciliary incision is made, and a blepharoplasty-type flap is turned down to expose the orbicularis. Subcutaneous tunnels are made medially toward the silicone rod.

On the paralyzed side, tunnels are made in the upper and lower lids. The extensor digitorum muscle bellies are dissected free of fascia, and the muscle bellies and tendons are separated into single units. One muscle is laid on the upper orbicularis and one on the lower. These are sutured to the normal muscles with catgut. The tendons are taken through the tunnel formed by the silicone rod and are led through the tunnels in the paralyzed lids. The upper muscle tendon goes through the lower lid and vice versa. These tendons are then tightened and sutured to the periosteum of the lateral orbital margin. All incisions are carefully closed (Fig. 45–11).

Hakelius[13] has modified this approach by using a vein graft with the endothelium against the silicone rod to form the nasal tunnel. This minimizes tendon adhesions. He now uses a muscle graft only from the normal lower lid to the paralyzed upper lid. Again, he finds this has reduced adhesions. For the ectropion of the lower lid, a tendon graft is used to provide support.

Results. Both Thompson[35, 36] and Hakelius[14] have reported very good results with this

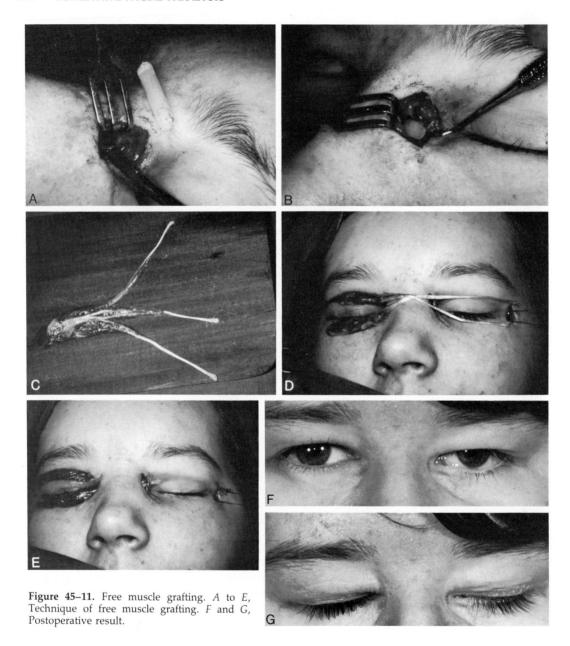

Figure 45–11. Free muscle grafting. *A* to *E*, Technique of free muscle grafting. *F* and *G*, Postoperative result.

technique, as have Mazzola and Antonelli.[20] This has also been our finding, but we feel that the simple gold weight can be just as satisfactory. The complications of free muscle grafting are adhesions in the nasal tunnel, which required tenolysis on one or more occasions, and nonfunctioning of the graft. Perhaps the biggest problem (before the dorsalis pedis vascular territory on the dorsum of the foot was charted) was delayed healing, sometimes with extensive skin necrosis, associated with the donor incision.

Free Vascularized Innervated Muscle Grafts

As described in Chapter 44, free vascularized muscle grafts reinnervated by suturing the muscle nerve to a cross-facial nerve graft could revolutionize the active treatment of lagophthalmos. Much work still needs to be done in relation to which muscle and how much should be transferred.

Lower Lid. The paralyzed orbicularis muscle of the lower lid will sometimes cause

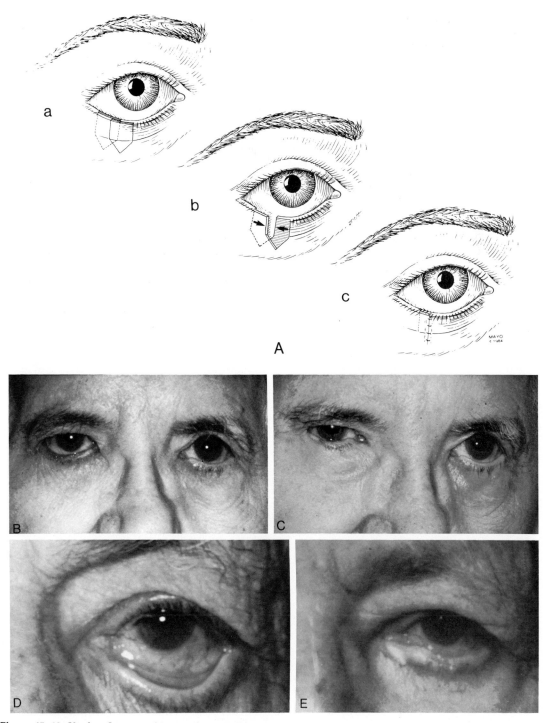

Figure 45–12. Kughnt-Szymanoski procedure. *A*, Diagram showing the steps of the Kuhnt-Szymanowski operation. *B* to *E*, Pre- and postoperative results.

ectropion and troublesome epiphora. As stated earlier, this is partly due to the punctum's being pulled away from the globe, but in addition is aggravated by the lack of the muscle suction pump mechanism that results from action of the orbicularis on the lower lid and encourages drainage of tears. There are four main methods of treatment:

Lateral Tarsorrhaphy. This has been described previously.

Fascial Sling. In this procedure, a strip of fascia is taken from the fascia lata.

TECHNIQUE. A tunnel is created through the lower lid parallel to the lid margin and about 0.5 cm from the margin. Using the lateral and medial canthal incisions, the fascial strip is passed through the tunnel. It is sutured laterally and medially under sufficient tension to hold the lid in correct position.

RESULTS. The results of this procedure are good, although with time the fascia tends to stretch. When this occurs, the symptoms tend to recur.

Lid Support. The support may be of cartilage or silicone.[2]

TECHNIQUE. A tunnel is dissected between the septum orbitale and the orbicularis and is taken up to the lid margin. A portion of the conchal cartilage or a carved piece of silicone is inserted and is secured to the soft tissue with fine nonabsorbable sutures.

RESULTS. In mild cases, lid support is successful, although skin edema has been reported in some cases of silicone implants.[3]

Kuhnt-Szymanowski Procedure. This old operation is a tightening procedure on the lower lid. If a simple wedge excision is performed, there may be problems of marginal notching and stretching with recurrence of symptoms.[18, 32] This technique attempts to address these problems.

TECHNIQUE. A pentagonal wedge is outlined on the middle area of the lid to provide the required tightness. This wedge is removed, taking only the outer half of the lid. A similar wedge is taken from the conjunctival aspect, but it is placed more laterally and takes only the inner half of the lid. The split lids are now moved together and sutured in position with deep catgut and superficial nylon (Fig. 45–12).

RESULTS. If this operation is performed correctly and the tension on the lower lid is satisfactory, the results are good. If there is some slackness of the lid in the long term, this procedure can be repeated. This is prob-

ably the technique of choice in patients with lower lid laxity associated with facial palsy. Occasionally, when the lower lid is very lax, the technique is modified by using the principle of the Bick procedure.[7] The wedge is moved laterally and the orbicularis and tarsal plate are dissected out and sutured to the lateral canthal ligament with fine nonabsorbable sutures. Some of the procedures described for lagophthalmos, e.g., silicone sling, magnets, temporalis transfer, and free muscle grafts, will also help the ectropion by virtue of their lower lid component.

CONCLUSIONS

Lagophthalmos can undoubtedly be greatly improved by surgery. Of the static methods, the gold weight is simple and reliable. Of the active methods, temporalis transfer gives good results in experienced hands, as do free muscle grafts.[16] Future management is clearly microsurgical, as replacement of nonfunctioning nerves and muscles with revascularization should solve the problem of lagophthalmos. However, that solution, in a reliable form, lies some way in the future.

References

1. Anderl, H.: Reconstruction of face through cross-face-nerve transplantation in facial paralysis. Chir. Plast., 2:17, 1973.
2. Anderl, H.: A simple method for correcting ectropion: preliminary report. Plast. Reconstr. Surg., 49:156, 1972.
3. Anderl, H., and Muhlbauer, W. D.: Surgery of facial palsy. In Jackson, I. T. (ed.): Recent Advances in Plastic Surgery. New York, Churchill Livingstone, 1981, p. 181.
4. Arion, H. G.: Dynamic closure of the lids in paralysis of the orbicularis muscle. Int. Surg., 57:48, 1972.
5. Arion, H. G.: Technique de fermeture dynamique des paupières dans les paralysies de l'orbiculaire. Ann. Chir., 23:847, 1969.
6. Barclay, T. L., and Roberts, A. C.: Restoration of movement to the upper eyelid in facial palsy. Br. J. Plast. Surg., 22:257, 1969.
7. Bick, M. W.: Surgical management of orbital tarsal disparity. Arch. Ophthalmol., 75:386, 1966.
8. Converse, J. M.: Facial paralysis. In Converse, J. M. (ed.): Surgical Treatment of Facial Injuries, Vol 2, 3rd Ed. Baltimore, Williams & Wilkins, 1974, p. 1235.
9. Erlacher, P.: Experimentelle Untersuchungen über Plastik und Transplantation von Nerv und Muskel. Arch. Klin. Chir., 106:389, 1915.
10. Freilinger, G.: A new technique to correct facial paralysis. Plast. Reconstr. Surg., 56:44, 1975.

11. Gillies, H., and Millard, D. R., Jr.: The Principles and Art of Plastic Surgery, Vol 2. Boston, Little, Brown & Co., 1957, p. 605.

12. Guy, C. L., and Ransohoff, J.: The palpebral spring for paralysis of the upper eyelid in facial nerve paralysis: technical note. J. Neurosurg., 29:431, 1968.

13. Hakelius, L.: Free muscle and nerve grafting in the face. In Rubin, L. R. (ed.): Reanimation of the Paralyzed Face: New Approaches. St. Louis, C. V. Mosby Co., 1977, p. 278.

14. Hakelius, L.: Transplantation of free autogenous muscle in the treatment of facial paralysis: a clinical study. Scand. J. Plast. Reconstr. Surg., 8:220, 1974.

15. Illig, K. M.: Eine Neue Operationsmethode gegen Lagophthalmus. Klin. Monatsbl. Augenheilkd., 132:410, 1958.

16. Jackson, I. T.: Surgical treatment of eyelid problems in facial palsy. In Tessier, P., Callahan, A., Mustarde, J. C., and Salyer, K. (eds.): Symposium on Plastic Surgery in the Orbital Region. St. Louis, C. V. Mosby Co., 1976, p. 389.

17. Jobe, R. P.: A technique for lid loading in the management of the lagophthalmos of facial palsy. Plast. Reconstr. Surg., 53:29, 1974.

18. Kuhnt, H.: Beiträge zur Operativen augenheilkunde. Jena, G. Fischer, 1883, p. 45.

19. Masters, F. W., Robinson, D. W., and Simons, J. N.: Temporalis transfer for lagophthalmos due to seventh nerve palsy. Am. J. Surg., 110:607, 1965.

20. Mazzola, R. F., and Antonelli, A. R.: Contribution to treatment of permanent facial paralysis by free muscle grafting based on 21 cases. Chir. Plast., 3:59, 1975.

21. McLaughlin, C. R.: Epiphora in facial paralysis. Br. J. Plast. Surg., 3:87, 1950.

22. McLaughlin, C. R.: Permanent facial paralysis: the role of surgical support. Lancet, 2:647, 1952.

23. Morel-Fatio, D.: Le ressort palpébral. Ann. Chir. Plast., 12:51, 1967.

24. Morel-Fatio, D., and Lalardrie, J.-P.: Palliative surgical treatment of facial paralysis: the palpebral spring. Plast. Reconstr. Surg., 33:446, 1964.

25. Muhlbauer, W. D., Segeth, H., and Viessman, A.: Restoration of lid function in facial palsy with permanent magnets. Chir. Plast., 1:295, 1973.

26. Rubin, L. R.: Reanimation of the Paralyzed Face: New Approaches. St. Louis, C. V. Mosby Co., 1977, p. 294.

27. Scaramella, L.: L'anastomosi tra l due nervi facciali. Arch. Otol., 82:209, 1971.

28. Smellie, G. D.: Restoration of the blinking reflex in facial palsy by a simple lid-load operation. Br. J. Plast. Surg., 19:279, 1966.

29. Smith, J. W.: Advances in facial nerve repair. Surg. Clin. North Am., 52:1287, 1972.

30. Smith, J. W.: A new technique of facial animation. In Hueston, J. T. (ed.): Transactions of the Fifth International Congress of Plastic and Reconstructive Surgery, Melbourne. London, Butterworths, 1971, p. 83.

31. Stranc, M. F.: Personal communication, 1973.

32. Szymanowski, J.: Handbuch der Operativen Chirurgie. Braunschweig, F. Vieweg u. Sohn, 1870, p. 243.

33. Tessier, P., Delbet, J.-P., Pastoriza, J., and Lekiefre, M.: Les paupières paralysées. Ann. Chir. Plast., 14:215, 1969.

34. Thagoraj, R. H.: The correction of lagophthalmos in leprosy. In Hueston, J. T. (ed.): Transactions of the Fifth International Congress of Plastic and Reconstructive Surgery, Melbourne. London, Butterworths, 1971, p. 59.

35. Thompson, N.: Autogenous free grafts of skeletal muscle: a preliminary experimental and clinical study. Plast. Reconstr. Surg., 48:11, 1971.

36. Thompson, N.: Treatment of facial palsy by free skeletal muscle grafts. In Hueston, J. T. (ed.): Transactions of the Fifth International Congress of Plastic and Reconstructive Surgery, Melbourne. London, Butterworths, 1971, p. 66.

37. Walsh, F. B.: Clinical Neuro-Ophthalmology, 2nd Ed. Baltimore, Williams & Wilkins, 1957.

38. Wilflingseder, P., and Anderl, H.: Indications for intermittent palliative surgical measures and long-term results with alloplasties in facial paralysis. Arch. Ital. Otol., 82:268, 1971.

39. Wood Smith, D.: Experience with Arion prosthesis. In Tessier, P., Callahan, A., Mustarde, J. C., and Salyer, K. (eds.): Symposium on Plastic Surgery in the Orbital Region. St. Louis, C. V. Mosby Co., 1976, p. 404.

46

Microsurgical Reanimation of the Eye Sphincter

■

Kenneth K. Lee, M.B.B.S., F.R.A.C.S.
Julia K. Terzis, M.D., Ph.D.

The problems of facial palsy can be arbitrarily divided functionally and anatomically into disorders of the upper and lower face. The dominant problem in the upper face is paralysis of the eye sphincter, which can occur in both partial and complete facial palsy. The resultant deformity and disability of the affected eye may vary from individual to individual. Ocular problems and complications occur secondary to lagophthalmos, paralytic ectropion of the lower eyelid, and decreased tear production.[20, 23] In particular, lagophthalmos will result in widening of the palpebral fissure and loss of protective function of the upper lid. Keratitis and corneal ulcerations may also occur. Paralytic ectropion of the lower eyelid will lead to epiphora and chronic inflammation and epidermidalization. Both conditions produce obvious esthetic deformities. Tear production may be decreased if the involvement of the facial nerve is proximal to the greater superficial petrosal nerve branch, which is the secretomotor nerve for the lacrimal gland. As in all facial nerve palsies, we should look for and exclude possible concomitant trigeminal nerve loss, which will produce the condition of neuroparalytic keratopathy. The aims in management are to protect the cornea, preserve vision, and then correct functional and esthetic deformities.

The methods of management can be nonsurgical or surgical. Nonsurgical measures are primarily protective and supportive and include ocular lubrication, lid taping, protective glasses and moisture chambers, pressure patches, soft contact lenses, scleral shells, physiotherapy, and exercises. Surgical procedures are usually required for long-standing and permanent paralysis. Various ingenious procedures have been devised in the past to provide esthetic support. Tarsorrhaphies have been the most common procedures, and these range from the simple eyelid suture to the two-pillar tarsorrhaphy to the improved lateral tarsorrhaphies of McLaughlin.[27] Tarsorrhaphies have reduced the complications of lagophthalmos, and some, such as the McLaughlin tarsorrhaphy, also attempt to support the lower eyelid. To correct paralytic ectropions, lid shortening and many different methods of canthoplasties have been designed. An excellent review of this has been done by Edgerton and Wolfort.[9]

These procedures are simple and functionally very effective in protecting the function of the eye and improving the appearance, especially at rest. Most of them, however, share a common problem of deterioration with time as a result of gravity or opposing forces and therefore require revisions. In addition to limiting the range of vision, they are esthetically unsatisfactory because they are fixed and tend to deform the normal appearance of the eye. As a result, dynamic procedures have been designed to improve appearance by providing lid blinking and more natural facial characteristics during repose and animation.

There are two main groups of procedures: those using synthetic implants and those using autogenous muscle transfer or transplantation. Synthetic implantations included lid loading,[36, 37] palpebral spring,[29] silicone encircling band,[2] and lid magnets.[31] Good results have been demonstrated by all these methods. However, as with all synthetic implants, particularly those exerting a force and situated close to the skin, complication rates are high. Complications include extrusion, migration, failure of the synthetic material, inflammatory, and infection. Furthermore, they tend to give an unnatural appearance to the eye, both at rest and during motion.

Autogenous muscle was first used as a motor unit for reinnervation of the eye by Gillies in 1934.[16] The muscle transferred was the temporalis, and various modifications of the original method have been described.[1, 25] As the temporalis muscles used are innervated by the fifth (trigeminal) nerve, action of the muscle on the eye is not coordinated or synchronous with action of the normal eyelid or facial expression. The most commonly used muscles for free muscle transplantation were the extensor digitorum brevis of the foot, innervated either by direct innervation of the orbicularis oculi muscle of the normal side or by nerve grafts.[17, 40] As well as causing deformities of the normal eye, all these procedures using autogenous muscle units exert their actions on the eyelid via two tendon-like bands situated in the upper and lower eyelids. This caused narrowing of the palpebral fissure into a slit at rest and deformity of the eye when the muscle contracted. That is, the eyelid tended to be pulled toward the side where the muscle belly lies.

More recently, in reanimation of the lower face by means of a microneurovascular motor unit, muscle strips were directed toward the eye for reanimation.[33] Such maneuvers result in action on the eye that is directly dependent on the action of the transplanted muscle on the lower face.

The dynamic procedures discussed so far all aim to give motion to the upper eyelid and usually fail to correct the lower eyelid problems and deformities. The therapeutic approach to reanimation of the eyelids so far has been a process of using consecutive procedures in ascending order of complexity, resulting in a combination of many methods, none of which has been totally satisfactory.

The advances in microreconstructive surgery have revitalized the management of the lower face in unilateral facial nerve palsy. In particular, the concept of free microneurovascular muscle transplantation, innervated by revised ipsilateral facial nerve stumps or sharing of contralateral facial nerve fibers via cross-facial nerves, has opened new horizons in surgery for reanimation of the lower face.[18, 32, 38] Since then, continuous progress has been made, not only in the search for a

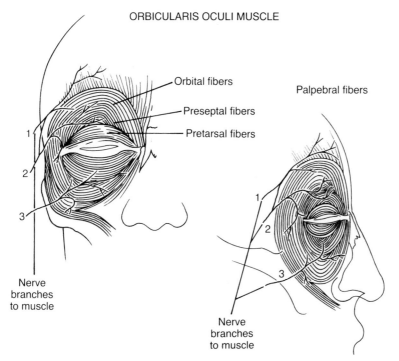

ORBICULARIS OCULI MUSCLE

Orbital fibers

Preseptal fibers

Pretarsal fibers

Palpebral fibers

Nerve branches to muscle

Nerve branches to muscle

Figure 46–1. The normal anatomy of the orbicularis oculi muscle. Note the division into pretarsal, preseptal, and orbital fibers and their innervation from frontal and zygomatic branches of the seventh cranial nerve.

better muscle as a motor unit, but also in the way the muscle is tailored and arranged to fit into the face and the site and method of attachment for the origin and the insertions in order to provide more natural reanimation of the paralyzed lower face. The pectoralis minor, serratus anterior, and tailored latissimus dorsi muscles have been used because of the multiple slips of muscle available in the former two muscles and the dual nerve supply present in the pectoralis minor muscle.[4, 39] In selected cases these muscles have given results superior to simple muscles, such as the gracilis.

Unfortunately, parallel advances have not been made in the reconstruction of the eye sphincter. Since 1980, our unit (the Microsurgery Research Center, Eastern Virginia Medical School) has commenced to address the problems of eye sphincter reanimation as one of its many projects. All patients with unilateral facial palsy admitted for reanimation by free microneurovascular muscle transplantations have multiple facial nerve grafts performed as the first stage. Attention is directed not only to having two or more nerve grafts available for reanimation of the lower face, but also to having one nerve graft available from branches of the frontal-zygomatic nerve on the normal side for reanimation of the upper face. Our search for a suitable muscle to reanimate the eye was carried out by reviewing all the available transplantable muscles in the body and progressing to available facial muscles on the normal side. The aim of our present study was to (1) examine the normal anatomy and function of the eye sphincter (Fig. 46–1) and (2) assess the suitability of two facial muscles, namely the platysma and frontalis, as neurovascular motor units for the replacement reconstruction of the paralyzed orbicularis oculi muscle.

MATERIAL AND METHOD

Cadaveric Dissections

Eighteen fresh cadavers were dissected. They were all white, and the male:female ratio was 10:8. The ages ranged from 49 to 85 years with a mean of 71 ± 10 years.

Dissection of these fresh cadavers commenced with the dissection of the facial nerve from its extracranial origin at the stylomastoid foramen to its terminal branches, and

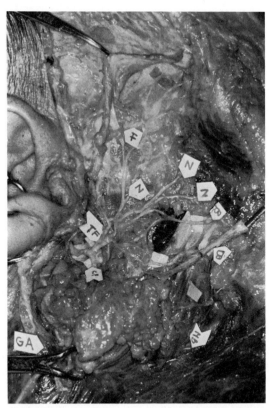

Figure 46–2. The extracranial course of the upper and lower divisions of the facial nerve was studied from the stylomastoid foramen to its muscular terminations. Labels depict the frontal (F), zygomatic (Z), buccal (B), mandibular (MB), temporofacial (TF), and cervicofacial (CF) branches. The greater auricular nerve (GA) is seen retracted to the left.

the nerve was carefully followed to its insertion into the frontalis, orbicularis oculi, and platysma muscles (Fig. 46–2). The skin and subcutaneous tissue overlying these three muscles were then carefully removed, using sharp scalpel dissection. The muscles were then elevated from their beds. The major vascular pedicles of the frontalis (supraorbital artery and vein) and the platysma (branches of the facial artery) were identified, followed, and measured, using a caliper with a linear scale. The motor nerve pedicles were also measured. In ten of the cadavers the following parameters of the three muscles were measured: (1) average fiber length, (2) width, (3) thickness, and (4) weight of the dissected muscles.

In six fresh cadavers extra care was taken to identify and follow the nerve fascicles going to each of the three muscles. These nerve fascicles were taken and immediately fixed in buffered formalin solution. Paraffin blocks were made and cross-sections were obtained with Luxol fast and Masson stains. Their corresponding muscles were also marked and fixed in buffered formalin solutions. Cross-sections of the muscles were made at the following specifications: (1) the frontalis at the junction of the caudal and middle third of the muscle belly, (2) the platysma at the junction of the cranial third and middle third of the muscle belly, (3) the orbicularis oculi, both upper and lower lids, at the midpoint of the palpebral fissure. These muscle cross-sections were processed in trichrome stain. The cross-section slides of the nerves and their corresponding muscles were then magnified and projected onto a wall screen with a light microscope projector. The number of myelinated nerve fibers and the number of muscle fibers were counted manually. This was done to give an indication of the muscle:nerve fiber ratio, that is, the density of innervation of these three muscles.

In six of the fresh cadavers the left side of the face was not dissected. The supraorbital arteries were identified, cannulated, and injected with barium suspension. A short section of the facial artery (measuring approximately 1 to 2 cm in length), where the direct muscular branch from the facial artery to the platysma and the submental branch of the facial artery emerged, was isolated, ligated at both ends, cannulated, and injected with a suspension of barium. After injection, the frontalis and platysma muscles were elevated from their bed. The overlying skin and subcutaneous tissue were then raised and discarded. The final specimens of injected muscle were taken to the Radiology Department where a xerogram was done to show the vascular pattern and to assess the adequacy of the arterial pedicles (Fig. 46–3). In another four of the fresh cadavers the supraorbital artery to the frontalis and the facial artery segment to the platysma were isolated, as just described. Freshly prepared colored acrylic solutions were injected. The cadavers were left overnight in order to have the acrylic solution solidify, and dissection of the muscle and the arterial pedicles was carried out the following day for demonstration purposes.

Functional Studies

Needle electromyography (EMG) was performed on six volunteers. The EMG needles

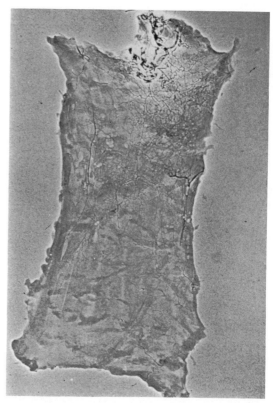

Figure 46–3. Xerogram of the vascular supply of the platysma muscle after injection of barium into a specified segment of the facial artery. Note that the intramuscular vasculature is voluminous in the upper two thirds of the platysma muscle, whereas there is a paucity in the lower one third.

were inserted into the upper eyelid at the middle of the pretarsal, preseptal, and orbital segment of the orbicularis oculi muscle (Fig. 46–4). Recordings were made with the subjects at rest, during automatic blink, during slow voluntary closure of the eyelid, and finally during forceful closure of both eyelids (Fig. 46–5). The tracings of the recordings were studied. Using a computerized digitized tablet, the amplitude and frequency of firing of the pretarsal, preseptal, and orbital segments of the orbicularis oculi muscles were calculated during blink, slow voluntary light closure, and forceful closure. The ages of the six volunteers ranged from 22 to 34 years with a mean of 27.5 years, and the male: female ratio was 4:2.

Another six volunteers, age range 16 to 32 years with a mean of 21.3 years, were involved in the next series of studies. By applying marking ink to the skin and measuring with a thread, the excursion of the orbicularis oculi, platysma, and frontalis muscles be-

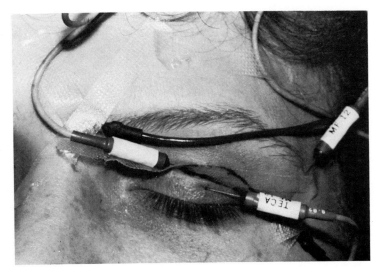

Figure 46–4. Position of the EMG needles in the pretarsal, preseptal, and orbital segments of the orbicularis oculi muscle.

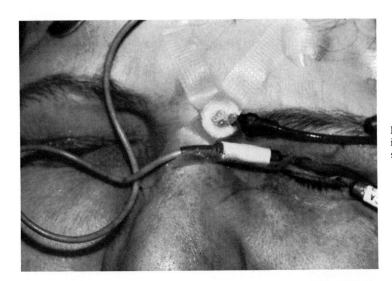

Figure 46–5. The needle EMG recording during forceful closure of the eye sphincter.

Figure 46–6. A force transducer records the force generated by movements of the upper lid in an otherwise immobile subject.

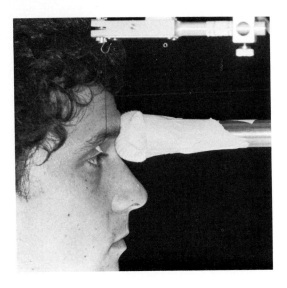

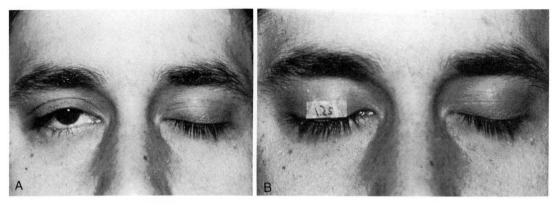

Figure 46–7. *A*, Temporary nerve blocks were carried out to the innervation of the right orbicularis oculi muscle. Note the inability to close the right eye. *B*, A 1.25-gm lead weight was needed to accomplish symmetrical closure of the right eye sphincter.

tween at rest and maximal voluntary action was measured. In order to measure the force generated by the upper lid in the direction of the action, which is at right angles to the direction of the muscle fibers, a thread is double taped at the mid-point of the eyelid. The head is positioned in the frame to prevent movement. The other end of the thread is connected to a force displacement transducer and recorder on a pencil meter chart. The amount of force generated when the subject performs involuntary blink, rapid forceful closure, and finally sustained forceful closure was recorded (Fig. 46–6).

Another six volunteers, age range 20 to 30 years with a mean of 25 years, were involved in the next set of studies. The frontal zygomatic nerve to the volunteer's right eye was blocked by means of an injection of 1% lidocaine (Xylocaine) with a 1:100,000 concentration of epinephrine (Fig. 46–7A). When the orbicularis oculi is paralyzed, which is shown by inability to raise the eyebrow as well as close the eyelids, a lead weight was used to load the upper eyelid until symmetrical closure of the eyelids was achieved. The amount of lead weight required was then recorded (Fig. 46–7B).

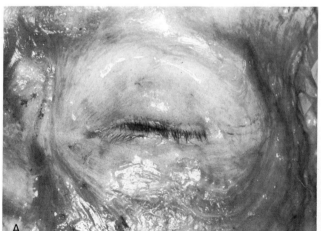

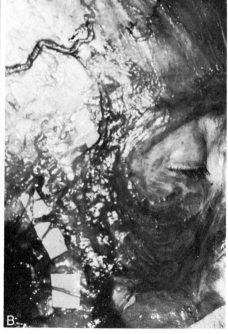

Figure 46–8. *A*, In all our dissections, the three parts of the orbicularis oculi muscle (the pretarsal, preseptal, and orbital) were present and easily identifiable. *B*, Note the extensive neural network entering the eye sphincter laterally. However, our microdissections could not depict dedicated innervation to each part.

RESULTS

Anatomy

All three muscles studied were present in all the dissections. In particular, all three portions, that is, the pretarsal, preseptal, and orbital portions of the orbicularis oculi, were identified (Fig. 46–8A), although partial or complete absence of these portions has been described.[41] The orbicularis oculi muscle is well vascularized by branches of the facial, superficial temporal, and internal maxillary arteries and has been described previously.[21, 41, 42] The motor nerve supply of the orbicularis oculi is by the frontal and zygomatic branches of the facial nerve. These branches divide into multiple small fibers, which freely com-

municate with each other before the insertion into the orbicularis oculi muscle (see Chapter 42) (Fig. 46–8B; see also Fig. 46–1). Identification of the nerve branches to the specific individual segments of the orbicularis oculi muscle could not be achieved in our microdissections (Fig. 46–8B).

In every case a constant dominant muscular branch to the platysma muscle was noted emerging from the facial artery just proximal to where the submandibular branch of the facial nerve crosses the facial artery. Of the 18 hemi-faces dissected for documentation of the vascular pedicle, 16 (88%) showed a direct branch emerging from the facial artery. In two cases (11%) this muscular branch shared a common trunk with the submental branch of the facial artery. This is illustrated in Figure 46–9A. Two basic patterns were

MUSCULAR BRANCH VARIATION

(N=18)

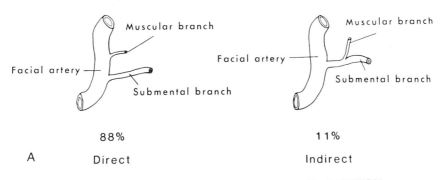

88%

A   Direct   11%

Indirect

CONSTANT MUSCULAR BRANCH PATTERN

(N=18)

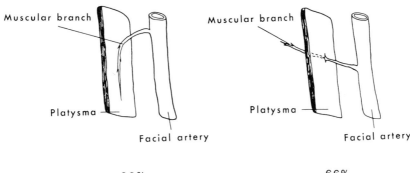

33%

B   Axial Pattern   66%

Perforator Pattern

Figure 46–9. *A,* diagrammatic depiction of the arterial supply to the platysma muscle from the facial artery. Note variation in the type of direct vs. indirect arterial supply. *B,* The arterial supply to the platysma can have a perforator pattern (66%) or an axial pattern (33%).

found. In all the male specimens and in two of the eight female specimens, the direct muscular branch is of the perforator pattern, which perforates the platysma muscle, giving off the branches in the substance of the muscle, and continues on to supply the skin and subcutaneous tissue. This perforator pattern accounts for 12 of 18 specimens. These arteries measured approximately 0.7 to 1.2 mm in diameter.

The remaining 6 of 18 specimens showed an axial pattern (Fig. 46–9B). That is, the direct muscular branch entered the deep surface of the platysma muscle and continued on this plane caudally and terminated at, or just close to, the point where the cervical branch of the facial nerve innervates the platysma muscle. The size of these arteries was comparatively smaller, as they measured 0.5 to 1 mm in diameter with a mean of 0.7 mm in diameter.

In both patterns the arteries were accompanied by a single vena comitans measuring approximately 0.8 to 1.5 mm in diameter with a mean of 1.2 mm. This single vein joins the submental vein before entering the facial vein. Injection with barium suspension and xerogram of the muscle showed that there is a vertically oriented plexus of arteries in the substance of the platysma muscle. With only the direct muscular branch and part of the

submental branch as pedicles, the cranial two thirds of the vascular plexus in the muscle can be well demonstrated (see Fig. 46–3). The dominant motor nerve supply in all cases was found to be the cervical branch of the facial nerve, which innervates the muscle at the junction of the cranial and middle third of the muscle, approximately 2 to 3 cm caudal to the direct muscular arterial branch. The available nerve pedicle measures approximately 3 to 5 cm with a mean of 3.5 cm (Fig. 46–10).

From the dissection of the 18 frontalis muscles, in every case the supraorbital artery was found situated in the supraorbital notch or tunnel, together with the sensory supraorbital nerve. The arteries are small and measure between 0.5 and 1 mm with a mean of 0.6 mm in diameter. The artery is accompanied by a number of veins. A dominant vein is always present close to, but lying outside, the supraorbital tunnel or notch and measures approximately 0.8 to 1.5 mm in diameter. Despite this small size, the adequacy of the supraorbital artery was demonstrated by the injection of barium suspension and a xerogram of the muscle. The motor supply of the frontalis muscle is small and difficult to identify (Fig. 46–11). Usually two to three small fascicles can be identified entering the lateral aspect of the frontalis muscle close to

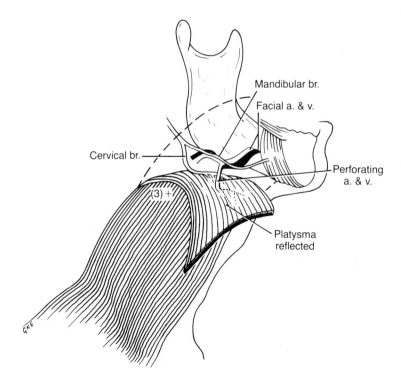

Mandibular br.

Facial a. & v.

Cervical br.

Perforating a. & v.

(3) +

Platysma reflected

Figure 46–10. The cervical branch of the facial nerve enters the platysma muscle 2 to 3 cm caudal to the entry of the direct muscular vessels, which corresponds to the proximal one third of the length of the platysma muscle.

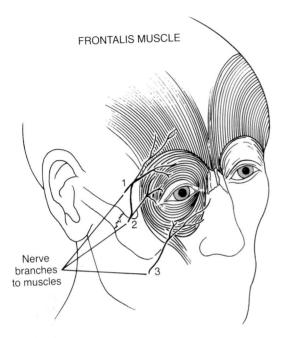

FRONTALIS MUSCLE

Nerve
branches
to muscles

Figure 46–11. The innervation of the frontalis and the orbicularis oculi muscles is shown diagrammatically. Branch No. 1 depicts branches to the frontalis and orbital portions of the upper eyelid. However, intraoperative single fascicular stimulation studies carried out in actual clinical cases disclose dedicated fascicles that innervate only the frontalis to the exclusion of orbicularis oculi muscle fibers. These dedicated frontalis fascicles can be identified only at the lateral border of the frontalis muscle. Branch No. 2 depicts the upper zygomatic neural outflow to the eye sphincter, while branch No. 3 suggests the innervation to the lower eye sphincter (see also Fig. 46–8B).

the junction between the interdigitations of the frontalis and orbicularis oculi muscles (see Fig. 46–8B). Other small fascicles are seen to innervate the orbital portion of the orbicularis oculi. The length of these tiny available branches is very small, measuring approximately 0.5 to 1 cm in all cases. The specificity of these fascicles in innervating the frontalis muscle was confirmed by the use of a nerve stimulator in our first clinical case report.

Table 46–1. MUSCLE DIMENSIONS (N = 10)

Muscle	Fiber Length (cm)	Width (cm)	Thickness (mm)
Orbicularis oculi	min. 3.52 max. 8.48	3.60*	1.03†
Platysma	16.21	7.40	1.05
Frontalis	9.00	5.62	1.23

*Upper half of orbicularis oculi.
†Mid-pretarsal segment.

Table 46–2. WEIGHT OF MUSCLE SPECIMENS

Muscle	Range	Mean (± 1 SD)
Orbicularis oculi	3.72–5.93	4.60 ± 1.50
Platysma	4.13–11.74	7.90 ± 2.35
Frontalis	2.18–7.09	3.73 ± 1.25

Parameters regarding fiber length, thickness, and weight of the dissected muscles were recorded in ten cases and are shown in Tables 46–1 and 46–2.

Data on the innervation density from three dissections are shown in Table 46–3. Cumulative data depicting the density of neural innervation of each muscle as represented by the muscle:nerve fiber ratio are shown in Table 46–4. It can be seen that the density of innervation of the frontalis and the platysma is similar and comparable to that of the orbicularis oculi muscle. The range between 10 to 26 is consistent with the findings of previous workers.[11]

Functional Studies

Needle EMG studies of each segment of the orbicularis oculi muscle of the six volunteers showed that the pretarsal and preseptal segments contract together and synchronously during blink and slow voluntary light closure as well as forceful closure. The orbital segment shows practically no activity at all during blink and slow voluntary light closure and is activated only during forceful closure of the eyelids (Fig. 46–12). In other words, the palpebral portion of the eye sphincter is concerned not only with the normal resting tone and support of the eyelids but is also the primary muscle involved in blinking and

Table 46–3. INNERVATION DENSITY (THREE DISSECTIONS)

Muscle	Muscle Fibers	Nerve Axons	M/N
First Dissection			
Orbicularis oculi	20,715	1,251	16.48
Platysma	15,341	806	19.03
Frontalis	15,060	1,043	14.44
Second Dissection			
Orbicularis oculi	23,518	908	25.90
Platysma	10,263	820	12.52
Frontalis	10,489	578	18.15
Third Dissection			
Orbicularis oculi	19,919	1,286	15.49
Platysma	3,709	753	4.93
Frontalis	9,612	848	11.33

BLINK

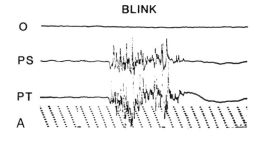

SLOW VOLUNTARY CLOSURE

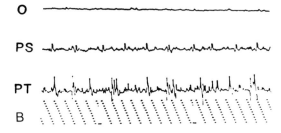

FORCEFUL CLOSURE

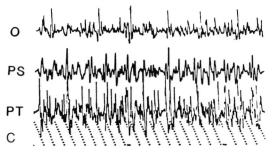

Figure 46–12. Needle EMG tracings of the pretarsal (PT), preseptal (PS), and orbital (O) segments or the orbicularis oculi muscle during (A) blink, (B) slow voluntary closure, and (C) forceful closure. Note that the orbital segment of the eye sphincter does not participate in the blink or slow voluntary closure activities and it is recruited only during forceful eye closure. In contrast, the pretarsal portion of the orbicularis oculi seems to be essential for all the eyelid functions.

Table 46–4. MUSCLE–NERVE FIBER RATIO

Specimen	Orbicularis Oculi	Platysma	Frontalis
A	15.49	4.93	11.33
B	25.90	12.52	18.15
C	16.48	19.03	14.44

light voluntary closure of the eye. Measurements of amplitude and frequency showed that the pretarsals have the highest values, followed by the preseptal segment and finally the orbital portion (Tables 46–5 and 46–6). This is similar to earlier findings reported previously.[13]

The force generated by the upper eyelid in the direction of closure is summarized in Figure 46–13. From the tracing we can see that in a normal blink approximately 2 to 3 gm of force is generated, whereas in a rapid forceful closure, up to 41 gm is generated. In sustained forceful closure, after the initial force equals the rapid forceful closure, the muscle settles into an average force of 21 to 42 gm. The difference between the rapid and the sustained forceful closure may be due to the fatigue of the fast-acting muscles. The slow-acting muscles are primarily responsible for the sustained forceful closure. The amount of force generated in the direction of the muscle fibers can be worked out by a simple formula involving work.

$$F = \frac{L \cdot X}{\Delta S}$$

where F = force in the direction of the muscle contraction, L = force generated in the direction of eyelid contraction, X = vertical displacement of the upper eyelid, and S = excursion at rest and at eye closure.

In our six volunteers who had the frontal zygomatic branch blocked with local anes-

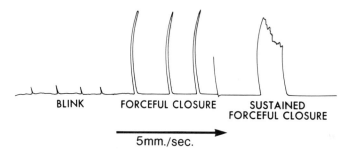

BLINK   FORCEFUL CLOSURE   SUSTAINED FORCEFUL CLOSURE

5mm./sec.

Figure 46–13. The force generated by the upper eyelid in the direction of forceful closure is depicted in this diagram.

Table 46–5. NEEDLE EMG STUDIES (N = 6)

	Mean Amplitude (mV)		
	O	PS	PT
Blink	62.88	461.16	933.40
Slow voluntary closure	100.46	254.14	405.60
Forceful closure	1,195.61	1,314.57	1,487.87

Table 46–7. MINIMUM FORCE REQUIRED TO CLOSE UPPER EYELID (N = 6)

Range	Mean (±1 SD)
1.00–1.25 (gm)	1.13±0.14 (gm)

thetic, the minimum amount of weight required to close the upper eyelid symmetrically with the normal side varied from 1 to 1.25 gm, with a mean of 1.13 gm (Table 46–7). This weight requirement is similar to that carried out by Smellie,[37] which was performed on patients with facial palsy.

The amount of excursion of each muscle from rest to maximum voluntary contraction is summarized in Table 46–8. It can be seen that the frontalis has the greatest range of excursion per centimeter of muscle compared with the pretarsal segment of the orbicularis oculi, which is greater than that of the platysma. However, the difference between the three muscles is very small, and the range of excursion of all three muscles is comparable.

DISCUSSION

We have reviewed the management available so far for the eye in facial paralysis. There has been no attempt to restore eye sphincter function by replacement reconstruction. Our aim is to replace the atrophied, paralyzed orbicularis oculi muscle with a comparable muscle that has intrinsic resting tone as well as a range for dynamic action. The replacement muscle is situated in and has action directly on both the upper and the lower eyelids. This motor innervation is either by revised ipsilateral nerve stumps or by sharing of contralateral facial nerve fibers that are specific for eye sphincter function.

An ideal replacement muscle should have the following qualities: (1) capability of being transferable or transplantable as a neurovascular unit, (2) adequate excursion, (3) ade-

quate tension, (4) adequate density of innervation, (5) comparable muscle type, (6) capability of being arranged into a sphincter configuration, and (7) minimal donor site morbidity.

Transferability

The vascular supply of the platysma muscle has been studied because of its relationship to the cervical skin flaps used in reconstructive surgery for head and neck cancer patients.[10, 24] Kambic and Sirca[22] injected red mercuric sulphice in gelatin in seven cadavers of newborns and showed that the arterial branches in the neck run vertically and supply segmentally. This is confirmed by studies performed by Freeland and Rogers,[12] who also showed that the platysma muscle is pierced by branches from multiple sources that form a vascular plexus in this substance, which also runs vertically. Cadenat et al.[5] studied cadavers of ten adults, three infants, and three fetuses and noted a significant contribution by a direct muscular branch to the platysma muscle from the superior thyroid artery. Advances in myocutaneous flaps led to the use of the platysma muscle.[14, 34] The flexibility and versatility of the platysma myocutaneous flap have been reported recently by Hurwitz et al.[19] and Coleman et al.[6] The flexibility was due to the abundance of direct branches to the platysma muscle from the facial, superior thyroid, occipital, posterior auricular, subclavian, transverse, or superficial cervical arteries.[19] Preservation of at least one region will supply the entire muscle. Direct branches from the facial artery to the platysma and its overlying skin were first described in 1936 by Salmon[35] and were men-

Table 46–6. NEEDLE EMG STUDIES (N = 6)

	Mean Frequency (msec)		
	O	PS	PT
Blink	10.50	33.83	39.83
Slow voluntary closure	18.33	32.83	35.67
Forceful closure	38.67	41.17	40.83

Table 46–8. EXCURSION STUDIES (N = 6): cm/cm RESTING LENGTH

Muscle	Range	Mean (±1 SD)
Orbicularis oculi	0.12–0.23	0.18±0.03
Platysma	0.10–0.17	0.14±0.03
Frontalis	0.19–0.31	0.27±0.04

tioned and shown in illustrations by many other authors.[5, 12, 19, 22, 26] From our dissection and injection studies, it is seen that this direct muscular branch from the facial artery is not only constant but of adequate size to nourish a large portion of the platysma muscle. The direct muscular branch may be used as the pedicle for anastomosis, or if a larger vessel is desired, the facial artery and vein may be used. The large caliber of the facial artery and vein is in keeping with the current trend of using a large vascular pedicle in free flap transplantation to decrease risk of failure. Furthermore, the cervical branch of the facial nerve, which is also constant in all our dissections, innervates the muscle at close proximity to the vascular pedicle. Based on these data, a large proportion of the platysma muscle is transplantable as a neurovascular free flap.

The idea of using the frontalis muscle as a pedicled transpositional flap to provide a neurovascular motor unit was initiated by the senior author (JKT) in her search to find a comparable muscle while simultaneously avoiding demanding microvascular anastomoses, which would allow wider clinical usage for this transfer. This search started by observing the many flaps that have been used successfully for nasal reconstruction. In particular, the supraorbital artery and vein were the major vascular pedicle for the up-and-down forehead flap advocated by Gillies,[15] the so-called loop-shaped supraorbital flap described by New,[31] and the midline vertical forehead flap proposed by Millard.[28] Further stimulus was provided by the use of the forehead island flap with a subcutaneous pedicle[7] and the use of the midline forehead flap in reconstructive procedures of the eyelids and the exenterated socket.[8] As determined by our anatomic dissections, the entire frontalis muscle can be raised as an island transpositional flap based on the supraorbital artery and vein. When transposed over the opposite eye, the muscle belly would cover the entire orbit and beyond. The adequacy of the supraorbital artery to supply the entire muscle despite the small size of the artery and the fact that the major trunk of the artery lies within the muscle have been demonstrated by the barium injection studies and xerograms. This was further confirmed by the use of a Doppler device during our first clinical case. Our anatomic studies also showed that the motor nerve supply to the frontalis muscle can be identified, dissected

out, and used as a motor nerve pedicle for the frontalis muscle flap.

Excursion and Tension

The potential excursion of a muscle is related to its fiber length.[3] From our measurements of the average fiber length, we have shown that the platysma and frontalis muscles have more than adequate fiber length for reconstruction of the eye sphincter. This is further demonstrated by our studies using volunteers, which show comparable excursion per centimeter of the muscle among all three muscles studied. The relative tension of the muscle has also been assessed to be proportional to the cross-section of the muscle. As the width of the replacement muscles will be equal to the width of the original atrophied orbicularis oculi muscle, the thickness of the muscle will determine the relative tension. From our dissections, the thickness of the muscle, in decreasing order, is (1) frontalis, (2) platysma, and (3) orbicularis oculi (measured at the mid-point of the pretarsal segment in the upper eyelid) [see Table 46–1]). Adequate excursion and tension of the donor replacement muscles are important to allow for the loss of the working capacity of the muscle after transplantation and reinnervation because, as has been shown by Terzis et al.,[39] even under optimal experimental conditions, free muscle transplantation would result in the loss of 75% of the previous working capacity of the muscle. Furthermore the force generated by the upper eyelid orbicularis oculi muscle can range from 0 to 50 gm. As the force generated by a normal involuntary blink is only approximately 2.6 gm, it is hoped that the reinnervated replacement muscles will retain enough working capacity to generate a varying range of forces for automatic blink and light voluntary closure, as well as moderately forceful closure, for both protection and animation. Attention to the muscle's normal resting tension during transplantation has also been emphasized.[39]

Muscle Type

The platysma and the frontalis muscles, like the orbicularis oculi, are facial muscles of expression. They have the same origin from mesoderm of the second brachial arch.[21] They are all innervated by branches of the facial nerve and are capable of automatic, involuntary, and voluntary as well as reflex actions. The platysma and frontalis are therefore two of the best muscles available for replacement reconstruction of the orbicularis oculi muscle.

Density of Innervation

The density of innervation for the platysma and frontalis muscles has been shown to be comparable to that of the orbicularis oculi muscle. The total number of myelinated nerve fibers to the orbicularis oculi muscle has also been shown to be nearly twice that of myelinated fibers innervating the platysma or frontalis. In all our cross-facial nerve grafting procedures, at least 50% of all the fibers to the normal eye sphincter are selected and used as donor nerve fibers to the cross-facial graft. The remaining 50% or less appear to be more than adequate to maintain normal function of the normal eye sphincter. The number of myelinated motor fibers available to reinnervate the transplanted muscles is also likely to be adequate. In the past, reinnervation of the frontalis muscle following trauma to its motor nerve had a low success rate and poor results. We feel that this was due more to the difficulties involved in identifying and isolating the specific motor fascicles of the frontalis than to a problem of low density of innervation of the frontalis.

Donor Site Morbidity

The platysma and frontalis muscles are minor muscles of facial expression and are not primarily involved with sphincter function. Taking of the platysma muscle does leave a permanent extra scar in the neck, although this can be minimized by having the scar lie in the transverse skin crease. Elevation of the muscle may interfere with the sensory supply to the overlying skin, as the sensory branches of the cervical plexus may be disturbed. However, such a deficit is minor and is limited only to the small areas equal to the amount of platysma required to reconstruct the eye sphincter. A short segment of the facial artery and vein may be sacrificed to be used as the pedicle for the muscle flap. This has little influence on the overall blood supply of the head and neck region. The limited function of the platysma as a muscle of facial expression will be lost, although this may be an advantage, to match the appearance of the neck on the paralyzed side.

For the frontalis muscle, a bicoronal scalp flap is used for access and will be hidden within the hair line. Sensory supply to the forehead of the donor site will be interfered with, as the supraorbital nerve is included with the vascular pedicle for the island frontalis muscle flap. This loss will be minimized by preserving the supratrochlear nerve, which lies more medially, as well as some of the direct cutaneous branches of the supraorbital nerve. Taking of the muscle will result in the loss of ability to elevate the eyebrow on the donor side and interference with some facial expressions. However, like the platysma, this may also be an advantage, to add symmetry to match the paralyzed side.

In addition to donor site morbidity, the major disadvantage of the free neurovascular platysma flap is that it is a long procedure that requires microsurgical techniques. It also has all the risks and complications of a free vascularized tissue transplantation. The frontalis neuromuscular unit does not involve microvascular anastomosis and is therefore much safer, although identification and preservation of the motor nerve to the muscle is a very difficult and tedious process.

Configuration

Functional EMG studies of the upper eyelid show that the pretarsal and preseptal segments of the orbicularis oculi muscle function together and synchronously to close the upper eyelid in normal automatic blink, voluntary light closure, and forceful closure. The orbital portion, however, is activated only in forceful closure. If the palpebral portion (which includes the pretarsal and preseptal segments) and the orbital portion have independent function and nerve supply, reconstruction of the entire orbicularis oculi muscle will require a muscle with at least a dual nerve supply with independent function. Moreover, it is not possible to identify and dissect separate donor nerve fibers that innervate the specific segments of the orbicularis oculi muscle. Our aim, therefore, is to

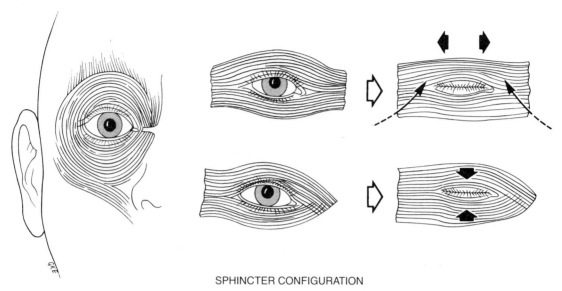

SPHINCTER CONFIGURATION

Figure 46–14. The sphincter configuration that we recommend is diagrammatically depicted in the lower part of the diagram. Note that the two muscular strips drape over the eyeball and overlap onto each other at the ends. This allows simultaneous support of the eyelid and an open position of the palpebral fissure. Eyelid closure then is achieved by vertical forces generated by contraction of the muscle fibers from a resting open position (lower right). The sphincter configuration depicted on the upper part of the diagram is to be avoided (see text).

reconstruct only the palpebral portion of the orbicularis oculi muscle. The muscle fiber configuration of inner parallel fibers of the pretarsal segment and outer concentric ellipses for the preseptal segment arranged in a thin sheet of muscle draped on the globular eyeball is unique.

An attempt is made to arrange the thin sheet of donor muscles (the platysma or the frontalis) into a configuration that will act as a sphincter similar to that of the orbicularis oculi. The neurovascular pedicle is kept intact on one end of the donor muscle sheet. The opposite end is split into two strips. The width of each strip is measured to correspond to the width of the palpebral segment of the eyelids to be reconstructed. The split is carried as close to the neurovascular pedicle as possible without disturbing the vascular and motor nerve supply to each strip. The two strips can then be draped over the globular eyeball and made to overlap onto each other at the free divided ends. In this way the replacement muscle will wrap around the globular surface of the eye with intrinsic muscle tone, which will support the eyelid and leave an open position of the palpebral fissure, as on the normal side. Contractions of the muscle will result in closure of the palpebral fissure from an open position.

Without this overlapped configuration, the two strips of muscle with this resting tone will cause narrowed palpebral fissure with a slit-like appearance. Furthermore, with both strips of muscle parallel to each other, contraction of the muscle will generate a force pressing directly down onto the eyelid. This concept is demonstrated in Figure 46–14.

Based on the above studies, the platysma and frontalis muscles have been shown to be potentially suitable for replacement reconstruction of a paralyzed eye sphincter. The indication for their use is to restore sphincter function to the eye in the case of a long-standing permanent complete or partial facial palsy. The prerequisite is loss of either the intact platysma or the frontalis muscle from the normal functioning side. Since 1981, the senior author (JKT) has successfully carried out two free platysma and eight pedicled frontalis muscle flaps for eye sphincter reanimation in unilateral facial palsy cases. These are being reported separately.

In addition, the platysma may be used as a free neurovascular motor unit to provide exact motion with limited tension excursion requirements. For example, it can be used to supplement defects of incomplete facial palsies. With the muscle innervated, the soft, pliable, well-vascularized, sheet-like platysma can be used to cover scalp defects or as cartilage frameworks for ear reconstruction. The frontalis as a pedicled island muscle flap has many potential uses, e.g., as a cover for exposed vital structures or a filler for contour defects around the orbital, periorbital, forehead, and nasal regions.

CONCLUSIONS

A study has been undertaken to better understand the anatomy and function of the normal eye sphincter. A new approach of replacement reconstruction using a neurovascular motor unit has been proposed to solve the orbital problems associated with unilateral long-standing permanent facial palsy. Two facial muscles were studied and proposed as suitable donor muscles. The platysma muscle can be used as a free neurovascular motor unit for transplantation, and the frontalis muscle can be used as a pedicled island neurovascular motor unit. The first respective clinical cases were carried out with success.

References

1. Anderson, J. G.: Surgical treatment of lagophthalmos in leprosy by the Gillies temporalis transfer. Br. J. Plast. Surg., 14:339, 1961.
2. Arion, H. G.: Dynamic closure of the lids in paralysis of the orbicularis muscle. Int. Surg., 57:48, 1972.
3. Brand, P. W., Beach, R. B., and Thompson, D. E.: Relative tension and potential excursion of muscles in the forearm and hand. J. Hand Surg., 6:209, 1981.
4. Buncke, H.: Personal communication.
5. Cadenat, J., Combelles, R., Closet, N., and Fabert, G.: Lambeaux cervicaux et cervico-dorsaux. Vascularization. Applications chirurgicales. Rev. Stomatol. Chir. Maxillofac., 79:227, 1978..
6. Coleman, J. J., III., Jurkiewicz, M. J., Nahai, F., and Mathes, S. J.: The platysma musculocutaneous flap: Experience with 24 cases. Plast. Reconstr. Surg., 72:315, 1983.
7. Converse, J. M., and Wood-Smith, D.: Experience with the forehead island flap with a subcutaneous pedicle. Plast. Reconstr. Surg., 31:521, 1963.
8. Dortzbach, R. K., and Hawes, M. J.: Midline forehead flap in reconstructive procedures of the eyelid and exenterated socket. Ophthal. Surg., 12:257, 1981.
9. Edgerton, M. T., and Wolfort, F. G.: The dermal-flap canthal lift for lower eyelid support. J. Plast. Reconstr. Surg., 43:42, 1969.
10. Ellis, M.: A surgical technique following irradiation of the neck. J. Laryngol. Otol., 77:872, 1964.
11. Feinstein, B., Lindegrad, B., Nyman, E., et al.: Morphologic studies of motor units in normal human muscles. Acta Anat., 23:127, 1954.
12. Freeland, A. P., and Rogers, J. H.: The vascular supply of the cervical skin with reference to incision planning. Laryngoscope, 85:714, 1975.
13. Furnas, D. W.: The orbicularis oculi muscle. Management in blepharoplasty. Clin. Plast. Surg., 8:687, 1981.
14. Futrell, J. W., Johns, M. E., Edgerton, M. T., Cantrell, R. W., and Fitz-Hugh, G. S.: Platysma myocutaneous flap for intra-oral reconstruction. Am. J. Surg., 136:504, 1978.
15. Gillies, H.: New free graft (skin and ear cartilage) applied to the reconstruction of the nostril. Br. J. Surg., 30:305, 1943.
16. Gillies, H. D.: Experiences with fascia lata grafts in the operative treatment of facial paralysis. Proc. Royal Soc. Med., 27:1372, 1934.
17. Hakelius, L.: Free muscle grafting. Clin. Plast. Surg., 6:301, 1979.
18. Harii, K., Ohmori, K., and Torii, S.: Free gracilis muscle transplantation with micro-neurovascular anastomosis for the treatment of facial palsy. Plast. Reconstr. Surg., 57:133, 1976.
19. Hurwitz, D., Rabson, J. A., and Futrell, J. W.: The anatomic basis for the platysma skin flap. Plast. Reconstr. Surg., 73:302, 1983.
20. Jelks, G. W., Smith, B., and Bosniak, D.: The evaluation and management of the eye in facial palsy. Clin. Plast. Surg., 6:397, 1979.
21. Jones, L. T., and Wobig, J. L.: Surgery of the Eyelid and Lacrimal System. New York, Aesculapius Publishing Company, 1976.
22. Kambic, V., and Sirca, A.: Die Vasculariztion der Haut des Halses und ihre Bedeutung fur die Schnittfuhrung dei der Radical Neck Dissection. Hals nas Ohren, 15:46, 1967.
23. Levine, R. E.: Management of the eye in facial paralysis. Otolaryngol. Clin. North Am., 7:531, 1974.
24. Martin, H.: Surgery in the treatment of head and neck cancer. Cancer, 13:65, 1963.
25. Masters, F. W., Robertson, D. W., and Simons, J. N.: Temporalis transfer for lagophthalmos due to seventh nerve palsy. Am. J. Surg., 110:607, 1965.
26. Mathes, S. J., and Nahai, F.: Classification of the vascular anatomy of muscles: Experimental and clinical correlations. Plast. Reconstr. Surg., 67:177, 1981.
27. McLaughlin, C. R.: Surgical support in permanent facial paralysis. Plast. Reconstr. Surg., 2:25, 1947.
28. Millard, D. R., Jr.: Hemirhinoplasty. Plast. Reconstr. Surg., 40:400, 1967.
29. Morell-Fatio, D., and Lalardrie, J. P.: Palliative surgical treatment of facial paralysis. The palpebral spring. Plast. Reconstr. Surg., 33:446, 1964.
30. Muhlbauer, W. D., Sageth, H., and Viessman, H.: Restoration of lid function in facial palsy with permanent magnet. Chir. Plastica (Berlin), 1:295, 1973.
31. New, G. B.: Total rhinoplasty using a forehead flap. Trans-Am. Soc. Plast. Reconstr. Surg., 13:33, 1944.
32. O'Brien, B. McC., Franklin, J. D., and Morrison, W. A.: Cross facial nerve grafts and micro-neurovascular free muscle transfer for long established facial palsy. Br. J. Plast. Surg., 83:202, 1980.
33. O'Brien, B. McC.: Personal communication.
34. Saito, H., Nishimurs, H., Matsui, T., Yamamichi, I., Tachibana, M., and Mizukoshi, O.: Primary reconstruction by modified island skin flap following resection of oral and pharyngeal cancer. Arch. Otolaryngol., 221:203, 1978.
35. Salmon, M.: Arteres des Muscles de la Tete et du Cou. Paris, Masson, 1936.
36. Sheehan, J. D.: Progress in correction of facial palsy with Tantalun wire and mesh. Surgery, 27:122, 1950.

37. Smellie, G. D.: Restoration of the blinking reflex in facial palsy by a simple lid load operation. Br. J. Plast. Surg., 19:279, 1966.

38. Terzis, J. K.: Personal communication.

39. Terzis, J. K., Sweet, R. C., Dykes, R. W., and Williams, H. B.: Recovery of function in free muscle transplants using micro-neurovascular anastomoses. J. Hand Surg., 3:37, 1978.

40. Thompson, N., and Gustavson, E. H.: The use of a neuromuscular free autograft with micro-neuro-anastomosis to restore elevation to the paralysed angle of the mouth in case of unilateral facial paralysis. Chir. Plastica, 3:165, 1976.

41. Whitnall, S. E.: The Anatomy of the Human Orbit and Accessory Organs of Vision. 2nd Ed. London, Oxford University Press, 1932.

42. Wolff, R., and Last, L. J.: Wolff's Anatomy of the Eye and Orbit. 6th Ed. Philadelphia, W. B. Saunders Company, 1968.

47

Facial Nerve Grafting in Acoustic Neurinoma

■

Madjid Samii, M.D.

The portion of the facial nerve in the cerebellopontine angle is compressed and lengthened by any space-occupying process. During the growth of neurinomas in the cerebellopontine angle and in the internal auditory canal, facial nerve function remains intact for a long time. The facial nerve around the tumor is mostly displaced in the ventral-caudal direction. Based on our own case material, we have never seen the course of facial nerve displaced posterior to the tumor. When a neurinoma is present, the individual fascicles of cranial nerves seven and eight are connected very closely to the tumor capsule. Therefore, the identification of the facial nerve has proved to be extremely difficult during tumor surgery.

The introduction of the operating microscope has strongly influenced our ability to preserve the facial nerve in tumor surgery involving the cerebellopontine angle as well as the internal auditory canal.[3-6, 9-11, 15] Three different microsurgical approaches for the treatment of acoustic neurinomas have been developed in the last 15 years: the middle fossa and translabyrinthine approaches (developed by otolaryngologic surgeons) and the lateral suboccipital approach (developed by neurosurgeons). With growing knowledge of the microanatomy of the cerebellopontine angle and internal auditory canal, the experience of the past few years has shown that the lateral suboccipital approach offers the best possible visibility to identify the facial nerve from the exit zone at the brain stem up to the fundus of the internal auditory canal. Therefore, this approach provides the best possible chance for preservation of the facial nerve. In addition, in most cases both continuity and function of the vestibulocochlear nerve can be preserved.[12-14] Our experience is based on 14 years of microsurgery in more than 200 cases of cerebellopontine angle lesions. In 85% of these cases we could preserve the continuity and function of the facial nerve. In those cases in which total removal of tumor necessitated sacrificing the facial nerve, the reconstruction of this nerve was accomplished in the same stage. However, instead of Dott's technique,[1] in 1975 we introduced a new method for facial nerve reconstruction in the cerebellopontine angle.

OPERATIVE TECHNIQUE

We operate upon cerebellopontine angle tumors with the patient in a semi-sitting position (Fig. 47–1). The head, supported in a special Mayfield holder, is anteflexed, fixed, and turned 30° to the contralateral side, with a slight upward tilt of the side to be operated on. This ensures good visibility of the cerebellopontine angle and strongly reduces the danger of air embolism compared with the usual sitting position. As an added precaution, the anesthetist introduces an intravenous catheter into the right atrium to enable aspiration of air in the rare event of an air embolism. Another advantage of the semi-sitting compared with the prone position is that with the former the operative field remains clearly visible without the need for continuous suction of blood and cerebro-

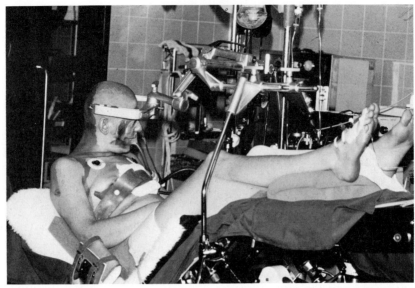

Figure 47–1. Semi-sitting position of patient. The head is fixed in the Mayfield holder apparatus, anteflexed, and turned 30° to the side of the lesion. Because of the positive venous pressure in this position, the danger of air embolism is eliminated.

spinal fluid. Therefore, the danger of traumatizing the brain stem as a result of continuous suction is reduced to a minimum.

After a vertical retroauricular, retromastoidal skin incision (Fig. 47–2), a craniectomy with a diameter of 2 to 3 cm is performed in such a way that the upper limit extends to the transverse sinus and the lateral limit to the sigmoid sinus. There is no need for opening the foramen magnum. The craniec-

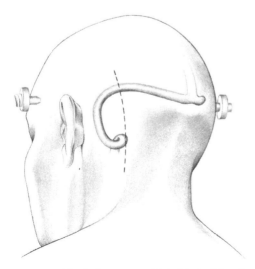

Figure 47–2. Vertical retromastoidal skin incision for a lateral suboccipital craniectomy between the transverse and the sigmoid sinus.

tomy must be performed far laterally, partly sacrificing the mastoid cells, if necessary, to gain an angle of 30 to 40° toward the cerebellopontine angle. The borders of the transverse and sigmoid sinuses must be exposed. Of special importance is the bipolar coagulation of the mastoid emissary vein and the use of a diamond drill and bone wax in the region of the mastoid cells. How far the pneumatic system of the mastoid has to be opened and removed depends on the position of the sigmoid sinus as well as the pneumatization of the cell system. By carrying out these steps, the surgeon can minimize the degree of bone opening and has optimal visibility to the brain stem.

The dura is opened at a 2-mm distance from the sinus by a medially pedicled flap. From this angle the self-holding retractor can be introduced without significant compression of the cerebellum, and the region of the cerebellopontine angle can be exposed after opening the pontocerebellar cistern and draining a sufficient amount of cerebrospinal fluid. At this point, the posterior wall of the tumor can be identified.

The caudal cranial nerves, which are often slightly compressed by the tumor, must be identified and freed from the tumor capsule. Immediate identification of the facial nerve in the cerebellopontine angle will be possible only in small tumors without brain-stem compression. In the case of a large tumor, the facial nerve is not visible at the brain stem or in the internal auditory meatus.

Starting from a 5- to 10-mm opening of the tumor capsule, reduction of tumor size is performed using the operating microscope. Thus, loss of primary tension of the tumor capsule occurs. By a gradual resection of the capsule, the facial nerve can be identified at the brain stem. Any direct manipulation of the facial nerve in the cerebellopontine angle will lead to postoperative loss of function. The nerve must not be detached from the tumor capsule, but the capsule itself must be dissected carefully from the nerve using microinstruments. Owing to an expansive compression, the nerve is often stretched around the tumor capsule as a very thin, broad band. The preservation of the continuity and function of the facial nerve in such a case is quite difficult, but not impossible.

If the facial nerve is injured in one area, the surgeon should still continue the careful preparation of the nerve. Because of tumor growth in the region of the cerebellopontine angle, the nerve becomes stretched, so that in the event of interruption of continuity and loss of substance of up to about 1 cm during tumor extirpation, an end-to-end suture without any tension can still be performed.

In patients with large defects of the facial nerve, an end-to-end-suture is impossible and a nerve graft has to be done. Identification of the distal nerve stump is very difficult when the tumor grows in a cone-shaped fashion into the internal auditory canal, and even electrostimulation cannot help to distinguish the distal stump of the facial nerve from the vestibulocochlear nerve. Dott[1] therefore recommended an intracranial-extracranial repair of the facial nerve using sural nerve grafts of 15 to 20 cm in length (Fig. 47–3). This technique is performed in two stages. The first stage is the suture of the graft to the central stump of the facial nerve. The nerve graft is directed out of the skull through the craniectomy and then passed through a tunnel below the mastoid between the sternocleidomastoid and the splenius capitis muscles. The distal end of the graft is marked with a silver clip and fixed in the retromandibular fossa. In a second stage, 3 months later, the distal end of the facial nerve is identified and anastomosed to the peripheral end in front of the stylomastoid foramen. We have used this method in a 46-year-old man with a large left acoustic neurinoma who

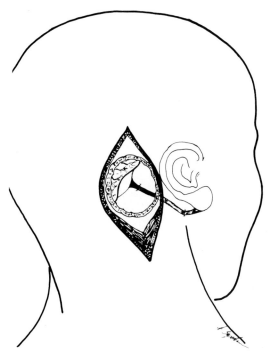

Figure 47–3. Operative technique as employed by Dott. (From Samii, M.: Clin. Plast. Surg., *11*:222, 1984.)

had previously undergone an enucleation of the left eye because of angiomatosis of the retina. We were able to achieve a good result 18 months after the operation in this patient.

In 1958, Dott[1] reported his results in four patients. He had achieved satisfactory results in two patients and excellent results in the other two. After performing the operation on five patients, Drake[2] was able to achieve good results in four. In 1962, Loew published a report of one patient whom he and Miehlke had operated upon with a good result. In 1967, Miehlke and Bushe[8] also achieved a good result using this technique in another patient.

It seems somewhat surprising after Dott's publication in 1958 that, in spite of the good results achieved with this method, we have found only seven reported cases over approximately the last 25 years. This is probably due to the fact that the exposure of the facial nerve at the brain stem in very large acoustic neurinomas is too difficult without the use of an operating microscope and microsurgical technique. Now that microsurgery has become somewhat routine, one can expect that in the future the operative treatment of cerebellopontine angle lesions will include reconstruction of the facial nerve.

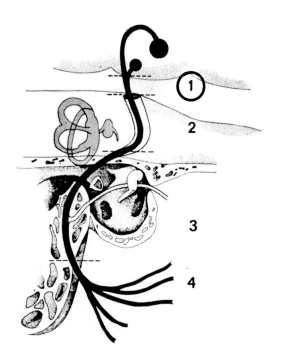

Figure 47–4. Scheme of intracranial-intratemporal grafting of facial nerve. *1*, Coaptation of the central stump of the facial nerve at the brain stem with a sural nerve graft. *2*, The graft is placed dorsal to the internal auditory meatus between the labyrinth and sigmoid sinus. *3*, The distal end of the sural nerve graft is coapted to the mastoidal part of the facial nerve. *4*, The facial nerve after its exit from the stylomastoid foramen. (From Samii, M.: Clin. Plast. Surg., *11*:222, 1984.)

As an alternative to Dott's surgical method, in 1975 we developed a technique of intracranial-intratemporal repair (Fig. 47–4) in cooperation with two otolaryngologic surgeons (Drs. Wigand and Draf). If the facial nerve cannot be preserved during extirpation of the tumor, we try to prepare the nerve at the brain stem in the region of the pontobulbar sulcus. In our experience it is possible to gain a stump of the facial nerve of at least 1 to 1.5 cm in length, even in huge tumors (Fig. 47–5*A* and *B*). Subsequently, an autologous nerve graft of about 5 cm in length is taken from the sural nerve and sutured to the central stump of the facial nerve at the brain stem with one or two epi-perineural sutures (Fig. 47–5*C*). The distal end of the graft is placed dorsal to the internal auditory meatus between the region of the labyrinth and the sigmoid sinus. The facial nerve is exposed in its mastoidal and tympanal course through a mastoid approach (Fig. 47–5*D*). Now the distal end of the graft can be transferred to the mastoid through a small incision in the dura just anterior to the sigmoid sinus. After transection of the facial nerve distal to the geniculate ganglion, the nerve stump is mobilized and anastomosed with the distal end of the graft (Fig. 47–5*E*). In this manner an intracranial-intratemporal reconstruction of the facial nerve is performed with a 5-cm nerve graft.

RESULTS

From 1975 to August 1982, we have accomplished reconstruction of the facial nerve in the cerebellopontine angle in 20 patients. In 15 patients the technique of intracranial-intratemporal nerve grafting has been used directly after the removal of acoustic neurinomas (Figs. 47–6 and 47–7). In one patient we used this technique 15 months after a translabyrinthine approach to remove an acoustic neurinoma (Fig. 47–8) and in another after translabyrinthine removal of an extensive cholesteatoma with sacrifice of the facial nerve proximal to the geniculate ganglion. We also performed intracranial-intratemporal nerve grafting in three patients with complete facial nerve paralysis after laterobasal fractures. In all three patients the exposure of the facial nerve in the intratemporal region had been attempted. However, the decompression and suture of the facial nerve in the intratemporal region did not result in any reinnervation of denervated muscles, despite a long period of follow-up. Dott's technique was performed in two patients.

In this chapter we are reporting the results of 12 patients who underwent surgery in which our technique was used with a follow-up from 1 to 7 years. In 11 patients the intracranial-intratemporal grafting of the facial nerve had been performed immediately

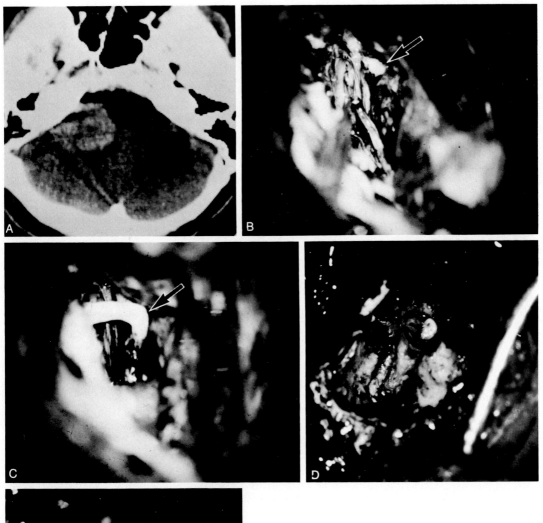

Figure 47–5. *A,* CT scan of a moderately large left-sided acoustic neurinoma. *B,* Condition after total removal of a large left-sided acoustic neurinoma, which resulted in sacrifice of the lateral part of the facial nerve. The central stump of the facial nerve of the brain stem is visualized (*arrow*). *C,* Sural nerve (*arrow*) is coapted to central stump of facial nerve. *D,* transmastoidal approach of facial nerve. *E,* The second end of the sural nerve is sutured to the mastoidal part of the facial nerve section distal to the geniculate ganglion. Note coaptation (*arrow*) between the sural nerve and the facial nerve.

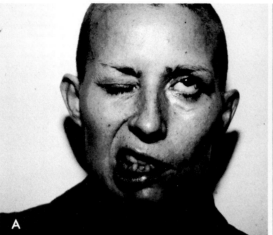
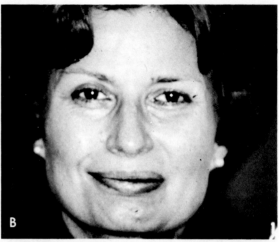
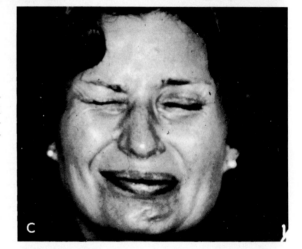

Figure 47–6. *A,* Appearance of face immediately after acoustic neurinoma removal requiring sacrifice of facial nerve. *B* and *C,* Functional result 13 months after intracranial-intratemporal grafting of facial nerve. (From Samii, M.: Clin. Plast. Surg., *11*:223, 1984.)

at the same stage after total removal of large acoustic neurinomas, and in one patient this operation had been done 15 months after translabyrinthine acoustic neurinoma surgery. Patient 12, a 57-year-old woman, had complete facial palsy for the preceding 8 years and was considered to have Bell's palsy until a CT scan was done, which demonstrated a cerebellopontine mass. An acoustic neurinoma was totally excised by us in 1981 and reconstruction of the facial nerve was done at the same stage. This patient, unfortunately but not unexpectedly, had not shown any recovery when reviewed 18 months after surgery.

Table 47–1 lists the results of individual patients. The first active muscle movement in the face was observed in all remaining 11 patients between 7 and 10 months after pri-

mary reconstruction of the facial nerve. In all these patients the face is symmetrical at rest and active movement of the face ranges from satisfactory to very good. It is interesting to note that even the frontal muscle has some reinnervation.

The satisfactory results in all remaining 11 patients operated upon justify the future use of this technique. The extra 1½ hours necessary for the operation entails minimal additional stress for the patient. It is our opinion that the reconstruction of the facial nerve in the cerebellopontine angle has a role in the modern concept of cerebellopontine angle surgery, and at present there is no other surgical technique for reconstruction of the facial nerve in patients with excised acoustic neurinomas that can give a comparable result.

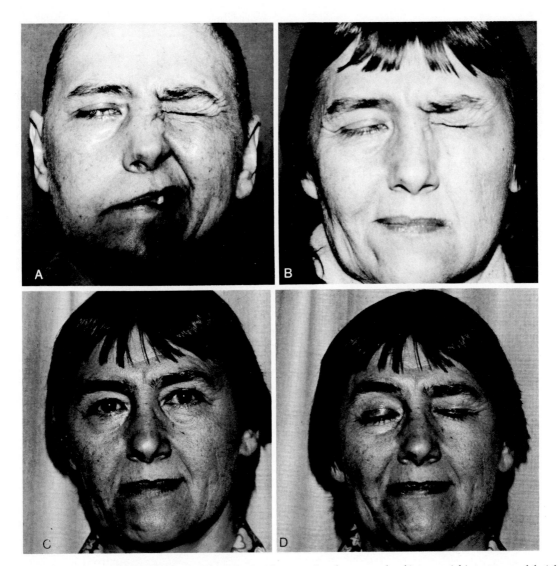

Figure 47–7. *A*, Postoperative paralysis of the right facial nerve. Another example of intracranial-intratemporal facial nerve repair. *B*, Satisfactory function already after 9 months after sural nerve graft. *C* and *D*, Further improvement of nerve function 15 months postoperatively.

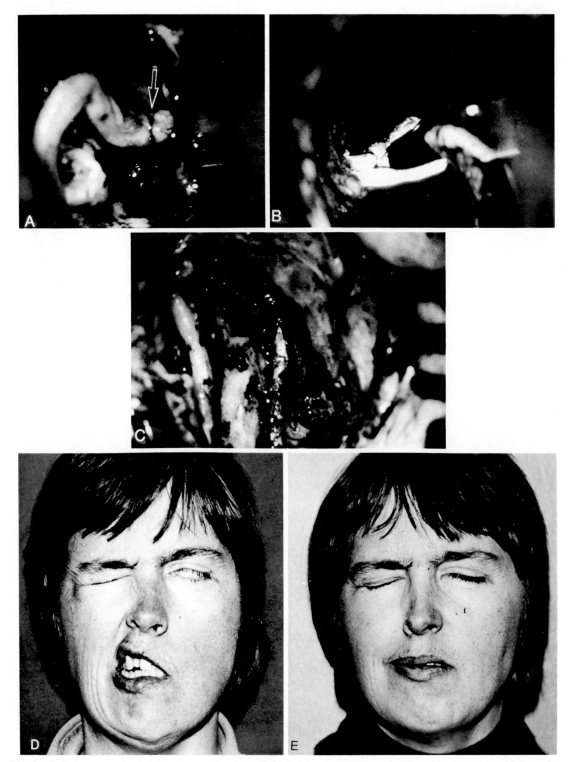

Figure 47–8. An example of delayed reconstruction of the facial nerve in the cerebellopontine angle. Fifteen months earlier an acoustic neurinoma was removed by the translabyrinthine approach, causing complete facial palsy. *A,* Exposure of the cerebellopontine angle. The central stump of the facial nerve is prepared and is being sutured to the sural nerve in the cerebellopontine angle. Note coaptation (*arrow*) between the facial nerve at the brain stem and the sural nerve graft. *B,* After a small incision in the dura in front of sigmoid sinus, the distal end of the sural nerve is being led out to the mastoidectomy. Shown are the distal end of the sural nerve, sigmoid sinus, and instrument for guiding the graft. *C,* The mastoidectomy, showing the exposure of the facial nerve. *D,* Complete left facial paralysis 15 months after translabyrinthine removal of an acoustic neurinoma. *E,* Twenty-two months after nerve grafting.

Table 47–1. RESULTS OF INTRACRANIAL-INTRATEMPORAL GRAFTING OF THE FACIAL NERVE IN 12 PATIENTS WITH ACOUSTIC NEURINOMA

Patient	Age	Year of Operation	First Active Muscle Movement (months)	Follow-up (months)	Symmetrical State of Rest and Active Muscle Movement	Frontal	Eye	Mouth
					Results, August 1982			
1	17	1975	10	87	Yes	×	× ×	× ×
2	24	1976	9	72	Yes	×	× ×	× ×
3	39	1976	10	69	Yes	×	× ×	× × ×
4	46	1977	8	67	Yes	×	× ×	× × ×
5	55	1979	7	42	Yes	×	× ×	× × ×
6	41	1979	8	39	Yes	×	× ×	× × ×
7	46	1979	8	39	Yes	×	× ×	× × ×
8	27	1979	7	38	Yes	×	× × ×	× × ×
9	42	1980	10	27	Yes	×	× ×	× ×
10	53	1981	10	20	Yes	×	× ×	× × ×
11	35	1981	7	9	Yes	×	× ×	× ×
12	57	1981	—	18	No	—	—	—

— = negative, × = weak, × × = good, and × × × = very good. (From Samii, M.: Clin. Plast. Surg., *11*:224, 1984.)

SUMMARY

The introduction of the operating microscope has strongly influenced our surgical possibilities for preserving and reconstructing the facial nerve during tumor surgery in the cerebellopontine angle as well as in the internal auditory canal. The lateral suboccipital approach offers the best possible visibility in order to identify the facial nerve from the exit zone at the brain stem up to the fundus of the internal auditory canal during surgery for tumors of different sizes. Since 1968 we have been using the operating microscope for surgery for cerebellopontine angle lesions. In 85% of these cases both the continuity and function of the facial nerve have been preserved. In the remaining cases the reconstruction of the facial nerve has been accomplished at the same stage.

In 1975 we introduced a new method for facial nerve reconstruction in the cerebellopontine angle. Since then, we have operated upon 20 patients by this technique of intracranial-intratemporal nerve graft; 15 of these procedures have been done directly after the removal of an acoustic neurinoma. Twelve of these patients have been followed over a period of 9 to 87 months. A 4- to 5-cm sural nerve graft was placed between the central stump of the facial nerve at the brain stem and the distal end of the facial nerve in a tympanal or mastoidal course after total removal of the acoustic neurinoma. This intracranial-intratemporal grafting of the facial nerve was used in one patient 15 months after translabyrinthine removal of an acoustic neurinoma. The results, demonstrated in this chapter, are highly encouraging. It is therefore recommended that this operative technique be included as one of the microsurgical procedures for cerebellopontine angle lesions.

References

1. Dott, N. M.: Facial paralysis. Restitution by extrapetrous nerve graft. Proc. Soc. Med., *51*:900, 1958.
2. Drake, C. G.: Acoustic neurinoma. Repair of facial nerve with autogenous graft. J. Neurosurg., *17*:836–842, 1960.
3. Fisch, U., and Weber, J.: Der diagnostische Wert der Pantopaque-Cisternographie. Med. Hyg., *30*: 1567–1568, 1972.
4. Fisch, U. Otochirurgische Behandlung des Acusticneurinoms. *In* Plester, von D., Wende, S., and Nakayama, N. (eds.): Kleinhirnbrückenwinkel-Tumoren, Diagnostic und Therapie. New York and Berlin, Springer-Verlag, 1978, pp. 196–214.
5. House, W. F.: Surgical exposure of the internal auditory canal and its contents through the middle cranial fossa. Laryngoscope, *11*:1363, 1961.
6. House, W. F.: Transtemporal microsurgical removal of acoustic neurinoma. Arch. Otolaryngol., *80*:597, 1964.
7. Loew, F.: Die kombinierte intrakranielle extratemporale Fazialisplastik nach Dott. Langenbecks Arch. Chir., *298*:934–935, 1962.
8. Miehlke, A., and Bushe, K. A.: Die operative Freilegung der mittleren Schädelgrube und des Porus acusticus internus zur Behandlung interlabyrinthärer Läsionen des Nervus facialis. Chir. Plast. Reconstr., *3*:37–46, 1967.

9. Rand, R. W.: Microneurosurgery for acoustic tumors. *In* Rand, R. W. (ed.): Microneurosurgery, 1st Ed. St. Louis, The C. V. Mosby Co., 1969.

10. Rand, R. W.: Microneurosurgery for acoustic tumors. *In* Rand, R. W. (ed.): Microneurosurgery, 2nd Ed. St. Louis, The C. V. Mosby Co., 1978.

11. Samii, M.: Neurochirurgische Gesichtspunkte der Behandlung der Akustikusneurinoma mit besonderer Berücksichtigung des N. facialis. Laryngol. Rhinol. Otol., *58*:97–106, 1979.

12. Samii, M.: Nerves of the head and neck. *In* Omer, G. F., and Spinner, M. (eds.): Management of Peripheral Nerve Problems. Philadelphia, W. B. Saunders Co., 1980, pp. 507–547.

13. Samii, M.: Preservation and reconstruction of the facial nerve in the cerebellopontine angle. *In* Samii, M., and Jannetta, P. J. (eds.): The Cranial Nerves. New York and Berlin, Springer-Verlag, 1981, pp. 438–450.

14. Sterkers, J. J.: Facial nerve preservation in acoustic neurinoma. *In* Samii, M., and Jannetta, P. J. (eds.): The Cranial Nerves. New York and Berlin, Springer-Verlag, 1981, pp. 438–450.

15. Yasargil, M. E.: Mikrochirurgie der Kleinhirnbrückenwinkel-Tumoren. *In* Plester, von D., Wende, S., and Nakayama, N. (eds.): Kleinhirnbrückenwinkel-Tumoren, Diagnostik und Therapie. New York and Berlin, Springer-Verlag, 1978, pp. 215–257.

INDEX

Note: Page numbers in *italics* indicate figures; page numbers followed by t indicate tables.